D0847233

The
FINE STRUCTURE
of the
NERVOUS SYSTEM:

The Neurons and Supporting Cells

ALAN PETERS

Waterhouse Professor of Anatomy, Department of Anatomy,
Boston University School of Medicine, Boston, Massachusetts

SANFORD L. PALAY

Bullard Professor of Neuroanatomy, Department of Anatomy,
Harvard Medical School, Boston, Massachusetts

HENRY deF. WEBSTER

Associate Chief, Laboratory of Neuropathology and Neuroanatomical
Sciences, National Institute of Neurological and Communicative Disorders
and Stroke, Bethesda, Maryland

The
FINE STRUCTURE
of the
NERVOUS SYSTEM:

The Neurons and Supporting Cells

1976
W. B. SAUNDERS COMPANY
Philadelphia • London • Toronto

W. B. Saunders Company: West Washington Square
                            Philadelphia, PA 19105

                            1 St. Anne's Road
                            Eastbourne, East Sussex BN21, 3UN, England

                            833 Oxford Street
                            Toronto, Ontario M8Z 5T9, Canada

Frontispiece
Various Aspects of Nerve Cells in Light Microscopic Preparations.

A. A small pyramidal cell from the visual cortex, Golgi method. The axon (*a*) descends from the cell body.

B. A small neuron in the dentate nucleus of the cerebellum, Golgi method. The axon (*a*) is represented only by its initial segment.

C. Protoplasmic (velate) astrocyte in the gray matter, Golgi method.

D. Oligodendrocyte in the white matter, Golgi method.

E. A motor neuron in the spinal cord showing the Golgi apparatus, osmium tetroxide impregnation.

F. A motor neuron in the abducens nucleus showing the distribution of mitochondria, Altmann-Kull method.

G. A motor neuron in the spinal cord showing the distribution of neurofibrils, Cajal's silver stain.

H. A motor neuron in the abducens nucleus showing the disposition of the Nissl bodies, thionin.

I. A dorsal root ganglion cell, showing the axon coiled about the perikaryon and dividing into central and peripheral fibers.

J. A myelinated peripheral nerve fiber, showing a node of Ranvier, Schmidt-Lanterman clefts, Schwann cell nucleus, and neurofibrils.

The Fine Structure of the Nervous System:
The Neurons and Supporting Cells   ISBN 0-7216-7207-8

Last digit is the print number: 9   8   7   6   5   4   3   2   1

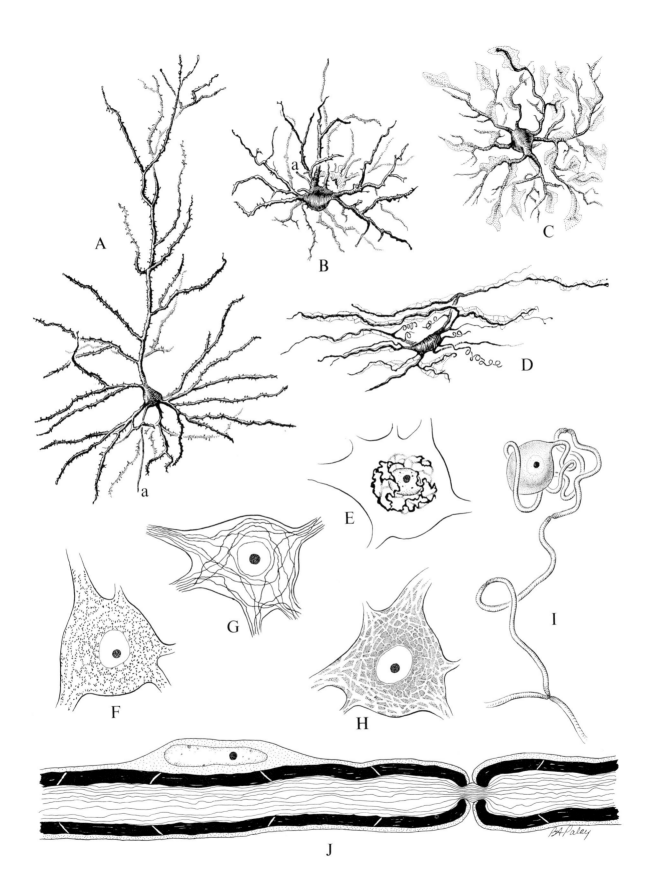

A

B

a

C

D

E

G

F

H

I

J

B.A.Paley

Dedicated to the Memory of

Jan Evangelista Purkinje	1787–1869
Louis-Antoine Ranvier	1835–1922
Camillo Golgi	1843–1926
Santiago Ramón y Cajal	1852–1934

CONTENTS

Chapter VI

THE CELLULAR SHEATHS OF NEURONS

Chapter VII

THE NEUROGLIAL CELLS

LIST OF PLATES

LIST OF ABBREVIATIONS
USED IN ILLUSTRATIONS

A	Artery	**Col**	Collagen
Al	Axolemma	**ct**	Crown-like array of threads
AlA	A face of freeze-fractured axolemma	**cv**	Coated vesicle
AlB	B face of freeze-fractured axolemma	**D**	Dense layer or undercoating
AM	Arachnoid mater	**Den**	Dendrite
As	Astrocyte	**DL**	Major dense line
AsA	A face of freeze-fractured astrocyte plasmalemma	**DM**	Dura mater
AsB	B face of freeze-fractured astrocyte plasmalemma	**En**	Endoneurium
AsP	Astrocyte process	**End**	Endothelium
At	Axon terminal	**Ep**	Epineurium
Ax	Axon	**ER**	Granular endoplasmic reticulum
B	Basal lamina	**f**	Fibrils or filaments
ba	Basket axon	**Fa**	Fat cells
bb	Basal body	**Fb**	Fibroblasts
Bv	Blood vessel	**fg**	Fibrogranular aggregates
C	Cytoplasm	**G**	Golgi apparatus
Cap	Capillary	**g**	Gap junction
Chr	Chromatin	**GC**	Growth cone
Ci	Inner cytoplasm	**gem**	Gemmule of dendrite
cil	Cilia	**GL**	Glia limitans
Co	Outer cytoplasm	**gly**	Glycogen

H	Axon hillock
I	Intermediate line of laminated body
IL	Intermediate or intraperiod line of myelin sheath
IS	Interstitial space
J	Intercellular junction
Lf	Lipofuscin granule
Ly	Lysosome
M	Microglial cell
m	Microtubule
Mes	Mesenchyme cells
mes	Mesaxon
mf	Microfilaments
mit	Mitochondrion
mv	Microvilli
mvb	Multivesicular body
my	Myelin sheath
N	Neuron
NB	Nissl body
ncl	Nucleolus
Nd	Node of Ranvier
NdA	A face of freeze-fractured axolemma at node of Ranvier
Nev	Nuclear envelope
nf	Neurofilaments
Nuc	Nucleus
O	Oligodendrocyte
Op	Oligodendrocyte process
p	Peroxisome
P	Paranodal cytoplasm

pa	Punctum adhaerens
PB	B face of Purkinje cell plasmalemma
pcp	Perichromatinic particle
Per	Perineurium
PF	Pars fibrosa
PG	Pars granulosa
PM	Pia mater
post	Postsynaptic membrane
pre	Presynaptic membrane
r	Ribosome
s	Synaptic junction
sa	Spine apparatus
SC	Satellite or Schwann cell
SCA	A face of freeze-fractured Schwann cell plasma membrane
SCB	B face of freeze-fractured Schwann cell plasma membrane
SM	Smooth muscle
sp	dendritic spines
SR	Smooth endoplasmic reticulum
SS	Subarachnoid space
sv	Synaptic vesicle
t	Thorn or spine of dendrite
T	External tongue process
tb	Tubules
v	Vesicle
vac	Vacuole
za	Zonula adhaerens
zo	Zonula occludens

PREFACE

The kind reception given our initial attempt "to present in words and pictures an account of the salient features of mammalian neurons and neuroglial cells" encouraged us to undertake a revised and enlarged version. The revision was started in the spring of 1973 when one of us (A.P.) was on sabbatical leave in Cambridge, England, and it has taken almost two years to complete the task.

Upon its completion we saw that we had so thoroughly redone the work and had so significantly added to its scope and detail that, with the agreement of our publisher, we decided that this justly should be thought of as an altogether new book rather than as a revision of the old. However, as a matter of historical interest we have included hereafter the *Preface to the First Edition* (1970, Harper & Row, Publishers).

We had not realized the explosion that had occurred in the volume of neurocytological literature during the four years since the writing of the original text. This increase in the amount of information is largely due to the proliferation of conventional fine structural studies, but the techniques of scanning electron microscopy and freeze-fracturing have added new dimensions to our understanding of cells in the nervous system. Hence we have included some of these results in our present account. The intervening years have also seen the beginning of the application of the high voltage electron microscope, but so far the use of this instrument has added little to our appreciation of the components of the nervous system. Most exciting is the introduction of the new tracing techniques employing labelled amino acids and horseradish peroxidase. Used in conjunction with the more established methods of Golgi impregnation and experimental degeneration, these techniques refine the structural analysis of the nervous system and extend the value of electron microscopy. We have tried to indicate how these techniques can be used. It will be evident that when we completed the manuscript about a year ago, we had not predicted the extent to which horseradish peroxidase and radioactive amino acids would be employed. They are now competing very strongly with the older technique of experimental degeneration. Even now, however, these tracers are not used very much in electron microscopy.

All of the chapters have been thoroughly rewritten in order to incorporate new information and to expand the scope of what was already included. To make our account of the nervous system more complete we have introduced new chapters on the ependyma, the choroid plexus, the blood vessels, the connective tissue sheaths of peripheral nerves, and the meninges. These new chapters have necessitated the use of many new illustrations. Only 30 plates of the original edition have been retained, and 88 new plates including four drawings have been added. While many of these new illustrations are from our own collections, a number of colleagues have supplied illustrations. We gratefully acknowledge the help given by D. J. Allen, Milton W. Brightman, Mary B. Bunge, Victoria Chan-Palay, M. W. Cloyd, Edward V. Famiglietti, Martin Feldman, James Kerns, Frank N. Low, Enrico Mugnaini, Tom Reese, Julian Saldanha, Bruce Schnapp, Constantino Sotelo, Deborah W. Vaughan, James E. Vaughn, Bruce W. Warr, and Raymond B. Wuerker.

Many of these colleagues and others have also generously given us information about their studies, some of which have not yet been published. We hope that we have interpreted their information correctly.

We are deeply grateful to the National Institute of Neurological and Communicative Disorders and Stroke, whose continued support of our laboratories in a very real sense made this book possible. The following grants are acknowledged: (A.P.) NS 07016; (S.L.P.) NS 03659.

We are also grateful to Miss Kathy Murphy, Miss Anna Marie Bellotti, Mrs. Mary Alba, and Mrs. Eleanor Dowling for typing the several versions of the manuscript and the many references to the literature. We are indebted to Howard Cook for photographic assistance and to Miss Betsy Palay for preparing the Frontispiece and diagrams. We wish to thank our new publisher and especially Mr. John Dusseau for his encouragement and help in the earlier phases of preparation of this book. The enthusiasm and skills of the staff at Saunders have made it very easy to bring this book to fruition, and for this, we are very grateful.

By no means last in importance, we also wish to pay tribute to our wives. Without their patience and understanding, we could not have completed this undertaking.

Boston, Massachusetts　　　　　ALAN PETERS
Bethesda, Maryland　　　　　　SANFORD L. PALAY
　　　　　　　　　　　　　　　HENRY deF. WEBSTER

PREFACE
To The First Edition

This book attempts to present in words and pictures the salient features of the fine structure of mammalian neurons and neuroglial cells. Naturally, the cells of the nervous system share with their counterparts in all other tissues the same structural elements—the nucleus, mitochondria, ribosomes, endoplasmic reticulum, filaments, microtubules, to name only a few. Indeed, many of these organelles, now known to be of general distribution, were first noticed in the nerve cell, for example, the Go gi apparatus and the mitochondria. The cells of the nervous system, however, have special characteristics that make it impossible to convey an adequate notion of their internal organization by means of a single electron micrograph or even a small collection of micrographs, as can be done for many other tissues. Three characteristics are especially pertinent to this point: the cells are all relatively large (even the smallest can have linear dimensions measured in millimeters); many are multipolar and highly irregular in shape, and they all display local differentiations in their internal structure. As a result, no single micrograph can be representative of the structure of any cell type. It should be remarked that these characteristics are true of the neuroglial and Schwann cells as well as of the neurons. In addition, the cells of the nervous system are functionally interdependent to a degree evinced in no other tissue, and this interdependence is correlated with precise and coherent morphological interrelations, which neuroanatomists have been at pains to unravel for the past century.

Electron microscop c investigations of the nervous system have not been systematic. Technical difficulties and the scarcity of investigators have hampered progress in this field of research more than in other branches of cytology. Nevertheless, a great deal of information has been garnered in the past 15 years, much of it scattered in various scientific journals and records of symposia, often inadequately documented by electron micrographs. We have endeavored to collect this information in a form convenient to students and research workers and to illustrate it with micrographs selected from our own studies. As most of the nervous system is still terra incognita so far as electron microscopy is concerned, our selection of illustrative regions is necessarily limited. We hope that this volume may serve as a base for further exploration.

In this place we wish to record our appreciation of the assistance of our colleagues in this country and abroad, many of whom may find their published opinions and observations echoed in this book without specific attribution. Drs. Milton W. Brightman, Raymond B. Wuerker, Constantino Sotelo, and James E. Vaughn have generously provided electron micrographs of structures that could not be illustrated from our own collections. We are deeply grateful to the National Institute of Neurological Diseases and Blindness, whose support of our laboratories has in a very real sense made this book possible. The following current grants are acknowledged: (A. P.) NB 07016; (S. L. P.) NB 03659 and NB 05591; (H. deF. W) NB 03789 and NB 07011. One of us (A. P.) has also received support from the United Cerebral Palsy Research and Educational Foundation (grant R-210). We are indebted to Mrs. Sylvia Colard Keene for the Frontispiece, and we are especially grateful to Mrs. Phoebe Franklin for typing the manuscript in its several versions and for preparing the bibliography.

ALAN PETERS
SANFORD L. PALAY
HENRY deF. WEBSTER

Boston, Massachusetts

The
FINE STRUCTURE
of the
NERVOUS SYSTEM:

The Neurons and Supporting Cells

Child! Do not throw this book about,
Refrain from the unholy pleasure
Of cutting all the pages out!
Preserve it as your chiefest treasure.

Hilaire Belloc, 1870–1953
Bad Child's Book of Beasts.

Therefore anything wrongly written in
is due to inadequate of knowledge
and is not to be taken as an insolent

George Simeon Mwase, 1880–1962

Chapter I

GENERAL MORPHOLOGY
OF THE NEURON

Anyone who has studied the early history of cytology cannot fail to be impressed by the slow development of the concept of the nerve cell. Most types of cells do not have a history. Once the idea was grasped, in the theory of Schleiden and Schwann, that cells are the architectonic units of living things, it was fairly quick work to recognize them in the various tissues and to proceed to the study of their contents, their interrelations, and their functions. But the nerve cell was more perplexing. It occasioned so much difficulty for its students that almost a century passed before they could agree upon its shape. At first it was thought to be an independent globular corpuscle suspended among nerve fibers, which looped and coiled about it and which it somehow nourished (Valentin, 1836). Later, when the continuity between the perikaryon and the nerve fibers was finally established (Remak, 1838 and 1841; Helmholtz, 1842; Hannover, 1844; Kölliker, 1844; Bidder, 1847; Wagner, 1847), then the nerve cell appeared to have no definite boundaries and seemed endless. Except for the fibers attached to organs in the periphery, the processes of all nerve cells seemed to be equivalent and to be confluent with one another. The nerve cells seemed to be only nodal points in an enormously intricate reticulum pervading the nervous system (Gerlach, 1858 and 1872). It appeared that the cell theory did not really apply to the nervous system; one had rather to speak of cell territories or spheres of influence surrounding nucleated centers.

It seems clear that one of the major obstacles to the appreciation of the cellular nature of the nervous system lay in the shape of the nerve cell itself and to some extent in its size. The medusa-like nerve cell, with its corona of seemingly endless processes, was bizarre. Other cells had relatively simple shapes — globular, cylindrical, squamous, fusiform, and so on. Some fitted one into the other like pieces of a jigsaw puzzle to form an epithelium; others lay free and definable in the tissue fluids. Many, such as cartilage or certain epithelial cells, were clearly circumscribed by walls. Only pigment cells, astrocytes, myoepithelial cells, and a few others had shapes even roughly approximating those of nerve cells. But aside from the fact that some of these examples were unknown in the early days, such cells could be easily encompassed in a single field or at least in a single preparation under the microscope. The multipolar nerve cell, however, with its meter-long axon did not fit into a single section and could not be easily plucked from its context or distinguished from its neighbors by the methods used for other cells. New methods had to be developed. And so a true cell theory of the nervous system did not emerge until the discovery and exploitation of special techniques that had the merit of bringing into view entire nerve cells as if dissected or isolated from the central nervous system.

Actually, the first successful method was microdissection of whole nerve cells from hardened specimens of brain and spinal cord. On the basis of experience with such isolated cells Deiters (1865) was able to distinguish between the numerous branching processes that we now call dendrites and the single process that slips into a myelin sheath to become the axis cylinder of a nerve fiber. Then toward the end of the nineteenth century very powerful techniques were developed that allowed the patient and discerning investigator to see the whole nerve cell *in situ* for the first time. Foremost among these new methods was the "black reaction" of Golgi (1873, 1882–1885, and 1891). This procedure involves hardening blocks of brain in potassium dichromate alone or in a mixture of potassium dichromate and osmium tetroxide followed by impregnation with silver nitrate. Whole nerve cells become selectively filled with silver chromate (Fregerslev, Blackstad, Fredens, and Holm, 1971; Chan-Palay, 1973h), which precipitates within the matrix of the cytoplasm. As the precipitate accumulates, it changes from a deep red fibrillar form to opaque blocky crystals, which appear black in transmitted light, especially at low magnifications (Chan-Palay and Palay, 1972a; Palay and Chan-Palay, 1973). For some unknown reason only a small proportion of the cells in a preparation are impregnated, so that they appear deep red or black against a transparent light golden background. The technique therefore results in a remarkable dissection *in situ*.

In the hands of Ramón y Cajal (1909–1911), this method provided the foundation for our understanding of the structure of the nervous system. From his studies of specimens prepared by the Golgi method, Cajal deduced that nerve cells are morphologically independent trophic and functional units and that a diffuse anastomosing network of nerve cell processes does not exist. Waldeyer in 1891 suggested the name *neuron* for the cellular units, and the generalization became known as the *neuron doctrine*. It was really an affirmation, 50 years late, that the cell theory applies to the nervous system as well as to other organs and tissues. Incidentally, it may be remarked that the term *doctrine* was an unfortunate designation. A doctrine often expresses a view superimposed by authority. Those who chose this word might have selected a term less suggestive of rigidity, such as the word *theory*, which is closer to the meaning of the German equivalent in *Neuronlehre*. A theory can be flexible and can assimilate new information that modifies and enriches it without contradicting its essence.

Although the neuron doctrine was well received by many of the leading microscopists of the day (see Barker, 1899), it was soon challenged by new observations of anastomoses between the processes of nerve cells, especially in the invertebrate nervous system. A passionate controversy arose, with Cajal as the protagonist (see, for example the Nobel prize lectures of Cajal and Golgi in 1906). A review of the issues with selected passages from the original writings of the principal disputants is given by Clark and O'Malley (1968) in their historical study of the nervous system. The details of the controversy are beyond the scope of this chapter, which is concerned rather with the development of a different theme. But it does reveal a second major reason for the long germination of a true cell theory for the nervous system, and this reason was more conceptual than technical in origin.

In order to understand this second aspect, we must return to the descriptions of Schleiden (1838) and Schwann (1839). For them each cell was a vesicle containing a nucleus and bounded by a cell wall or a membrane. Among animal cells, those in the notochord and in cartilage and certain epithelia conform readily to this botanical prototype. In the preparations of the nineteenth century, however, most animal cells possessed no discernible cell wall or surface membrane. Indeed, Max Schultze (1861) considered that when a distinct membrane appeared, it was an early sign of retrogression, for the cell could no longer divide. Schwann himself did not insist on the presence of a visible cell wall; although he could see none surrounding the corpuscles of pus and mucus or around myoblasts, he nevertheless regarded them as cells (see Florkin, 1960). Before the middle of the nineteenth century it was recognized that the analogy between the surface of a cell and the cell wall of plants was fallacious, and emphasis was soon transferred to the protoplasmic contents rather than the limiting membrane. By the late 1860's the familiar definition of Max Schultze became the generally accepted starting point for thinking about cells: a cell is a lump of protoplasm containing a nucleus. The surface of the cell was imagined as a naked interface between the protoplasm and its environment. By the end of the century, Verworn could write in his well-known textbook (p. 65) on general physiology, "Hence, since Max Schultze's establishment of the protoplasm theory, the idea that the cell-membrane is a general cell constituent has completely disappeared." It remained invisible until the advent of electron microscopy, despite the experiments of astute cytologists like Robert Chambers (see his review, 1949).

For students of the nervous system Max

Schultze's definition seemed admirably suited to the known facts. Not only did it agree with the prevailing image of the nervous system as a vast and intricate reticulum punctuated by nucleated nodal points, but it also fitted in with the prevailing concept of the nature of the nerve impulse and its conduction from place to place, in which intervening cell membranes were perceived as undesirable obstacles. Thus, as van der Loos (1967) reminds us, Deiters saw no difficulty in having a second system of small axons originate from the dendrites by means of triangular or pyramidal bases, which must surely have been the *boutons terminaux* of modern terminology. This type of image formed the prevailing background for the resistance to the neuron doctrine: all nerve cells interconnected through some or all of their processes, with protoplasmic continuity and without clearly defined cell limits, even, according to some, at the peripheral end-organs.

The early acceptance of Cajal's conclusions in the 1890's must therefore be seen as only a temporary diversion created by the clarity of his preparations and his drawings and by the authenticity of his genius. For Cajal had made a series of brilliant deductions. His evidence was only indirect and circumstantial, as indeed it had to be before the invention of the electron microscope. At that time the actual interface between nerve cells or between nerve ending and muscle could not be visualized, even though Cajal (1888a and b) had recognized characteristic terminals of nerve fibers in his first investigations of the central nervous system and a decade later, by using aniline dyes to stain the neuronal cytoplasm, Held (1897) and Auerbach (1898) had demonstrated the intimate attachment of nerve endings to nerve cell bodies and their processes. Soon afterward Sherrington (Foster and Sherrington, 1897) introduced the concept of the synapse to denote the point where the nerve impulse must be transferred from one cell to another. The structure of this critical interface remained hidden for another 50 years.

With the appearance of Apáthy's work on the ganglia of the leech in 1897, the comfortable idea of a continuous network returned in full force. Apáthy proposed that the neurofibrils within the nerve cells and their processes were continuous from one cell to another and that the nervous currents followed the paths laid out by them. Experiments by Bethe (1897–1898, 1900, and 1904) seemed to show that, far from playing an essential role in nervous function, the perikaryon could be dispensed with altogether. The deprecation heaped upon the neuron doctrine increased steadily in its severity. Held withdrew his support (1909); Nissl (1903) published an influential book of acerbic criticism. Cajal complained in his introduction to Marinesco's book (1909) that, whereas other scientists could discuss theories and hypotheses, neuroanatomists could not even agree upon the facts.

One of the principal reasons why the reticular concept of the nervous system was so attractive during the period from about 1840 to 1935, and why it seems almost incomprehensible today, is that the biologists of that time had an entirely different understanding of the cell surface from ours. It seemed much more plausible to them that the nerve impulse could pass from cell to cell along the bundles of neurofibrils, like a current in a wire, than that it could cross an intercellular gap. As the cell surface was merely a phase boundary between the cytoplasm and the environment, there was no obstacle to the confluence of two cells when they came close together, or more important, as Nissl proposed, the neurofibrils could traverse open intercellular spaces and re-enter the cytoplasm of another cell without transgressing any physiological or structural rules.

Because of this attitude, the marshalling of evidence for the morphological, embryological, and functional integrity of the nerve cell engaged biologists for a long time. The most suggestive evidence is provided by Cajal's own work (summarized in the monographs of 1909–1911, 1929, and 1934 among others): his codification of the types of synapses, his meticulous studies of the embryological development of the brain and spinal cord, his patient exposition of the logic of the central nervous system in analyses of the cortex and hundreds of lower centers. But none of it alone was compelling. The observation that nerve fibers could grow out of nerve cells in the absence of Schwann cells finally disposed of the notion that axons were produced by the fusion of a chain of Schwann cells and proved that the axons were independent of the sheath (Harrison, 1907 and 1924; Levi, 1916). The dependence of the axon on the cell body was demonstrated by countless variations on the early experiments of Waller (1850 and 1852a, b, and c), in which the distal fragment of a severed axon degenerates whereas the proximal stump regenerates. Furthermore, in most cases injury or death of a nerve cell does not affect the neighboring cells, nor does it produce a deleterious effect upon more distant cells connected by synapses. And as far as the intercellular continuity of neurofibrils is concerned, it could be seen in Cajal's improved silver preparations that they do not even enter the terminals in most instances. In very large synapses a limiting membrane, the synaptolemma, could be seen separating the two components, and in carefully prepared specimens it could be shown that the neurofibrils did not cross this barrier (Bartelmez and Hoerr, 1933; Hoerr, 1936; Bodian, 1937 and 1942). Concurrently the accumulating evidence of neurophysiology required an interruption at the synapse in order to account both for the time course of a reflex circuit and for the chemistry of transmission. Finally, electron microscopy of synapses demonstrated the integrity of the two components separated by a shallow interstice and thus completed the evidence with direct visualization (see Palay, 1956a and b and 1958b). During the same period, the cell membrane was transformed from a mere interface into a special phase of the protoplasm with quite specific chemistry and enzymatic machinery and with a complex role of the utmost importance in the economy of the cell.

Today the evidence for the neuron doctrine seems overwhelming. The integrity of the neuron has become so readily acceptable that any discussion of the evidence for it seems almost banal. Like most received ideas, it seems to have been true since the beginning of time. Nevertheless, it is worth while to dwell on the special significance of the cell theory for an understanding of the nervous system.

When we say that the nervous system contains independent functional and morphological entities called neurons, we are saying much more than what appears at first sight. For unlike the cells in most other tissues, the components of the nervous system are not equivalent, are not interchangeable parts. Each neuron is unique, and its singularity resides in its specific position in the nervous system. That position is given by its peculiar synaptic connections with other neurons and, either directly or indirectly, with the periphery. As the pattern of these connections is reflected in a rigorous fashion by the form of the neuron, its shape is its most properly *neural* feature. Thus, the form of a neuron provides the key to its role in the nervous system.

In most neurons three distinct regions can be recognized: a cell body containing the nucleus; a number of tapering, twisting, and ramifying dendrites; and a single, smooth, and relatively straight axon that extends farther away from the cell body than the dendrites and may acquire a myelin sheath. If the axon and its

branches are followed to their terminal arborizations, a wide variety of formations is encountered. There are small bulbous endings, calyciform endings, small varicosities linked together in a chain, and many others. These terminals are attached to the cell bodies, dendrites, or even to axons or axon terminals of other neurons, and in the periphery they may be incorporated into a sense organ or attached to a muscle cell. It was one of Cajal's marvelous insights to conceive of the neuron as topographically polarized so that its cell body and dendrites receive impulses from the axonal endings impinging upon its surface while the axon conveys the response of the cell away toward its terminal arborizations. Although it is now clear that this "law of conduction" depends upon a more fundamental polarization of the synaptic junction and the differential properties of the axonal and dendritic surface membranes, it remains correct as a description of the roles of the three different regions of the cell.

Of the two receptor regions, the dendrites are vastly more important in most neurons. For example, in the average pyramidal cell of the cat's somatosensory cortex, only 4 per cent of the surface area of the cell is taken up by the cell body, whereas 43 per cent of the surface area is accounted for by the dendritic spines alone (Mungai, 1967). In the cat's reticular formation the ratio between the surface areas of the cell body and the dendrites of certain giant cells is 1:5 (Mannen, 1966). The dendrites seem to be a device for vastly increasing the surface area and, therefore, the receptor area of the cell. But the dendrites have a more subtle function than merely increasing surface area. The form of the dendrites and the pattern of their arborizations permit the neuron to make specific contacts, to receive from certain axons. The dendrites appear to be reaching out toward the axonal terminals and, reciprocally, the axons appear to ramify in such a way as to terminate in synapse with certain dendrites and on specified parts of dendrites. Since the efficacy of synapses must vary with, among other factors, their distance from the initial segment of the axon, the form of the dendritic tree provides a topographic map of the world as seen by a particular cell. The shape of the cell body and particularly the dendritic tree is an expression of the receptive field of the neuron. A cell with widespread dendrites must receive information from fibers of diverse origins and functions. A cell with a small, closely ramifying dendritic tree must receive from a smaller, more homogeneous pool of sources. Between these two extremes lie all sorts of variations. For example, a cell with short, radiating dendrites could also receive from a variety of afferents, if it is appropriately located at a strategic intersection. It could make high resolution comparisons between two types of input on different dendrites. The significance of the dendritic pattern must, therefore, be sought in its relationship to the functional pattern of its afferent fibers.

At the other pole of the neuron, the axon is a device for distributing to other neurons or effector cells the activity of the neuron as modified by its environment. The form of the axon, like that of the dendritic tree, reflects its relations to other neurons. It gives the addresses to which impulses are directed and the routes over which they are delivered. Thus, the originally baffling and difficult shape of the neuron leads directly into an understanding of its role as an integral element in the complicated organization of the nervous system.

Ten years ago, when electron microscopy provided the final proof of the discontinuity of the cells in the nervous system, it seemed that the neuron doctrine would need no further defense and could be accepted henceforth without apology. But it is hardly to be expected that any simple conception concerning the fundamental architecture of the nervous system could remain inviolate for long. New information is bound to modify it, if only by forcing a redefinition of the terms in which it is expressed. In recent years both morphological and physiological results have been brought forward that invite a re-examination of the basic tenets of the neuron doctrine, especially of the law of dynamic polarization. Unlike the ancient controversy which Cajal had to deal with, the new challenges come not from old prejudices and confusions but from a new set of clear observations which were made with highly sophisticated techniques and about which there are no real disagreements. The questions that have been raised are directed at the fundamental nature of the parts of the nerve cell and at the correlation between function and structure that lies at the root of so many recent discoveries in neurocytology. These challenges have been most clearly and systematically articulated in a number of publications by Shepherd (1972 and 1974). There are really two points at issue: first whether the principle of true discontinuity between nerve cells can be maintained in view of the growing catalogue of electrically coupled neurons, and second, whether a consistent and dependable definition of axon and dendrite can be constructed in view of the existence of processes that exhibit the structure and function of both.

In order to discuss these issues it is necessary to review the essential features of the synapse, which will be described in greater detail in Chapter V. The concept of the synapse is central to the neuron doctrine. Without it the neuron doctrine would be no more useful in understanding the nervous system than the reticular theory. Since, under the neuron doctrine, nerve cells are seen as independent morphological, trophic, and functional units, contiguous but not continuous, they must interact through intercellular mechanisms. These mechanisms are provided by the synapses, intercellular junctions which are specialized for the transmission of nerve impulses. The concept of the synapse is therefore both morphological and physiological in origin. It implies first of all a discontinuity between nerve cells generally, an intercellular gap that must be bridged by some specific agency, electrical or chemical, in order for the nerve impulse to pass from one cell to another. It implies also the existence of specialized loci, junctions between nerve cells where transmission can take place. Third, it implies a distinct polarity such that one member of the junction is equipped with the apparatus for dispatching the nerve impulse while the other member is equipped with the apparatus for receiving it. This is the polarity that gives an apparent orientation to the flow of impulses through the whole neuron. Finally, the concept of the synapse implies some degree of specificity in the articulation between two cells, since the synaptic terminals in many systems are known to be distributed according to precise patterns. All these implications direct attention to the apposed surfaces of the articulating partners for the sites of important specializations.

In considering this aspect of synaptic morphology it is useful to recall that the nervous system is a derivative of the surface epithelium of the embryo and that it retains many epithelial characteristics even in the mature individual. For example, it contains relatively little intercellular space, it rests upon a continuous basal lamina, and it has a free surface covered with microvilli and cilia (the ependymal lining of the ventricles). Among these epithelial traits is the tendency of neighboring cells to stick together, and the synapse can be considered primarily as a site of attachment or adhesion between two nerve cells. In most epithelia adjacent cells adhere to one another by means of a variety of devices, which have come to be understood only since the introduction of fine structural studies. The most comprehensive investigation is that of Farquhar and Palade (1963), who presented a systematic nomenclature for junctional specializations that has proved quite useful even though it has had to be modified in the light of more recent information. There are four common specializations: (1) the macula adhaerens, or desmosome, (2) the zonula adhaerens, (3) the zonula occludens, or tight junction, and (4) the nexus, or gap junction. In their original catalogue, Farquhar and Palade did not differentiate the last two, but more recent analyses, especially with electron-opaque tracers and with freeze-fracturing techniques, have clearly distinguished between them.

The *macula adhaerens* is a complex spot-like junction characterized by thick pads of fine filaments inserted symmetrically into the cytoplasmic faces of the plasmalemmas of the apposed cells. The interstitial cleft is noticeably widened in the macula, and it is often bisected by a thin, dense lamella running parallel with the plane of the confronted plasmalemmas. This type of intercellular junction is seldom, if ever, encountered in the nervous system.

The *zonula adhaerens* resembles the macula in having symmetrical deposits of filamentous material on the cytoplasmic surfaces of the apposed surface membranes and in having a thin dense lamella running through the interstitial cleft, but there are several important differences. Although the interstitial cleft is widened, the confronted plasmalemmas diverge less than in the macula. The pads of filaments adherent to the cell membranes are less complex than those in the macula, consisting merely of close-packed tufts, and the whole junction is shaped like a ribbon or girdle as the name *zonula* implies, rather than a round spot. The zonula adhaerens occurs in the nervous system, particularly between ependymal cells (Brightman and Palay, 1963), where it forms part of the terminal bar complex near the apices of the cells. A miniature version of this junction—named the punctum adhaerens because of its punctate form—is found very commonly between nerve cells and their processes and between neuroglial cells, and even sometimes between neuroglial cells and neurons. For example, tiny symmetrical junctions of this type, consisting of one or two paired tufts of filaments, occur frequently between adjacent dendrites of granule cells in the cerebellar cortex (Gray, 1961b; Palay, 1961b;

Palay and Chan-Palay, 1974). Similar, but somewhat more extensive puncta adhaerentia are found along the synaptic interfaces of certain large boutons against the perikarya of Deiters cells in the lateral vestibular nucleus (Sotelo and Palay, 1970).

The *zonula occludens* is characterized by the obliteration and sealing off of the interstitial space and by coaptation of the apposed plasmalemmas. Dense filamentous aggregates may line the cytoplasmic faces. Freeze-fractured preparations show that this junction comprises a network of intersecting linear fusions of the confronted plasmalemmas. In the nervous system it occurs commonly between cells in the choroid plexus and in the ependyma, and in the mesaxon of the myelin sheath and between adjacent paranodal myelin loops. The endothelial cells of most capillaries in the central nervous system parenchyma are bound to one another by apparently complete, delicate zonulae occludentes, which thus provide the morphological basis of the blood-brain barrier.

The *nexus* or *gap junction* is an extensive ribbon-like or spot-like junction in which the intercellular space is much reduced but not completely obliterated. In the nervous system such junctions are very common between ependymal cells; between neuroglial cells, especially astrocytes, and between nerve cells of certain kinds. There are few known examples of interneuronal gap junctions in the mammalian nervous system (mesencephalic nucleus of trigeminal nerve, lateral vestibular nucleus, and the inferior olive), but they have been found frequently in lower vertebrates and in invertebrates (for example, ciliary ganglion of chick, Mauthner cell of fishes, spinal cord of lamprey, giant motor synapses of crayfish).

Of these four types of symmetrical adherent devices, the nervous system apparently makes use of only two in forming synapses between neurons: the zonula adhaerens, usually as some variant of the punctum adhaerens, and the nexus or gap junction. By far the most common of these two is the punctum adhaerens. In many interneuronal but nonsynaptic contacts, as along crossing or parallel dendrites, or between dendrites and adjacent neuronal somata it occurs in an unmodified form as small symmetrical tufted points, spotted here and there along the apposed surfaces. It also occurs at many axo-dendritic and axo-somatic synaptic interfaces without being the actual site of transmission. An example is given in Figure 5–19, in which an extensive set of puncta adhaerentia marks the synaptic interfaces without being associated with synaptic vesicles. It seems that in all these instances, the puncta are merely adhesive points, which ensure the integrity and the stability of interneuronal relationships.

The zonula or punctum adhaerens is further modified in the formation of the so-called "synaptic complex" (Palay, 1956b) or "active zone" (Couteaux, 1961), the most highly specialized part of the interneuronal junction, believed to be the precise site of impulse transmission. In these foci the intercellular or synaptic cleft is somewhat widened, and the filamentous material condensed on the cytoplasmic faces of the apposed cell membranes is asymmetrically disposed. The material on the presynaptic side is often set out in a regularly arranged, tufted grid with synaptic vesicles lodged in its openings. On the postsynaptic side the dense material is more continuous, comprising a plaque attached to the inner side of the membrane. Fine filaments cross the cleft and a thin laminar density of unresolved structure often bisects it. Because of the clearly demonstrable intercellular cleft and the presence of synaptic vesicles in the presynaptic terminal, junctions of this description have been consistently associated with chemical transmission. The vesicles discharge their load of transmitter into the cleft, the transmitter diffuses across the cleft and is taken up by receptor molecules in the postsynaptic membrane with a resultant alteration in its permeability, and the production of either an excitatory or inhibitory postsynaptic potential ensues. The structural and physiological asymmetry of such junctions carries the polarity of the nerve cell to its ultimate boundaries and substantiates the neuron doctrine as it is usually conceived.

Synapses that are based upon the gap junction, however, may be considered as challenges to the neuron doctrine. These junctions are structurally symmetrical, and although an intercellular cleft exists, it is filled with an array of "gap" subunits, which apparently serve as direct conduits for the intercellular passage of ions and experimentally introduced tracer molecules (Asada and Bennett, 1971; Bennett, 1973; Pappas, Asada, and Bennett, 1971; Payton, Bennett, and Pappas, 1969; Peracchia, 1973a, and b). The electrotonic coupling of neurons that are united by such junctions can be regarded as evidence of intercellular continuity, thus contradicting the neuron doctrine. But it has to be admitted that the connection of a few, select nerve cells by means of gap junctions is a far cry from the reticulum envisaged by the old opponents of the neuron doctrine. Each cell is still bounded by its proper cell membrane, each has its own nucleus and its independence. Gap junctions are not indiscriminate corridors between cells; they are specializations in the surface membrane. They provide a high speed, low resistance pathway that may be useful in coordinating and synchronizing certain nerve cells. The essential individuality of the cells is not impugned by such junctions, and the neuron doctrine is not threatened by the discovery of their existence.

A more fundamental challenge is presented by the recent discovery of several types of synapse that were not anticipated by the classical authors. Cajal's lists of synaptic varieties are all axo-dendritic and axo-somatic articulations, in keeping with the law of dynamic polarization, and his descriptions are primarily concerned with morphological variations in the terminal ramifications of axons (Cajal, 1909 and 1934). Synapses between axons and synapses between dendrites were not recognized and were considered to be specifically prevented by the proliferation of neuroglial fibers running between components of the nervous system. Indeed the one axo-axonal synapse that Cajal discovered, the articulation of the descending collaterals of basket cell axons with the initial segment of the Purkinje cell axon, was cited by him (Cajal, 1909, p. 94) as indicating the dendritic nature of that part of the Purkinje cell. Thus, he upheld the purity of the functional and morphological distinctions between axons and dendrites. For if the law of dynamic polarization was to have any validity there would have to be recognizable differences between these two processes of the nerve cell. As was mentioned above, the morphological distinction goes back to Deiters (1865), who differentiated two classes of neuronal processes: (I) the "protoplasmic extensions" (*Fortsätzungen*), which have since come to be called *dendrites*, and (2) the axis cylinder, or *axon*. Each cell was furnished with numerous dendrites, which originated as radiating, tapered prolongations of the perikaryon and ramified by repeated bifurcations during their course, subdividing into finer and finer branches. In contrast, each nerve cell emitted only one axon, a smooth, thin, unbranched process of nearly uniform caliber, which was eventually traceable into a "true" (myelinated) nerve fiber. It was left to later investigators to realize that not all axons are myelinated and that even dendrites may be myelinated. Golgi (1886), having discovered the recurrent collateral branches of axons, pointed out that dendrites habitually branch at acute angles, whereas axons branch at right angles; and Cajal (1894) saw regularity and functional significance in the observation that axons normally terminate upon the cell bodies and dendrites of nerve cells. Furthermore, an internal distinction was provided by Nissl (1894) who showed that the basophilic masses bearing his name occur in the cell body and extend into the dendrites of large neurons but never into the axons (see Chapter II). More recently electron microscopy has elaborated these characteristics by demonstrating differences in the internal architecture of the two processes (Palay, 1956a; Peters, Palay, and Webster, 1970). For example, large axons generally contain a high proportion of longitudinal neurofilaments, whereas dendrites of similar caliber display a high proportion of microtubules (see Chapters III, IV, and IX).

Thus a set of purely morphological criteria was developed for distinguishing between axons and dendrites. These criteria were consistent with the law of dynamic polarization. Since only dendrites and perikarya could receive the terminals of axons, dendro-dendritic and axo-axonal synapses were forbidden. And these criteria seemed to be validated by the electrophysiological distinctions that were discovered during the second quarter of the twentieth century: dendrites were capable of producing only graded potentials, whereas axons generated all-or-none action potentials (Eccles, 1961).

When the earlier edition of this book was written, the morphological and physiological distinctions between axons and dendrites appeared to be clear enough to support the traditional definitions. Even at that time, however, there were indications of ambiguity, and with the subsequent more intensive investigations of the nervous system the examples of apparent exceptions to the earlier generalizations have multiplied. Although early papers on the fine structure of the central nervous system maintained the clear differentiation of axons and dendrites, later reports warned that identification of profiles in electron micrographs must be founded on a solid knowledge of the architecture of the specific region under investigation at the light microscope level, since the form of nerve cells varies so much from region to region. Examples of axons that behave like dendrites in one respect or another and of cells lacking either clearly identifiable axons or dendrites were already well known (see Bodian, 1962). The dorsal root ganglion cell, with its central and peripheral processes both morphologically and physio-

logically behaving like axons, is a case in point. And amacrine cells in the retina and granule cells in the olfactory bulb are only two of many cell types in the central nervous system that have no morphologically definable axons. The fact is that the distinction between axons and dendrites, and with it the law of dynamic polarization, is based upon an idealized nerve cell exemplified by the mammalian ventral horn motor neuron. In such a cell there is no difficulty in differentiating between the two kinds of processes, and for the vast majority of the nerve cells in the vertebrate central nervous system this paradigm still holds true. It is impossible to describe either their structure or their physiology without reference to their major parts: the cell body, dendrites, and axon.

The situation is quite different, however, in invertebrates. In these animals, nerve cell bodies are usually located at the periphery of a ganglion with their processes extending into a neuropil at the center. The cells are typically unipolar, and dendrites and axons branching from the primary process are not readily distinguishable by their form. Thus the distinction between axons and dendrites seems equivocal in invertebrates. The historical importance of the invertebrate ganglion in the heated controversy over the neuron doctrine is an indication of the power of this ambiguity. The noncommittal term *neurite* can be adopted in situations in which neither axon nor dendrite is satisfactory. Yet if we apply the old criteria demanded by the law of dynamic polarization to the invertebrate neuron, certain branches of the primary neurite become clearly dendritic, since they receive synaptic input, while other branches become clearly axonal, since they conduct impulses away to other cells. The antecedent ambiguity is to some extent attributable to inadequate information, for the synaptic organization of invertebrate ganglia remains largely obscure. The form of the invertebrate neuron, however, demonstrates that dendrites can be collateral branches of axons and need not be widely separated as in the model of the vertebrate neuron. This circumstance indicates that dendritic form and function can be intermingled with those of the axon like the pieces in a mosaic.

The example of the invertebrate neuron brings into focus the essential characteristics of dendrites and axons: dendrites are those processes of a nerve cell that receive inputs, while axons are those processes that conduct and transmit. From the morphological point of view this means that the mere form of a process would be less useful in identification than the presence of the cytological apparatus associated with either reception or conduction and transmission, for example, appendages like thorns or spines, postsynaptic densities, synaptic vesicles, a myelin sheath. The terms *axon* and *dendrite* would then designate functional entities with which certain structural features are consistently correlated. The difficulties in identification (definition) have arisen because the nerve cell has been conceived in fairly gross histological terms instead of in terms of effective structure. Consequently, the discovery of the forbidden dendro-dendritic and axo-axonal synapses, reciprocal synapses, dendrites that can propagate action potentials over part of their course, dendrites coated with thin layers of myelin, and other unexpected conditions are perceived as paradoxical. It must be evident that the paradigm of the vertebrate motor neuron does provide a useful standard for the description of structure and function in most nerve cells, but it represents one extreme of the spectrum of possibilities, in which axonal functions and structure are distinctly separated topographically from those of dendrites. The amacrine cell of the retina, the granule cell of the olfactory bulb, and typical invertebrate neurons lie at the other extreme, in which axonal and dendritic functions and structure are intermingled.

The mosaic construction of the nerve cell implicit in this intermingling is only a somewhat coarse expression of the chemical mosaic nature of the cell membrane and of the separation of functions distributed among the organelles within the cell. The typical internal fine structure of a dendrite or an axon is very likely related not to the specific function of the process but rather to the maintenance of anisotropy, axoplasmic flow, protein synthesis, and the necessity of making specific connections with other nerve cells and their processes. In contrast, the fine structure at those points of connection is directly related to the specific functions of reception or transmission, which are carried out by the special apparatus located there, such as the synaptic vesicles, the mitochondria, the components of the pre- and postsynaptic membranes, and so on. Thus, although a process can by its shape and branching pattern have the appearance of a proper dendrite at the level of the light microscope and may be identifiable as a dendrite by virtue of its receiving numerous synaptic terminals, such a process can still have axonal foci dispersed along it as evidenced by synaptic vesicles and other presynaptic structures clustered against its surface. Similarly a process that is an axon by all the usual criteria of morphology

and physiology can have segments of postsynaptic structure intercalated along its course, such as typical postsynaptic thorns projecting from the initial segment or postsynaptic membrane specializations at a node of Ranvier. Such deviations from the paradigm appear less paradoxical and less contradictory if the nerve cell is recognized as a mosaic, a patchwork of functions, the pattern of which is variable but characteristic of each cell type.

Finally there is the question of the independent action of neuronal processes united by dendro-dendritic synapses or certain complicated synaptic arrangements involving both axons and dendrites. Unquestionably such synaptic junctions offer the opportunity for direct interaction between synaptic components without the participation of the normal axonal action potential and the activation of the long-distance signalling mechanism. This circumstance has been viewed as undermining the neuron doctrine since the unit of operation is considered to be a synaptic pair or a complex synaptic articulation. This argument is similar to the old claim (Nissl, 1903; Bethe, 1904) that since the cell body is not involved in the propagation of impulses through the invertebrate ganglion, there is no basis for the unitary nerve cell. In the case of the new kinds of synaptic junction they are still articulations between two (or more) cells. It would seem, however, that the law of dynamic polarization is not applicable in these instances, since the whole cell is not induced to discharge. These are mechanisms for subtle alterations in the local activity of the synaptic partners. Long-distance signalling is not involved, although it may ultimately be influenced or regulated by the results of the local interactions produced at these unusual synapses.

Despite the apparent contradictions that exist, the basic terms *dendrite* and *axon* still need to be retained, for although a process may have both receptor and transmitting portions it would be clumsy and confusing to refer to it as a *neurite*, for example. Thus, dendrites will be considered to be those processes that are essentially extensions of the perikaryon and contain the same catalogue of organelles. Such processes may be multiple and are primarily receptive in function. Axons are unique processes, are not usually multiple, do not contain ribosomes, and are mainly concerned with transmission and conduction. On this basis, neurons that have a number of similar processes, but no one unique, would be considered anaxonal or amacrine. The salient features of these two types of processes are given in Table 1–1.

TABLE 1-1 *Characteristics of Axons and Dendrites*

Axon	Dendrite
1. Extends from either cell body or dendrite	1. Extends from cell body
2. Begins with a specialized initial segment (except dorsal root ganglion cell and autonomic ganglion cell)	2. At least in proximal portions, continues cytoplasmic characteristics of cell body
3. May be absent	3. Usually has irregular contours and specialized appendages
4. Unique in most cells, but there are some examples of multiple origin	4. Usually multiple
5. May be myelinated or unmyelinated	5. Rarely myelinated (and if so, only thinly)
6. Almost never contains ribosomes (except in initial segment)	6. Usually confined to the vicinity of the cell body
7. Usually has smooth contours and cylindrical shape	7. Microtubules predominate in the larger stems and branches
8. Usually thinnest process of the cell at site of origin	8. Usually originates as a thick tapering process
9. Ramifies by branching at obtuse angles	9. Ramifies by branching at acute angles
10. Usually gives rise to branches of the same diameter as parent stem	10. Usually subdivides into branches smaller than parent stem
11. Capable of generating action potentials, propagating them, and transmission	11. Conducts in a decremental fashion, but may be capable of generating action potentials
12. May extend long distances away from cell body	12. If cell body lies in central nervous system, dendrites remain entirely within central nervous system
13. Primarily concerned with conduction and transmission	13. Primarily concerned with receiving synapses

As the form of a nerve cell can hardly be appreciated in electron micrographs of thin sections, it may seem paradoxical to begin this book on fine structure with a discussion emphasizing the importance of that form. Yet it is not irrelevant. The fine structure of the neuron cannot be understood without a conception of the neuron as an entity. Just as no other cell displays such significant polymorphism as the neuron in the several parts of the nervous system, so no other cell displays such a variety of regional differentiations within its own boundaries as does the neuron. The perikaryon and its processes have each a characteristic internal structure that permits the microscopist to recognize them in extremely small samples and with minimal clues. In electron micrographs, the base of a dendrite is appreciably different from the axon hillock, and parts of the axon—the initial segment, the preterminal, and the terminal—are all distinctive and recognizable. Similarly, proximal and distal stretches of the dendrite are distinguishable. Thus, although most of the nervous system has still not been explored by electron microscopy, a pattern for the internal structure of the neuron seems now to be established, and it can be expected to hold good for all neurons. Much of this book is devoted to describing and illustrating this pattern of fine structure.

Armed with these morphological criteria for recognizing the neuron and its parts, the cytologist is prepared to begin the next important task: namely, to analyze the interrelations of the nerve cells. For this task an understanding of the form of the neuron is crucial. At first sight it might appear that electron microscopy is not a very appropriate tool for the study of interneuronal connections. The more traditional techniques, such as the various silver stains, and the more recently developed autoradiographic and enzymatic methods for tract tracing may seem more fitted to this purpose. Further reflections, however, will disclose that these methods applied at the light microscope level are not adequate by themselves and that electron microscopy is necessary for the analysis of the interrelations among cells. Electron microscopy offers two advantages not shared by the other morphological methods (Palay, McGee-Russell, Gordon, and Grillo, 1962). First, in properly prepared specimens all the different cells and their processes are visible in place at the same time in a single section. Second, the limits of each cell are clear because its surface membrane is visible. These two advantages make it possible to define precisely the morphological interrelations of cells. With this knowledge an understanding of the organization of the nervous system begins.

Chapter II

THE NEURONAL CELL BODY

Neurons are generally recognized in conventional histological preparations by their multangular shape, their large vesicular nuclei, and the Nissl bodies in their cytoplasm. Special stains and special modes of fixation are required to show not only the rest of the cell—for only the cell body is identified by these features—but also the other organelles that are disposed within its limiting membrane. Our image of the nerve cell at the light microscope level is like a collage of many overlapping views, patiently accrued during a century of study. Methods that display the Nissl bodies and the nuclei leave the rest of the cell uncolored, while methods that stain the mitochondria give only a pale rendition of the Nissl bodies, and methods that bring out the neurofibrillae reveal neither mitochondria nor Nissl bodies (see Frontispiece). The result is an image put together from various techniques and highly dependent on the methods commonly used for teaching histology and neurology. This restricted image must be reconciled with the dynamism of the crowded cytoplasm seen in the living nerve cell under cultivation *in vitro* and with the even richer, but unfortunately static cytoplasm seen in electron micrographs. The explication of these images is best made in conjunction with the light microscopy of fixed and stained preparations. Because of the size and shape of the nerve cell, constant cross reference between the two levels of microscopy is essential for orientation. Therefore in this and the following chapters, the description of cytological features will relate light microscopic findings to fine structure wherever possible.

The cell body, or soma, is the globular or polyhedral part of a neuron which comprises the nucleus and the surrounding cytoplasm and which gives rise to the processes of the cell. The cytoplasm contained in the cell body is known as the perikaryon. Although all three terms—cell body (soma), perikaryon, and neuron (nerve cell)—are often used interchangeably as if they were synonymous, each has a precise and distinct meaning. *Cell body* or *soma* includes both nucleus and cytoplasm; *perikaryon* refers only to that part of the cytoplasm surrounding the nucleus and excluding that part lying in the processes. *Neuron*, or *nerve cell*, should be reserved for the whole nerve cell, including the cell body, processes, and terminal arborizations.

THE PERIKARYON

THE NISSL SUBSTANCE

In light microscope preparations stained with basic dyes such as toluidine blue, cresyl violet, and methylene blue the cytoplasm of neurons displays an intensely basophilic component known as the Nissl substance (Frontispiece). This component is most striking in the large motor neurons of the spinal cord and brain stem, because in these cells the Nissl substance

11

has the form of large rhomboid blocks separated from one another by lighter-staining cytoplasm. In other neurons, such as those of the sensory ganglia, the Nissl substance occurs as small bodies of different sizes and shapes. In the smaller ganglion cells the Nissl substance appears as dust-like particles dispersed throughout the cytoplasm, whereas in the larger ganglion cells it is arranged as small granules concentrated at the periphery of the perikaryon. Between these two extremes of dust-like and block-like Nissl substance lie the Nissl patterns of most neurons in the central nervous system. Most commonly the Nissl bodies are basophilic masses of small to intermediate size (Nissl, 1894).

The different patterns of the Nissl substance are, however, regular characteristics of different types of neurons. At one time elaborate classifications of neurons were attempted on the basis of minute differences in the size, shape, and distribution of the Nissl bodies, but such classifications are no longer in fashion. Since both the intensity of cytoplasmic basophilia and its distribution are highly susceptible to postmortem and fixation artifacts, it is difficult to evaluate how significant many of these differences are. Certain categories may originate entirely during the postmortem processing of the tissue. Nevertheless, different neuronal types display distinctive and consistent Nissl patterns, which are probably correlated with the particular dynamics of their metabolism and protein production.

Although small neurons always contain dust-like Nissl bodies, there seems to be little correlation between the size of the Nissl bodies and the size of the perikaryon in larger neurons. Among large neurons, the spinal cord anterior horn cells with their block-like masses of Nissl substance must be compared with other equally large neurons, such as the Purkinje cells of the cerebellar cortex and the Deiters cells of the lateral vestibular nucleus, all of which possess

small Nissl bodies. In extremely large cells, like the Mauthner cell of teleost fishes, the Nissl substance is so widely dispersed that it hardly forms recognizable aggregates. In the cerebral cortex of primates, the giant Betz cell displays large, blocky Nissl bodies, while the equally large Meynert cell displays only small and diffuse granules (Chan-Palay, Palay, and Billings-Gagliardi, 1974).

Apparently each type of neuron has its characteristic Nissl pattern, which not only contributes an important identifying feature to its appearance but also reflects in some complex way its usual metabolic state. When this state is seriously disturbed, the Nissl pattern may be altered. For example, under various noxious conditions, such as excessive stimulation or interruption of the axon, certain large neurons undergo a sequence of changes in their Nissl pattern which is known as chromatolysis. This process was first reported by Nissl (1892), who described how the basophilic pattern of neurons in the facial motor nucleus of the rabbit changes after avulsion of the seventh cranial nerve. A detailed account of these changes is given in a classic paper by Bodian and Mellors (1945) on motor neurons in the anterior horn of the monkey's spinal cord. According to these and similar experiments, the parent cell body exhibits no obvious sign of reaction during the first few days after division of its axon. During this period, however, the nerve terminals synapsing on its surface are displaced through the activity of the surrounding neuroglial cells (Blinzinger and Kreutzberg, 1968; Torvik and Söreide, 1972; Cull, 1974 and 1975; Sumner, 1975). Regeneration of the severed axon already begins during these first few days while the cell body appears quiescent. But after three or four days the perikaryon begins to swell and the nucleus becomes eccentric. At the same time the Nissl bodies begin to fragment, a process that results in increasing pallor as the basophilic

Figure 2–1.   **The Cell Body of a Small Pyramidal Neuron.**

In the center of the field is the perikaryon of a pyramidal neuron from layer II of the rat cerebral cortex. Emerging from the perikaryon are the apical dendrite (Den_1), a basal dendrite (Den_2), and the axon (Ax). Most of the perikaryon is occupied by a large, rounded nucleus (Nuc), which contains a nucleolus (ncl) and homogeneously dispersed karyoplasm. The cytoplasm surrounding the nucleus is confined to a rim containing a few Nissl bodies (NB). One relatively large Nissl body lies at the base of the apical dendrite. The perikaryal cytoplasm also contains elements of the Golgi apparatus (G), which is most obvious at the bases of the processes of the neuron. In addition there are mitochondria (mit), free ribosomes (r), lysosomes (Ly), and microtubules (m) in the cytoplasm. The microtubules funnel into each of the processes in which they form parallel arrays. A number of axon terminals (At) synapse with the neuron, which is indented on one side by a capillary (Cap).
Cerebral cortex from adult rat. × 11,000.

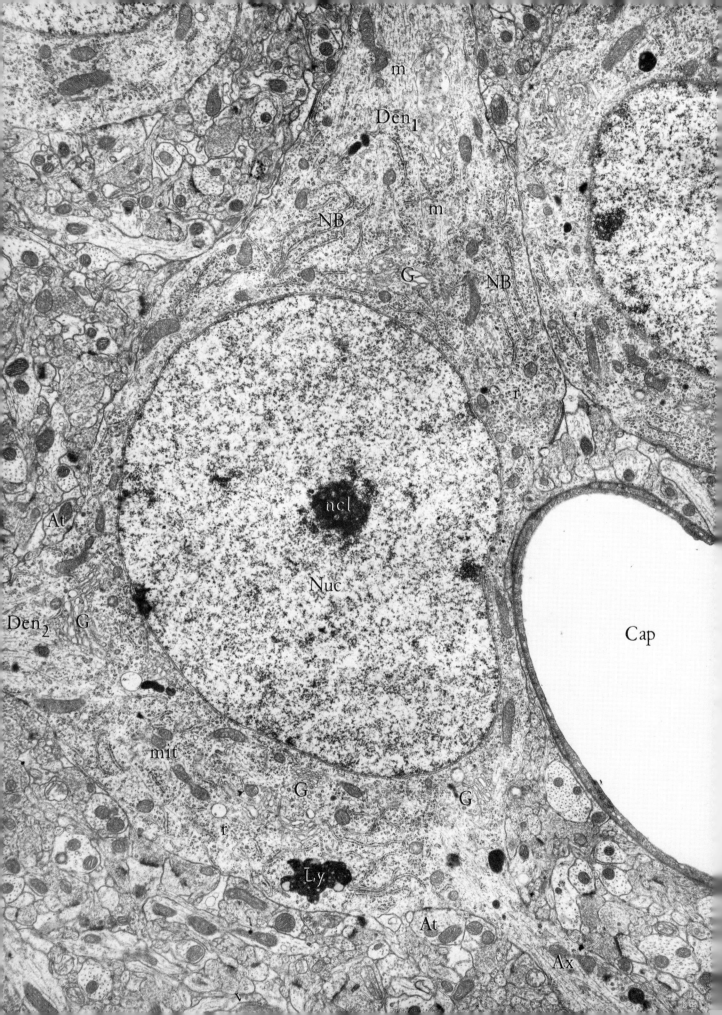

material becomes generally diffused throughout the cytoplasm. By the end of a week the Nissl bodies have disappeared from the central zone of the cytoplasm and are confined to a marginal region at the periphery of the cell body. If the cell succumbs to the injury, this process goes on to complete lysis, but if the cell is destined to survive, recovery is usually signalled by the appearance of basophilic material capping the pole of the nucleus that faces the center of the cell. During the second week the amount of basophilia in the cytoplasm progressively increases and the nucleus returns to its normal position. Nissl bodies first reappear as small, irregular particles, and these gradually increase in size until the normal pattern for the cell type is re-established over a period of four to twelve weeks. At this time regeneration can still be active at the damaged end of the axon, but apparently the neuronal cell body has recovered its equilibrium. The response of the basophilic material in this classic experiment reveals that the typical Nissl pattern of a neuron reflects the dynamic relation between the Nissl substance and the protein-synthesizing activity of the cell, rather than some conveniently fortuitous artifact of histological procedures. The fine structure of these changes will be considered in some detail later in this chapter.

The Nissl substance is not confined to the perikarya of neurons, for it is also present in dendrites. It is, however, absent from the axon, and at least in large neurons, a reduction in the amount of Nissl substance can already be observed within the axon hillock (see page 90).

Consequently, in preparations stained with basic dyes the axon hillock appears as a pale region at one pole of the perikaryon, giving a clue to the site of origin of the axon, which itself is not stained in such preparations.

Both in the light microscope and in the electron microscope it can be observed that the Nissl bodies do not have sharply defined limits but have wispy projections and sometimes stout arms extending to neighboring bodies. Connections between Nissl bodies are easy to find. It was just this appearance in fixed and sectioned material that led many cytologists to regard the Nissl bodies as nothing more than artifacts of precipitation (see Bensley and Gersh, 1933). But since it has been amply demonstrated that Nissl bodies are visible in living neurons, their existence is no longer called into question (Deitch and Murray, 1956; Deitch and Moses, 1957). Nevertheless, it is important to note that the Nissl bodies are not completely independent and separate cytoplasmic organelles like mitochondria or centrioles. They are more properly to be regarded as nodal points in an extensive reticulum that pervades almost the entire cytoplasm of the perikaryon and the major dendrites. This structure, of complex composition, is the exact counterpart of the basophilic substance, or ergastoplasm, of glandular cells, and it is the principal protein-synthesizing apparatus of the cytoplasm.

The electron microscope correlate of the Nissl substance is the granular or rough endoplasmic reticulum (Palay and Palade, 1955). In the most striking form of the Nissl substance, for

---

Figure 2–2.   **A Purkinje Cell.**

This large nerve cell displays all the organelles found in neurons. The nucleus (*Nuc*) is generally smooth but presents a wrinkled surface to the origin of the main dendrite, which passes out of the field at the left margin of the picture. The nucleus contains a fairly smooth dispersal of fine chromatin filaments and a large, dense, eccentric nucleolus (*ncl*). Well-organized granular endoplasmic reticulum (*ER*) and clouds of ribosomes in polysomal array form a rim around the nuclear envelope and stuff the infoldings in its apical surface. Smaller and less well ordered clumps of endoplasmic reticulum are distributed in the rest of the perikaryon. The Golgi apparatus (*G*) appears as an array of Golgi complexes disposed in the middle region of the perikaryon encircling the nucleus. Mitochondrial (*mit*) profiles of various sizes are grouped in clusters, and occasional microtubules (*m*) are visible. In the upper left corner, at the edge of the Purkinje cell, two mitochondria can be seen which approach very close to the surface membrane but are separated from it by subsurface cisternae. Other elements of the hypolemmal cisterna can be seen elsewhere beneath the surface membrane. At the bottom of the field a broad terminal (*ba*) of a basket cell axon approaches the surface of the Purkinje cell and forms a long synaptic junction with it. The terminal contains many flattened synaptic vesicles, and the approaching preterminal axon contains neurofilaments. A granule cell is evident at the bottom of the field.
Cerebellar cortex of adult rat. × 15,000.

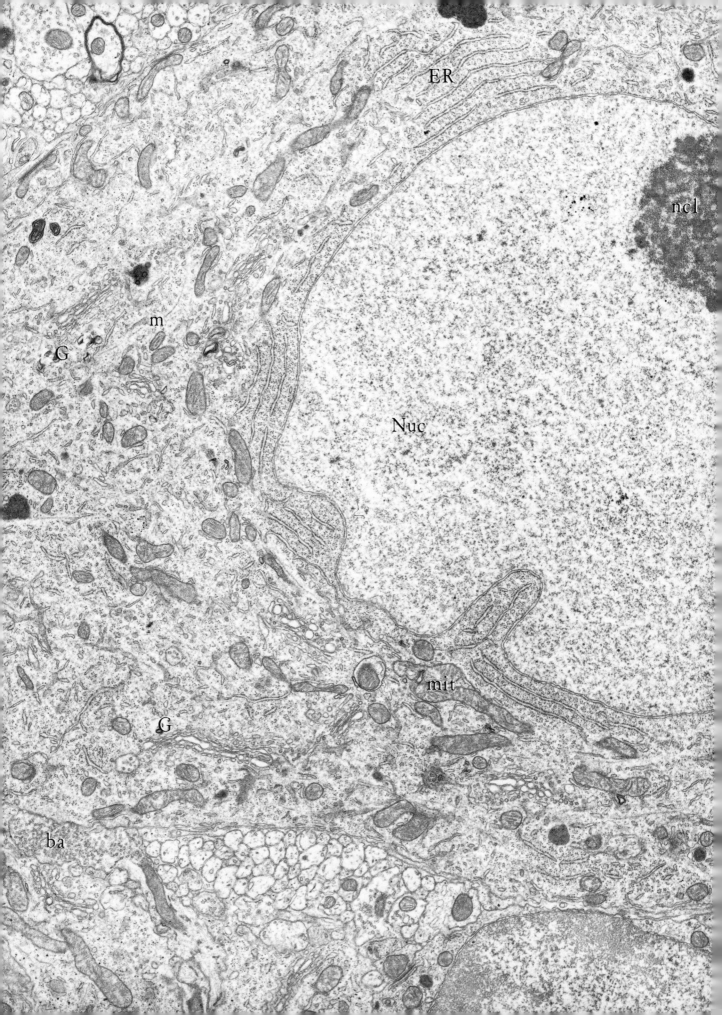

example, in the large, blocky Nissl bodies of motor neurons (Figure 2–8), the endoplasmic reticulum is disposed in orderly arrays of nearly parallel, broad cisternae, stacked one on top of another like pancakes, with fairly regular intervals of 0.2 to 0.5 micron intervening between them. As can be seen in Figures 2–2, 2–6, and 2–7, anastomoses between cisternae are frequent, and in addition, many cisternae are fenestrated. The result is a three-dimensional reticular structure of a complexity found in few cell types outside the nervous system.

The external surfaces of the membranes limiting these cisternae are studded with ribosomes arranged in rows, loops, spirals, or clusters (Figures 2–2 and 2–5 to 2–9). Some of these formations can be rather long, consisting of as many as 32 ribosomes. Careful inspection of the membranes shows that the ribosomes are not uniformly distributed and that large stretches of the cisternae are devoid of these embellishments. Consequently, in nerve cells it is not difficult to demonstrate continuity between the granular and agranular forms of the endoplasmic reticulum.

Ribosomes also lie free in the cytoplasmic matrix between the cisternae of the reticulum. They tend to be arranged in small clusters or rosettes of five or six granules surrounding a central one. These small free polysomes are characteristic of nerve cells. Even in perikarya with large and well-ordered Nissl bodies, a close examination of their construction reveals that most of the ribosomes are set into polysomal rosettes suspended in the intervals between cisternae rather than attached to the surface of the endoplasmic reticulum (see Figures 2–2, 2–5, 2–8, and 2–9). Accordingly, the structure of the Nissl bodies in nerve cells differs importantly from the structure of the ergastoplasm in protein-producing gland cells. Thus, in the exocrine pancreatic cell, for example, the cisternal membranes are regularly decorated with attached polysomes and only a small proportion of them are free. Although the significance of these dif-

ferences in the architecture of protein-producing structures is unknown at present, the following correlations may be pertinent:

1. The polysomal pattern apparently is related to the size and complexity of the protein molecules assembled in the cell, for both polysomal size and protein molecular size are dependent on the same messenger ribonucleic acid (Warner, Knopf, and Rich, 1963). If the differences in this respect between neurons and gland cells are to be considered significant, then the less obvious, but nevertheless discernible, differences in polysomal patterns among neurons of various types may also be taken seriously (see Sotelo and Palay, 1968). The existence of such differences among nerve cells suggests that neurons produce some proteins that are specific for their cell type or, at least, a specific mixture of proteins.

2. In gland cells the predominant pattern of attached ribosomes can be correlated with the production of protein that is deposited in the lumen of the endoplasmic reticulum and destined to be released from the cell as secretory droplets. In most neurons probably only a minor part of the protein production is devoted to secretory activity of this sort. The largest part of the proteins synthesized by neurons must be devoted to the maintenance and renewal of the protoplasm, including its organelles, especially the large fraction of it included in the axon. For example, more than 98 per cent of the protein in synaptic terminals originates in the perikaryon, from which it is conveyed to the nerve endings by means of fast axonal transport (Droz, 1973; Droz, Koenig, and Di Giamberardino, 1973; Koenig, Di Giamberardino, and Bennett, 1973; see also Chapter IV). The rate of this synthesis is thought to be exceptionally high in neurons. On the basis of regeneration rates it has been estimated that a large neuronal perikaryon renews one-third of its protein content each day. In the view of some, the large amount of Nissl substance and the high rate of protein synthesis are to be correlated with more specifi-

---

Figure 2–3.   **Pyramidal Neuron.**

This picture shows the apical pole of the perikaryon. The nucleus of the cell occupies the lower left portion of the field. In the cytoplasm are a few cisternae of endoplasmic reticulum (*ER*) and clusters of free ribosomes (*r*), while at the base of the apical dendrite (*Den*) are portions of the Golgi apparatus (*G*). Microtubules (*m*) funnel from the perikaryon into the dendrite to become oriented in parallel array. Between them are longitudinally arrayed mitochondria (*mit*) and profiles of smooth endoplasmic reticulum.

Note the lysosomes (*Ly*) in the cytoplasm and the axon terminals (*At*) that synapse with the neuron.

Cerebral cortex of adult rat. × 20,000.

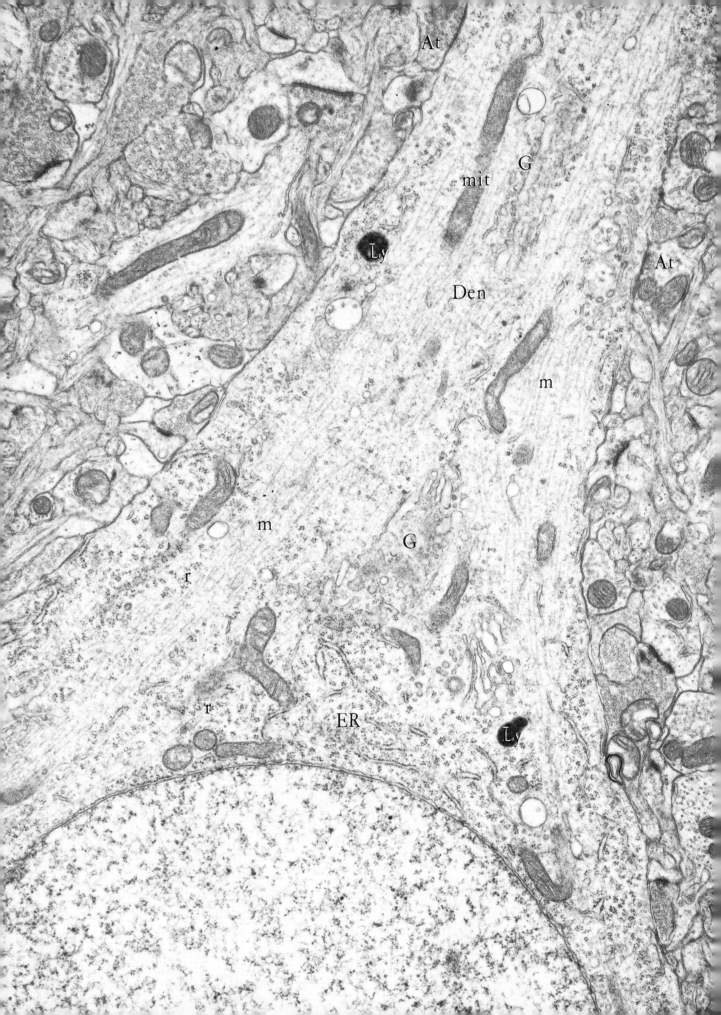

cally neural functions, such as the chemical encoding of previous events. Be that as it may, the important point to be noted here is that the ribosomes of the Nissl substance are probably concerned with synthesizing proteins destined for local use, within the neuron, rather than for exportation.

Neuronal perikarya lacking polysomal arrays have recently been noted in the visual cortex of the monkey *Macaca mulatta* (Palay, Billings-Gagliardi, and Chan-Palay, 1974). In these cells, mostly stellate and small pyramidal cells, the pattern of cytoplasmic organelles appears to be simplified. The endoplasmic reticulum consists of a single branched cisterna (or at most a few cisternae), wandering through the cytoplasm and delimiting broad fields, which are filled with ribosomes. The particles are set out individually, with no perceivable order. Even those attached to the outer surface of the endoplasmic reticulum appear to be randomly arranged. Some of the neuronal perikarya contain a few polysomes among the randomly dispersed ribosomes. The existence of such intermediate cells suggests that these cortical neurons undergo a cycle of protein-synthesizing activity in which transient cessation of protein synthesis is correlated with a dispersed ribosomal pattern, while decline or recovery is reflected by the appearance of a few polysomes in the fields of monoribosomes. Thus far, similar ribosomal patterns have not been found in any other neurons, and it remains to be seen how important this highly unusual configuration is. Electron micrographic studies of chromatolytic neurons have shown that although the aggregates of the granular endoplasmic reticulum decrease markedly in size (corresponding to the fragmentation of Nissl bodies visible in the light microscope) and although the great majority of the ribosomes detach from the cisternal membranes, the free ribosomes retain their polysomal clustering pattern (Pannese, 1963; Bodian, 1964; Kirkpatrick, 1968; Byers, 1970; Lieberman, 1971b and 1974b; Price and Porter, 1972). Only slow cell death (Schlüter, 1973; O'Connor and Wyttenbach,

1974) and injection of L-dopa (Munro, Roel, and Wurtman, 1973) are known to produce disaggregation of brain polysomes as complete as that seen in these cells of the monkey visual cortex. But these conditions are accompanied by severe degenerative changes in the other cellular organelles, which are not seen at all in these cortical neurons of normal monkeys.

In addition to the orderly arrays of the granular endoplasmic reticulum found in large motor neurons, small disorderly arrays and even individual isolated cisternae occur. These are most common in small neurons, which display small or ill-defined Nissl bodies in light microscopic preparations. But disorderly arrays also occur in the large cells, such as dorsal root ganglion cells (Figures 2-6 and 2-7). In the small and medium-sized pyramidal neurons of the rat's cerebral cortex the granular endoplasmic reticulum is arranged either as isolated cisternae or as small clumps concentrically disposed in the narrow rim of cytoplasm surrounding the nucleus (Figures 2-1 and 2-3). In the granule cells of the cerebellar cortex, the granular reticulum is hardly more than a few membrane-limited tubules associated with clusters of ribosomes (Figure 2-4).

It is these small, disorderly arrays of the granular endoplasmic reticulum that dominate the Nissl pattern of neuronal perikarya undergoing chromatolysis (Pannese, 1963; Bodian, 1964; Kirkpatrick, 1968; Byers, 1970; Lieberman, 1971b and 1974b; Torvik and Skjörten, 1971; Price and Porter, 1972). Furthermore, the proportion of free ribosomes markedly increases, while the amount of ribosomes attached to the cisternal membranes diminishes. Thus, there is an increase in the amount of agranular endoplasmic reticulum and a redistribution of the ribosomes that corresponds to the migrations of the Nissl substance seen in the light microscope. In mammals the Nissl substance tends to marginate at the periphery of the cell body, whereas in the cockroach ganglia, it accumulates around the nucleus in a distinctive ring (Cohen and Jacklet, 1965; Byers, 1970). As already mentioned, how-

---

Figure 2-4. **The Cell Bodies of Granule Cells.**

The perikarya of granule cells are usually clustered together, and their plasma membranes are often closely apposed (*arrowheads*). As these neurons are small, most of the cell body is occupied by the nucleus (*Nuc*), which displays several chromatin aggregates (*Chr*). The perikaryal cytoplasm is confined to a thin shell. The few cisternae of the granular endoplasmic reticulum (*ER*) and the free ribosomes (*r*) are not aggregated to form well-defined Nissl bodies, as in larger neurons. Other cytoplasmic organelles seen here are the mitochondria (*mit*) and the Golgi apparatus (*G*). *Cerebellum of adult rat.* × 22,000.

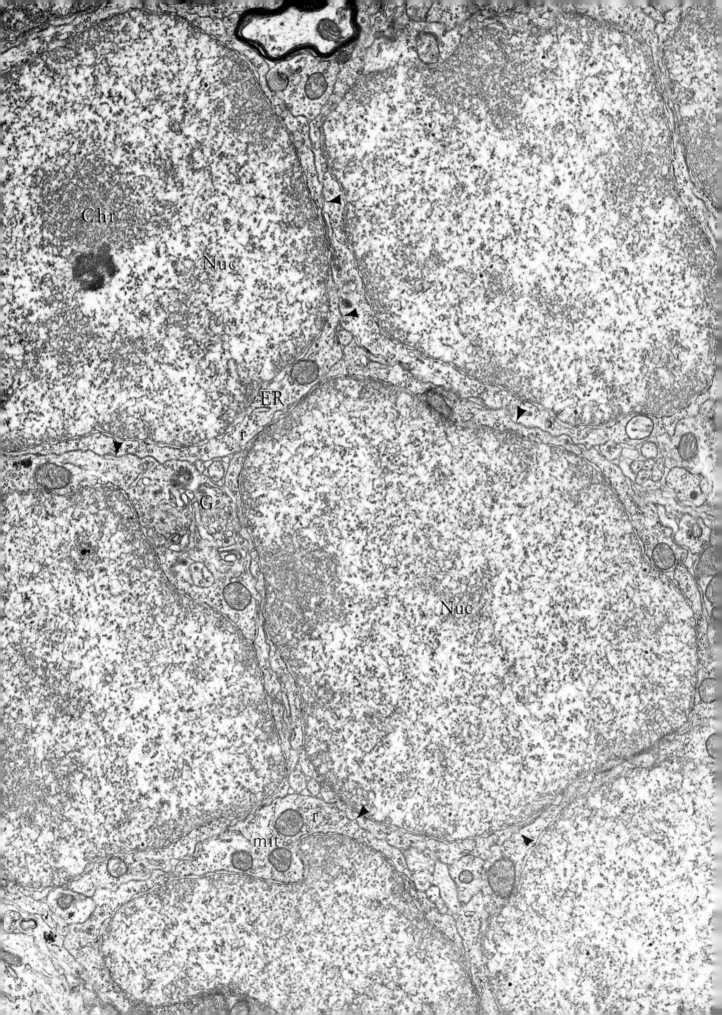

ever, the ribosomes in these rearranged Nissl bodies still appear in polysomal clusters. This morphological feature correlates very well with the seemingly paradoxical cytochemical analysis of chromatolytic perikarya, which shows that the amount of ribonucleic acid within the cell body has not declined during this process (Brattgård, Edström, and Hydén, 1957 and 1958). On the contrary, the first response of hypoglossal neurons to the interruption of their axons is a heightened nuclear RNA synthesis, which reaches a peak in the first three days (Watson, 1965 and 1968). This response is reflected in enlargement of the nucleolus and is accompanied by a rise in the cytoplasmic RNA to as much as twice the normal amount. The nuclear cap of basophilia, which Bodian and Mellors (1945) recognized as an early sign of recovery, is related to this increased transfer of RNA into the cytoplasm. Most of the RNA exists in the form of ribosomes, and associated with its increase is an intensification of cytoplasmic protein synthesis. As Bodian and Mellors (1945) noted, acid phosphatase also increases in the cytoplasm, and this is correlated with enlargement of the Golgi apparatus and increased numbers and complexity of lysosomes (Matthews and Raisman, 1972). In view of all these reconstructive changes, the chromatolytic response to axonal damage should be considered not a degenerative phenomenon ("retrograde degeneration," "Nissl's degeneration") but a restorative process aimed at reconstituting the neuron in its original state. The close coordination of the chromatolytic sequence in the perikaryon with regeneration of the axon at its severed end is thus more comprehensible.

THE AGRANULAR RETICULUM

The irregular distribution of ribosomes attached to the membranes of the endoplasmic reticulum, mentioned earlier, leads to an indefinite distinction between the granular (rough) and the agranular (smooth) endoplasmic reticulum. In neurons the continuity between the two types can easily be demonstrated. The agranular reticulum is, however, a prominent component of many neurons. For example, in the Purkinje cell (Figure 2–5) it occupies much of the space between the characteristically small Nissl bodies, giving the cytoplasm a dense appearance in electron micrographs that is not matched in stained preparations viewed with the light microscope. In the perikarya of large motor cells and pyramidal cells, it supplies a pervasive membranous network that becomes more noticeable at the bases of the processes, where the Nissl bodies dwindle and recede from prominence. The agranular reticulum consists of both tubular and cisternal elements, dispersed haphazardly and branching irregularly. Sometimes the cisternae are broad, fenestrated sheets with microtubules passing through the openings in them. Elements of the agranular reticulum extend into the dendrites and axon (Figures 2–1 and 2–3), where they are drawn out into sparsely branching tubules that meander in a roughly longitudinal direction. In some cell types the cisternae cross the general longitudinal traffic nearly at right angles and at fairly regular intervals along the length of these processes. A cross-striated appearance in the profile results. The fleshy axons of the cerebellar basket cells provide

---

Figure 2–5.   **The Cytoplasm of a Purkinje Cell.**

This field shows a region of the perikaryon that is particularly rich in Nissl substance. The nuclear envelope is just visible at the lower left edge, and the perikaryal surface appears at the lower right edge of the picture. The granular endoplasmic reticulum (*ER*) exhibits a rather disorderly organization with many anastomosing and branching cisternae. The agranular reticulum (*SR*) is widely distributed as individual tubular and cisternal elements and forms the hypolemmal cisterna just beneath the plasmalemma. The Golgi apparatus (*G*) with its associated vesicles, tubules, multivesicular bodies (*mvb*), and lysosomes (*Ly*) winds its way through the middle zone of the cytoplasm. The difficulty of deciding which aspect of the Golgi apparatus should be termed the forming face and which the maturing face is well shown in this figure. A cisterna of the granular endoplasmic reticulum clearly joining the Golgi apparatus through an agranular segment is shown in the lower right Golgi complex (*arrow*). Clustered mitochondrial profiles (*mit*) and relatively rare microtubules are also shown. Note the occasional dense-cored vesicles associated with the Golgi complexes.
Cerebellar cortex of adult rat. × 25,000.

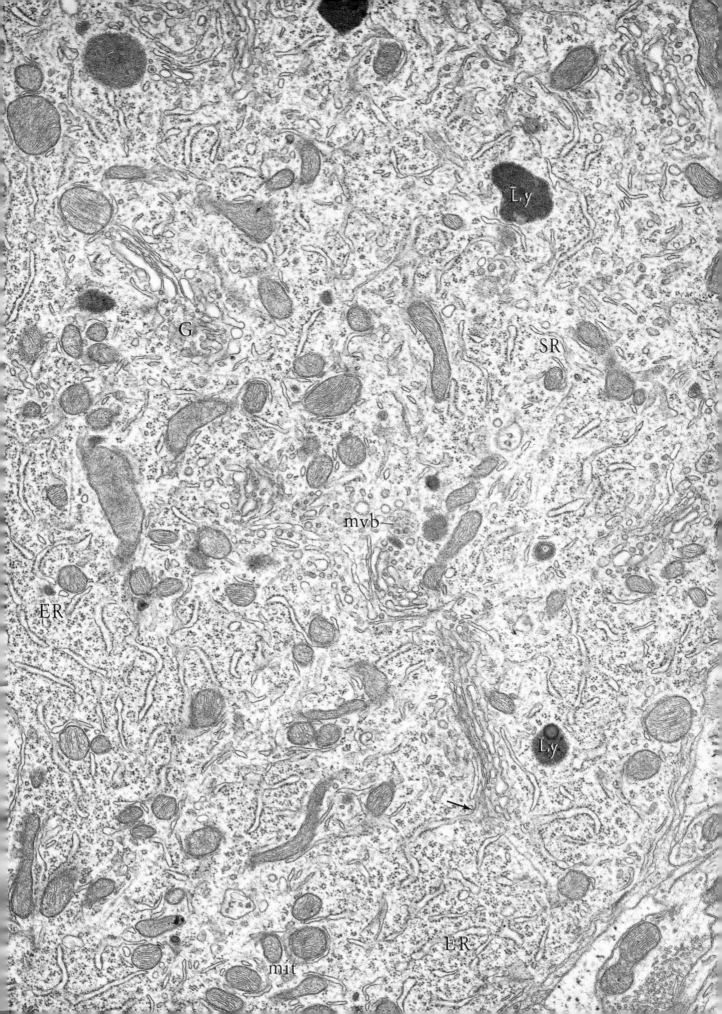

good examples of this appearance (Eccles, Ito, and Szentágothai, 1967; Palay and Chan-Palay, 1974). In traversing the axoplasm a cisterna must either circumvent the longitudinal elements or allow them to penetrate through it. In either case the cisterna is converted into a lacy curtain stretched across the axon, but it is no obstacle to the axoplasmic stream since the neurofilaments, microtubules, mitochondria, and matrix can all pass through the holes in it.

A somewhat peculiar modification of the agranular reticulum has been described by Rosenbluth (1962b) in cortical neurons and acoustic ganglion cells, by Nathaniel and Nathaniel (1966) in posterior horn cells of the spinal cord, and by many later authors. These authors have described stacks of agranular cisternae deep within the cytoplasm, in which the cisternae are arranged parallel to each other, and since their lumina are almost entirely obliterated, the appearance is that of a series of parallel and evenly spaced lines. At the edges of the stacks the cisternae may be dilated and may become confluent with one another or with the granular endoplasmic reticulum. Although these stacks of agranular cisternae somewhat resemble the spine apparatus in the dendritic spines of cortical neurons (see pages 81 to 82), it is not clear how much their existence is due to fixation artifacts or premortem anoxia.

As the agranular reticulum pervades the neuronal cytoplasm, it extends into the peripheral, or ectoplasmic, zone and approaches very close to the plasmalemma. Here it expands into a broad, flat, highly perforate cisterna that lies about 60 nm beneath the surface membrane. It runs consistently parallel to the plasmalemma, giving off streamers that turn inward and join the deeper elements of the granular or agranular reticulum. This hypolemmal cisterna was first recognized in the Purkinje cells of a mormyrid fish (Kaiserman-Abramof and Palay, 1969) and has since been noted in a large variety of nerve cell types. It is probably a characteristic of nerve cells generally. In most neurons the hypolemmal cisterna is represented by only a few

flattened cisternal profiles close to and parallel with the surface, but in the Purkinje cells of all animals so far examined (including fishes, amphibians, and mammals) it forms a conspicuous and characteristic secondary membranous boundary beneath the plasmalemma (Figures 2–2 and 2–5; Palay and Chan-Palay, 1974). In these cells it is so highly developed that it can be used to identify isolated profiles of the perikarya, dendrites, and axons of Purkinje cells in thin sections, since it extends into all these parts. Tangential as well as serial sections demonstrate that it is a continuous, although highly fenestrated (or reticular) cisterna. The existence of the hypolemmal cisterna indicates that the agranular reticulum has a much broader distribution in the cytoplasm of neurons than the granular (rough) endoplasmic reticulum and belies the adjective "endoplasmic," which has been attached to this system of membranes since the concept was introduced (Porter, 1953; Palay and Palade, 1955). The granular or rough reticulum, represented in the neuron by the Nissl substance, almost never approaches the surface membrane. It can, therefore, be readily considered as "endoplasmic." In contrast, the agranular reticulum suffers no such restrictions. Therefore, the term "endoplasmic" should probably be eliminated from its name.

A specialized variety of the hypolemmal cisterna was, in fact, the first part of this structure to be discovered. In 1962 Rosenbluth (1962b) drew attention to large, flattened vacuoles that were closely applied to the inner aspect of the plasma membrane of neuronal cell bodies and proximal dendrites. No other organelles intervene between the plasma membrane and such vacuoles, so that the two can be only 10 nm apart and the interval may be bisected by a faint intermediate line similar to that occurring in myelin (see page 192). Rosenbluth referred to these vacuoles as subsurface cisternae. Examples are visible in Figures 2–2, 2–3, and 2–4. Although these subsurface cisternae may occur singly, it is not uncommon for several cisternae to be aligned one beneath the other in a stack. Com-

---

Figure 2-6.   **The Cytoplasm of a Dorsal Root Ganglion Cell.**

At the right is the double-layered envelope (*Nev*) surrounding the nucleus of a sensory nerve cell. The envelope has pores that appear as circular profiles (*arrow*) where the nucleus is sectioned tangential to its surface.

In the perikaryal cytoplasm are small Nissl bodies (*NB*) composed of granular endoplasmic reticulum (*ER*) and many clusters of free ribosomes (*r*). In this type of neuron the areas of cytoplasm surrounding the Nissl bodies are rich in microtubules, neurofilaments, and mitochondria (*mit*). Note that in this neuron the cristae of the mitochondria are mainly oriented transversely. Also present in the cytoplasm are a few lysosomes, which have dense, granular contents.
Dorsal root ganglion of adult rat. × 36,000.

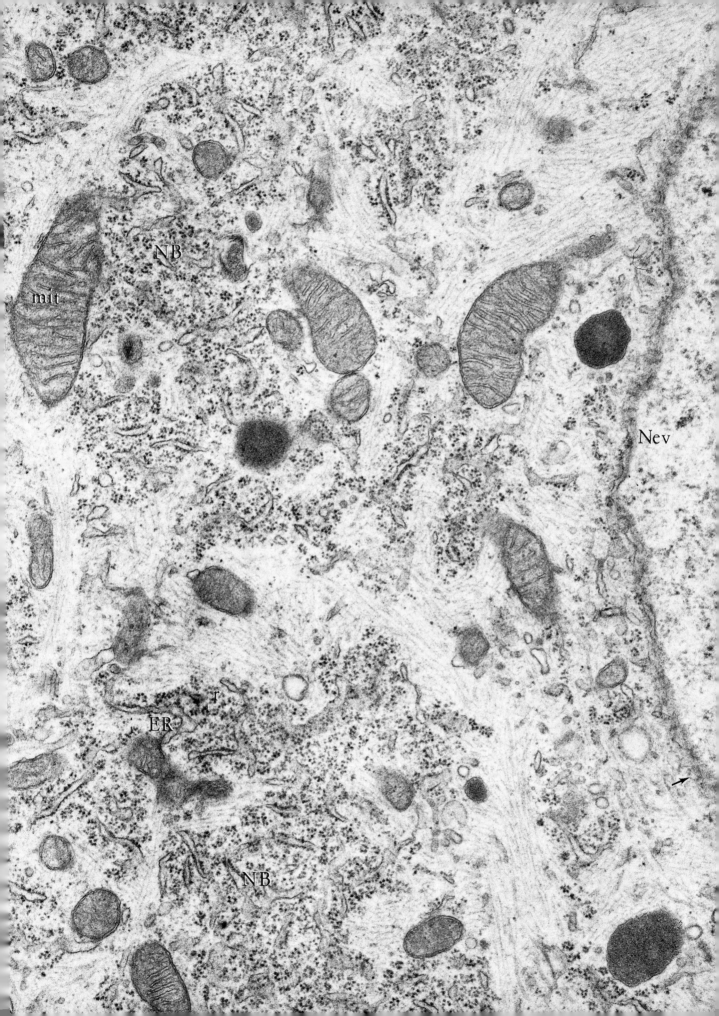

monly, the cisternae are dilated at their ends, and continuities have been demonstrated between them and components of both the granular and agranular reticulum, as with the hypolemmal cisterna in general. Further, the deep surface of the subsurface cisternae is sometimes studded with ribosomes. A peculiarity of subsurface cisternae in Purkinje cells is that they are often in close apposition to mitochondria, so that a subsurface cisterna sandwiched between a plump mitochondrion and the plasmalemma forms a distinctive complex (Figure 2–2; see Herndon, 1963; Siegesmund, 1968; Palay and Chan-Palay, 1974).

The functional role of the agranular reticulum in general, and of the hypolemmal and subsurface cisternae in particular, is difficult to envisage with the inadequate information available. The diffuseness of its distribution on the one hand and its intimate relationships to cell surfaces and the granular endoplasmic reticulum on the other all suggest that it would be a suitable structure for the rapid and wide dissemination of substances from their sites of synthesis or uptake. This expectation is encouraged by autoradiographic studies which provide indications that both proteins and glycoproteins are transported rapidly from the perikaryon to nerve endings by way of the agranular reticulum (Droz and Koenig, 1970; Schonbach, Schonbach, and Cuénod, 1971; Droz, 1973; Droz, Koenig, and Di Giamberardino, 1973; Koenig, Di Giamberardino, and Bennett, 1973; Droz, Koenig, and Rambourg, 1974). Furthermore recent work with horseradish peroxidase as a tracer demonstrates more strongly that the agranular endoplasmic reticulum is the pathway for retrograde transport of exogenous substances from the nerve endings toward the cell body (Sotelo and Riche, 1974; Nauta, Kaiserman-Abramof, and Lasek, 1975).

Indeed, the demonstration that all the reticular membranous organelles contain concanavalin binding sites—an indication of the presence of glycoproteins—seems to confirm a general chemical uniformity of the entire system and to relate it to the surface of the cell (Wood, McLaughlin, and Barber, 1974). The hypolemmal cisterna displays an intense affinity for concanavalin A, which suggests that it may contain a reservoir of glycoprotein for use at the plasma membrane. Rosenbluth (1962b) suggested that since subsurface cisternae lie close to the neuronal plasma membrane, whose contours they follow, the cisternae may be sites where material is taken up from the surrounding medium. This mechanism would allow ions and substrates to be channeled directly into the granular and agranular endoplasmic reticulum by way of the connections with the subsurface cisternae. It must also be mentioned that it is not uncommon to find subsurface cisternae lying beneath synapses, but whether the association of these two structures is significant or accidental is not clear, as subsurface cisternae can also occur where other types of processes approach a neuron (e.g., see Bodian, 1966a).

THE GOLGI APPARATUS

A special configuration of the agranular endoplasmic reticulum is identified with the "internal reticular apparatus" discovered by Golgi (1898a and b and 1899). In neurons examined by light microscopy, this apparatus appears as a tangled skein of tortuous, anastomosing strands and small vacuoles disposed around the nucleus like a garland or a shell (see Frontispiece). Golgi described this structure in a variety of neuronal types in a number of different animal species (not merely in the Purkinje cell of the barn owl, as is usually stated). It was quickly recognized that the apparatus is ubiquitous in plant and animal cells of all types, and after more than half a century of vexatious disputation, it is now generally agreed to be a genuine organelle, although of somewhat enigmatic function (Palay, 1958a; Novikoff and Goldfischer, 1961; Novikoff, 1967a; Beams and Kessel, 1968).

The electron microscopic equivalent of the

Figure 2–7.   **The Cytoplasm of a Dorsal Root Ganglion Cell.**

The cytoplasm of this cell contains well-defined Nissl bodies separated by spaces containing many microtubules (*m*) and neurofilaments (*nf*). Some of the ribosomes in the Nissl bodies are arrayed in rows attached to the outer surfaces of the cisternae of the granular endoplasmic reticulum (*ER*). Others (*r*) lie free in the intervening cytoplasmic matrix. In this picture most of the free ribosomes appear as rosettes of six or more members.

In the top left corner is part of the Golgi apparatus (*G*). This contains long, parallel cisternae with which many vesicles are associated. Part of the nucleus (*Nuc*) occupies the bottom of the field.

Dorsal root ganglion of adult rat. × 49,000.

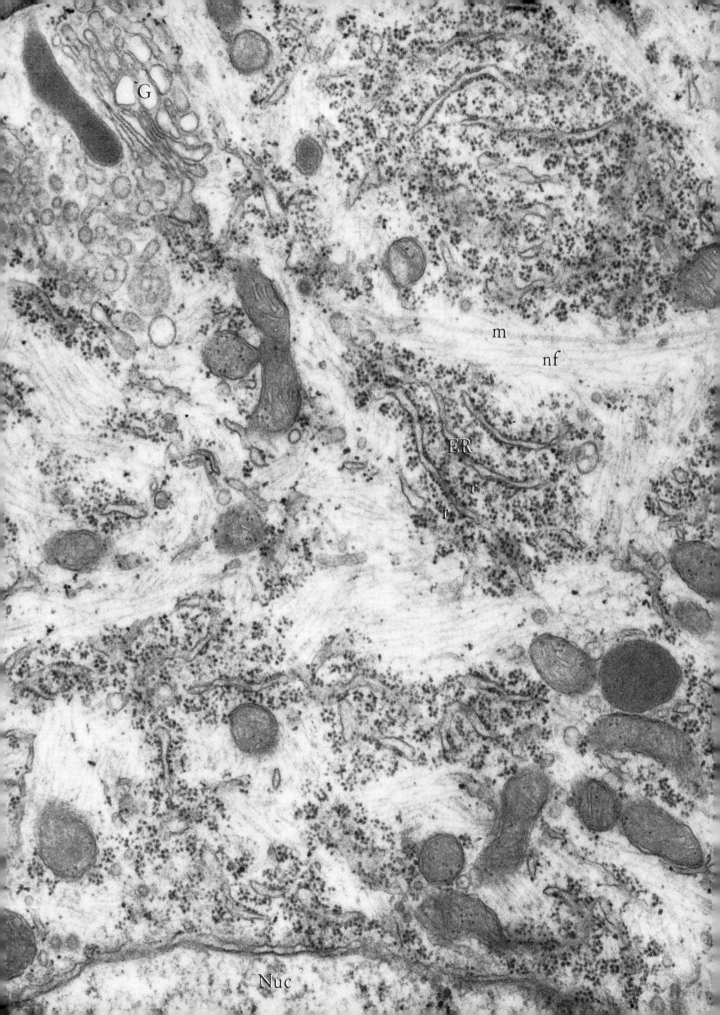

Golgi apparatus is a complex of broad, flattened cisternae together with a throng of various small vesicles (Figures 2–2, 2–5, and 2–8 to 2–11). In accordance with the location of the Golgi apparatus in light microscopic preparations, this aggregation of cisternae is usually disposed in the middle zone of the perikaryon, halfway between the nuclear envelope and the plasmalemma. The Nissl bodies tend to be concentrated in the cytoplasm on either side of this zone, thereby forming an inner, perinuclear zone and an outer, peripheral zone. Many neuronal cell types display such a concentric disposition of the more diffuse organelles, which are, perhaps, ordered by the course of the microtubules and neurofilaments through the cytoplasm.

As seen in the electron micrographs of thin sections, the cisternae of the Golgi apparatus are usually set out in curved arrays several microns in extent. Each of these arrays is known as a *Golgi complex.* In small to medium-sized cells such arrays can often be followed within a single thin section halfway or more around the nucleus, but in larger cells the complexes form apparently independent masses of cisternae and vacuoles. The reason for this discontinuity is that the thin section misses the connecting links that would tie the isolated masses into the continuous, loose-meshed network seen in the light microscope. Reconstructions from serial thin sections and high voltage electron microscopy of single thick sections (Favard and Carasso, 1973; Rambourg, Marraud, and Chretien, 1973) prove the soundness of this interpretation.

In each Golgi complex, the large cisternae are usually piled one atop another in stacks of five to seven with very little space between them (Figures 2–2, 2–5, 2–8, and 2–9). The close packing of the cisternae and the absence of ribosomes, either attached or free, distinguish Golgi complexes from the rest of the agranular reticulum on the one hand and from the Nissl substance on the other. Each cisterna is usually shallow, but some are widely dilated, especially at the edges of the complex (Figures 2–2, 2–8, and 2–11) or in its depths (Figures 2–2, 2–5, and 2–9). The cause of this dilation is uncertain; sometimes it is clearly artifactitious, but in some instances it seems to be related to function, as will be indicated presently. Although the cisternae ramify and their branches then join one another, there is very little anastomosis between cisternae at different levels within a stack. This is another distinction between the endoplasmic reticulum in the Golgi apparatus and that in the rest of the cell.

Morphological and histochemical studies on both neural and other tissues indicate that the Golgi complex is not homogeneous but that, instead, its cisternae display differential characteristics depending upon their location in the stack. In the first place each complex tends to have a curved outline, either completely enclosing a cytoplasmic space or, more frequently, opening like an archway toward the nucleus. The geometry of this form allows two surfaces to be distinguished in each stack of cisternae: a convex or external face and a concave or internal face.

Second, the character of the cisternae changes as one proceeds from the external to the internal face. The cisternae of the external face, especially the outermost one, are highly fenestrated, while those deeper in the stack display few interruptions. Thin sections that graze the outer surface of a Golgi complex show regularly spaced circular apertures in the cisternae (Figure 2–11). In contrast, sections that pass perpendicular to the surface show a chain of clear, circular or oval profiles that represent the membrane-bound lumen of the cisternae (Figures 2–2, 2–5, 2–8, and 2–9). In the latter plane, the cisternae appear to be discontinuous on account of the fenestrae which were shown *en face* in the grazing sections. Reconstruction of a short series of sections in the perpendicular plane easily demonstrates the continuity of the cisternae around these fenestrae. Fortunate cross fractures of neuronal cytoplasm in freeze-fractured mate-

---

Figure 2–8.   **A Nissl Body of an Anterior Horn Cell.**

Most of the field is occupied by a large Nissl body containing flattened cisternae of granular endoplasmic reticulum (*ER*). For the most part these cisternae form groups in which they are oriented parallel to each other. Between the cisternae are clusters of ribosomes (*r*) and small areas of cytoplasm containing a few microtubules (*m*) and neurofilaments (*nf*). The cytoplasm surrounding the Nissl body also contains neurofilaments and microtubules, in addition to mitochondria (*mit*).

In the lower left is part of the Golgi apparatus (*G*); its composition can be compared with the structure of the Nissl body.
Spinal cord of adult rat. × *31,000.*

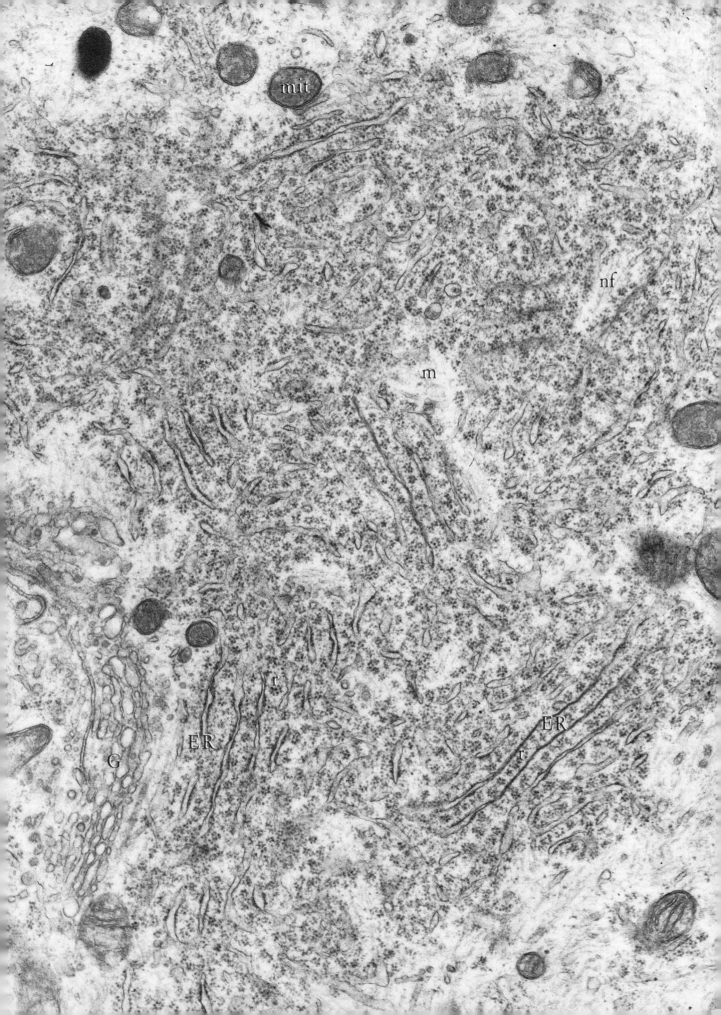

rial also confirm the continuity of the cisternae (Figure 2–10). Here the fenestrae can appear as regularly spaced pits if the fracture plane grazes the surface of a cisterna, or as broken columns of cytoplasmic matrix if the fracture plane splits off the roof and exposes the lumen of a cisterna (Figure 2–10). In either case the integrity of the cisterna is well shown. Another way of describing the same fenestrated cisternae was adopted by Rambourg, Marraud, and Chretien (1973) in their high voltage electron microscope study of the Golgi apparatus after osmium tetroxide impregnation. According to these authors the cisternae consist of "a tubular polygonal network," the fenestrae therefore being the openings in a two-dimensional lattice of connected tubules. Since the geometry of the fenestrated Golgi cisternae resembles that of the nuclear envelope and the annulate lamellae and since the fenestrae may well be transient or mobile features, it seems preferable to use a descriptive mode that emphasizes the larger, continuous, cisternal unit rather than its sometimes tubular form between fenestrae.

The deeper cisternae in the middle of the stack have few fenestrations and tend to be collapsed into thin discs, except at their perimeters, where, as already mentioned, they are frequently dilated. The deepest cisternae, on the concave or internal face of the Golgi complex, are often expanded into vacuoles, which in some instances bear a dense content. Associated with these are throngs of smaller vesicles, some clear and some dense-centered, some smooth-surfaced and some coated or alveolate. The field enclosed by the Golgi complex also contains some less well ordered membranous components, smooth-surfaced cisternae, and tubules that appear to be intermediate between the Golgi apparatus and the general agranular reticulum. These have been designated a part of the GERL system (Golgi apparatus, smooth endoplasmic reticulum, and lysosomes) by Novikoff (1967a) in order to suggest their intimate relation to the synthetic and condensing activity of the Golgi apparatus.

Third, the cisternae display differential cytochemical properties depending upon their location within the Golgi complex. The cisternae on the outermost, convex face of a stack are preferentially impregnated with heavy metal when the Golgi apparatus is visualized by the osmium tetroxide procedure. It is the one or two outer cisternae that become impregnated first (Friend and Murray, 1965; Friend and Farquhar, 1967; Friend, 1969; Rambourg, Marraud, and Chretien, 1973); only later do the deeper cisternae darken, making the whole apparatus appear coarse in light microscopic preparations. The deeper cisternae and vacuoles of the concave inner face fail to become impregnated with osmium, but can be shown to contain a variety of hydrolytic enzymes: acid phosphatase, thiamine pyrophosphatase, and AMPase (Osinchak, 1964; Friend and Farquhar, 1967; Novikoff, 1967a; Friend, 1969; Holtzman, 1971; Farquhar, Bergeron, and Palade, 1974). These cisternae also contain glycoprotein (Neutra and Leblond, 1966a and b; Rambourg, Hernandez, and Leblond, 1969; Weinstock and Leblond, 1971; Bennett, Leblond, and Haddad, 1974). Cytochemical studies on Golgi membrane fractions isolated from gland cells have shown that they contain glycosyltransferase, which catalyzes the attachment of terminal sugar residues onto the glycoproteins that are apparently concentrated by the Golgi apparatus (Fleischer, Fleischer, and Ozawa, 1969; Ehrenreich, Bergeron, Siekevitz, and Palade, 1973; Bergeron, Ehrenreich, Siekevitz and Palade, 1973). The recent demonstration that the Golgi apparatus of nerve cells is rich in binding sites for concanavalin A (Wood, McLaughlin, and Barber, 1974) suggests that in nerve cells, too, this organelle is concerned with

---

Figure 2–9. **The Golgi Apparatus and the Nissl Substance of a Purkinje Cell.**

In the upper half of the picture the Nissl substance is displayed in a fairly typical configuration. The granular endoplasmic reticulum (*ER*) extends in imbricated cisternae with free polysomes suspended in the voluminous matrix between. The plane of section first appears normal to the plane of the cisternae in the upper left corner and then becomes progressively tilted across the field so that in the lower half of the figure, the section is almost parallel with the membranes of the cisternae. This tilting allows the disposition of the attached polyribosomes to be seen. These polysomes appear in rows, spirals, circles, and rosettes.

Between the two masses of Nissl substance an elongated Golgi complex (*G*) stretches diagonally across the field. This shows narrow and dilated cisternae, fenestrated and nonporous cisternae, and numerous vesicles with and without alveolate coatings. Many mitochondria (*mit*) appear as clusters of small profiles, indicating that they are various sections of single digitate organelles. Finally, a few lysosomes (*Ly*) are visible, some of which are complex enough to be considered lipofuscin granules (*Lf*).

Cerebellar cortex of adult rat. × 23,000.

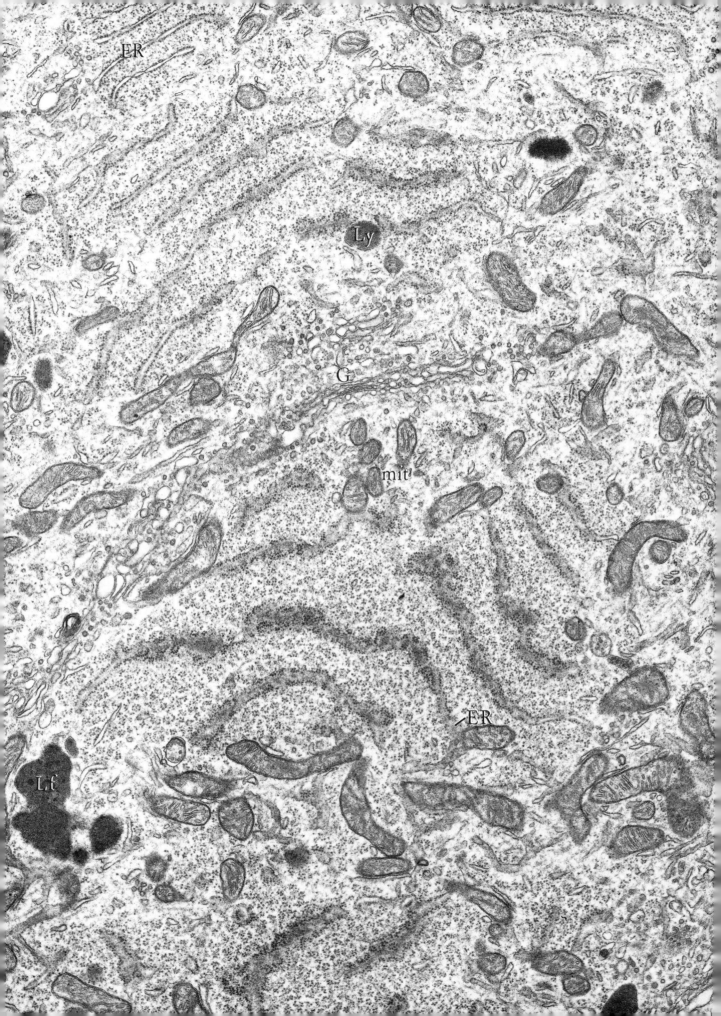

glycoprotein assembly. Although nearly all the investigations dealing with the cytochemistry of the Golgi apparatus have been done on gland cells, especially liver and pancreatic cells, enough histochemical observations have been made on nerve cells to indicate that their Golgi apparatus serves the same general function as in other cells (Osinchak, 1964; Holtzman, Novikoff, and Villaverde, 1967; Novikoff, 1967a; Holtzman, 1971; Novikoff, Novikoff, Quintana, and Hauw, 1971; Sotelo and Palay, 1971; Holtzman, Teichberg, Abrahams, Citkowitz, Crain, Kawai, and Peterson, 1973; Bennett, Leblond, and Haddad, 1974).

On the basis of morphological observations on plant cells, Mollenhauer and Whaley (1963) proposed that the formation of secretory vesicles involves a progressive movement of secretory product through the stack of cisternae in such a way that cisternal fragments separate as vesicles from the maturing, concave aspect of the Golgi complex while new cisternae are continually added at the opposite, forming face. Although Mollenhauer and Whaley performed no experiments to substantiate their interpretation, the polarization of the Golgi apparatus, along with the implied translocation of cisternal membrane from one side to the other, rapidly entered the standard descriptive terminology of the Golgi apparatus. A certain amount of evidence has accumulated which indicates that at least with respect to gland cells it may be substantially correct. For example, in an autoradiographic study of intestinal goblet cells Neutra and Leblond (1966a and b) showed that tritiated glucose or galactose migrates from the cisternae of the Golgi apparatus to the mucus droplets forming along the inner face. Similarly Weinstock and Leblond (1971), in a more detailed examination of the Golgi apparatus in ameloblasts, demonstrated that the labelled precursor (tritiated galactose) first appears in the cisternae of the form-

ing face, then in the maturing face, and finally in the secretory droplets. Claude (1970) analyzed the progressive accumulation of lipoprotein particles in the Golgi cisternae of the liver after a dose of alcohol and concluded that there was a progressive translocation and concentration of the secretory product from the forming face to the maturing face of the Golgi complexes. The cytochemical studies on isolated subfractions of Golgi complexes from liver also lend some credence to the hypothesis of polarization, since the fractions isolated from the more central parts of the complex have a different enzymatic content from that of the more peripheral parts (Ehrenreich, Bergeron, Siekevitz, and Palade, 1973). Nevertheless, as these authors have remarked, in the liver the Golgi apparatus is not so clearly polarized as it is in the goblet cells or in the epididymal epithelium (Flickinger, 1969), and therefore it is difficult to be sure that the apparent origins of the subfractions are correctly identified.

So far as nerve cells are concerned it must be admitted that the polarization of the Golgi apparatus is even less clear than in the liver cell. Although roughly circular and arching arrays are common configurations, vacuoles, small vesicles, and alveolate vesicles are not consistently disposed on only one aspect of the stack, so that it is often difficult to decide which face should be considered as the forming face or the maturing face. In neurons the Golgi apparatus is not only widely dispersed in the cytoplasm as a circumnuclear reticulum but it is also prolonged into the dendrites, at least as far as the first branching (Figure 2–2). It does not, however, extend into the axon (Figure 2–1). As a result of this dispersal, the neuronal Golgi apparatus lacks a single morphological center of reference. Furthermore, since the formation of secretory droplets is not a common activity of the neuronal Golgi apparatus, there is usually no visible cli-

---

Figure 2–10.   **Two Views of the Golgi Apparatus in a Freeze-Fractured Preparation.**

The **upper panel** is a portion of the nuclear envelope (*Nev*) and perikaryal cytoplasm of a granule cell in the cerebellar cortex. A number of mitochondria (*mit*) and cisternae of the endoplasmic reticulum (*ER*) appear in relief or are cross-fractured. The Golgi apparatus (*G*) is represented by the outermost cisterna, which has been broken open and shows an array of pillar-like protrusions (*arrows*) that correspond to the fenestrations seen in conventional electron micrographs. Similarly in the nuclear envelope, where both the inner and outer membranes are seen, the nuclear pores appear either as projecting mounds (▼) or as rounded craters (△). *Cerebellar cortex of rat.* × 90,000.

The **lower panel** shows a cross-fracture of a Golgi complex and displays the fenestrated character of the outer three cisternae in contrast to the broad continuity of the inner cisternae. *Arrows* point to some of the perforations in the cisternae. Small vesicles appear at the ends of the cisternae and within the circle of the complex. *Cerebellar cortex of rat, Golgi cell.* × 98,000.

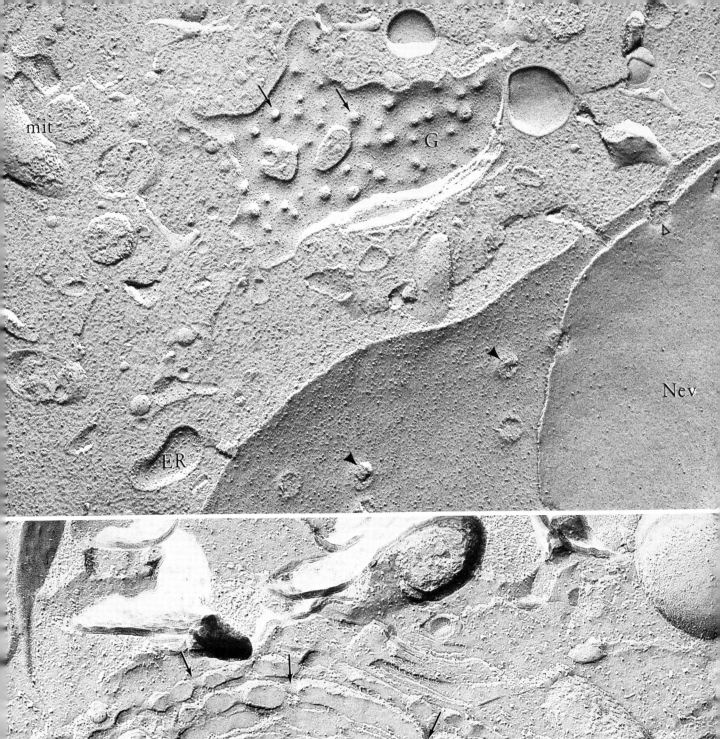
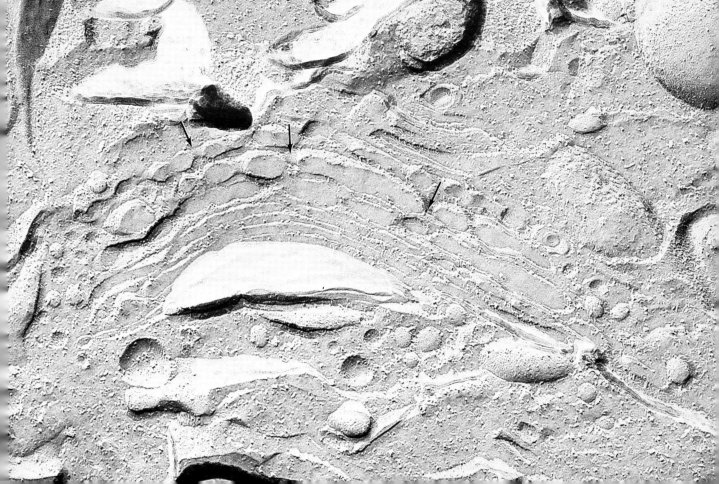

max to the supposedly orderly progression of Golgi vesicles. Indeed, the differences between the two faces of the Golgi complexes are not so regular as they are reported to be in other cell types. At least in some nerve cells, sugar residues (as detected by concanavalin A binding sites) are not selectively restricted to the inner maturing face, as has been suggested for other types of cells (Wood, McLaughlin, and Barber, 1974). Consequently the proposed polarity of the Golgi apparatus may be obscured in nerve cells, even though maturation of individual cisternae and their content may occur. For example, in neurosecretory cells, which do form droplets, the dense neurosecretory material can appear within cisternae that lie deep within a Golgi complex and are not clearly associated with either face.

Finally, the Golgi apparatus is not nearly so homogeneous and exclusive a structure as the Nissl substance. It shares its cytoplasmic precinct with a variety of other organelles—mitochondria, multivesicular bodies, lysosomes, granular vesicles, and alveolate vesicles—some of which seem to be directly related to it and others of which appear unrelated. In most epithelial cells this heterogeneous assemblage is concentrated in a single region, usually near the apical pole of the nucleus, with the closely packed cisternae forming a kind of enclosure around the small vesicles, lysosomes, centrioles, and other bodies and constituting with them a specialized zone, called the centrosphere. In some small neurons this arrangement is reproduced at the base of one or another dendritic process, but generally the Golgi apparatus is dispersed throughout the intermediate zone of the cytoplasm, as has been mentioned. This reticular form and diversified composition make it difficult to ascertain which organelles and inclusions in the intermediate zone really belong to the Golgi apparatus and which are intruders. Continuity with the more diffuse agranular endoplasmic reticulum also makes the margins of the region somewhat arbitrary. For these reasons histochemical and functional characterizations of the components of the Golgi region, for example, the alveolate vesicles and the lysosomes, have been especially illuminating.

The swarms of small vesicles associated with the Golgi complexes vary considerably in size, shape, and other properties. They range from 20 to 60 nm in diameter and are generally round or elliptical. Most of them have a smooth limiting membrane like that of the cisternae, but many of them bear a furry coat that marks them as a special class of vesicle (Figure 2–5). These "coated" vesicles are generally 50 to 60 nm in diameter and are distinguished by having regularly spaced striae, about 15 nm long, extending radially from the outer surface of their limiting membrane. Although the striae have been referred to as "spines" and "bristles," surface views and oblique sections suggest that they actually are the vertical walls of contiguous hexagons that cover the surface of the vesicles like a honeycomb (Palay, 1963b; Bowers, 1964; Friend and Farquhar, 1967; see also Chapter V). For this reason the name "alveolate vesicles" was proposed for them (Palay, 1963b). In 1969 Kanaseki and Kadota reported their successful isolation of coated or alveolate vesicles from synaptic terminals of guinea pig brain and carried out a careful high resolution study on the nature of

---

Figure 2–11.   **Golgi Apparatus, Lysosomes, Nematosomes, and Fibrillary Inclusions.**

The **upper picture** shows part of the cytoplasm of a neuron. In the middle of the field is part of the Golgi apparatus (*G*) to show the appearance of the cisternae sectioned in different planes. Toward the bottom, the profiles of the cisternae are cross-sectioned (*asterisk*) so that their typical stacking is apparent. Elsewhere the cisternae have been grazed in a plane parallel to their long axes and display the regularly spaced, circular apertures (*arrows*) by which they intercommunicate. In addition to the Golgi apparatus the picture shows granular endoplasmic reticulum (*ER*), ribosomes (*r*), microtubules (*m*), and multivesicular bodies (*mvb*). There are also some lysosomes (*Ly*) and a lipofuscin granule (*Lf*).
Cerebellar cortex of adult rat, Purkinje cell. × 27,000.

The **lower left picture** is of a nematosome (*arrow*) which has a finely filamentous matrix with some particles, so that the structure resembles a nucleolus. Near the bottom of the micrograph is another inclusion (*arrowhead*) that is more homogeneous and does not have its contents aggregated into small clusters like the nematosome.
Ventral cochlear nucleus of rat. × 40,000.   *Micrograph by M. L. Feldman.*

The **lower right picture** is a fibrillary inclusion. Bounding the inclusion (*arrow*) is a wall composed of finely filamentous material that forms a network containing tubules, so that it has a honeycombed appearance. The contents of the inclusions are slender filaments (*f*) arranged in a skein. Note the lysosome (*Ly*) in the field.
Ventral cochlear nucleus of rat. × 30,000.   *Micrograph by M. L. Feldman.*

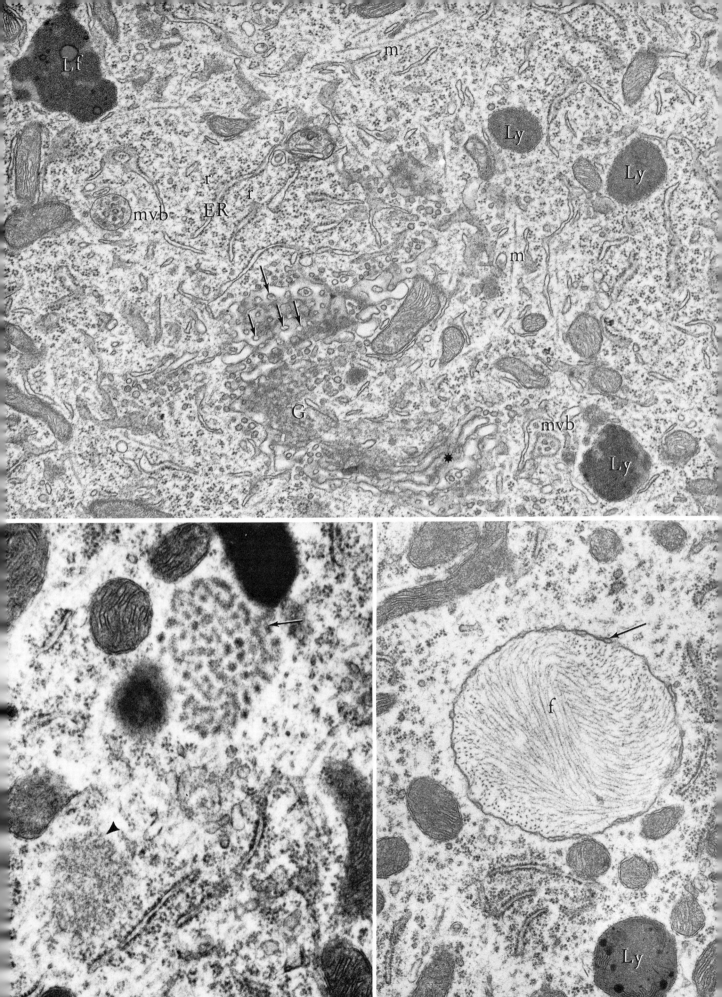

the coat in both sectioned and negatively stained specimens. They concluded that all the images seen in thin section could be accounted for by projections onto a single plane of a kind of cage work composed of hexagonal and pentagonal units within which the vesicle is freely suspended. Consequently they described the coated vesicle as "a vesicle in a basket." Although this term has not been widely adopted since it is too cumbersome for ordinary usage, the essential correctness of their analysis has been generally recognized. The encompassing "basket" has even been considered a completely independent structure that can slip off the vesicle and survive intact in the cytoplasmic matrix (Gray and Willis, 1970; Heuser and Reese, 1973 and 1974). But in recent publications Gray (1972 and 1973) regards the "basket" as part of the "cytonet," a filamentous protein reticulum that pervades the cytoplasmic matrix.

The ideas that the "basket" is independent of the vesicle or that it is continuous with a pervasive fibrillar reticulum are both difficult to reconcile with the prevalent notion that the coating specifically marks certain kinds of membrane or membranous organelles. For example, similarly coated membranes are frequently encountered at the ends of the Golgi cisternae and even as bud-like protuberances from the main bodies of the cisternae, especially in regions where they are fenestrated (Figures 2–5 and 2–7). Images such as these suggest that alveolate vesicles originate from or coalesce with the Golgi cisternae. Histochemical work at the electron microscope level (Osinchak, 1964; Holtzman, Novikoff, and Villaverde, 1967; Friend and Farquhar, 1967; Lane, 1968, among many others) indicates, however, that whereas only the innermost Golgi cisternae contain acid phosphatase, the alveolate vesicles of the region are full of this hydrolytic enzyme. Thus the alveolate vesicles qualify for the second name "primary lysosomes" (Friend and Farquhar, 1967). In recent years the concept has been gradually developed that the alveolate vesicles are derived from the Golgi elements and that they are concerned with the transport of hydrolases to the multivesicular bodies and other lysosomal inclusions (see, for example, Novikoff, 1967b; Friend and Farquhar, 1967; Holtzman, Novikoff, and Villaverde, 1967).

In some cells there is another type of alveolate vesicle, about 100 nm in diameter, which has been shown to contain no hydrolases and to derive from the cell surface by a process of invagination or pinocytosis. Vesicles of this type are much less common in neurons than the small vesicles of the Golgi region, but they can be found at the surface of the perikaryon and its processes and occasionally in the cytoplasm. Such vesicles evidently ingest protein and carry it into the cell, where it is deposited in the multivesicular bodies, or "secondary lysosomes," for digestion (see Roth and Porter, 1964; Rosenbluth and Wissig, 1964; Graham and Karnovsky, 1966; Friend and Farquhar, 1967). The fact that these vesicles are much more common in nerve terminals than in the cell body (see Chapter V) has become the basis for a valuable new method for tracing nervous connections in the central nervous system (La Vail and La Vail, 1972; La Vail, Winston, and Tish, 1973). Exogenous horseradish peroxidase injected into the nervous tissue is preferentially taken into the terminals by these pinocytotic vesicles and transported to the smooth endoplasmic reticulum within which it is conveyed back to the parent cell body (Sotelo and Riche, 1974; Nauta, Kaiserman-Abramof, and Lasek, 1975). Cells of origin for terminals in almost any region can be conveniently and precisely labelled in this way (Figure 11–6). Cell bodies in the immediate area of the injection site are not labelled unless they have been previously damaged or are mechanically injured by the injection (Lynch, Gall, Mensah, and Cotman, 1974).

In nearly all nerve cells some of the larger smooth-walled vesicles associated with the Golgi apparatus contain a single dense spherical granule (Figure 2–5). These are termed large granular vesicles and their significance has been the subject of a long-standing debate. The best single review of this subject has been published by Bloom (1973). Since similar large, dense-cored vesicles appear in nerve terminals in varying numbers throughout the nervous system, it was reasonable to search for correlations between the presence of these vesicles and the existence of certain neurotransmitters. Because of their frequency in sympathetic ganglia (Grillo and Palay, 1962; Grillo, 1966; Bloom and Barrnett, 1966) and in certain regions of the brain known to contain catecholamines, large granular vesicles were quickly taken to be storage vesicles for catecholamines (Pellegrino de Iraldi, Farini Duggan, and De Robertis, 1963; Aghajanian and Bloom, 1966; Pellegrino de Iraldi and Etcheverry, 1967; De Robertis, 1967). They were present along with small granular vesicles (see Chapter V) in the nerve endings of the pineal gland, which Wolfe, Potter, Richardson, and Axelrod (1962), in the first study of its kind, had shown to be capable of taking up exogenous tritiated norepinephrine and thus of being labelled for electron microscopic autoradiography. An early success in concentrating large granular vesicles in a subfraction of brain homogenates that was enriched with norepinephrine seemed to substantiate the claim that these vesicles were catecholamine storage sites (De Robertis, Pellegrino de Iraldi, Rodriguez de Lores Arnaiz, and Zieher, 1965). While this surmise was undoubtedly correct in some instances, attempts to correlate the incidence of large granular vesicles in electron micrographs of brain sections with the biochemical estimates of the concentration of catecholamines in the same regions met with conflicting evidence from other methods such as formaldehyde-induced fluorescence (Fuxe, Hökfelt, and Nilsson, 1965; Fuxe, Hökfelt, Nilsson, and Reinius, 1966; Dahlström and Fuxe, 1964; Hökfelt, 1967a and b). The resulting disagreements led to confusion and a mistrust in the putative relation between large granular vesicles and catecholamines that was summed up in the earlier edition of this book with the words "Clearly, more information is needed."

Doubts that they had any significant relation were strengthened by two studies published in the early 1970's. In an autoradiographic investigation with tritium-labelled exogenous norepinephrine, Descarries and Droz (1970) could find no correlation between the location of the labelled transmitter and the presence or absence of vesicles of any kind in the cells of the locus coeruleus and the griseum centrale pontis, centers with high concentrations of endogenous norepinephrine. Similarly, Sotelo (1971b), in a study of the substantia nigra and the area postrema, found that axonal profiles devoid of any granular vesicles (although filled with small, round, clear vesicles) could be richly labelled with radioactive norepinephrine, while terminals containing large granular vesicles could be unlabelled. Thus, the conclusion seemed inescapable that the presence of large granular vesicles was not necessarily a sign of catecholamine storage. In neither of these studies was the possibility explored that the large granular vesicles might be incapable of taking up exogenous norepinephrine and therefore failed to be labelled although containing endogenous transmitter.

As more regions have been studied, and as the techniques for identifying and differentiating transmitter *in situ* have become more sophisticated, the nature of the large granular vesicles has begun to clarify, but much work must still be done to dispel the confusion of the initial period. Clearly, the source of the confusion is the simplifying assumption that all large granular vesicles in neurons are alike. That this is not true is indicated by their wide range of sizes, from 80 to 200 nm in diameter. The largest of these vesicles, 120 to 200 nm in diameter, are found only in the cells of the hypothalamic neurosecretory nuclei, the supraoptic and paraventricular nuclei, and in their axons and terminals in the neurohypophysis. Early or immature neurosecretory granules, occurring in the Golgi regions of the parent cell bodies, are, however, likely to be smaller, and therefore they resemble the ordinary large granular vesicles found generally in neuronal perikarya. In addition, some of these vesicles, 80 to 120 nm in diameter, may be early lysosomes since they may contain acid phosphatases. Vesicles of this type could not be expected to undergo depletion under the influence of reserpine or repletion in the presence of catecholamine analogues such as 5-hydroxydopamine and so would fail to correlate with the titer of catecholamines in the region.

In the peripheral nervous system there are nerve cell bodies that contain numerous large granular vesicles together with a high content of biogenic amines. These are the perikarya in the sympathetic ganglia, which use norepinephrine as a transmitter, and include the small, intensely fluorescent cells also found in these ganglia, which in some cases, for example, in the rat's superior cervical ganglion, use dopamine as a transmitter. The latter cells are filled with large granular vesicles. In the central nervous system, neuronal perikarya that are well supplied with biogenic amines have been found in the hypothalamus, locus coeruleus, the reticular formation, and the basal ganglia (striatum and substantia nigra), but by and large, these cells exhibit few or no granular vesicles. For example, the cells of the locus coeruleus, one of the richest sources of catecholaminergic fibers in the brain and an avid acceptor of exogenous norepinephrine, contain only rare large granular vesicles (Ramón-Moliner, 1974). Similarly the cell bodies in the nucleus of the dorsal raphe, which are rich in serotonin (5-hydroxytryptamine, 5-HT), an indolamine, also contain few, if any, large granular vesicles (Bloom, Hoffer, Siggins, Barker, and Nicoll, 1972; Chan-Palay, 1975), while their axonal terminals characteristically contain many large granular vesicles of a variably dense sort as well as many small clear vesicles. On the other hand, the cells of the arcuate nucleus in the hypothalamus contain numerous large granular vesicles that apparently are associated with biogenic amines (Brawer, 1971). The question of the significance that should be ascribed to the different kinds of dense-cored vesicles in synaptic terminals will be taken up again in a later chapter (Chapter V), where their relation to small granular vesicles will also be discussed.

It is clear that the diversity of situations in which large granular vesicles appear within neuronal perikarya and axonal terminals militates against forming any firm generalizations about their significance until a large variety of situations has been thoroughly explored by morphological, cytochemical, metabolic, and autoradiographic techniques. Even then the vesicles may remain enigmatic in particular cases because they fail to participate in known mechanisms. In relation to the Golgi apparatus it is only pertinent to remark that large dense-cored vesicles are not a homogeneous population and that they differ in chemical content in different regions of the nervous system, in different species, and even perhaps in different parts of the same neuron. They must therefore be examined independently by pharmacological and cytochemical means in each site and in each species where they are discovered. The explanation of their rarity in the somata of known bioamine-containing cells in the central nervous system may have to be sought in the particular characteristics of these cells—perhaps in the rate of production of such vesicles in the Golgi apparatus, or in the rate of axoplasmic transport so that the vesicles are quickly removed and not stored in the cell body, or in the peculiarly efficient uptake and recycling mechanisms available at the axonal terminals which make prepackaging in the Golgi apparatus superfluous.

Before leaving the topic of the Golgi apparatus it seems desirable to review its role in the neuron. In gland cells, in which it has been most thoroughly studied by cytochemical methods, the Golgi apparatus plays a pivotal role in the condensation and segregation of the secretory product for export out of the cell. It also appears to be a nodal point in some of the interchanges between the granular endoplasmic reticulum and the plasmalemma, exchanging membrane components with the former on one face and with the latter on the opposite face. It also has a function in completing the assembly of glycoproteins, which may be later incorporated into the plasmalemma or attached to its outer surface. Finally, it has a part to play in the formation of lysosomes, at least to the extent that acid hydrolases are deposited within the lumina of its cisternae and then transported to definitive lysosomes.

Although corresponding cytochemical studies have not been specifically carried out in nerve cells, except for extensive work on the stages of lysosome production, it may be safely assumed that the Golgi apparatus has a similar cluster of related roles in the metabolic economy of nerve cells. Can any of these roles be regarded as especially neuronal in nature or as contributing specifically to the economy of neurons in their capacity as *nerve* cells rather than merely in their capacity as living cells? Of course, there are well-known examples of neurons that produce visible secretory droplets containing polypeptide hormones, and in these neurosecretory cells there is morphological evi-

---

Figure 2–12. **Lipofuscin Granules, Cilia, and Centrioles.**

The **upper picture** shows part of the perikaryal cytoplasm containing three lipofuscin granules (Lf_1–Lf_3). These dense, membrane-bound granules increase in both number and size as the animal ages. Because of their density, the internal structure of the granules is often difficult to interpret. However, as shown here, the granules are usually vesiculated and commonly contain grains, in addition to a few membranous arrays (see Lf_2). It seems likely that the major constituent of the granules is produced by a partial degradation of unsaturated lipids and that lipofuscin granules are residual bodies derived from lysosomes.

Also in the field is a small lysosome (Ly), which contains dense grains. The extension of the bounding membrane projecting to the right (*arrow*) suggests that the lysosome is in continuity with the smooth endoplasmic reticulum.
Cerebral cortex of rat, pyramidal neuron. × 45,000.

The **lower left picture** shows a longitudinal section of a cilium arising from a neuron. At the base of the cilium is a basal body (*bb*), which has a parabasal body (*arrow*) attached to its side. In neurons the tubules or fibrils (*f*) in the center of the cilium have a 9 + 0 configuration. These fibrils continue into the basal body. The cilium is bounded by an extension of the plasma membrane of the neuron.
Cerebral cortex of rat. × 42,000.

The **lower right picture** is part of the perikaryon of a cerebellar granule cell containing two longitudinally sectioned centrioles (*arrows*). Each centriole is a cylinder whose wall is formed by nine triplets of short tubules arranged parallel to its long axis.
Cerebellar cortex of rat. × 33,000.

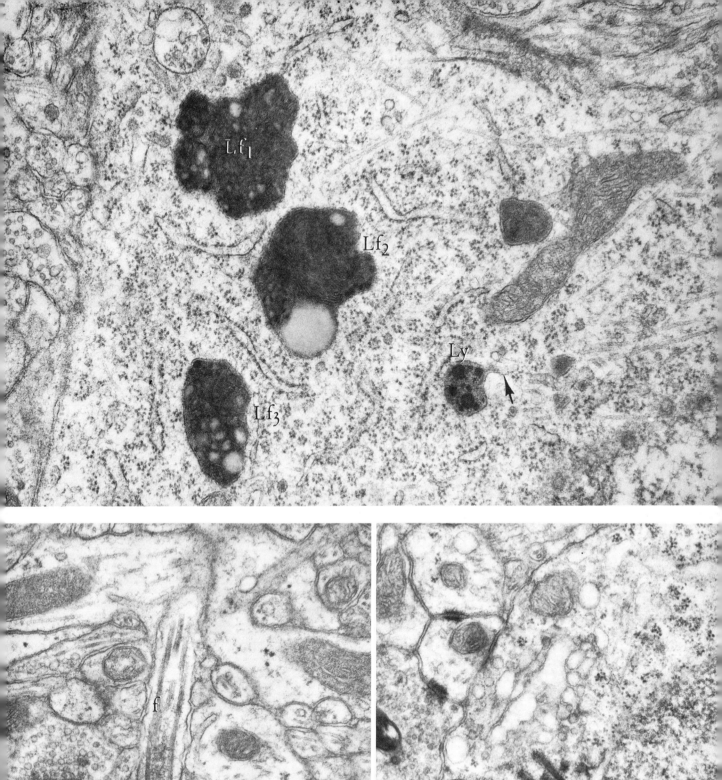
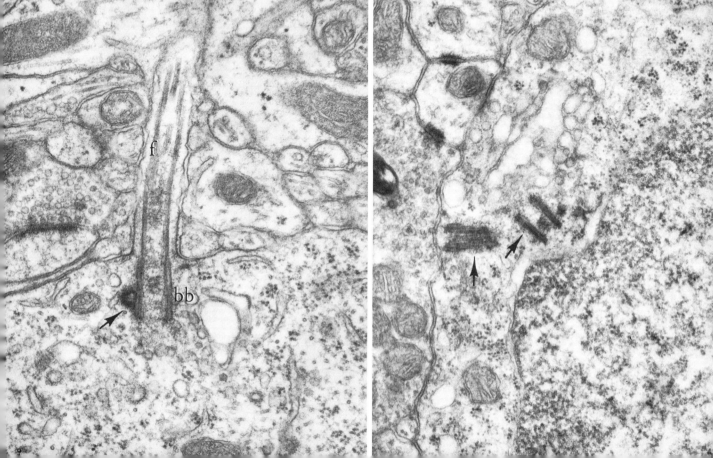

dence that the droplets originate in the meshes of the Golgi apparatus as in other glandular cells (see review by Dellmann, 1973). There are other neurons which produce secretory products of a different order, not usually conceived of in the same way. These are cells which produce biogenic amines and send vesicles containing a protein carrier together with certain specific enzymes and catecholamines or serotonin down the axons to their synaptic terminals. These vesicles can be discharged and apparently recharged several times in the terminals, but eventually they must be renewed by a supply originating in the cell body, perhaps in the Golgi apparatus. If this paradigm is correct for these two systems, there is no reason to expect it to be incorrect for nerve cells that synthesize other kinds of transmitters, such as acetylcholine, γ-aminobutyric acid, and certain amino acids. In these, the transmitter molecule itself is probably not a Golgi product since it can be synthesized or recycled in the terminal, but the segregation of enzymes—like acetylcholine synthetase, necessary for producing the transmitter in the terminal—may well occur in the Golgi apparatus. Furthermore, it should not be forgotten that the membrane of the vesicle itself is very likely a Golgi product even if it may ultimately spend a part of its existence in the surface membrane of the terminal to which it is consigned (see Chapter V).

To these considerations it should be added that the relation between the Golgi apparatus and the surface membrane of the nerve cell is likely to be significant. The presence of glycoproteins in the Golgi apparatus of nerve cells as in gland cells suggests that the Golgi apparatus may be an essential way station in the supplying and replenishing of the surface coat of the nerve cell, which should have a large role in the distribution of charges across the surface membrane. Furthermore, the Golgi apparatus may have a part in supplying or repairing the critical permeability mechanisms that underlie the operation of the nerve cell in both its synaptic and its electrogenic regions. In this latter role the agranular reticulum probably acts as an intermediary through its hypolemmal and subsurface cisternae.

In connection with these suggested links to the surface membrane it may not be too speculative to note that certain elements in the operation of the Golgi apparatus reappear in the hypotheses used to describe the operation of nerve terminals. As will be better appreciated when the chapter on synapses (Chapter V) has been read, vesicular membrane in nerve endings is thought to shuttle between the synaptic vesicles and the presynaptic surface. As in the perikaryon, the vesicles containing a specific product (transmitter) are transported to the surface, where they join the plasmalemma, discharge their content, and after some translocation laterally are taken up again as coated vesicles, which rejoin the smooth endoplasmic reticulum of the nerve ending. This "secretory" discharge can be repeated several times but cannot continue indefinitely without sustenance from the perikaryon, as is shown by the loss of function that follows interruption of the axon. Apparently, as in the perikaryon, replacement of vesicles depends in some way upon the function of the Golgi apparatus. Considered from this point of view, the nerve terminal can be regarded as a distant outpost of the Golgi apparatus.

MULTIVESICULAR BODIES

Multivesicular bodies were first described by Palay and Palade (1955). These spherical bodies, which are about 0.5 micron in diameter, are limited by a unit membrane (Palay, 1963a). They contain a variable number of small spherical and ellipsoidal vesicles (Figures 2–5 and 2–11) and an assortment of other inclusions among which may be filaments, granules, irregular dense masses, and membranes. The matrix in which inclusions are embedded can be either clear or dark, but there are many gradations between these two extremes (Palay, 1960b). One side of the multivesicular body is flattened, and in this site a plaque of fuzzy or radially striated material is attached to its outer surface (see Pappas and Purpura, 1961). This plaque is about 30 nm thick and is usually separated from the limiting membrane by a light zone (Rosenbluth and Wissig, 1964).

Although multivesicular bodies occur throughout the perikarya of neurons and in the dendrites and axons, they are most commonly found in association with the Golgi complex, often in clusters of three or more. The limiting membrane of a multivesicular body frequently sends out a tubular projection toward the Golgi cisternae. Such images suggest that multivesicular bodies and the smooth endoplasmic reticulum can at times be directly confluent, or at least linked by vesicular intermediaries. But direct connections between these two membranous organelles have not been recorded.

Rosenbluth and Wissig (1964) have shown that when ferritin is introduced into the spinal ganglia of adult toads, the particles are engulfed by the neurons and become enclosed within alveolate vesicles 0.1 to 0.2 micron in diameter that are derived from the surface membrane of the cell. Thereafter, the ferritin appears to be segregated within the multivesicular bodies. Since the coated vesicles and the multivesicular bodies are the only two components in the cell that possess coated limiting membranes, Rosenbluth and Wissig suggested that either (1) the alveolate vesicles are multivesicular bodies in the process of forming, or (2) a number of alveolate vesicles coalesce with one another or with existing multivesicular bodies, adding their surface membranes and discharging their content into the lumen.

Investigations of Friend and Farquhar (1967), on the absorption of horseradish peroxidase by cells of the vas deferens, support the ideas of Rosenbluth and Wissig (1964) and others that material taken up by cells from the surrounding medium is sequestered within alveolate vesicles and then discharged into multivesicular bodies. As mentioned earlier, Friend and Farquhar have further shown that there is a second and smaller type of alveolate vesicle which is derived from the Golgi apparatus. This smaller coated vesicle contains hydrolytic enzymes (Holtzman, Novikoff, and Villaverde, 1967) which it transports to the multivesicular bodies and empties into them, thus converting them into lysosomes (see Novikoff, 1967b).

LYSOSOMES

Lysosomes were first recognized as a separate category of cytoplasmic particles by de Duve and his collaborators in 1955 (see de Duve, 1963). The name reflects the localization of acid phosphatase and other hydrolytic enzymes in these particles. From the morphological standpoint acid phosphatase activity has been their most important identifying characteristic, for, as it can be demonstrated histochemically at the electron microscope level (see Novikoff, 1967b), it provides an unequivocal functional mark.

All neurons contain numerous lysosomes. They are visible in the light microscope even in unstained preparations of living nerve cells. Because of this ready visibility they have been confused with neurosecretory granules, with mitochondria, and with the Golgi apparatus (see Palay, 1960b). The relation between them and the Golgi apparatus is evident from the many studies of Novikoff and his colleagues (see Novikoff and Shin, 1964; Novikoff, Essner, and Quin-

tana, 1964; Holtzman, Novikoff, and Villaverde, 1967; Novikoff, Novikoff, Quintana, and Hauw, 1971). A direct involvement of the Golgi complex in the formation of lysosomes is also suggested by Friend and Farquhar (1967), Moe, Rostgaard, and Behnke (1965), and Brandes (1965). Electron microscopy and especially high resolution histochemical techniques are the only ways to prevent erroneous identification of lysosomes with other cytoplasmic organelles or inclusions (Osinchak, 1964).

Most of the particles identified as lysosomes in electron micrographs are between 0.3 and 0.5 micron in diameter. They are usually spherical or oval bodies bounded by a single unit membrane and filled with a finely granular content. There is, however, a great diversity of size and form (Figures 2–5, 2–6, and 2–11). In neurons, larger lysosomes, 1 to 2 microns across, are not uncommon. Elongated, bent, and cup-like shapes are frequent (Figure 2–7). In many cell types lysosomes also have a variegated content: membranes in stacks or whorls, granules of various sizes and densities, and lucent vacuoles. But in neurons of young adult animals the homogeneity of the lysosome population is striking. Almost all the lysosomes have a homogeneously dense granular texture. As the animal ages, or if the nervous system is subject to disease or trauma, the lysosomes become more heterogeneous and many of them appear to develop into lipofuscin granules (Figure 2–12).

LIPOFUSCIN GRANULES

Lipofuscin is generally considered to be a wear-and-tear pigment since the amount of this material in nerve cells increases with age (e.g., Toth, 1968; Hasan and Glees, 1972; Glees and Gopinath, 1973; Nanda and Getty, 1973; Sekhon and Maxwell, 1974; Mann and Yates, 1974). In unstained preparations viewed in the light microscope the pigment appears yellow to brown. At times such cytoplasmic organelles as mitochondria (e.g., Hess, 1955; Duncan, Nall, and Morales, 1960), the Golgi apparatus (e.g., Bondareff, 1957), lysosomes (e.g., Essner and Novikoff, 1960; Toth, 1968; Samorajski, Keefe, and Ordy, 1964; Sekhon and Maxwell, 1974), and the GERL complex, that is, a combination of the Golgi apparatus, the endoplasmic reticulum, and lysosomes (e.g., Novikoff, 1967a), have been considered to be involved in the genesis of lipofuscin.

Perhaps the most widely accepted concept is that lipofuscin granules are derived from lysosomes, and a probable sequence of changes leading to the formation of lipofuscin granules has been presented by Sekhon and Maxwell (1974). These workers studied the sequence of changes of membrane-bound granules in the cervical anterior horn cells of aging mice. They found that the neurons of young mice contain only a few rounded granules that resemble lysosomes. These granules, which measure 0.12 to 0.5 micron are bounded by a membrane, have homogeneous dark contents, and tend to occur in the vicinity of the Golgi apparatus. Other membrane-bound granules resemble primary phagosomes, for their dark matrix contains small dense bodies and bands of dense material. Such granules show less affiliation with the Golgi apparatus and are larger than the lysosomes, being 0.5 to 1.5 microns in diameter. With advancing age, a third set of granules, lipofuscin granules, begin to appear. These lipofuscin granules are also bounded by a single membrane and are larger than the previous two types of granules, being 1.5 to 2.5 microns. An important feature of lipofuscin granules is that they have one or two peripherally located vacuoles, the rest of the granule being filled with a heterogeneous mixture of dense particles and bands.

A fact made clear by the studies of Nandy (1971) is that lipofuscin granules do not form a homogeneous population. Thus, Nandy (1971) has demonstrated at least two kinds of lipofuscin granules. The granules which predominate in young rats are scattered singly in the cytoplasm. They are easily stained with Sudan black B and the periodic acid—Schiff reaction, and have a greenish-yellow autofluorescence. On the other hand, the lipofuscin granules of older animals tend to occur in clumps and are more easily stained with Nile blue and the ferric-ferricyanide methods, while their autofluorescence is golden yellow.

A point emphasized in the review by Hasan and Glees (1972) is that the deposition of lipofuscin in neurons does not occur at the same time in all parts of the nervous system. Thus, in the guinea pig, for example, Wilcox (1959) reported that the mesencephalic neurons are the first to show the pigment. This occurs at the age of about two years. At three years of age the pigment appears in the motor nuclei of cranial nerves, but the pigment fails to appear in the cochlear nuclei even in the oldest animals. In the human brain (Buttlar-Brentana, 1954), the hypothalamic nuclei, and in particular the nucleus supraopticus and nucleus paraventricularis, fail to show pigmentation with age. Also in the human brain, in neurons of the inferior

olivary nucleus and the anterior horn of the spinal cord, Mann and Yates (1974) find that lipofuscin accumulates steadily throughout life. Initially this accumulation appears to be without detriment to the cell, but when a certain point is reached there is a progressive reduction in the amount of cytoplasmic ribonucleic acid.

While the factors leading to the increase in lipofuscin with age are not known, there is some suggestion that inactivity of neurons accelerates lipofuscin accumulation. On the other hand, treatment of animals with centrophenoxine (Nandy and Bourne, 1966; Nandy, 1968) and vitamin E (Miyagishi, Takahata, and Lizuka, 1967) seems to protect neurons against lipofuscin accumulation, as do kavain and magnesium orotate (Varkonyi, Domokos, Maurer, Zoltan, Csillik, and Földi, 1970).

MITOCHONDRIA

Neuronal mitochondria are generally described as small, rounded granules or slender rodlets about 0.1 micron in diameter. Although this is the prevalent appearance on superficial view, they are really quite variable in size and shape, as a glance at Figures 2–2, 2–5, and 2–7 will show. Even within a small field, some of the mitochondria are plump, sausage-shaped organelles 0.5 micron or more in width, whereas others are elongated threads 0.1 micron in diameter and several microns long. Branching forms are not uncommon (Figures 2–3 and 2–7). Karlsson (1966b) estimated that about one-third of the mitochondria in the perikarya of the lateral geniculate nucleus in the rat are of this branching type. In single sections it is often impossible to demonstrate branching, but in a field like that of Figure 2–5, where small mitochondrial profiles appear clustered together in the neighborhood of one or two large profiles, the presence of a single mitochondrion of complex spidery shape may be suspected. In the processes of neurons, the mitochondria tend to be of simpler shapes, usually rodlets about 0.1 micron across and 1 micron or more long. In smaller dendrites and axons slender mitochondria predominate except in the synaptic terminals, where small globular mitochondria are the most common. However, in the tenuous preterminal axons and in dendritic tips (see below and Figure 3–10) extremely long and slender mitochondria are frequently encountered. In such places some as long as 20 microns have been measured.

In the perikaryon the mitochondria are usually distributed apparently at random throughout the cytoplasm. Curiously, however, they are to a large extent excluded from the Nissl bodies, to the margins of which they adhere like the prickles on a burr (Figures 2–8 and 2–9). They are thus closely associated, as in many other cell types, with organelles that require the adenosine triphosphate (ATP) generated by their oxidative activity. They are not, however, so intimately related to the Nissl substance as to be enfolded into the ribosome-studded endoplasmic reticulum, as mitochondria frequently are in the cells of liver, pancreas, or intestinal epithelium. Mitochondria in neurons are only rarely encountered deep in the Nissl substance.

Cinematographic observations on neural tissues in culture chambers show that, as in other cells, the mitochondria of neurons are in constant motion, changing their shape and size and, most impressively, changing their position in the cell (Pomerat, Hendelman, Raiborn, and Massey, 1967). These organelles tend to migrate at variable rates from one region to another in the cytoplasm, from the perikaryon into one process or another and back again. They move with slow writhing or rapid saltatory movements that result in linear progress within spatially confined paths, as if their freedom of movement were restricted to definite and enduring channels in the cytoplasm. Although such channels cannot be identified with certainty in electron micrographs, it appears most likely that they correspond to the *Plasmastrassen* (Andres, 1961) or "roads" (Bunge, Bunge, Peterson, and Murray, 1967) that run among the Nissl bodies as was described earlier (see page 12) and as may be seen in Figure 2–6. The long parallel microtubules and neurofilaments in these "roads," as well as the longitudinal elements of the agranular endoplasmic reticulum, would tend to confine the mitochondria and other granules such as the lysosomes to longitudinal channels from which they would not easily escape. The mechanism of propulsion and longitudinal progression is still not understood, although the neurofilaments and microtubules are probably involved in some way (see Barondes, 1967).

The basic architecture of neuronal mitochondria is the same as that of mitochondria in all other vertebrate cells (Palade, 1953; Fawcett, 1966a). Each organelle is bounded by a smooth unit membrane which encloses a second, highly folded membrane. The inner membrane circumscribes an internal space, the inner mitochondrial compartment, filled with a dense matrix, while the space between the two membranes, the outer mitochondrial compartment, generally has a lucent content. The two membranes display important differences in structure, chemical composition, and function. For example, the inner face of the inner membrane is studded with stalked knob-like projections, about 9 nm in diameter, whereas the outer membrane is smooth on both faces. All the cholesterol and all the monoamine oxidase of the mitochondrion is located in the outer membrane while all the cardiolipin, all the respiratory electron transport mechanisms, and many of the dehydrogenases are located in the inner membrane. The dissection of the mitochondrion, structurally and biochemically, is one of the more exciting chapters in the history of cell biology during the past 10 years (see, among others, Fernández-Morán, Oda, Blair, and Green, 1964; Kagawa and Racker, 1966; Lehninger, 1967 and 1968; Fernández-Morán, 1967; Schnaitman and Greenawalt, 1968).

So far as is known, mitochondria have the same molecular structure and metabolic role in the neuron as they have in other cells. They display certain differences, however, that are interesting although of unknown significance. Mitochondria separated from brain and deprived of adenosine diphosphate (ADP) fail to exhibit the large amplitude swelling and contraction characteristic of mitochondria extracted from other organs. Whether this resistance to large amplitude swelling is related to structural peculiarities of neuronal mitochondria is unknown. In neurons, elongated mitochondria are common, as previously mentioned, and it is frequently seen in electron micrographs that they contain longitudinally oriented cristae (Palay and Palade, 1955). This feature is most prevalent in the long slender mitochondria found in the processes. As these mitochondria are very thin, it is not uncommon to see a single crista running the length of the organelle, and in transverse sections the crista appears to float in the dark matrix, unattached to the inner membrane of which it is a projection. Figure 3–10, which shows an enormous number of mitochondria mostly in transverse section, provides an opportunity to study the variety of forms taken by the cristae in neuronal mitochondria.

A second peculiarity of the mitochondria in neurons is that they contain few dense matrix granules. These granules (Peachey, 1964) are apparently deposits of hydroxyapatite sequestered by the oxidative activity of the mitochondrion in the presence of calcium ions (see Lehninger, 1967). Although they are extremely common in any random section of mitochondria from liver, kidney, or muscle, they are much less common in sections of neuronal perikarya or processes (Brightman and Palay, 1963; Bunge, Bunge, and Peterson, 1965). Whether this reflects an agonal change in neurons during the early stages of fixation, or a peculiarity of neuronal metabolism with respect to calcium ions is unclear at present. Perhaps the paucity of mitochondrial granules is linked to the low reserves of energy and the high requirements for glucose and oxygen that are characteristic of brain.

MICROTUBULES AND NEUROFILAMENTS

Two other conspicuous elements in the cytoplasm of the perikaryon are microtubules and neurofilaments (Figures 2–1, and 2–5 to 2–7). The microtubules appear in electron microscope preparations as long tubular elements 20 to 26 nm in diameter. When they are sectioned transversely, each one shows a dense wall about 6 nm thick surrounding a lighter core in which a centrally placed dense dot may be visible. Thus, the microtubules in neurons resemble those in all other cells (Porter, 1966). Neurofilaments are more slender than microtubules. They are only about 10 nm in diameter, but again, at high resolution their appearance is that of a tubule rather than a filament, for in cross sections they show an outer dense layer, about 3 nm thick, surrounding a lighter core (see Palay, 1964; Peters and Vaughn, 1967; Peters, 1968; Wuerker and Palay, 1969; Wuerker and Kirkpatrick, 1972).

In the neuronal perikaryon, neurofilaments and microtubules occupy most of the space not pre-empted by the larger and more prominent organelles. But although their extent appears to be indefinite, only short lengths are usually visible in high magnification electron micrographs. Such micrographs also give the impression that the microtubules and neurofilaments run randomly throughout the cytoplasm. At lower magnifications it is apparent that, although their orientation is not completely orderly, these organelles tend to run parallel to one another in loose bundles that course, like the traffic in city streets, around the more agglomerated organelles, such as the Nissl substance and the mitochondria. These bundles funnel into the bases of the dendrites and axon (Figures 2–1 and 2–3), where the microtubules and neurofilaments form parallel arrays and where, because of the relative sparsity of other organelles, they become more prominent than they are in the perikaryon. For this reason, a detailed description of the microtubules and neurofilaments will be

delayed until the structure of the axon is considered (see page 96).

The general distribution of the microtubules and neurofilaments within the perikarya of neurons is very similar to that of the much thicker neurofibrils of light microscopy (see Frontispiece). Indeed, from various studies that have been carried out (reviewed in Gray and Guillery, 1966), it seems likely that the neurofibrils of light microscopy probably represent clumped microtubules and neurofilaments (see page 102 for further comments on this subject).

CILIA AND CENTRIOLES

Cilia arising from neurons have been described in many different regions of the central nervous system. For example, Palay (1961a) has described them in the preoptic nucleus (goldfish), Gray and Guillery (see Dahl, 1963) in the lizard forebrain, Dahl (1963) in the fascia dentata of the hippocampus (rat), Duncan, Williams, and Morales (1963) in the dorsal columns of the spinal cord (rat), Allen (1965) in the bipolar and ganglion cell layers of the retina (pig and man), and Karlsson (1966b) in the lateral geniculate nucleus (rat). They also occur in the substantia gelatinosa of the cat (Peters, unpublished) and in the pyramidal cells of the rat neocortex (Figure 2–12). Karlsson (1966b) found that in the two neurons he serially sectioned, each had only one cilium.

In most tissues of the body cilia contain nine longitudinal doublets of microtubules arranged to form a cylinder surrounding a central pair of microtubules (see Fawcett, 1961). This "standard" arrangement has been termed the 9 + 1 pattern. The members of a peripheral doublet share a common wall where they are in contact with each other, but the central pair of microtubules are separate from each other and are apparently linked only by cross bridges. In neuronal cilia the central pair of microtubules are missing, so that the cilia are characterized by a 9 + 0 pattern. As the doublets extend distally toward the tip of the cilium, however, one doublet loses its place in the peripheral cylinder and becomes shifted inward. Beyond the site of this displacement the remaining eight doublets adjust their positions so that they become evenly spaced. Thus, more distally, a cilium appears to have an 8 + 1 pattern, although the aberrant doublet does not occupy the true center. This pattern is the one most commonly encountered in transversely sectioned profiles of cilia in the neuropil. Although thin and short connections may sometimes be observed between members of neighboring doublets, no arms, spokes, or other accessory structures appear to occur in neuronal cilia.

The basal bodies of neuronal cilia resemble those of other cells. They consist of nine evenly spaced triplets of microtubules arranged longitudinally to form a short cylinder. Both Allen (1965) and Dahl (1963) have described thin rootlets radiating from the basal body into the surrounding cytoplasm. These resemble small ladders, since they are composed of strands of fine filaments with regularly spaced, dark cross striations. A parabasal body may also be present (see Figure 2–12).

Allen and Dahl have both shown that a neuronal cilium can have an associated centriole suspended in the cytoplasm at right angles below the basal body. The centriole also has a 9 + 0 pattern formed by nine triplets of microtubules. Sometimes (Figure 2–12) two centrioles occur in a neuron. In that case, the neuron appears to be nonciliated. Consequently, it may be suspected that when a cilium is present, one of the centrioles has become the basal body.

Although cilia with a 9 + 1 configuration seem always to be motile, those with a 9 + 0 configuration appear to be nonmotile. It is indeed difficult to believe that a cilium enmeshed in the neuropil of the central nervous system could be motile when it is so closely surrounded by interwoven processes of other neurons and neuroglial cells that it could have no freedom to beat. Barnes (1961) has suggested that these nonmotile cilia may have a sensory function, and supports this idea by giving a number of examples of receptors in which such cilia occur. This concept is also discussed by Fawcett (1961), Dahl (1963), and Allen (1965). Perhaps the best-known example of a cilium involved in a sensory structure occurs in the retina, in which the outer segments of the rods and cones are formed by modified and enlarged cilia (see De Robertis, 1956b; Sjöstrand, 1961; Tokuyasu and Yamada, 1959). Allen (1965) proposes that the cilia of the bipolar and ganglion cells may detect deformations and changes in the osmolarity and composition of the immediate environment of the cell. A more tempting suggestion concerning the cilia of neurons in the central nervous system proposes that they are vestigial and functionless structures which owe their existence to the epithelial origin of the parent cells.

Milhaud and Pappas (1968) have shown that in certain areas in the brains of adult cats treated with pargyline, which is an inhibitor of mono-amine oxidase, there is an increase in the number of cilia. The increase is most marked in the habenular nuclei, and the cilia have a 9 + 1 pattern. Most of the cells that form additional cilia appear to be neuroglia, however. Milhaud and Pappas suggest that the increase in cilia is due to stimulation of centriole formation in the absence of any subsequent cell division.

CYTOPLASMIC INCLUSIONS

A prominent feature of the cytoplasm of the neuronal perikarya in the lateral geniculate body of the cat is a structure that Morales, Duncan, and Rehmet (1964) have termed a *laminated body* (Figure 2–13). This structure has also been described by Smith, O'Leary, Harris, and Gay (1964), Peters and Palay (1966), Barron, Doolin, and Oldershaw (1967), and Doolin, Barron, and Kwak (1967). A similar structure is present in other nuclei of the thalamus (Herman and Ralston, 1970) and has been encountered in the stellate cells of the cat cerebellar cortex (Morales and Duncan, 1966; Mugnaini, 1972), in neurons of the cat deep cerebellar nuclei (Sotelo and Angaut, 1973), and in neurons of the monkey striate cortex (Kruger and Maxwell, 1969). The laminated bodies are up to 5 microns in diameter and may occur either in the perikaryal cytoplasm or in large dendrites. Probably there are not more than one or two of them per neuron. At low magnifications the bodies have a striking appearance because of their regular pattern of alternating dark and lighter zones, which are arranged in whorls. At higher magnification (Figure 2–13), however, it is evident that each dark line represents a sheet of parallel tubules (*tb*), which are quite regularly spaced, adjacent sheets being 70 to 100 nm apart. The tubules are each about 25 nm in diameter and because of this size they were originally regarded as microtubules. It is now clear that the walls of the tubules do not display the subunits typical of microtubules. Instead their 7 nm thick walls show the trilaminar pattern characteristic of a membrane.

At the edges of laminated bodies the tubules of the sheets connect with cisternae of endoplasmic reticulum (Figure 2–13, *ER*) and it seems that a number of tubules arise as extensions, somewhat like the fingers of a glove, from each cisterna.

A material of moderate density lies between, and alternates with, the sheets of tubules. Halfway between neighboring sheets this material (Figure 2–13, *IL*) is concentrated to form an intermediate line which at higher magnifications can be seen to consist of a pair of layers. Small islands of ordinary cytoplasm are usually included in the laminated bodies and a number of mitochondria frequently accompany them, often indenting their surface. Histochemical studies of the laminated bodies by Doolin, Barron, and Kwak (1967) demonstrate that the bodies contain a considerable amount of protein, some lipid, and perhaps polysaccharide, but no nucleic acid.

Arrays of tubules also form the basic element of bodies which occur in the cytoplasm of neurons in the lateral geniculate body (Karlsson, 1966b) and other thalamic nuclei (Lieberman, Špaček, and Webster, 1971) of the rat. In these bodies there are several sheets of tubules. The tubules are larger than those in the cat and have diameters of 30 to 50 nm. Another complex structure found in these neurons is more difficult to interpret. It appears to consist of a skein of convoluted tubules embedded in an amorphous dense material. Both of these organelles are in continuity with the cisternae of the granular endoplasmic reticulum.

Le Beux (1972b) distinguishes these laminated bodies from the *lamellar bodies* that also occur in the cytoplasm of neurons. The lamellar bodies are composed of stacks of unperforated cisternae derived from the granular endoplasmic reticulum. The cisternae are spaced at intervals of about 30 to 40 nm, and as they become involved in the stacks they often collapse. Ribosomes are only retained on the outer faces of the cisternae that form the upper and lower layers of the stacks. *Subsurface cisternae* have a similar form and are essentially distinguished from the lamellar bodies by their position beneath the plasma membrane. In this case ribosomes occur only on the outer face of the deepest cisterna of the stack, for the outermost cisterna lies very close to the plasma membrane. In both lamellar bodies and subsurface cisternae ribosomes stud the surfaces of the cisternae as they emerge from the edges of the stacks and dilate before passing into the adjacent cytoplasm. The same is true of the connections of the tubules of laminated bodies with the cisternae of the granular endoplasmic reticulum. Another parallel is the finely granular or filamentous material that forms laminae alternating with the sheets of cisternae or tubules. Hence it may be speculated that these organelles are variations on a common pattern, and it may be pertinent that Doolin, Barron, and Kwak (1967) referred to small lamellar bodies as presumptive stages in the genesis of laminated bodies. The same pattern of tubular components alternating with granular material is also displayed by the spine apparatus and the cisternal organelles (see page 81). However, it appears that these organelles are derived from the smooth, rather than the granular endoplasmic reticulum.

At present, the function and significance of all these bodies are unknown.

Another type of organelle involving stacks of cisternae has been described by Pannese (1969) in the perikarya of spinal root ganglion cells of the guinea pig and rabbit. These organelles are infrequently seen and consist of stacks of smooth-surfaced cisternae aligned in parallel arrays and alternating with sheets of glycogen particles. Similar organelles have been described in many other types of cells (see Pannese, 1969, for references), but seem to be relatively rare in neurons.

In the giant cells of Deiters from the lateral vestibular nucleus of the rat, Sotelo and Palay (1968) have described unusual inclusions 0.1 to 6 microns in diameter (Figure 2–11). These inclusions appear in sections as circular areas filled with fine, slender filaments each about 10 nm in diameter. These filaments seem to be identical to neurofilaments, and Sotelo and Palay consider that in three dimensions their configuration is rather like a knot of coarsely twisted twine. In addition to this densely concentrated population of neurofilaments, some of the inclusions contain a few ribosomes and small vesicles.

Figure 2–13. Laminated Inclusion Body.

The striped appearance of this inclusion body is due to the presence of regularly spaced sheets of tubules embedded in a dense matrix. Because of the swirling of these sheets some of the tubules are sectioned transversely *(tb₁)* and others longitudinally *(tb)*. At the edges of the sheets the tubules seem to expand into cisternae of granular endoplasmic reticulum *(ER)*. Midway between adjacent sheets of tubules the dense matrix is condensed so that in sections it appears as an intermediate line *(IL)*. A number of mitochondria *(mit)* frequently occur in the vicinity of these bodies, which usually contain small islands of cytoplasm *(arrows)*.
Lateral geniculate body of cat, dorsal nucleus. × 80,000.

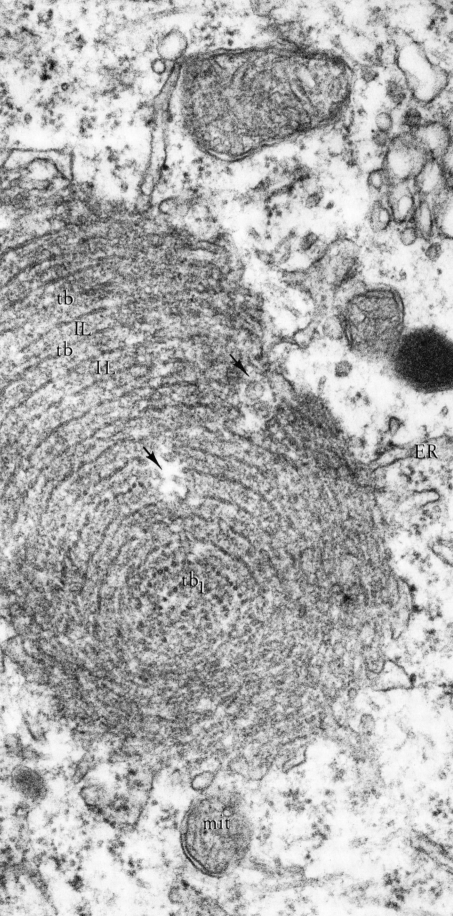

Delimiting these fibrillary inclusions from the cytoplasmic matrix is a wall of variable complexity. In the simplest examples the wall consists of a continuous single membrane about 7 nm thick, but in many inclusions it consists entirely or partially of a tubular network composed of a fine filamentous material that gives the wall a honeycombed appearance. Similar inclusions also occur in the ventral cochlear nucleus (Feldman, 1974, personal communication), the spinal cord, and the posterior colliculus (see Sotelo and Palay, 1968) and substantia nigra (Le Beux, 1972a), but so far they have only been found in the rat. The significance of these inclusions is completely unknown. Le Beux (1972a) refers to them as reticular nematosomes and regards them as nematosomes that have been excavated in their centers to accommodate neurofilaments, although the reasoning behind this assumption is not too apparent.

The fine structure of *nematosomes* was first elucidated by Grillo (1970) in the sympathetic neurons of adult rats. In their form these cytoplasmic inclusions resemble nucleoli and were originally observed by light microscopists because of their basophil staining properties. They are ball-like structures, about 0.9 micron in diameter, and lack a limiting membrane (Figure 2–11). Structurally, nematosomes appear to be composed of tightly packed, fine filaments and particles, with some ribosomes apparently attached to them by means of fine filaments that radiate from their peripheries (e.g., Le Beux, 1972a and 1973). Hence in their characteristics they bear some resemblance to the fibrous component of nucleoli, and cytochemically, nematosomes seem to consist of nonhistone proteins and some ribonucleic acid (Grillo, 1970). Although nematosomes usually lie free in the cytoplasm, often in association with smooth-surfaced and coated vesicles, they may also be associated with the postsynaptic densities of synapses (Grillo, 1970; Le Beux, 1972a). As mentioned above, Le Beux (1972a) considers that associations of the nematosomes with neurofilaments produce the fibrillar inclusions described by Sotelo and Palay (1968). Nematosomes have now been described in a number of different neuronal types, including those from the sympathetic ganglia (Grillo, 1970), substantia nigra, supraoptic nucleus, and medial vascular prechiasmatic gland (Le Beux, 1971; Le Beux, Langelier, and Poirier, 1971; Le Beux, 1972a), arcuate nuclei (Brawer, 1971; Santolaya, 1973), and cultured rat spinal cord (Bunge, Bunge, and Peterson, 1965). A useful table giving the full range of occurrence of nematosomes can be found in the article by Santolaya (1973).

A quite different type of cytoplasmic inclusion has been described by Fraser, Smith, and Gray (1970) in the thalamus of aging mice. These round, oval, or disc-shaped bodies are as large as 25 microns in diameter and consist of parallel arrays of fibrillar material. The fibrils appear to be proteinaceous and composed of identical macromolecules, for they have a crystalline appearance and an electron-dense banding which repeats at 15 nm. While the bodies seem to represent material that accumulates with age, nothing is known of their nature.

This list by no means exhausts the inventory of cytoplasmic inclusions that can be found in apparently normal neurons. The number increases as the coverage of more areas of the nervous system and of different species expands. Recently a variety of previously unknown inclusions have been found in the pyramidal cells of the cerebral cortex in monkeys—interlocking honeycombed bodies and densely coiled tubular and vesicular masses (Kohno, Chan-Palay, and Palay, 1975). These new structures have in common with all the inclusions already mentioned a completely enigmatic function and morphogenesis.

THE NUCLEUS

GENERAL MORPHOLOGY

Typically, neurons have a large, round nucleus located in the center of the cell body. In small neurons the nucleus occupies most of the cell body with only a thin husk of cytoplasm surrounding it. In larger neurons it floats free in the cytoplasm, circumscribed by a thin nuclear membrane and often separated from the other organelles by a distinct clear halo. Cinematographic recordings of cultured neurons from cerebellar cortex and sensory root ganglia show that the nucleus slowly rotates just as it does in many other types of cell (Pomerat, Hendelman, Raiborn, and Massey, 1967).

The karyoplasm of neurons is distinguished by its lack of chromatin particles and its typically clear vesicular appearance. It must, however, be pointed out that this description applies only to the largest neurons, and even in them the nucleus can contain a few deeply stained, irregular bodies. In many of the small cells—for example, the granule cells in the cerebellar cortex—the nucleus appears as speckled as that of any respectable plasma cell or lymphocyte. Thus, as is the case with the cytoplasm, defining the typical pattern is possible only if one ignores the largest number of neurons, whose baffling variety in external form and cytological characteristics is but the counterpart of their individuality in function. A good example of this variety is the shape of the neuronal nucleus, which is classically described as being spherical, ellipsoidal, or polyhedral with rounded edges to fit the shape of the perikaryon enclosing it. But many neurons have nuclei with complex shapes that are not related to the overall form of the perikaryon. The nucleus of the anterior horn cell is generally perfectly spherical, as are the nuclei of the giant cells in Deiters nucleus. But the medium-sized and small cells of this group, with the same general form as the giant cell, have irregular creased nuclei. In the Purkinje cell the nucleus nearly always has deep folds on its external aspect facing the origin of the main stem dendrite (see Figure 2–2). The nuclei of pyramidal cells in the cerebral cortex generally have a crease on one side running parallel with the long axis of the cell. In the giant isolated cells of Meynert, in the visual cortex of primates, the nucleus displays deep folds on its basal aspect, facing the origin of one of the basal dendrites (Chan-Palay, Palay, and Billings-Gagliardi,

1974). The nuclei of supraoptic neurons are irregularly creased on the side facing the origin of the main process, and in addition these nuclei are eccentrically located as in chromatolytic cells. Superimposed on this variety there are profound differences in nuclear shape in different classes of animals. In amphibia most neurons appear to have spherical nuclei, whereas in fishes the large neurons tend to have nuclei of bizarre shapes.

The creases and folds in the nuclear surface are usually filled with basophilic cytoplasm resembling the Nissl substance. In a neuron like the Purkinje cell this basophilic material is heaped up to form a distinctive cap overlying the top of the nucleus (Figure 2–2). In other cells, like the pyramidal neuron of the cerebral cortex (Figures 2–1 and 2–3), the basophilic material is merely a thin sheet or finger-like invagination that contributes to the staining density of the nuclear membrane and may in certain views suggest an intranuclear inclusion. Colonnier (1965) proposed that such invaginations stuffed with Nissl substance are the counterparts of Cajal's *bâtonnets intranucléaires* or the rodlets of Roncoroni. Although this may be the correct explanation of these structures in some instances, many nerve cells contain true intranuclear inclusions in the form of rods or sheets of ordered filaments, which are described in a later section of this chapter.

It is difficult to reconcile the regular location of creases and folds in the nuclear outline and its associated Nissl substance with the observations that the nuclei are constantly rotating. Since these observations have usually been made on young sensory ganglion cells without nuclear folds, they may not apply to more mature neurons. Possibly, however, the whole nucleus does not rotate, but only a certain few components, like the nucleolus, revolve within it. In that case it is even more difficult to understand how such a body can make its rounds through the meshwork of extended chromatin in which it is immersed.

In all types of neurons, except the smaller granule cells, the nucleus is marked by a conspicuous, large, spherical nucleolus. According to measurements by Marinesco (1909) in a variety of nerve cell types in several mammalian species, the diameter of the nucleolus, 3 to 7 microns, can be one-third to one-fourth that of the nucleus. The nucleolus of the Purkinje cell in the rat is 2.1 to 3.1 microns in diameter, which is about one-sixth that of the nucleus of this cell (Armstrong and Schild, 1970; Palay and Chan-Palay, 1974), while in the cat, the nucleolus is much larger, 3.6 microns in diameter, although the nucleus is about the same size as in the rat (Palkovits, Magyar, and Szentágothai, 1971). Usually there is only one nucleolus in mammalian neurons, but occasionally there are two or more. It is common to find clear round vacuoles or open spots in the otherwise dense and deeply stained nucleolus.

In mature cells the nucleolus lies free in the karyoplasm, almost unencumbered by particles or scales of heterochromatin (see LaVelle, 1956, for developmental stages in the maturation of the nucleolus). There is one important exception to this generality. In female animals of many species (e.g., cat, rat, mouse) a small spherical mass of heterochromatin about 1 micron in diameter often appears attached to the nucleolus (Barr, Bertram, and Lindsay, 1950; Moore and Barr, 1953). In male animals this nucleolar satellite is not usually seen, and in some species (e.g., man and other primates) it is attached to the inner side of the nuclear membrane instead of to the nucleolus. When a large motor cell in a female cat undergoes chromatolysis the nucleolar satellite migrates from its paranucleolar position toward the nuclear membrane, and during recovery it returns to its normal position. These migrations are what first brought the satellite to the attention of its discoverers. Because of its occurrence in female animals and its content of deoxyribonucleic acid, the nucleolar satellite is believed to represent one of the X chromosomes (see the review by Barr, 1966).

The incidence of nucleolus-associated heterochromatin in Purkinje cells of a variety of species has recently been re-examined by Chan-Palay (given in Palay and Chan-Palay, 1974, pp. 20–22) in order to see whether it would correlate with the suppositional polyploidy of these cells (see below). The results of this study indicate that considerable diversity exists in the number, position, and size of nucleolus-associated chromatin bodies between representatives of a single cell type, within an individual animal, between the sexes, and among species. For example, in female rats the Purkinje cell usually has one or two bodies attached to the nucleolus. When two are present each is about 1 micron in diameter, and when only one is present it tends to be large, 1.3 microns in diameter. In male rats single heterochromatic bodies are much less common, and double bodies are

quite rare. In the mouse both males and females have a high incidence of nucleolus-associated bodies, 84 and 98 per cent of the cells, respectively. The average size of these bodies in the mouse is quite impressive, 1.3 microns across when paired and 1.9 microns when single. In contrast, only about 40 per cent of the Purkinje cells in the female cat display a heterochromatic mass attached to the nucleolus and in the male hardly any cells do this. In a male monkey no nucleolus-associated chromatin was found in the Purkinje cells. The pattern of nucleolus-associated chromatin in these nerve cells depends strongly on species and is not consistently sex-related; perhaps it reflects the metabolic state of the cell and its nucleus at the time of death.

It is important to apprehend that mature nerve cells do not divide and increase in number. Although the generation of nerve cells continues for a short time after birth in a few regions of the central nervous system, for example, the cerebellar cortex (Miale and Sidman, 1961) and the dentate gyrus (Angevine, 1965), in general the full complement of neurons is determined early in postnatal development. Thus, the population of neurons is not renewed during the lifetime of an individual animal. And there is no turnover of deoxyribonucleic acid (DNA) in the brain after the end of the growth period (Bennett, Simpson, and Skipper, 1960). On the contrary, during the early development an excessive number of nerve cells is apparently produced and then eliminated by cell death. This procedure plays an important role in the final modelling of the central nervous system (Schlüter, 1973; O'Connor and Wyttenbach, 1974; Hamburger, 1975).

It was, therefore, of considerable interest to learn that some nerve cells have twice the usual complement of DNA; that is, they are tetraploid. Purkinje cells in the cerebellar cortex (Sandritter, Nováková, Pilny, and Kiefer, 1967; Lapham, 1965 and 1968), pyramidal cells in the hippocampus (Herman and Lapham, 1968), and a variety of other nerve cells, including Betz cells and anterior horn motor cells, have been shown by microspectrophotometry of Feulgen-stained sections to have twice as much DNA per nucleus as cerebellar granule cells, neuroglial cells, or other somatic cells. These startling results were confirmed by the use of the same methods in a number of laboratories in America, Europe, and Russia. Although at first it was postulated that the excessive amount of DNA was related to the large size of these neurons and their nuclei, it soon became clear that the size was not important, for even larger cells, such as the giant cells of Deiters in the lateral vestibular nucleus of rats (Sandritter, Nováková, Pilny, and Kiefer, 1967) and the giant cells of Mauthner in *Xenopus* larvae (Billings and Swartz, 1969), have merely the normal complement of DNA. Sandritter and his coworkers (1967) showed that in the rat's Purkinje cell the amount of DNA gradually increases from the diploid to the tetraploid amount during the third week postnatally. Lentz and Lapham (1970) found that the change occurs about two weeks earlier. These changes in nuclear DNA were thought to correlate well in time with either the beginning or the completion of the maturation of the extensive Purkinje cell dendritic tree.

In the past three or four years, however, the methods and interpretations of these studies have been subjected to devastating criticism. Several investigators have noted that the ratios of Purkinje cell to neuroglial cell DNA content obtained by microspectrophotometry are not 2 or more, which would be required for tetraploidy, but vary between 1.6 and 1.9. Although the discrepancy has been explained away by out-of-focus effects, Mann and Yates (1973) repeated these measurements on sections and smears of human cerebellum, taking care to measure nonspecific light loss through the Purkinje cell cytoplasm. They were unable to confirm the finding of tetraploidy. Indeed the ratio of DNA content for Purkinje cells and neuroglial cells was 1.11. The discrepancy between these and the earlier results was ascribable to the considerable nonspecific light loss in the beam passing through the cytoplasm around the Purkinje cell nucleus in sections. Concurrently, in a number of laboratories it was discovered that during the supposed period of DNA doubling, from the fifth to the twenty-first postnatal day, Purkinje cells fail to incorporate tritiated thymidine into their nuclei as detected by autoradiography (in the rat, Manuelidis and Manuelidis, 1972 and 1974; in the mouse, Mareš, Lodin, and Šácha, 1973). Consequently, unless there is some specific peculiarity of Purkinje cells that prevents their uptake of thymidine during the development of tetraploidy, it must be concluded that DNA synthesis does not occur during this period.

The discrepancy between these autoradiographic results and the microspectrophotometric results of Lapham and other workers (including themselves) prompted Cohen, Mareš, and Lodin (1973) to attempt a direct biochemical analysis of the DNA in Purkinje cells. They carried out a bulk separation of Purkinje cell perikarya from the cerebella of 8- to 10-week old mice by means of a velocity sedimentation technique. This method provided them with a fraction consisting of 60 to 80 per cent Purkinje cells. When they analyzed this fraction, enriched in Purkinje cells, for DNA content per cell, they found that there was no significant difference between the ratio in this fraction and that in the original total cell suspension, which consisted largely of granule cells. Thus, even concentrating the Purkinje cells failed to increase the DNA content per cell. These results were followed up by Mareš, Schultze, and Maurer (1974), who showed that mouse Purkinje cell nuclei labelled with tritiated thymidine during the prenatal period of proliferation and examined autoradiographically from the eighth to the ninetieth postnatal day displayed complete constancy in the grain counts per nucleus when corrected for the increasing nuclear volume with age and for self-absorption in the material of the sections. Similar results were obtained in the hippocampal pyramids of the same animals. Finally the doubts about the earlier results were substantiated by Fujita (1974), who carried out an extensive microspectrophotometric survey of human cerebella and spinal cords in various stages of development, from an 8-week embryo to a 68-year-old man. The DNA content of neuroblasts and neurons, including Purkinje cells and large anterior horn cells, showed no significant deviation from the diploid amount. A similar study on Purkinje cells and granules in the developing rat produced consistent results (Fujita, Hattori, Fukuda, and Kitamura, 1974). Therefore, the earlier results appear to be simply the elaboration of a technological error. Consequently, we have stronger evidence than before of the fundamental constancy of DNA in the nucleus of nerve cells during the life of the organism.

Despite the collapse of the case for polyploidy in mammalian neurons, there is still credible evidence for polyploidy in certain invertebrate neurons. For example, nerve cells in the cerebral ganglia of the fruit fly *Drosophila virilis* have been estimated by microspectrophotometry to have as much as 16 times the haploid amount of DNA for the species (Swift, 1962), and certain giant neurons in the abdominal and pleural ganglia of the marine snail *Aplysia californica* may have up to 32 times the haploid amount for this species (Coggeshall, Yaksta, and Swartz, 1970). Although both of these estimates depend on microspectrophotometric data, the strictures directed against the mammalian data do not apply because of the enormous size of the nuclei. In fact Lasek and Dower (1971), acting on a suggestion by Coggeshall (1967) and unpublished observations by Strumwasser (cited on page 140 in Bullock and Quarton, 1966), directly measured the DNA in the individual nuclei of 140 giant cells of *Aplysia*. They found that the amount of DNA per nucleus varied from 0.02 to 0.27 μg. Frequency histograms of the data indicated that there were two populations of cells with mean DNA contents per nucleus of 0.067 and 0.131 μg respectively. These amounts correspond to 67,000 and 131,000 times the haploid amount in this species, and the larger value indicates that the diploid complement had been doubled 16 times. Such high polyploidy may parallel the enormous size of these neurons, since it appears to increase by quantal multiples of 2 in pace with the growth of the animal (Coggeshall, Yaksta, and Swartz, 1970).

In the previous paragraphs we have reviewed the characteristics of the neuronal nucleus as seen in the light microscope. The fine structure of this nucleus has not been studied thoroughly and, like that of other interkinetic nuclei, is not yet well understood. For a discussion of the structure of nuclei in general, reference should be made to such accounts as those of Wischnitzer (1960) and Fawcett (1966a). Some aspects of the fine structure of nucleoli and chromosomes are to be found in the volume on the nucleus edited by Dalton and Haguenau (1968) and a review by Stubblefield (1973).

THE NUCLEAR ENVELOPE

Although Cajal (1909–1911) depicted the neuronal nucleus as being enclosed in a membrane of double contour, it was not until the advent of electron microscopy that the complexity of the nuclear envelope was appreciated. It cannot be decided now whether Cajal was merely recording a common diffraction image produced by refractile material adherent to both sides of the nuclear boundary or whether he saw the true nuclear envelope somewhat enlarged by inadequate preservation. In any case it occasioned no particular comment by his contemporaries, and the double contour of the boundary between nucleus and cytoplasm remained for the early electron microscopists to discover its significance (Hartmann, 1953; Sjöstrand and Rhodin, 1953; Watson, 1955).

The morphology of the nuclear envelope has been repeatedly studied in various types of cells, particularly in gland cells, in connection with the mitotic cycle, with meiosis, with oögenesis and spermiogenesis, and with the transformations of unicellular organisms. In addition, the past decade has seen the development of efficient techniques for the isolation of the nuclear envelope in bulk from selected populations of nuclei, and both cytochemistry and morphology have profited from the new approaches that have become feasible with such methods. The subject has recently been dealt with exhaustively by Franke (1974a and b) in detailed and comprehensive reviews. Unfortunately almost none of these advances have been applied specifically to the study of the neuronal nuclear envelope, and so we are obliged to assume that since it resembles that of other cell types morphologically, so fundamental a structure must have similar chemistry and functions. A like comment can be made with respect to the other parts of the nucleus. Yet, as indicated in earlier sections, the neuronal nucleus exhibits certain special charac-

Figure 2–14. **The Nuclear Envelope, Nissl Bodies, and Golgi Apparatus.**

The picture shows part of the nucleus and perikaryon of an anterior horn cell. In the cytoplasm are small Nissl bodies and parts of the Golgi apparatus caught in different planes of section. The fenestrations in the cisternae of the Golgi apparatus can be seen in surface view near the center and in transverse section near the right edge of the picture. Lysosomes (*Ly*) of diverse sizes and shapes are collected near the nucleus.

The nucleus is bounded by a double-layered envelope, which arches across the lower third of the picture. The inner membrane of the envelope is smooth, while the outer membrane undulates irregularly, and periodically they come together to form the walls of pores (*arrows*), each bridged by a diaphragm (see insets). Notice that ribosomes are only rarely attached to the outer (cytoplasmic) surface of the nuclear envelope and that the chromatin does not approach very close to its inner aspect. The karyoplasm seems to consist of a diffuse, cottony matrix in which small chromatin masses (*Chr*) and perichromatinic particles (*pcp*) are suspended.
Spinal cord of adult rat. × 34,000.

The **insets** at the lower edge of the picture are enlargements of the left half of the nuclear envelope. The thin fibrous lamina (*triangles*) adherent to the inner surface of the envelope, the nuclear pores with their diaphragms, and their crown-like array of threads (*ct*) are shown. See text for description.
Spinal cord of adult rat. × 91,000.

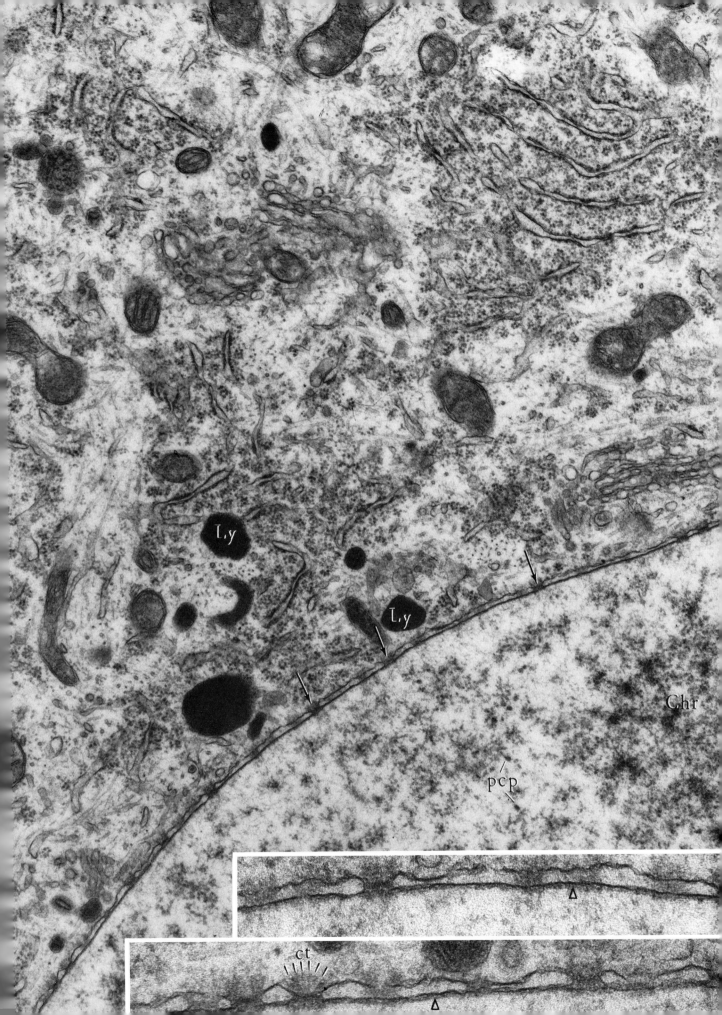

teristics that commend it for detailed study, for example, the loss of potential for mitosis, the high dilution of the chromatin in a large nuclear volume, and a high potential for protein synthesis. Admittedly the problem of collecting large quantities of neuronal nuclei from the heterogeneous cell populations of the vertebrate brain is an impediment, but it does not seem insuperable, since progress has been made in separating certain cell types from favorable tissues (Cohen, Mareš, and Lodin, 1973; Cohen, Dutton, Wilkin, Wilson, and Balász, 1974).

In the present account the morphological description of the nuclear envelope and the other parts of the neuronal nucleus are taken directly from electron micrographs in our collections. As may be seen in Figure 2–14, the nuclear envelope appears to consist of two membranes. Each is about 7 nm thick and is separated from its partner by a narrow space of varying depth. Whereas the inner membrane is quite smooth, the outer membrane is irregular or ruffled in appearance, and indeed at several points (*white arrows*) it seems to join the inner membrane. Thus, although it is often convenient to speak of the nuclear envelope as a double membrane, it is actually but a single membrane surrounding a space, the perinuclear cisterna. It is, furthermore, not difficult to show that in several places this cisterna is continuous with the cisternae of the endoplasmic reticulum that permeate the cytoplasm. Therefore, the nuclear envelope can be regarded as a specialized portion of endoplasmic reticulum which forms the boundary between the cytoplasm and the karyoplasm (Watson, 1955; Palay, 1960a). In keeping with this concept is the presence of ribosomes on the cytoplasmic surface of the nuclear envelope. But in neurons generally the nuclear envelope is not heavily decorated with ribosomes. Again, reference to Figure 2–14 will show that, although ribosomes in their polysomal clusters can approach the nuclear envelope, they are not usually attached to it.

On the inner (karyoplasmic) surface of the nuclear envelope there is in most cells a thin fibrous lamina of variable thickness (Fawcett, 1966b). This curious lamina consists of poorly resolved, extremely fine filaments arranged in a dense meshwork that runs parallel with the surface. In certain invertebrate neurons, for example, the ganglion cells of the leech (Gray and Guillery, 1963a; Fawcett, 1966b), this fibrous lamina is well developed and easily noticed, but in mammals it is almost entirely lacking. The

fibrous lamina is evident, however, on close inspection of the nuclear envelope in the vicinity of the nuclear pores (Figure 2–14) and here and there beneath the membrane between pores. Generally it stains rather poorly with the heavy metals used in electron microscopy. Even where it is apparently lacking there is still a thin interval, 5 to 8 nm thick, which is interposed between the inner membrane of the nuclear envelope and the cortical heterochromatin. According to cytochemical work in the leech, this lamina is composed almost entirely of acidic proteins (Stelly, Stevens, and André, 1970).

Both sectioned and freeze-fractured specimens show that the neuronal nuclear envelope, like that of other cell types, is fenestrated by numerous circular pores. These pores are often disposed in expansive arrays, which are best displayed in freeze-fractured specimens, but which can also be encountered in sections that graze the surface of the nucleus (Figure 2–15). The pores are about 65 nm in diameter and are set out in rows with a center-to-center spacing of about 150 nm. The distance between rows is also about 150 nm. Since the pores in adjacent rows are staggered, alternating rows are in register with each other. The result is a roughly hexagonal array of pores, similar to that found in other cells, e.g., the rat's kidney tubule epithelium (Maul, Price, and Lieberman, 1971) or *Xenopus* oöcytes (Kartenbeck, Zentgraf, Scheer, and Franke, 1971). However, the lattice is frequently incomplete, since many of the positions may be occupied by nonporous membrane. The array can be so defective or so fragmentary that it appears to be random. The pores exhibit enormous variability in their frequency, not only among different cell types and among cells of the same type, but even from spot to spot on a single nucleus.

Many large neurons, like the Purkinje cells in the cerebellar cortex and large pyramidal cells in the cerebral cortex, show numerous closely spaced nuclear pores in random sections through their nuclear envelopes. Often the pores are much more numerous in the region of the nuclear envelope that lines the deep invaginations of the nuclear cap (Figure 2–2) than on the smooth rounded surface. But it is difficult to be sure that this high incidence does not merely result from the higher frequency of tangential sectioning in this region, since this increases the opportunities for the section plane to include ranks of pores. Smaller neurons often show few pores, or occasionally none, in random sections through the nuclear envelope. This low incidence is also noticeable in freeze-fractured material. Such variability may be related to the synthetic activity of the cells at the time of fixation, since there are indications from studies on oöcytes (Franke and Scheer, 1970) and on lymphocytes (Maul, Price, and Lieberman, 1971) that the pore frequency increases when the nucleus is actively engaged in RNA synthesis. Pore frequency is, however, also subject to variations in the preparative method. Certainly, success in fixation, as estimated by the condition of the other organelles, would be necessary for any comparisons between different cell types or between different metabolic states.

In the past few years general agreement on the detailed structure of the nuclear pores has apparently been reached among investigators of a variety of cell types (Franke, 1974a and b). Their structure is best seen in negatively stained spreads or in thin sections from isolated nuclear envelopes. But the nuclear pores of neurons have not been studied to the same extent. The only detailed account in the literature was derived entirely from thin sections of cells *in situ* (Peters, Palay, and Webster, 1970). The following description expands that account and brings it into line with current descriptions in other cell types.

As can be seen in Figure 2–14, a pore is formed where the inner and outer nuclear membranes become confluent, thus obliterating the perinuclear cisterna (Palay and Palade, 1955). The circular aperture thus produced is, however, not a true perforation, for in places where the section passes perpendicularly through the envelope it is evident that the pore is closed by a dense material of indefinite composition. The material obturating the pore is known as the pore complex. Upon study with high resolution techniques (reviewed by Franke, 1974a and b), the pore complex has proved to have a complicated but regular plan of construction and intricate connections both with the nuclear envelope and with the nucleoplasm and cytoplasm on either side. The pore complex consists of (1) inner and outer annuli of globular units, (2) a ring of peripheral inner pore granules, (3) a central granule, and (4) various kinds of axial and internal filaments. The inner annulus comprises eight globules, each 10 to 25 nm in diameter, which are arranged in eightfold radial symmetry (Fabergé, 1973 and 1974) about the inner (karyoplasmic) margin of the pore. A similar annulus of eight globules is attached to the outer (cytoplasmic) margin in register with those of

the inner annulus. Between the two annuli, the wall of the pore is coated with a diffuse material from which the inner pore granules project like cones pointing toward the center of the pore, where a single, large, central granule is lodged. The projecting inner pore granules are also in register with the globules of the inner and outer annuli. Consequently when a nuclear pore is viewed *en face*, as in sections passing tangentially through the nuclear envelope (Figures 2–14 and 2–15), the diffuse material lining the pore, together with the superimposed inner and outer annuli and the inner pore granules, results in the appearance of a thick, dense wall about 20 nm thick, which seems to encircle the pore. In such sections, the connections between the central granule and the more peripheral granules or annuli are often invisible because of their extreme tenuity and lack of contrast. But in negatively stained preparations they can be made out (see Franke, 1974a and b). In sections passing normal to the nuclear envelope the peripheral inner pore granules are frequently fused to the central granule so that the pore appears to be closed by an equatorial diaphragm (Figure 2–14). Fine filaments reportedly extending in a spoke- or net-like fashion from the margin of the pore also contribute to this image. On the inner (karyoplasmic) side of the nuclear envelope a fine filamentous mat (Figure 2–14, *triangles*), can be seen bridging loosely across the pore and forming a second inner diaphragm. At the margins of the pore this mat appears to be continuous with the thin fibrous lamina, which is tightly applied to the inner surface of the nuclear envelope and which accounts for the apparently greater thickness of the inner nuclear membrane compared with the outer membrane.

Extending from the annular globules and the central granule are fine filaments, 3 to 6 nm thick, which stretch axially like wisps into the karyoplasm on one side and into the cytoplasm on the other. In sections these threads appear as tufts outlining a clear channel that passes from the karyoplasm through the pore into the cytoplasm. Such channels are less obvious in neurons than in other cells, such as lymphocytes, because the usually dilute chromatin does not aggregate in thick masses against the inner surface of the nuclear envelope (see below). But in cerebellar granule cells, which have a great deal of condensed chromatin, the clear channels are conspicuous (Figure 2–4). According to many high resolution studies, the fine filaments extending inward from the inner annulus and the central granule appear to link up with the periphery of the nucleolus, while those extending into the cytoplasm from the outer annulus and the central granule link up with polyribosomes near the nuclear envelope. These filaments appear to be related to the ribonucleoprotein network of the nucleus. According to RNA determinations correlated with quantitative electron microscopic studies (Scheer, 1970 and 1972), the nuclear pore complex contains a concentration of RNA higher than that of the nucleolus and almost half as great as that of polyribosomes. The association of pore complexes with RNA is strengthened by repeated observations, in amphibian oöcytes during the lampbrush chromosome stage, of dumbbell-shaped figures of dense granular material apparently in the course of passing through the pores from nucleus to cytoplasm (see Franke, 1974a and b; Frank and Scheer, 1970 and 1974). Such images strongly suggest that only the very center of the pore, about 15 nm across, is available for the translocation of material between the nucleus and the cytoplasm. Thus far, images of this sort have not been reported for neuronal nuclei.

THE KARYOPLASM

As already mentioned, the neuron possesses an interkinetic nucleus, and most of its chromatin is in an extended form. The chromatin is best studied in the nuclei of small neurons (Figure 2–4) in which the aggregates are more easily distinguished from the other components of the karyoplasm. In these cells it can be seen that the chromatin consists of a fairly homogeneous population of fine strands about 20 nm in diameter. On close examination many of these strands appear to be hollow with a circular cross section, and in side view their profiles are distinctly serrated. Such appearances, together with repetitive diagonal cross markings, strongly suggest

that these strands consist of one or more finer filaments helically wound around a central core of lesser density. These helical strands are agglomerated into irregular masses (chromatinic areas), some attached to the nuclear envelope and others suspended in the center of the nucleus. Clumps of the same composition surround the nucleolus and attach it to the nuclear envelope. In the granule cells of the cerebellar cortex, the condensation of the chromatin is so marked that the nuclei resemble those of lymphocytes or plasma cells. The most peripheral chromatin appears in sections normal to the nuclear envelope as a regularly spaced row of granules, usually separated from the envelope by the tenuous fibrous lamina or by a thin clear interval. In sections that graze the nuclear envelope and include a sector of the marginated chromatin, these granules are seen to be transverse sections of the helical strands, laid out in discrete undulating lines and snarls against the inner nuclear envelope (Figure 2–15). In larger cells (Figures 2–1, 2–3, 2–14) these helical strands appear to be widely dispersed throughout the nucleus and are not usually collected into masses except in the vicinity of the nucleolus. Only a thin layer of chromatin is condensed against the nuclear envelope and even this may be so slight as to be inconspicuous or absent altogether. This difference in the distribution of the chromatin is consistent with the vesicular appearance of the nuclei of large cells which stands in contrast to the spotted appearance of the nuclei of certain small cells, as given in light microscope preparations. This difference also supports the identification of the helical strands as chromatin.

Even in the small nuclei, however, the helical strands are not confined to the irregular blocks of chromatin but are scattered unevenly throughout the nucleus, mingling with the nu-

---

Figure 2–15. **Nuclear Pores.**

The blurred circle in the center of the field is the nuclear envelope of a small pyramidal cell in the cerebral cortex. The section just grazes the nucleus so that the nuclear pores appear as dark circles embedded in fine grainy mist that represents the membranous component of the nuclear envelope. In the middle of some of the pores is a dense dot, the central granule of the pore complex. The pores along the inner margin and in the middle region of the nuclear envelope display other components of the pore complex, such as the inner annulus of globular units and the peripheral inner pore granules. These are most clearly seen in the pores marked with *arrows*, in which eight globular units can be counted. Other pores both on the inner margin and on the outer margin of the envelope show only their circular boundary. Fine chromatin filaments attached to the inner surface of the nuclear envelope are laid out across the small bit of karyoplasm included in the section. The surrounding area of cytoplasm contains mostly ribosomes in small clusters and a few microtubules.
Visual cortex (area 17) of monkey (Macaca mulatta). × 95,000.

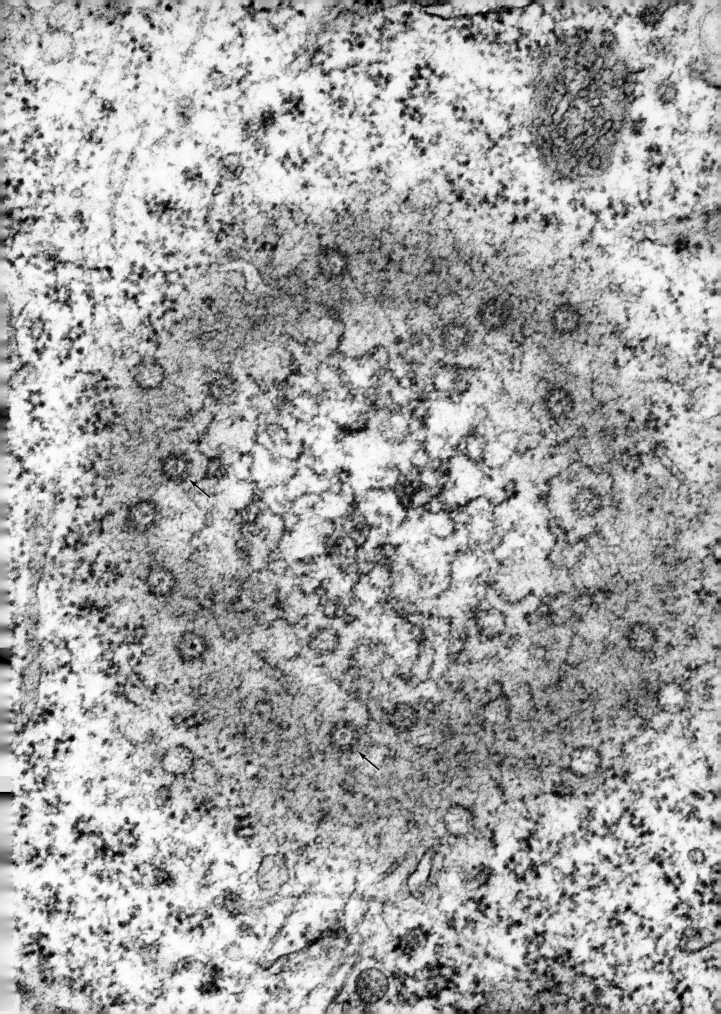

merous fine, twisted filaments that form a cottony matrix in the background. It has not been possible to ascertain whether the helical strands are continuous with the matrix filaments. In these interchromatinic zones there are also dense granules about 20 to 25 nm in diameter—the interchromatinic granules—that occur as single particles or in small clusters and rows, suggestive of ribosomes. Still larger dense particles, the perichromatinic particles (30 to 35 nm), can be seen here and there (Figures 2–1 and 2–3). The mingled strands and granules of different sizes, densities, and degrees of aggregation impart a variegated appearance to the nuclei of the large neurons. A fine cottony matrix pervades the whole nucleus, in which generally small, highly irregular collections of helical strands are suspended. Dense clusters of interchromatinic and a few perichromatinic granules stand out against the loose agglomerations of chromatin, increasing the impression of confusing heterogeneity.

Probably because of the great dilution of the nucleoprotein, the neuronal nucleus has been more difficult to preserve adequately for fine structural studies than have most other nuclei. In fact, it is more difficult to preserve the karyoplasm of neurons than their cytoplasm. Smooth, homogeneous distribution of the granulofibrillar material in the nucleus is a good criterion for satisfactory fixation. Although the introduction of glutaraldehyde (Sabatini, Bensch, and Barrnett, 1963) and especially of glutaraldehyde-formaldehyde mixtures (Karnovsky, 1965) have greatly improved the preservation of the karyoplasm, artifactitious clumping of the nuclear contents with intervening open and structureless spaces is still a common fault in electron micrographs of nervous tissue.

THE NUCLEOLUS

In electron micrographs (Figure 2–16) the nucleolus of a neuron appears as an extremely dense, large, roughly spherical mass clearly demarcated from the rest of the karyoplasm, just as it is in the light microscope. The nucleolus is a composite structure consisting of two principal components: (1) extremely dense granules about 15 to 20 nm in diameter and (2) very fine filaments that are difficult to define because of their low density and close packing. A third component usually seen in other cell types, consisting of chromatin surrounding and invading the nucleolus proper, does not contribute significantly to the neuronal nucleolus except in the female of some species in which the heterochromatic X chromosome is attached to its surface (see below).

The dense granules and fine filaments are segregated to some extent so that we can divide the nucleolus into a *pars granulosa*, composed of granules and filaments, and a darker *pars fibrosa*, composed of condensed filaments and only a few accompanying granules (Hay, 1968; Bernhard and Granboulan, 1968; Lafontaine, 1968). In many somatic cells, the pars granulosa surrounds the pars fibrosa, but in neurons the two parts are usually tangled together. The pars granulosa and the pars fibrosa both seem to be arranged in the form of knotted and contorted strands intertwined with each other so that the nucleolus resembles a hopelessly tight snarl of yarn. Furthermore, both parts contain ribonucleoprotein, as can be demonstrated by enzymatic digestion and histochemistry at the electron microscope level (Bernhard and Granboulan, 1968). In the pars granulosa the dense granules, which resemble ribosomes, are the more promi-

---

Figure 2–16.   **The Nucleolus and the Nucleolar Satellite.**

The most conspicuous object in the nucleus of the typical nerve cell is the nucleolus, which is usually large, dense, and spheroidal, like the one pictured here from an anterior horn cell. It often appears to be vacuolated because of entrapped masses of karyoplasm, which is considerably less dense. The nucleolus consists of two components: dense ribosome-like granules and fine filaments. The two components are incompletely separated from each other into a pars granulosa (*PG*), in which the granules predominate, and a pars fibrosa (*PF*), in which the filaments predominate. In several places the pars fibrosa is so highly condensed that the resultant structure is difficult to analyze.

Next to one such area at the surface of the nucleolus is a body with a different texture *(arrow)*. It consists of extremely dense, coarse, coiled fibrils. This body is the nucleolar satellite, or the sex chromatin, and it is characteristically found in this paranucleolar position in the neurons of females in certain species.
Spinal cord of adult female rat. × 35,000.

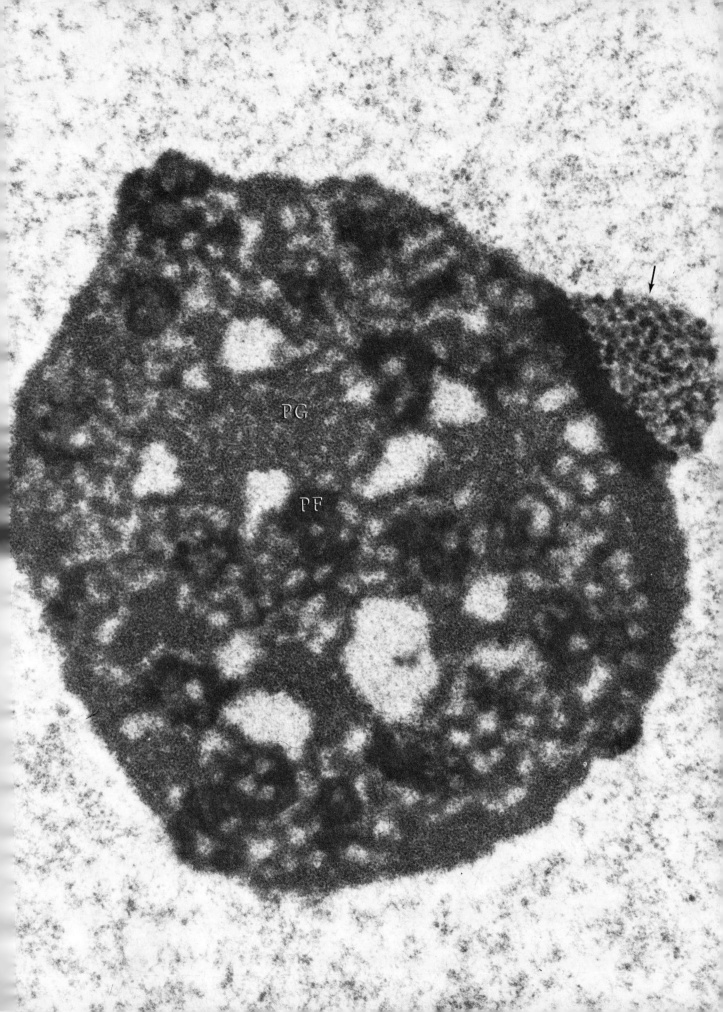

nent constituent. They appear to be laid out like beads entrapped in a complicated matting formed by the filaments. In the pars fibrosa the dense granules are much less numerous and the meshes of the matting are greatly condensed, so that the pars fibrosa appears extremely dark, with the individual filaments and granules almost entirely obscured. In the interstices between the tangled strands are lighter zones which seem to be entrapped karyoplasm with included matrix filaments and some chromatin threads. These regions, which are usually small in neuronal nucleoli, are sometimes large enough to be seen in the light microscope; in that case the nucleolus appears to be vacuolated. Such regions may be considered equivalent to the *pars chromosoma*, the third component of the nucleolus in other cell types.

As already noted, the heterochromatic X chromosome in females of certain species is condensed into a rounded nubbin attached to the nucleolus. This nucleolar satellite (Figure 2–16) is composed of extremely dense, coiled fibrils, rather tightly wound into a tangled mass. In Figure 2–16 the satellite is attached to a particularly compact segment of the pars fibrosa, but it can occur anywhere along the surface of the nucleolus. In the course of a fine structural study of the development of the Purkinje cell in the albino rat, Radouco-Thomas, Nosal, and Radouco-Thomas (1971) and Nosal and Radouco-Thomas (1971) refer to the formation and maturation of an intranuclear "spotted body," the function of which is unknown. In some of their pictures this "spotted body" strongly resembles the complex of tightly coiled fibrils attached to the nucleolus, which we have identified (Figure 2–16) as the nucleolar satellite or the heterochromatic X

chromosome. In others of their pictures it looks like an incompletely compacted portion of the pars fibrosa of the nucleolus. Radouco-Thomas and his coworkers equate the "spotted body" with a "coiled body" described by Monneron and Bernhard (1969) in various non-neural nuclei and thought to contain ribonucleoprotein. Our identification of this mass in Figure 2–16 and numerous other neuronal nuclei, is based upon its correspondence to the images seen in Feulgen preparations with the light microscope, its size, its close spatial relationship to the nucleolus, and its composition which is clearly different from that of the nucleolus. Besides, it is regularly present in female animals and no other condensed structure appears in such close and consistent relation to the nucleolus. Although the presence of RNA in such a body would not be surprising, specific cytochemical studies on these bodies in neuronal nuclei would be desirable before ruling out the possibility that they contain DNA and are chromatinic in nature.

NUCLEAR INCLUSIONS

Intranuclear rods were known to light microscopists (Figure 2–17A) and the presence of filaments in these rods has been shown by electron microscopy. Such inclusions have been described in a variety of neurons and are relatively widespread. In some parts of the central nervous system such as the cat olfactory system (Willey and Schultz, 1971) and the rat cochlear nucleus (Feldman and Peters, 1972), they are quite common, while in others, such as the hippocampus and thalamus (Chandler and Willis, 1966) and lateral vestibular nucleus (Sotelo and Palay, 1968) they are quite rare. The inclusions

---

Figure 2–17.   **Intranuclear Inclusions.**

A, Light microscope picture of silver-stained neurons. The nucleus of each neuron contains a nucleolus *(ncl),* an intranuclear rod, and a small fibrillogranular body *(arrow)* with staining properties similar to the nucleolus.
Cochlear nucleus of rat. × 2600.

B, Electron micrograph of part of an obliquely sectioned nuclear rod that consists of a single bundle of filaments *(f).* Each filament is about 7 nm thick. At the top left is the granulofibrillar body *(fg)* associated with this rod.
Cochlear nucleus of rat. × 55,000.

C, Electron micrograph of a portion of a sheet-like inclusion formed by crossing layers of filaments. At *a* the filaments are seen in vertical array and at *b* more horizontally arranged filaments are apparent. At the two ends of the inclusion the filaments in alternating layers cross each other at about 60° to form a lattice.
Cochlear nucleus of rat. × 55,000.

D, Electron micrograph of an intranuclear rod which is composed of bundles of filaments *(f).* The bundles seem to twist as they cross the field. A granulofibrillar body *(fg)* is closely associated with the rod.
Cerebral cortex of rat. × 55,000.

Material provided by M. L. Feldman.

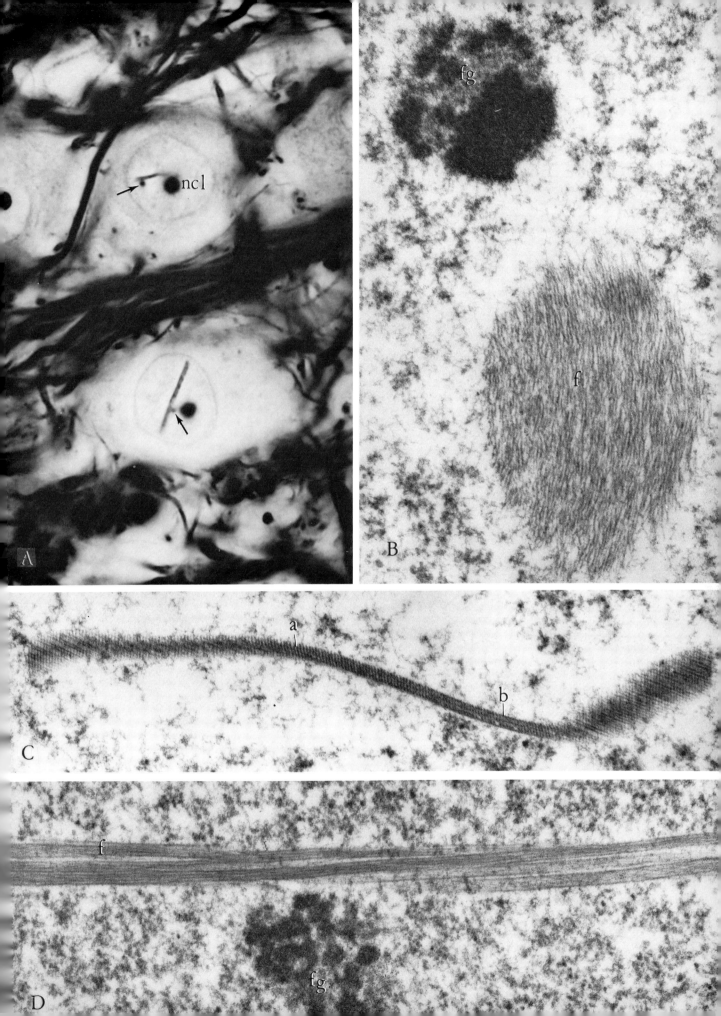

are of two types: rods and sheets (Figure 2–17). An intranuclear rod (Figure 2–17B) consists of one or more bundles of parallel filaments, each about 7 nm thick. They have been encountered in structures such as the olfactory bulb (Willey and Schultz, 1971), cerebellum, and cerebral cortex (Siegesmund, Dutta, and Fox, 1964; Gambetti and Gonatas, 1967; Andrews and Sekhon, 1969), lateral geniculate nucleus (Karlsson, 1966b), lateral vestibular nucleus (Sotelo and Palay, 1968), cochlear nucleus (Feldman and Peters, 1972), and sympathetic neurons (Masurovsky, Benitez, Kim, and Murray, 1968 and 1970; Seïte, 1970; Dixon, 1970; Seïte, Escaig, and Couineau, 1971). The rods appear to be proteinaceous in nature and probably have small amounts of bound lipids, but do not seem to contain either RNA or DNA (Kim, Masurovsky, Benitez, and Murray, 1970), and while some rods, as in the cochlear nucleus and chicken sympathetic neurons, consist entirely of filaments, others, as in the stellate ganglion of the cat and the lateral vestibular nucleus, may have microtubules associated with the filaments, usually forming a layer on the outside of the core of 7-nm filaments.

Small dense bodies resembling nucleoli are often associated with the rods, and in the sympathetic neurons of the chicken Masurovsky, Benitez, Kim, and Murray (1970) have noted that such granulofibrillar bodies are between 0.4 and 0.8 micron in diameter (Figure 2–17B). The granulofibrillar bodies appear as relatively small intranuclear structures early in development of the chick, and precede the appearance of the bundles of filaments by a week or more. In the early formative stages, the rods consist of sparse clusters of aligned filaments, but as neuronal maturation proceeds, the bundles become larger and the filaments arranged into well-ordered parallel arrays. The fact that the fibrils of granulofibrillary bodies enter the rods suggests that these bodies may be involved in the elaboration of the filaments. The granulofibrillary bodies themselves probably take origin from the nucleolus.

In most instances there appears to be only one rod per nucleus, although Mugnaini (1967) found instances of two or more rods in the same nucleus in the hagfish, *Myxine*. An additional feature described by Masurovsky, Benitez, Kim, and Murray (1970) is the extension of filaments of the intranuclear rod through the nuclear envelope into the cytoplasm. This observation does not appear to have been confirmed by others, although the rods frequently approach close to the inner side of the nuclear envelope.

The other type of inclusion encountered is a sheet of filaments (Figure 2–17C). These have been encountered in the cerebral cortex (Field and Peat, 1971; Gambetti and Gonatas, 1967; Andrews and Sekhon, 1969), sympathetic ganglia (Seïte, Escaig, and Couineau, 1971), lateral vestibular nucleus (Sotelo and Palay, 1968; Johnson and Miquel, 1974), hippocampus and thalamus (Chandler and Willis, 1966), olfactory system (Willey and Schultz, 1971), cochlear nucleus (Feldman and Peters, 1972), and retina (Magalhães, 1967). Again, the filaments are about 7 nm thick. The sheets they form consist of at least two parallel layers of filaments and are generally from 40 to 180 nm thick. In alternate layers the filaments of the sheets are all aligned in the same direction, and the angle subtended between the filaments of adjacent sheets is most commonly about 60 degrees, although it may vary from 40 to 80 degrees (Chandler and Willis, 1966; Seïte, Escaig, and Couineau, 1971; Willey and Schultz, 1971; Feldman and Peters, 1972). Because of this regular arrangement of the filaments, an almost crystalline pattern appears in sections of intranuclear sheets. In fact, the layers of filaments seem to be arranged in pairs, for as Feldman and Peters (1972) point out, there is an even number of layers in a sheet, and when the number of layers changes, as often happens when the sheets become thinner at their edges, the change involves pairs of layers and not single layers. Frequently the sheets are domed so that in sections passing in a tangential plane, ring-like profiles may be obtained. As with rods, microtubules may be associated with the filaments, and they form layers on the flat surfaces of the sheets. Sheets may also have a granular body associated with them and a bundle of microtubules passing close by (Seïte, Escaig, and Couineau, 1971).

It has become apparent that the intranuclear inclusions are not so unusual as was once considered. They have now been found in a wide range of neuronal locations, although their frequency of occurrence varies from place to place, and may be age-dependent, as shown by Field and Peat (1971), Feldman and Peters (1972), and Johnson and Miquel (1974). Clearly, the two kinds of inclusions have many features in common and they may be related to the activity of neurons for Seïte and Mei (1971) and Seïte, Mei, and Couineau (1971) have shown the frequency of intranuclear inclusions in the neurons of the stellate ganglia of cats to be increased by a factor of between 1.5 and 13.6 times after 15 minutes of electrical stimulation of the neurons followed by 10 minutes of rest.

Indeed, after stimulation, almost every neuron examined by these authors was found to contain inclusions. This increase in the number of inclusions is not inhibited by cycloheximide, which is an inhibitor of protein synthesis (Seïte, Mei, and Vuillet-Luciani, 1973) and so the inclusions induced by stimulation are probably constructed from pre-existing protein subunits. This relationship between neuronal activity and numbers of inclusions is also pointed out by Feldman and Peters (1972), who indicate that the inclusions are most common in neurons of the auditory and olfactory systems, which, unlike other sensory systems such as the visual and vestibular ones, are never "turned off" and probably remain active even during sleep.

It should be pointed out that these inclusions are not confined to neurons. They have been encountered in ependymal cells (Hirano and Zimmerman, 1967), neuroglial cells (Mugnaini, 1967), endothelial cells (Gambetti and Gonatas, 1967), and cells in the pancreas (Dahl,

1970; Boquist, 1969) and gastric mucosa (Tusques and Pradal, 1968).

There have been a number of reports linking the intranuclear inclusions with viral disease and other abnormal conditions (see Willey and Schultz, 1971; Feldman and Peters, 1972, for references), but it seems that while the inclusions may increase in number under abnormal conditions, they are not to be regarded as pathological entities.

Whether any of these inclusions correspond to Cajal's *bâtonnets intranucléaires* (Cajal, 1909–1911), as Siegesmund, Dutta, and Fox (1964) have suggested, is not clear, although Masurovsky, Benitez, Kim, and Murray (1970) consider the rods and *bâtonnets* to be equivalent. As noted previously, Colonnier (1965) has suggested that the *bâtonnets* probably correspond to the deep clefts that frequently indent the nuclear membrane, and ultimately, of course, any assumed correlation must rest upon how one interprets Cajal's drawings.

THE PLASMA MEMBRANE

Like all cells, the neuron is surrounded by a thin, continuous membrane, the plasmalemma or plasma membrane, which clearly defines its boundary. This membrane cannot be seen in the light microscope, although its presence is indicated by the well-known incongruity of the cytoplasmic organelles in neighboring cells. As has already been discussed in Chapter I, it was the invisibility of the cell membrane at the level of the light microscope that led to so much controversy over the morphological independence of neurons. In low power electron micrographs of thin sections, the plasma membrane appears as a fine, dark line bounding the cytoplasm and separating it from the extracellular space. At higher magnifications, especially if the section is exactly normal to the plane of the membrane, this line can be resolved into three layers—two limiting dark layers separated by a lighter layer, the so-called unit membrane (Robertson, 1959a). The overall thickness of the plasma membrane in such preparations is 7 to 8 nm and each of the three layers is 2.5 to 3 nm thick. The exact appearance of the membrane, however, varies somewhat according to the method of preparation and staining. In material fixed in potassium permanganate (Robertson, 1957) the two dark

layers of the plasma membrane have approximately the same thickness and density. But in material fixed either directly in osmium tetroxide or in aldehydes followed by osmium tetroxide, a somewhat different result obtains. Then the outer dark layer is thinner and lighter than the inner one, so that the membrane appears asymmetrical. Under the same conditions, the plasma membrane of other cell types, such as neuroglial cells, has a symmetrical appearance.

When the unit membrane was first proposed by Robertson in 1959(a), it became the subject of a prolonged debate, which revolved around the significance of the trilaminate image. The controversy has since been partially settled by consensus and to some extent deflected by newer data and more attractive models of membrane substructure. These subjects have been thoroughly discussed recently in a number of symposia and reviews, to which the reader is directed for details and primary references (Lehninger, 1968; Singer and Nicholson, 1972; Singer and Rothfield, 1973; Oseroff, Robbins, and Burger, 1973; Edidin, 1974; Oschman, Wall, and Gupta, 1974; Schmitt, Schneider, and Crothers, 1975).

The original exposition of the unit mem-

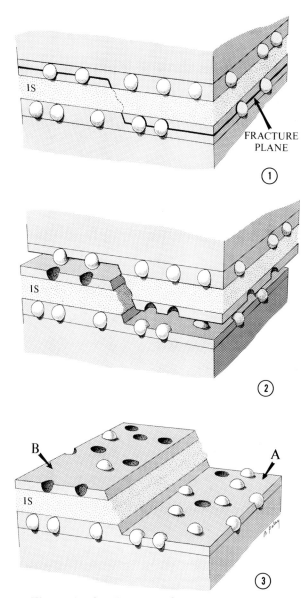

Figure 2–18. **Diagram of Freeze-Fracturing.**

These three panels show the development of the fracture plane within the plasmalemma and across the interstitial space *(IS)* between adjacent cells. In panel **1**, the fracture plane is indicated as a potential crack within the lower plasmalemma at the right and within the upper plasmalemma on the left. The spherical objects are intramembranous particles, usually regarded as globular protein assemblies within the membrane. In panel **2**, the fracture has been completed and the two fragments are separating. As can be seen in panel **3**, the lamina of membrane attached to the cytoplasm (A face) retains most of the intramembranous particles, while the outer lamina (B face) of the adjacent cell remaining at the left covers over the true external face of the lower cell and retains few intramembranous particles. *Not drawn to scale.*

brane concept derived its persuasiveness from its agreement with the then-current Davson-Danielli model of the cell membrane. According to this model the plasma membrane consisted of a bimolecular leaflet of lipid sandwiched between two continuous layers of protein. In the electron micrographs of stained sections, the two dark layers of the unit membrane were at first equated with the layers of protein themselves. Later, after much controversy, it became evident that the dark layers only signified the positions of the polar head groups of the lipid molecules in the bilayer, which are oriented along the inner and outer surfaces of the membrane. The nonpolar, hydrophobic tails of the lipids point into the membrane and, taking up little osmium, compose the light layer in between.

In the past four or five years this model of membrane structure has been seriously modified in the light of important new information from studies on both natural and artificial membranes. A fundamental skeleton consisting of a bilayer of lipid remains, but it is no longer covered with continuous layers of protein. Instead, globular proteins are selectively intercalated into the lipid bilayer and some 60 to 80 per cent of its surface is considered to be bare. The more hydrophilic proteins are weakly associated with the lipid layer and remain near its surface (peripheral proteins), while the more hydrophobic proteins extend across much of the bilayer (integral proteins). Proteins with hydrophilic ends and large hydrophobic portions could extend through the whole bilayer and protrude into the cytoplasm or into the extracellular space. In addition, sugar residues linked to the proteins (glycoproteins) or the lipids (glycolipids) extend beyond the bilayer to form a glycocalyx, which is more or less highly developed on all cells. On the inner side of the bilayer the proteins can be anchored to microtubular or actin-like filaments in the cytoplasm. The lipid bilayer itself is considered to be a fluid, with the polar head groups relatively fixed at the surfaces of the membrane and the nonpolar tails mobile and flexible. Regional variations in viscosity occur because of local specific interactions between lipid and protein and because of ordered, paracrystalline lipid arrays. In this fluid bilayer the protein components are allowed relatively free movement in the plane of the membrane.

The plasma membrane is therefore conceived of as a mosaic of globular proteins imbedded in a fluid lipid matrix (Singer and Nicholson, 1972). The chemical composition of the whole assemblage varies according to place and time on any individual cell. Since this fluid-mosaic model is much richer and more flexible than any previous model, it accommodates a much larger range of observational data. It admits considerable chemical variety in the cell membrane and allows for changes in membrane structure and composition during the life of the cell. It provides not only for the transport of ions, water, and lipid-soluble molecules through the membrane but also for the localization of recognition sites and immune interactions at the cell surface. Finally, as an ironic aside, the fluid mosaic model does not invalidate the unit membrane concept, despite some attempts to discard it (Singer and Nicholson, 1972), because the unit membrane is simply a morphological description of an electron microscopic image and is not a chemical statement. That the unit membrane concept is compatible with the new model is shown by the successful adaptation of both ideas in the explanation of the images seen in freeze-fractured tissues.

In the freeze-fracture method the specimen is frozen at liquid nitrogen temperatures and then cracked by a knife in a vacuum. Carbon-platinum replicas of the fracture faces are prepared by shadowing at narrow angles and digesting away the tissue. When such replicas are examined in the electron microscope it is seen that the fracture not only breaks open cells and processes, but also cuts across the interstitial space and does not run within it. However, cell membranes caught in the cleavage plane are split down the middle of their lipid bilayers, exposing one of two complementary faces: the A face, which represents the external aspect of the inner, cytoplasmic leaflet of the plasmalemma, and the B face, which represents the internal aspect of the outer leaflet. The course of the cleavage plane and the formation of the two complementary faces are explained diagrammatically in Figure 2–18. The true inner and outer faces of the plasmalemma are not exposed by this method, but they may be disclosed by subliming away some of the ice from the cytoplasmic matrix or the interstitial space by a process called freeze-etching. Although the cleavage plane follows the hydrophobic lipid

matrix of the unit membrane, the globular protein components remain with one or the other face and appear in the replicas as round particles, 6 to 10 nm in diameter, strewn about in random or ordered arrays. The patterns of the particles are characteristic for the region of the membrane and in some instances even characteristic for the group of animals. For example, in mammals the particles generally adhere to the A face, while in arthropods they adhere to the B face. On the complementary face the pattern of the particles is matched by a reciprocal pattern of small pits into which the particles would fit, as indicated in Figure 2–18. In many instances the pits suggest that the particles extend through the whole thickness of the plasmalemma. Orderly arrays of particles and their complementary pits are usually taken to signify the presence of a specific substructure in the plasma membrane, such as might occur at intercellular junctions and synapses. In fact this method has been most useful in elucidating the structure of intercellular junctions and for this reason has contributed new insights into the molecular architecture of the myelin sheath (Chapter VI) and the synapse (Chapter V).

Although the fundamental structure of the neuronal plasmalemma can be assumed to be similar to that of other cells, the peculiar functional and morphological specializations of the neuron indicate that its surface membrane cannot be uniform. The neurophysiologist finds different electrical properties in a postsynaptic membrane compared with the rest of the dendrite, in a dendritic membrane compared with an axon, and in a cell body compared with an axon hillock and initial segment. The neurochemist finds a differential distribution of receptor molecules over the surface, conferring sensitivity to different transmitters at different sites. Freeze-fracture studies to be described in Chapter V show a differential distribution of membrane particles in the pre- and postsynaptic membranes. Furthermore, at electrically coupled junctions the membrane particles display a characteristic aggregation and symmetry. These differential properties show that the neuronal membrane is a mosaic and is readily understood in terms of the fluid mosaic model.

Figure 2–19. **The Edge of a Purkinje Cell, Freeze-Fracture Preparation.**

The lower left third of this field is occupied by the edge of a Purkinje cell *(N)*, and the upper right third is occupied by a neuroglial cell (Golgi epithelial cell). In between course two thin unmyelinated axons *(Ax)* and several highly attenuated sheets of neuroglial cytoplasm *(AsP)*. Within the neuron lie several mitochondria *(mit)*, while most of the neuroglial cell is occupied by its nucleus. The rough fracture plane discloses the complementary faces of the apposed surface membranes in a fashion that exemplifies the diagram in Figure 2–18. Starting near the middle of the field, the first membrane exposed is the B face of the Purkinje cell plasmalemma *(PB)*. It is characterized by relatively sparse, randomly arranged intramembranous particles. The next membrane appears after an intercellular space of varying width. It is the A face of the plasmalemma limiting a sheet of neuroglial cytoplasm. The fracture then cuts across this sheet and cracking through the opposite surface membrane, leaves a slim remnant of A face and exposes a broader expanse of the B face *(AsB)* of this plasmalemma. The two axons lie between this sheet of neuroglial cytoplasm and the next. Both axons are fractured in the same way, exposing the A face *(AlA)* of their plasmalemma on the near side and the B face *(AlB)* on the far side. The next sheet of neuroglial cytoplasm is bounded by the A face *(AsA)* of the plasmalemma, which displays numerous large intramembranous particles. Some of them are arranged in quadrangular clusters *(arrows)*. The fracture plane proceeds across a rather featureless cytoplasm until it reaches the nuclear envelope *(Nev)*, which appears as two parallel membranes with two nuclear pores.
Cerebellar cortex of adult rat. × 88,000.

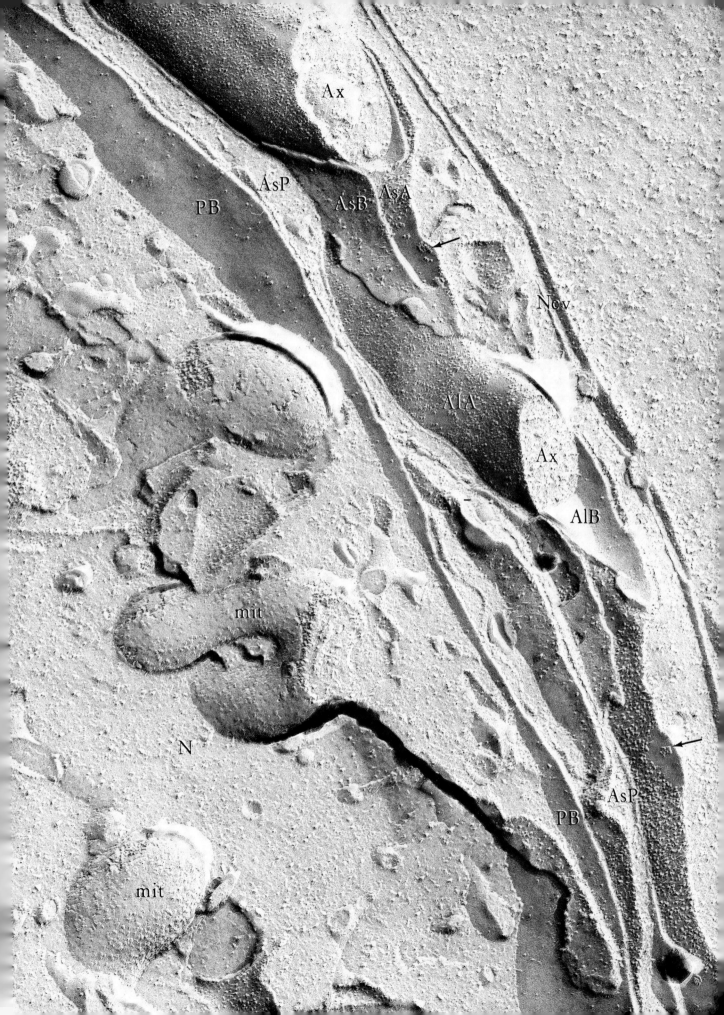

Chapter III

DENDRITES

GENERAL MORPHOLOGY

A dendrite is usually one of several similar processes that issue from the perikaryon of a neuron. Like the main branches growing from the trunk of a tree—whence their name—dendrites appear to be extensions continuous with the perikaryon. In fact in many neurons it is impossible to tell exactly where the perikaryon leaves off and the dendrites begin. In neurons like the so-called Lugaro cells of the cerebellar cortex and many cells in the medullary reticular formation, the whole cell is shaped like a spindle, with gradually diminishing tips, and the point at which the perikaryal extensions should begin to be called dendrites is purely a matter of taste. It is difficult to tell, even in electron micrographs, since dendrites contain the same organelles as the perikaryon, at least in their proximal parts. Furthermore, both can have similar populations of nerve terminals synapsing on their surfaces and can be enclosed in a similar or continuous neuroglial sheath. But this distinction becomes more easily made with increasing distances from the cell body; certainly there can be no confusion by the time the first branch point is reached. Actually, determining the point of onset of a dendrite is not of much consequence unless one is trying to estimate the dimensions of cell body or dendrite, since physiologically and morphologically they both have similar properties.

It is more critical to distinguish between axons and dendrites, as has been intimated in Chapter I. In general, dendrites taper gently as they extend away from the perikaryon, and their contours tend to be somewhat irregular, with protuberances, spines, thorns, hairs, spikes, or leaf-like or fungoid appendages projecting from their surfaces in patterns characteristic of the cell type. In both Golgi preparations and electron microscopic sections, dendrites sometimes display regular ovoid distentions along their course, which produce the effect of a string of pearls. It is generally agreed that this beaded appearance is artifactitious. Dendrites usually branch by bifurcating at relatively acute angles. Occasionally several branches are given off close together as a spray or tuft. Collateral branches tend to be thinner than the parent stem, and at bifurcations one of the branches, usually the shorter one, also is thinner than the other. In contrast to dendrites, axons have rather smooth contours and maintain a fairly uniform caliber once they have passed the thin initial segment. Axons do not exhibit appendages like those on dendrites, and they show distentions or varicosities only in the terminal parts of their arborization. They tend to branch at obtuse or, often, right angles, and their branches have the same caliber as the parent stem. As a general rule, dendrites ramify within a limited field rather close to, and often enclosing, the cell body. Axons usually generate their full arborization at some distance away from the cell body. However, the axons of many cell types give off recurrent collaterals close to their origin which return to the region immediately surrounding the perikaryon. There is also a class of cells—Golgi type II cells—which are characterized by axons that ramify within their own dendritic field. Furthermore, axons differ from dendrites in lacking Nissl bodies, although ribosomes can appear in the initial segment. Finally, axons can be either myelinated or unmyelinated, and the presence of the myelin sheath can generally be taken as a diagnostic characteristic. Quite in contrast, dendrites are as a rule not myelinated. Recently, however, thinly myelinated dendrites have been encountered in the olfactory bulb (Pinching, 1971; Willey, 1973), but such examples are decidedly rare and are not widespread enough in the nervous system to engender serious confusion in identification.

Most neurons give rise to a number of dendrites and for this reason are said to be multipolar. Others have only two main trunks, normally extending from opposite poles of the cell body. A few neuronal types, like the Purkinje cells in the cerebellar cortex of the cat, have only one major dendritic trunk, which generates the entire, complex arborization of smaller dendrites. A few cells in vertebrates lack proper dendrites, for example, the dorsal root ganglion cells, which typically possess a single myelinated trunk that subdivides into two myelinated processes, one that passes into a peripheral nerve and another that enters the central nervous system in a dorsal rootlet. Both the trunk and the two processes of these cells display all the characteristics of axons. In the invertebrates, nerve cells with a similar "pseudounipolar" shape are the rule, and dendrites can be branches of either the main trunk or of axons. But in the vertebrate central nervous system, in which adendritic nerve cells are virtually unknown and multipolar cells are the most common, a dendrite frequently gives rise to the axon. The shapes of a few neuronal cell types are displayed in the Frontispiece.

As was explained in Chapter I, the form of the dendritic tree is a major criterion for characterizing a nerve cell. Golgi preparations provide the best material in which to observe the overall form and ramification of dendrites. On the basis of such observations Ramón-Moliner (1968) has made an interesting attempt to classify neurons according to their dendritic arborizations. He recognizes three main groups of dendritic patterns: isodendritic neurons distinguished by relatively straight dendrites which radiate in all directions and bear relatively few spines; allodendritic neurons characterized by shorter, highly branched, tufted dendrites which pursue a more or less wavy course within a somewhat constrained territory; and idiodendritic neurons,

a heterogeneous group with peculiar dendritic trees absolutely characteristic of the location. Isodendritic neurons are best exemplified by the large ventral horn cells of the spinal cord, while an example of the allodendritic group is the pyramidal cell of the cerebral cortex. The idiodendritic group includes such diverse and distinctive types as the giant Purkinje cell in the cerebellar cortex, the small clustered cells of the inferior olive with highly wavy, recurved dendrites, and the principal cells of the ventral cochlear nucleus with highly tufted dendrites. Each of these cell types is so distinctive in form and so restricted in distribution that the view of even a small portion of its dendritic tree in a Golgi preparation is sufficient to identify the region in which it may be encountered.

Such attempts to rationalize the enormous range of dendritic form by gathering the highly individual dendritic trees into categories can be no more than descriptive devices. The inconclusiveness of Ramón-Moliner's scheme is evident in the diversity of cell types included in his third category, the idiodendritic cells, in which no common principle of form can be discovered. But since a nerve cell receives most of its input through its dendrites, an appreciation of the form of the dendritic tree provides some insight into the role of the cell in the nervous system. For example, the large, isodendritic motor cells in the spinal cord or the large isodendritic cells in the reticular formation of the brain stem receive a great number of afferents from a wide variety of sources. They are, therefore, highly integrative neurons. In contrast, the allodendritic cells with short, tufted, sinuous (or wavy) dendrites, like those found in the secondary sensory nuclei or, as an extreme example, the idiodendritic cells in the inferior olive, receive afferents from only one or, at most, a few sources and are concerned with processing information of a more limited compass. The form of the dendritic tree must reflect to some degree the connections made by a cell with its afferents.

How this form comes about is one of the great unsolved questions of neurocytology. Rakic (1962) has proposed that in the molecular layer of the cerebellar cortex, the form, spread, and orientation of the dendrites of the small neurons (the basket and stellate cells) reflect their sequential differentiation within the grid of parallel fibers, which are laid down at the same time. The neurons in the deeper, older parts of the molecular layer develop dendrites that generally radiate upward through the entire thickness of the layer, those in the middle have dendrites that radiate in all directions, while those near the top have dendrites that radiate downward. It appears as if the growth of the dendrites were directed toward unoccupied, or at least uncommitted, synaptic sites on the afferent axons and were deflected from sites already stabilized by earlier settlers.

Many embryological studies indicate that the growth of afferent axons into a developing region evokes or coincides with the differentiation of dendritic trees on the resident neurons (Morest, 1969a and b; Sidman, 1970b and 1974; Kornguth and Scott, 1972; Rakic, 1972b and 1973). Apparently there is some coordination between the development of the pre- and postsynaptic partners which ensures that the two come together appropriately. Whatever the mechanism for establishing these relationships, now very imperfectly understood, the partnership is highly selective and specific, to the degree that particular parts of the dendritic tree are precisely and reliably linked to particular afferent pathways. This architectural principle is most thoroughly exemplified by the distribution pattern of afferents on the dendritic tree of the Purkinje cell in the cerebellar cortex and on the pyramidal cells in the hippocampus. Detailed mapping of the connections in various parts of the central nervous system has brought many other examples to light.

The form of the dendritic tree also bears a significant relation to its electrical properties. In this respect the angle of branching and the curvature or course of the dendrite have no significant influence since the entire neuron is considered to be in an isopotential extracellular matrix. Its electrical properties are conditioned by the active and passive characteristics of the surface membrane and the diameter and length of the dendritic branches. Such considerations have been treated mathematically by Rall and his coworkers (Rall, 1970a and b; Rall and Rinzel, 1973) in order to obtain expressions for the effect of synaptic activation in various parts of the dendritic tree on the amount of depolarization reaching the cell body. The form of the dendritic arborization of any particular cell must therefore be taken as complementary to the size, location, and dispersion of synapses made by its afferent fibers. From this standpoint the simple location of a synaptic terminal within the dendritic tree should be understood as one of the parameters which control its influence, a parameter as important, perhaps, as the frequency with which it is activated or the potency of its transmitter (Barrett and Crill, 1974).

Cogent examples to illustrate the relevance of location to synaptic efficiency are offered by the cells in the cerebellar cortex. In this cortex, the Purkinje cell, a large and distinctive neuron with a highly complicated dendritic arborization (see Frontispiece), receives excitatory afferents only upon its thorns, whereas it receives inhibitory terminals directly upon the dendritic shafts. The excitatory input to the thorns of the more distal branches is provided by thousands of parallel fibers, thin unmyelinated axons, each of which has little influence on the depolarization of the cell body and initial axon segment, where the nerve impulse is generated. The high input resistance of the thorns and of the small dendrites, together with the long path over which the depolarization must spread in order to reach the cell body, all serve to attenuate the effect of discharges in any individual parallel fiber. In contrast, the excitatory input to the thorns projecting from the larger dendrites meets with relatively little input resistance and exercises an enormous influence on the responses of the cell body. This input is provided by a single climbing fiber, which supplies an elaborate terminal plexus to the trunks of the Purkinje cell dendritic tree. Similarly, the location of the inhibitory inputs determines the range of their effectiveness. Stellate cell axon terminals situated here and there on the distal branches can neutralize

---

Figure 3-1. **Apical Dendrite of a Pyramidal Neuron.**

Passing obliquely across the field is the apical dendrite *(Den)* of a small pyramidal neuron. At its base lies part of the Golgi apparatus *(G)* and Nissl substance *(NB)* of the perikaryon, which displays a portion of the nucleus *(Nuc)*. Microtubules *(m)* funnel into the dendrite to become arranged longitudinally and parallel to one another. Between the microtubules are varicose profiles of the smooth endoplasmic reticulum *(SR)* and mitochondria *(mit)*. More of the ribosomes *(r)* lie beneath the plasma membrane, and clusters of them *(r_1)* are located at the angle of bifurcation of the dendrite. At this site, the microtubules of the apical dendrite enter into one or the other of the secondary dendrites *(Den_1 and Den_2)*.

In the picture, a few axon terminals *(At)* synapse on the dendrite. The majority of axons in the cerebral cortex synapse with the dendritic spines *(t)*.
Cerebral cortex of adult rat. × 15,000.

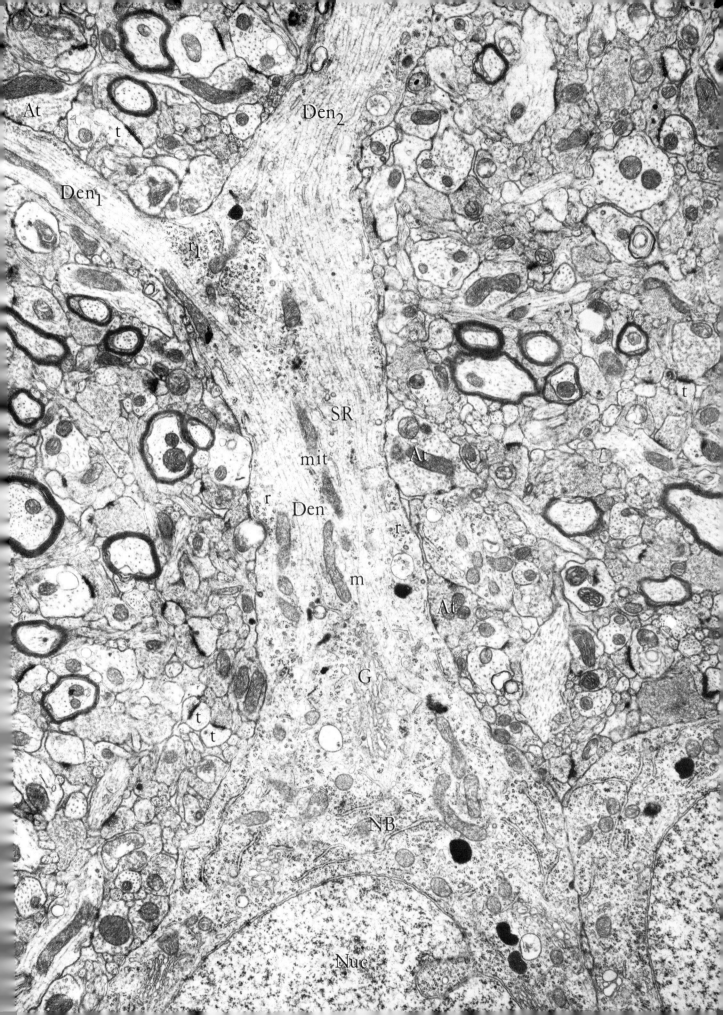

the local excitatory effects of a few parallel fiber-thorn synapses, but basket cell axons clambering over the more important branch points of large dendrites can eliminate the activation resulting from thousands of parallel fibers, synapsing on the more distal reaches of the dendritic tree beyond those branch points. If the dendrite is capable of generating propagated potentials from these branch points, the strategic location of inhibitory terminals, just at these critical sites, becomes even more pertinent. Thus, the location of a nerve ending at a particular place in the dendritic tree may not only influence the specific efficiency of that ending as an inhibitor or activator but also enhance disproportionately the power of an inhibitory ending to select or control which part of the dendritic field will be included in the integrative action of the neuron in question. These examples, taken from the connections of a single cell type, underscore the importance of detailed topographical and morphological analyses in any attempt to understand how a nerve cell behaves.

In many regions of the central nervous system, neurons are oriented with respect to such criteria as the axes of the body, the surfaces of the brain, or the prevailing course of fiber bundles. This orientation usually manifests itself in the direction and spread of the dendrites. For example, in the cerebral cortex there is a predominant radial or vertical orientation with the great majority of the pyramidal cells pointing their apical dendrites toward the pial surface. In the cerebellar cortex the molecular layer displays a strikingly rectilinear pattern resulting from repetitive dendritic trees of the Purkinje, basket, and stellate cells all spread out like fans in the parasagittal plane. Each layer in the gray matter of the spinal cord shows a characteristic

dendritic orientation. Further examples are given by the superior olive, inferior colliculus, medial geniculate body (Cajal, 1911; Morest, 1965). Recently, orientation patterns have been discovered in the central cerebellar nuclei (Chan-Palay, 1973a). Such dendritic patterns, of course, signify that there must be a complementary pattern in the axonal plexuses of these regions. The analyses of these dendritic and axonal patterns are among the most elegant investigations in modern neuroanatomy (Cajal, 1899, 1909–1911; Morest, 1965; Scheibel and Scheibel, 1968b; Chan-Palay, 1973a and d).

In addition to these cellular orientation patterns there is often a related aggregation of neurons in which nerve cell bodies are arranged in strands or columnar arrays, as a result of which their parallel dendrites are brought into close association. These have been most thoroughly studied in the cerebral cortex (Peters and Walsh, 1972; Fleischhauer, Petsche, and Wittkowski, 1972; Massing and Fleischhauer, 1973; Peters and Feldman, 1973; Fleischhauer, 1974; Scheibel, Davies, Lindsay and Scheibel, 1974), and in the ventral horn of the spinal cord (Scheibel and Scheibel, 1970 and 1973a and b; Kerns and Peters, 1974). The precise significance of such dendritic bundles is not yet understood. It is obvious that a certain economy in the distribution of afferent plexuses is achieved by the fasciculation of the postsynaptic elements and that a single fiber may be enabled to influence individual dendrites in the bundle at different levels in their course. But whether there is any specific advantage to the fasciculation remains an unanswered question. The Scheibels (1973a) have speculated that the close apposition of dendrites within a bundle permits various degrees of

---

Figure 3–2. **Dendrite of a Purkinje Cell.**

A large secondary dendrite ascends through the center of the field. The cytoplasmic components are nearly all aligned parallel with the axis of the dendrite. Microtubules *(m)*, mitochondria *(mit)*, and agranular reticulum *(SR)* are the most prominent organelles. Small aggregates of Nissl substance appear here and there, mostly as collections of free ribosomes *(r)*. The entire shaft of the dendrite is ensheathed in neuroglia *(AsP)*. Two terminals of basket cell axon collaterals *(ba)* synapse upon the surface of the dendrite. Note their flattened synaptic vesicles and the neurofilaments in the preterminal parts of the axons. Many of the neuroglial processes contain clusters of glycogen particles *(gly)*.
Cerebellar cortex of adult rat. × 22,000.

Inset. A transverse section of a smaller Purkinje cell dendrite. The mitochondria and agranular reticulum are largely marginated, while the microtubules are relatively evenly distributed throughout the cross section.
Cerebellar cortex of adult rat. × 26,000.

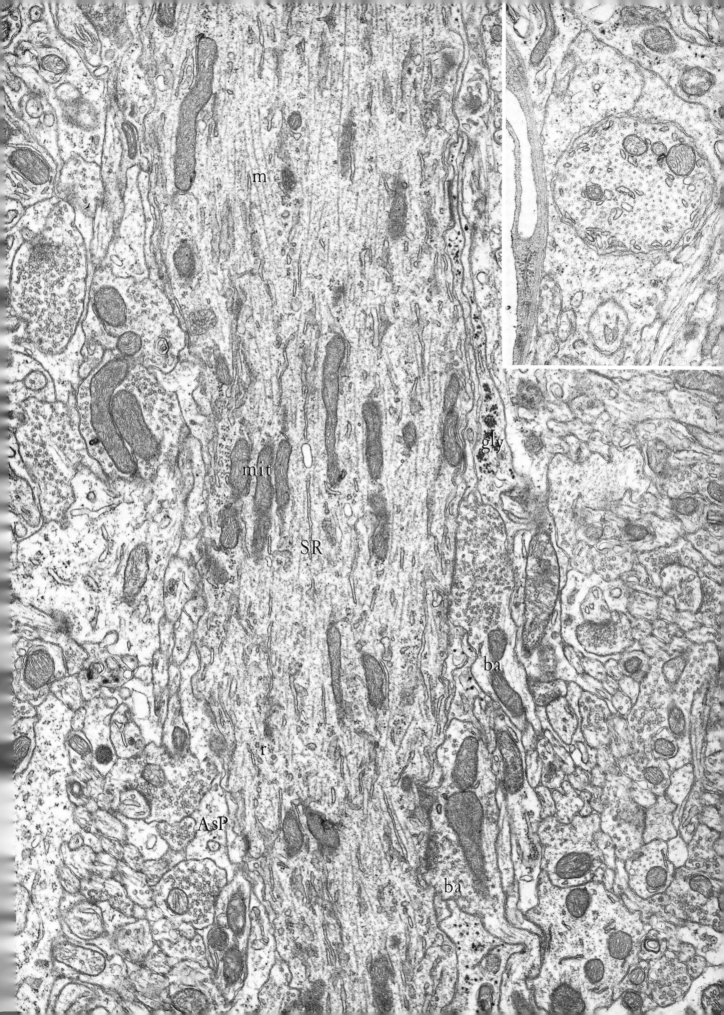

interaction between them, so that the activity in one dendrite may alter the environment of its neighbors, or even their membrane potentials, through presumed dendro-dendritic gap junctions. The dendritic bundles might then encode certain programs for emergent functions of the whole neuronal aggregate.

THE CYTOPLASM OF DENDRITES

In tissues prepared for conventional light microscopy and colored with the usual staining procedures, dendrites cannot be followed very far from their origins because they contain little stainable material. The Nissl bodies, which are the main colorable component of the perikaryon, extend into the dendrites but become progressively smaller and less conspicuous with increasing distance from the cell center. The more distal branches can be completely free of Nissl substance, except for the small triangular masses occupying branch points (Cajal, 1896 and 1909). As a result, the larger trunks of the dendritic tree can disappear into the clear and colorless neuropil in which they course. Even in silver-stained preparations dendrites can seldom be traced beyond one or two bifurcations, since with successive subdivisions they become indistinguishable from the background. In thick plastic sections of osmicated tissues, stained with toluidine blue, the smaller components of the neuropil produce a blue background. Against this background the colorless dendrites can be followed for much longer distances than in conventional Nissl preparations.

As would be expected from its form and the appearance of its content in light microscopic preparations, the initial part of the dendrite appears in electron micrographs to be merely a continuation of the neuronal perikaryon. It has the same organelles in roughly the same proportions. No special structure or deficiency marks the beginning of the dendrite, in contrast to the specializations that announce the initial segment of the axon. The only sign of the beginning of a dendrite, besides its tapering shape, is the gradual orientation of all elongated organelles into a line parallel with the axis of the process (Figure 3–1). It appears as if all the cytoplasmic structures in the perikaryon were streaming into the neck of a funnel or were being combed into parallel longitudinal array. The most prominent of the organelles are the neurofilaments, microtubules, mitochondria, and tubules of the agranular endoplasmic reticulum. But Nissl bodies (granular endoplasmic reticulum) and the Golgi apparatus also extend into the dendrites, and depending upon the diameter of the process, they are also more or less elongated.

The penetration of the Golgi apparatus into dendrites varies greatly in extent from cell to cell. Besides, it may run out into some dendrites and not others from the same cell. The streaming movements seen in living neurons in tissue culture suggest that this organelle is plastic and to some extent mobile. It is probably capable of slipping in and out of the dendrite in compliance with unknown commands. In electron micrographs of small neurons, which have relatively little perikaryal cytoplasm, the Golgi apparatus extends far into the principal dendrites. This is seen particularly well in small pyramidal and stellate cells of the cerebral and cerebellar cortices. The apparatus occupies the core of the dendrite and its cisternal elements are arrayed parallel to the longitudinal axis. Of all the organelles in dendrites, the Golgi apparatus is the first to disappear with advancing distance from the perikaryon. It hardly ever reaches beyond the first bifurcation.

Figure 3–3.   **Dendrite of a Purkinje Cell.**

A large secondary dendrite appears in the lower half of the field. The membranous components of the cytoplasm are prominent in this micrograph. The agranular reticulum *(SR)* is clearly continuous with the hypolemmal cisterna *(arrows)* at several sites. The mitochondria *(mit)* are all peripherally disposed, but small aggregates of ribosomes *(r)* appear here and there. The microtubules *(m)*, as usual, are dispersed throughout the dendrite. Two basket fibers *(ba)* terminate on the surface of the dendrite with Gray's type 2 synaptic junctions. In the surrounding neuropil parallel fibers form type 1 synaptic junctions with the thorns *(t)* of small Purkinje cell dendrites.
Cerebellar cortex of adult rat. × 36,000.

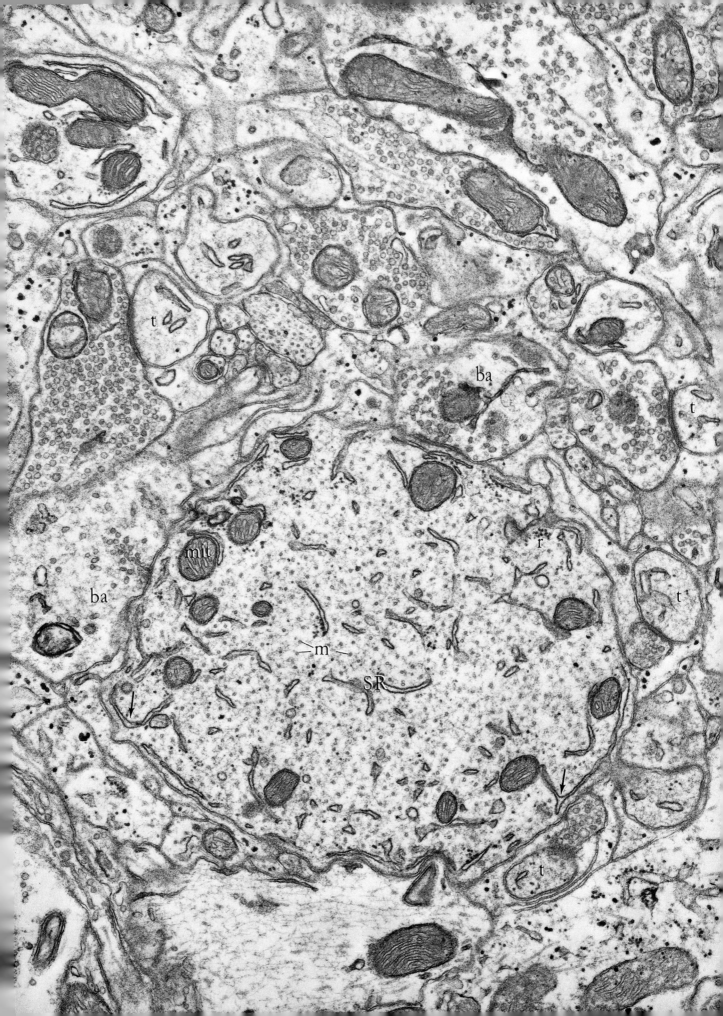

In contrast, the Nissl substance penetrates into the farthest subdivisions of the dendritic tree, although in steadily diminishing quantities. It does not enter into the thorns and other narrow appendages, however. In the proximal, larger dendrites the Nissl bodies have the same construction as they have in the perikaryon, that is, groups of anastomosing cisternae of the granular endoplasmic reticulum associated with polyribosomes lying free in the cytoplasmic matrix between them (Figure 3–5). In the base of the dendrite such masses appear either in the axial core or more peripherally. Farther out preferred locations for them are outpocketings or bulges in the contour of the dendrite and especially bifurcations, as already noted by light microscopy. With successive branchings of a dendrite into its arborization, the character of the granular endoplasmic reticulum gradually changes. Clumps of imbricated cisternae are not commonly encountered in small dendrites. Isolated cisternae or bent and branching tubular profiles become the most prevalent forms (Figures 3–2 and 3–4). A twisted tubule in the midst of a small cloud of ribosomes is the typical appearance of the Nissl substance in the distal parts of the dendritic tree. But even these representatives of the granular endoplasmic reticulum become infrequent in the smallest dendrites. This progressive diminution in the size and incidence of the Nissl bodies with increasing distance from the perikaryon accounts for the early clearing of stainable material in dendrites examined with the light microscope, since the smaller clumps of granular endoplasmic reticulum and associated free ribosomes do not retain enough color to be detectable with the light microscope.

The diminution in the amount of the Nissl substance sometimes leads to difficulties in distinguishing small axons from small dendrites in electron micrographs. If the axonal profiles lack synaptic vesicles and the dendritic profiles lack ribosomes, they can look very much alike, for both types of processes contain similar populations of other organelles. The fact that some dendrites also contain synaptic vesicles and prove to be presynaptic to other dendrites seriously complicates the problem of identification in certain parts of the central nervous system, such as the olfactory bulb and the thalamus. In general, however, dendritic profiles, even if small, can be identified by their irregular shapes, the presence of thorns or other appendages, their long fleshy mitochondria, numerous microtubules, and postsynaptic specializations. In addition the smallest dendritic profiles are almost never as small as the axonal profiles that might be confused with them on the basis of internal structure. In some instances tracing through serial sections to a larger more definitive profile may be necessary, and comparison with the form of Golgi-impregnated specimens is essential in most cases. It should be emphasized that the presence of clustered ribosomes, especially in association with cisternae or tubules of the granular endoplasmic reticulum, is usually a sufficient condition to secure the identity of a neural process as a dendrite. The only exception to this point is the initial segment of an axon, but in this case there are additional identifying features (see Chapter IV).

The agranular endoplasmic reticulum, which is often inconspicuous at the beginning of a dendrite, becomes more noticeable as the cytoplasm clears with progressive distance from the perikaryon. It is never very voluminous, but as the Nissl substance decreases distally, it becomes the principal membranous system in the dendrite. It forms a continuous network with its congener in the perikaryon and extends throughout the dendritic tree, even into the spines. It consists of wandering cisternae and tubules of various dimensions, expanding here

---

Figure 3–4. **Dendrites in Longitudinal and Transverse Section.**

In this picture from the neuropil of the anterior horn are two dendrites *(Den₁* and *Den₂)* sectioned longitudinally and a third one *(Den₃)* sectioned transversely. In the upper dendrite *(Den₁)* something of the extent of the individual microtubules *(m)* and neurofilaments *(nf)* may be seen. These structures have regular outlines which contrast with the more varicose outlines of the tubules of the smooth endoplasmic reticulum *(SR)*, with which clusters of free ribosomes *(r)* are often associated. Such large numbers of neurofilaments in groups are characteristic of the dendrites arising from large anterior horn cells and are not seen in dendrites generally.

With the exception of ribosomes, the same organelles are also present in the transversely sectioned dendrite *(Den₃)*. This smaller dendrite has two axon terminals synapsing upon its surface. In the upper terminal the synaptic vesicles are spherical, while in the lower one they are mostly ellipsoidal. Extending around the axon terminals and the postsynaptic dendrite is an astrocytic sheath *(As)*.
Spinal cord of adult rat. × 44,000.

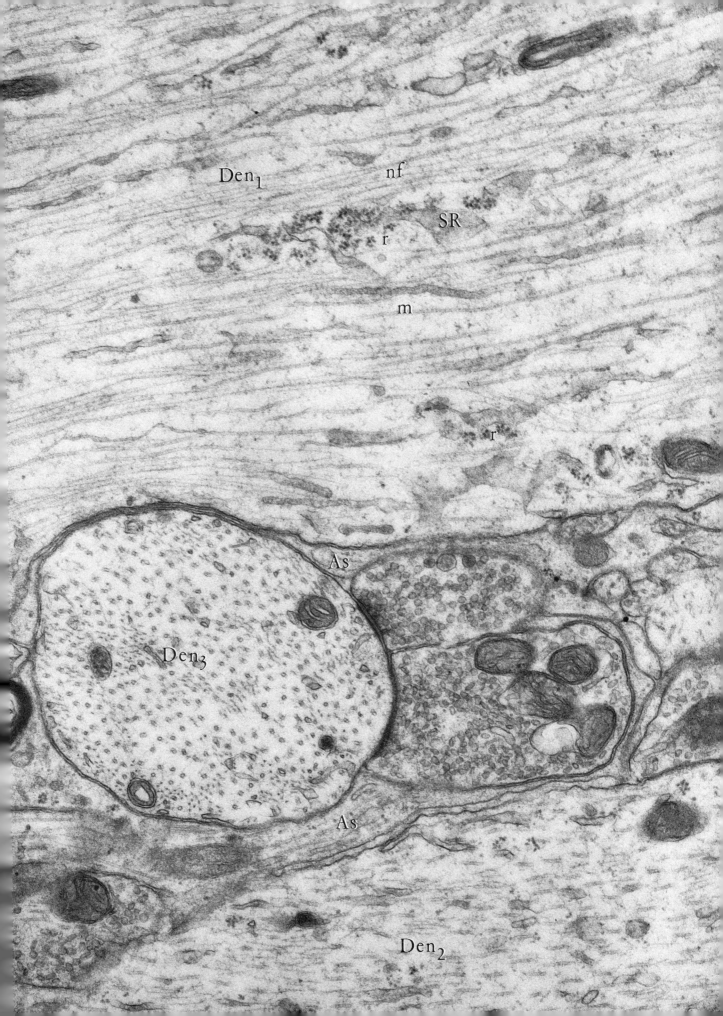

and there into broad lakes and constricting into narrow channels that twist in and out among the other organelles (Figures 3–2 to 3–4). In some places the cisternae lie athwart the longitudinal array of microtubules that pervades the dendritic cytoplasm. Such cisternae are curiously fenestrated in a regular way, and the microtubules pass straight through the pores.

A specialized part of the agranular reticulum is the hypolemmal cisterna, which was described in a previous chapter. As in the perikarya, it is developed to various degrees in the dendrites of different cells. The Purkinje cell provides the most elaborate example known (Kaiserman-Abramof and Palay, 1969; Palay and Chan-Palay, 1974). In this cell the hypolemmal cisterna underlies the plasma membrane of the entire dendritic tree. It occurs in every branch and even extends into the dendritic spines. Like other parts of the agranular endoplasmic reticulum it is actually a network of broad pools communicating with one another through narrow channels. The hypolemmal cisterna regularly lies about 60 nm beneath the plasmalemma, the undulations of which it follows quite faithfully. Here and there it sends off an anastomosing tubule or cisterna deeper into the cytoplasm to join the ordinary granular or agranular reticulum (Figure 3–3). On the other hand, the cisterna also approaches the plasmalemma in some places much more closely, so that barely 10 or 20 nm intervene between the two. In such places the cisterna may be collapsed and its lumen obliterated except at the ends. These constitute the subsurface cisternae, first described by Rosenbluth (1962a and b) in cell bodies of acoustic and vestibular ganglion cells. Such subsurface cisternae may be reduplicated so that a stack of broad, flattened cisternae, appressed together, underlies the plasmalemma (Rosenbluth, 1962b; Kerns and Peters, 1974). As in the perikarya of many cell types, the subsurface cisternae may be the only representatives of the hypolemmal cisterna in the dendrites.

The role of these membranous organelles in the function of dendrites is unknown. Since the speculations concerning them were discussed in the previous chapter and apply equally well here, they will not be repeated. It should be recalled, however, that Wood, McLaughlin, and Barber (1974) detected an interesting chemical difference between the hypolemmal cisterna and the deeper elements of the endoplasmic reticulum in the dendritic tree of the Purkinje cell. In the dendrites they found that the hypolemmal cisterna preferentially bound concanavalin A (which demonstrates the presence of mannose- or glucose-containing glycoproteins) while ordinary endoplasmic reticulum in the core of the dendrite did not. And this distribution differed from that in the perikaryon of the same cell, where all types of endoplasmic reticulum—including the granular, agranular, nuclear envelope, hypolemmal cisterna, and the Golgi apparatus—contained concanavalin binding sites. These results suggest that, in the dendrite, either the hypolemmal cisternal membrane has a higher concentration of glycoprotein in its composition than does that of the deeper endoplasmic reticulum or the hypolemmal cisterna actually contains glycoprotein in its lumen. Wood and his coworkers (1974) offered several hypothetical functions for the hypolemmal cisterna. It might be a storehouse of reserve glycoprotein for renewal of the plasmalemmal glycoprotein. It might be the preferred path for migration or transport of glycoproteins along dendrites. This suggestion is in harmony with the speculation of Kreutzberg and his coworkers (Kreutzberg, Schubert, Tóth, and Rieske, 1973; Kreutzberg and Tóth, 1974) to the effect that dendrites serve as secretory pathways for the perikaryon and secrete proteins into the perivascular space whence they pass into the blood stream. This speculation is interesting in itself as a curious inversion of Golgi's original proposal that dendrites are the conduits of nutrition from the blood vessels to the nerve cell body.

Figure 3–5. **A Dendrite in the Neuropil of the Anterior Horn, Transverse Section.**

In the center of the field is a large, transversely sectioned dendrite from an anterior horn cell. Scattered throughout its cytoplasm are relatively evenly spaced microtubules (*m*) interspersed with groups of neurofilaments (*nf*) and profiles of tubular smooth endoplasmic reticulum (*SR*). Most of the mitochondria (*mit*) are located at the periphery of the dendrite, as are the Nissl bodies (*NB*). Also present are two multivesicular bodies (*mvb*).

A number of axon terminals (*At*) surround the dendrite, and some of them synapse (*arrows*) on its surface.

In the upper right corner of the field is a node of Ranvier. At this node the axon (*Ax*) contains synaptic vesicles and forms a synapse (*s*) with a dendrite (*Den*).
Spinal cord from adult rat. × 23,000.

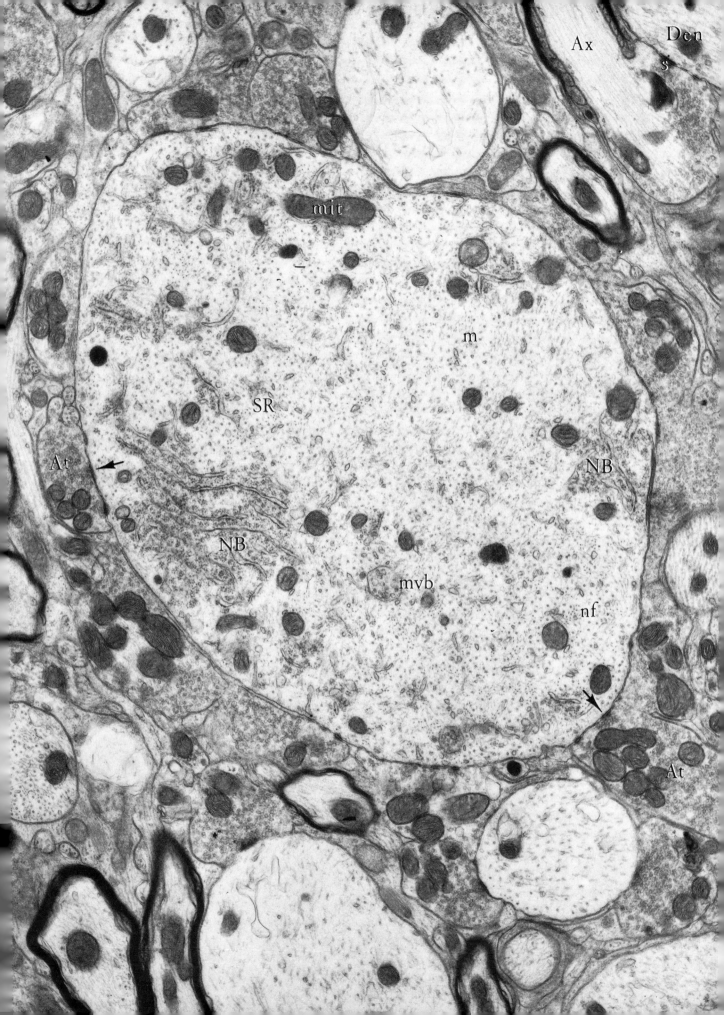

Because of the striking and consistent proximity of the hypolemmal cisterna to the surface membrane, it seems more plausible that the functions of these two structures are closely interdependent.

The mitochondria of dendrites are usually oriented longitudinally. Some of them can be very long. For example, Pappas and Purpura (1961) depict a mitochondrion 9 microns long in a dendrite from the superficial cortex of a cat. Small, rounded, and plump forms also occur, as in the cell body, and Y-shaped or branched configurations are not infrequent. In larger dendrites the mitochondria tend to slip toward the peripheral cytoplasm, leaving the core to the microtubules and the endoplasmic reticulum. As successive bifurcations reduce the size of the dendrites the mitochondria drift into the axial stream surrounded by parallel microtubules and sometimes encircled by the endoplasmic reticulum. It has been noted (Palay, 1964; Palay and Chan-Palay, 1974) that although the microtubules, neurofilaments, and elements of the endoplasmic reticulum are apportioned among the numerous branches of a dendrite, the mitochondria appear to become more concentrated. The number of mitochondrial profiles per unit of cross-sectional area increases in the smaller dendritic branches so that mitochondria appear much more numerous in small dendrites than in large ones.

Microtubules are the most prominent elements in the cytoplasm of large dendrites, and they funnel into the base of the dendrite to become arranged parallel to its principal axis (Figures 3–1, 3–2, and 3–4). In transverse sections (Figures 3–2 to 3–4) the microtubules appear to be regularly disposed with almost crystalline orderliness. The only distortions of this pattern are produced by the intrusion of other organelles, especially mitochondria. Often the mitochondria, as indicated above, appear to be wrapped in a basket of parallel microtubules. A network of fine, wispy, twisted threads extends radially from each microtubule and attaches to its neighboring microtubules as well as to nearly all other organelles in the vicinity (Wuerker and Palay, 1969; Tani and Ametani, 1970; Wuerker and Kirkpatrick, 1972; Hinkley, 1973; Metuzals and Mushynski, 1974). The nature of this material is obscure. It may be unpolymerized microtubular protein or some associated filamentous protein. It may also be protein of heterogeneous types, artifactitiously precipitated into an indiscriminate network. The attachment of these threads to both microtubules and other organelles has suggested to some investigators that they are important in the movement of vesicles, mitochondria, and other particles up and down the dendrite (Barondes, 1967; Hinkley, 1973; Metuzals and Mushynski, 1974).

Neurofilaments appear only in small numbers in the vast majority of dendrites. Usually they are single longitudinal threads running among the microtubules, or they may be collected into small bundles (Figures 3–4 and 3–5). They are less rigid than microtubules and shift their relative positions suddenly from point to point along their course. They too are surrounded by the network of fine cottony threads, which seems to bind them to the microtubules and other adjacent organelles with rather loose strands. A few cell types are now known that have unusually large numbers of neurofilaments in their dendrites. In large motor neurons of the rat and cat (Wuerker and Palay, 1969) and in the Betz cells of the cat, fascicles of neurofilaments are regular components of the large dendrites (Kaiserman-Abramof and Peters, 1972). The fascicles contain anywhere from 3 to 40 filaments all running approximately parallel with one another and close together. In their course the fascicles generally twist gradually, so that the filaments are not perfectly parallel with one another. In the giant Meynert cells of the primate visual cortex neurofilaments are unusually conspicuous components of all the dendrites,

---

Figure 3–6. **Dendrites in the Neuropil of the Cerebral Cortex.**

In this tangentially oriented section three large dendrites (*Den₁–Den₃*), which form part of a cluster, are apparent. Their cytoplasm contains regularly spaced microtubules (*m*), mitochondria (*mit*), and profiles of smooth endoplasmic reticulum (*SR*). A coated vesicle (*cv*) is being formed at the surface of one dendrite (*Den₂*). Other transversely sectioned dendrites (*Den₄–Den₆*) are smaller. One dendrite (*Den₇*) is sectioned longitudinally and this shows a coil of ribosomes (*r*).

Although only one dendritic spine (*sp₁*) is seen to be in continuity with its parent dendrite (*Den₈*), the neuropil shows many profiles of dendritic spines (*sp*), some of which contain a spine apparatus (*sa*). These spines form synapses with axon terminals (*At*).

At the bottom right is a section through the paranode of a myelinated axon (*Ax*). *Visual cortex of rat.* × 30,000.

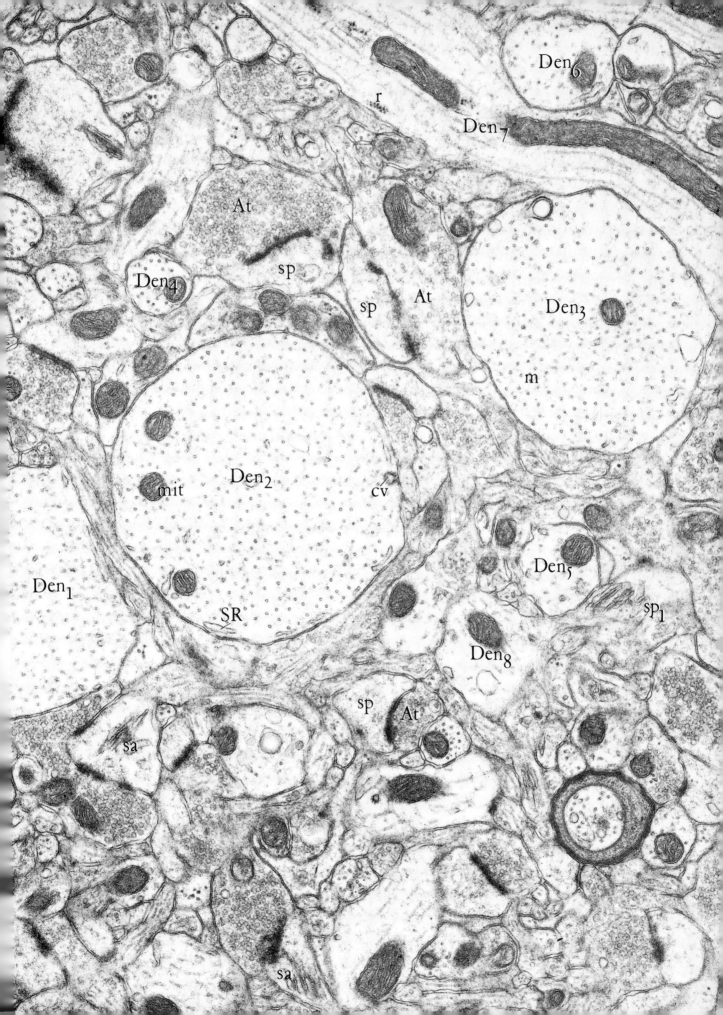

even the smaller subdivisions (Chan-Palay, Palay, and Billings-Gagliardi, 1974). In contrast to those in motor neurons and Betz cells, these neurofilaments are not fasciculated, but run as more widely spaced individual threads throughout the cross section. Although it might be thought that the presence of neurofilaments is related to the large size of all these cell types, there are other cells, equally large, such as Purkinje cells, that do not display extraordinary numbers of neurofilaments in their dendrites. There is, however, an interesting correlation with argyrophilia, since the dendrites of all three of the large cells containing neurofilaments stain well with silver.

Both neurofilaments and microtubules appear to be coextensive with the lengths of the processes in which they run. At each bifurcation it can be seen that the filaments and microtubules bend into the resultant branches and are apportioned according to the cross-sectional area of the daughter branches. The interfilamentous and intertubular distances remain fairly constant throughout the dendritic tree. There are, however, occasional observations of microtubules that loop from one branch into another without following the parent stem. Since microtubules, like neurofilaments, are single threads lacking any tendency to branch, these examples of microtubules looping between the dendritic branches must be independent of the tubular complement originating in the perikaryon. In view of the well-known propensity of microtubules to depolymerize and reassemble, it is really astounding that more erratic microtubules are not seen.

THE DENDRITIC SPINES

It is upon the surfaces of dendrites that most synapses occur. They are formed either directly upon the dendritic stems or upon the spines or thorns that project from them. A review of the literature on the dendritic spines up until 1968 has been presented by Scheibel and Scheibel (1968a). Perhaps the best-known examples of spines are those that emanate from the dendrites of pyramidal cells in the cerebral cortex (Figures 5–5, 5–6, and 11–3) and Purkinje cells in the cerebellum (Figures 3–8, 5–7, and 11–2), but they also occur in such regions as the substantia gelatinosa, vestibular nucleus, thalamus (Figures 5–18 and 11–4), olfactory bulb (Figure 3–7), and subfornical organ. Moreover, spines are not confined to dendrites, for they may also project from neuronal perikarya, as for example, in the vestibular, cochlear (Figure 5–14), cuneate, oculomotor, and red nuclei, and even from the initial segments of axons of pyramidal cells in the cerebral cortex (Westrum, 1970).

In the cerebral cortex few spines arise from dendritic shafts before the origins of the first branches. Along the length of the apical dendrites of pyramidal neurons in layer V of the human cerebral cortex, Marin-Padilla (1967) has shown that there is an initial increase in the density of spines as the distance from the perikaryon increases. Maximal numbers of dendritic spines are attained at about the midpoint along the length of the apical dendrite, and further distally the density of spines decreases again. In the visual cortex of mice the distribution of the spines appears to be rather different. Thus, Valverde has found that the apical dendrites of the layer V pyramidal neurons display an exponential increase in the concentration of spines as the distance from the cell body increases, and a mathematical model expressing the growth of spines with age of development has been introduced by Valverde and Ruiz-Marcos (1969). A similar conclusion about the distribution of dendritic spines has been drawn by Mungai (1967), who studied the cerebral cortex of the cat. He has shown that in pyramidal neurons the number of spines per 100 square microns of dendritic (apical and basal) surface is 0 to 2 on the main stem dendrite, 5 to 25 in the branching zone (the zone between the first and most peripheral bifurcations), and 10 to 37 in the terminal zone. In terms of total numbers of spines per cell within the three zones, Mungai (1967) gives figures of 5 to 18, 200 to 758, and 1337 to 3427, respectively. Of further interest is the estimate that these spines (some 4000 per pyramidal neuron) account for about 43 per cent of the total surface area of the perikaryon plus dendrites.

It should not be concluded, however, that all dendrites of a neuron necessarily have the same distribution of dendritic spines along their lengths. Thus, Globus and Scheibel (1966 and 1967a) have shown that different dendrites of pyramidal cells in the rabbit's cerebral cortex show different spine concentrations. They calculated that apical dendrites have an average of 0.75 spine per micron of length, oblique and terminal branches of apical dendrites have 0.40 spine per micron, and basal dendrites have 0.30 spine per micron.

A similar estimation of dendritic spine distribution has been made for the Meynert cell with somewhat different results (Chan-Palay, Palay, and Billings-Gagliardi, 1974). This cell is a giant, isolated pyramidal neuron in layer V of the visual cortex of primates. In the Meynert cell of the monkey the vast majority of the spines (over 77 per cent) occur on the basal dendrites, with a concentration of almost 3 per micron length. The apical dendrite is very stout and gives off few branches before its terminal bifurcation. Its proximal portion, about 30 to 35 microns long, is smooth, but thereafter it becomes extremely spiny, showing 5.6 spines per micron of length. This part of the apical dendrite accounts for only 4 per cent of the total length of the dendritic tree, but 3523 spines protrude from it, almost 10 per cent of the total number of spines on the entire dendritic tree. As the apical dendrite ascends through layers IV and III, the spine density decreases rather abruptly and progressively. Less than 2.5 per cent of the spines project from this part. In layer II the dendrite subdivides into a spray of tapering branches that spread out into layer I. The spine density rises again but not so high as in the basal dendrites or in the spiny part of the apical dendrite. The number of spines per micron on the terminal dendrites varies between 0.8 and 1.3. The total number of spines on a typical Meynert cell was estimated as 35,865, which may be compared to Cragg's estimate of an average of 60,000 synapses per pyramidal cell in the monkey's motor cortex. These numbers are far in excess of the numbers of spines reported for pyramidal cells in the earlier studies noted above.

The fine structure of dendritic spines in the cerebral cortex was first described by Gray (1959), Gray and Guillery (1963b), and Pappas and Purpura (1961). They showed that most spines consist of two portions, a narrow neck, or stalk, and an ovoid bulb (Figures 3–8 and 5–7). On the basis of measurements of dendritic spines in the pre- and postcentral cortex of the rat, squirrel monkey, and man, Jacobson (1967) concluded that in each species the overall length of spines is the same, about 2.0 microns. Spines of different dimensions and shapes in addition to those considered by Jacobson certainly exist, at least in the rat. Thus, Peters and Kaiserman-Abramof (1970) showed that the spines

on the pyramidal neurons of layers II and III in the rat parietal cortex are of three basic types. The most common ones have long, thin stalks and small end-bulbs. The least common have a mushroom shape, with a short, stout stalk ending in a large bulb, while the other spines are little more than stubby protrusions of the dendrite and lack a stalk. Somewhat similar conclusions have been drawn by Jones and Powell (1969b), who examined the dendritic spines of pyramidal neurons in the somatosensory cortex of the cat. They showed a range of morphological variations of spines and came to the conclusion that while spines of every shape and size may emanate from a pyramidal cell dendrite, there is a tendency for the largest spines to protrude from the smallest dendrites and vice versa. In this same vein, Laatsch and Cowan (1966a) have shown that in the dentate gyrus the dendritic spines on the larger and proximal branches of the granule cell dendrites are short and receive the terminals of commissural afferents, while those probably related to other afferent systems project from the smaller dendrites and tend to be long and thin.

In the electron microscope it is found that the spines in the cerebral cortex are filled with a fluffy material that seems to consist of fine and indistinct filaments, and this material is so characteristic that isolated profiles of the bulbs of spines can be readily recognized in the neuropil (Figures 5–5, 5–6, and 11–3). Identification of such isolated profiles may be further aided by the fact that the spines receive very distinct asymmetrical synapses. These criteria are important, for it is only rarely that the section passes through both the bulb of a spine and its stalk connecting it to the parent dendrite. The microtubules and neurofilaments in the dendritic stems pass by the stalks of the spines and do not enter them, and mitochondria and ribosomes are only rarely encountered in the spinal cytoplasm, although a few vesicles may be present.

Indeed the only organelle that seems to enter the cortical dendritic spines from the cytoplasm of the dendritic shaft is an extension of the smooth endoplasmic reticulum (Peters and Kaiserman-Abramof, 1970). Thus, it is not uncommon for a small enlargement of the smooth endoplasmic reticulum to occur at the base of a dendritic spine, and for this enlargement to give off a small tubular cisterna that passes through the stalk into the bulb of the spine. There the tubular cisterna may become confluent with the most conspicuous structure in the cytoplasm of a spine, the spine apparatus (Figure 5–5, *sa*). In its typical form this apparatus occurs only in the cerebral cortex (Gray, 1959; Gray and Guillery, 1963b). It consists of two or three membrane-bound sacs, alternating with thin laminae of dense material. Although a spine apparatus is not encountered in every section through a spine, it is very common, and in the larger spines, two or even three apparatuses may appear. The function of these structures is not known, and they are not unique to dendritic spines, for similar organelles have also been encountered in the axon initial segment (Peters, Proskauer, and Kaiserman-Abramof, 1968) and dendritic stems (Kaiserman-Abramof and Peters, 1972) of pyramidal neurons.

The spines of Purkinje cell dendrites (Herndon, 1963; Palay, 1964; Palay and Chan-Palay, 1974), like most spines of the pyramidal neurons in the neocortex, have a stalk that expands into a bulb (Figure 5–7). While a typical spine apparatus is not present, a simplified version invariably lies in the bulb. This consists of a diminutive cisterna or two connected by means of a tubular extension with the hypolemmal cisterna in the parent shaft of the dendrite (Figure 5–7).

Dendrites of other neurons, such as those of the anterior horn cells in the spinal cord, have simpler spines. They consist of little more than finger-like evaginations from the dendrite filled with a fluffy filamentous material. Similar spines also arise from the dendrites of the principal cells in the lateral geniculate body. In addition, these dendrites have "grape-like" protrusions (for example, see Szentágothai, 1963; Peters and Palay, 1966; Famiglietti and Peters, 1972) which are up to 5 microns long and consist of a short stem expanding into a terminal bulb. Similar protrusions occur in many regions of the thalamus, and they seem to enter into the synaptic glomeruli (see Chapter V).

The spines on any particular neuron can vary considerably in size, shape, and style. Even along the surface of a single dendrite some can be stalked, others sessile, some twisted, others rigidly straight, and some simple, others branched. In some cases the shape and size of the spine are specifically elaborated to match a particular kind of axonal terminal. For example, the pyramidal cells of the hippocampus have not only the relatively simple spines of the usual cortical neuron but also a set of larger, foliate spines attached to the apical dendrite near its origin. These spines invaginate into the large axon terminals of the mossy fibers and bear many small projections, or spinelets, each containing a spine apparatus and forming a separate synaptic junction with the terminal (Hamlyn, 1962; Blackstad, 1967).

An interesting fact to emerge in recent years is that the dendritic spines are sensitive barometers of change in their environment. Most of our information about these changes has been derived from a study of Golgi-impregnated material of the cerebral cortex. A few examples of these findings will now be considered.

Globus and Scheibel (1967a and b) found that when the afferent axons supplying axon terminals to the visual cortex are affected either by enucleation or by lesions in the lateral geniculate body, there is some loss of spines along the proximal three-fifths of the apical shafts of pyramidal neurons in the visual cortex. On the other hand, cutting callosal fibers brings about a diminution in the numbers of spines only from the oblique branches of the apical dendritic shafts (Globus and Scheibel, 1967c).

Valverde (1968) has also shown that unilateral eye enucleation at birth produces a significant decrease in the dendritic spines of those segments of apical dendrites that traverse layer IV of the contralateral visual cortex in the mouse. A parallel loss is brought about by rearing mice in complete darkness from birth (Valverde, 1967). From the analysis of a number of experiments, Valverde (1971) concluded that during development there are some dendritic spines whose growth is not dependent upon the presence of visual stimuli, but that a second group is dependent and that it is this group which does not grow if animals are reared in dark-

---

Figure 3–7. Olfactory Bulb.

The field contains a number of mitral cell dendrites *(Den₁)* surrounded by the dendrites *(Den₂)* and gemmules *(gem)* of granule cells. Like dendrites elsewhere, those of mitral cells *(Den₁)* have microtubules *(m)* and mitochondria *(mit)* in their cytoplasm, but in addition they contain synaptic vesicles *(sv)*. Synapsing with these dendrites are the gemmules *(gem)* of granule cells, which are filled with synaptic vesicles. The gemmules arise from dendrites *(Den₂)* which are thinner than those of mitral cells and have few, if any, synaptic vesicles in their cytoplasm.

Passing through this dendritic neuropil are the irregular processes of astrocytes *(As)*.

Rat olfactory bulb. × 40,000.

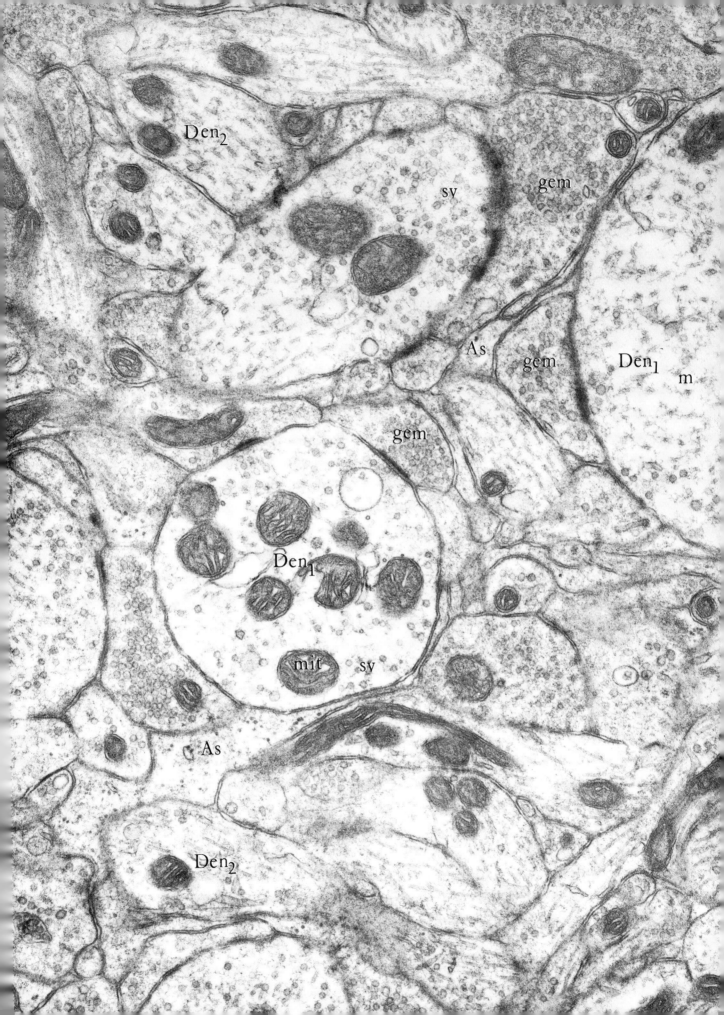

ness. If the animals are removed from the darkness after eyelid opening and allowed to live
under normal conditions, some apical dendrites
do not recover, but others attain a normal complement of dendritic spines.

In an ultrastructural study of visual deprivation induced by suturing one eyelid Fifková
(1970) has found that the mean density of synapses from layer II through layer V in the visual
cortex supplied by the deprived eye is 20 per
cent less than in the cortex of the control side.

A regrowth of dendritic spines also takes
place in the hippocampus (Parnavelas, Lynch,
Brecha, Cotman, and Globus, 1974). Following
lesions in the entorhinal cortex of adult rats
there is an initial loss of spines from those portions of the dendrites of pyramidal neurons that
enter the outer molecular layer of the hippocampus. Five days after the lesion these portions of the dendrites have lost about 30 per cent
of their spines. By 20 days the spine density returns to 80 per cent of the normal value, and by
60 days it has attained the normal value. The authors suggest that this regrowth of spines may be
attributed to collateral sprouting of surviving
axons in the area and that these newly sprouting
afferents replace the degenerated ones, thereby
inducing dendritic spines to re-form.

Subjecting the cerebral cortex to x-irradiation can also bring about a loss of dendritic
spines (Schadé and Caveness, 1968), and Westrum, White, and Ward (1964) found that the
production of epileptic foci by the application of
alumina cream induces a spine loss.

In a quite different type of study Marin-
Padilla (1974) has found that in the motor cortex
of a newborn girl with trisomy 13–15 (Patau
syndrome) not only is the number of neurons in
the cortex decreased, but there is a reduction in
the number of dendritic spines. Furthermore,
the spines appear abnormal in Golgi preparations, for they are very long and hairy, with irregular forms and, seemingly, they are dis-
oriented. Purpura (1974) has also found similar

long spines along the apical dendrites of cortical
neurons in retarded children with normal karyo-
types. Some of these spines may be 4 to 8
microns long.

In the cerebellar cortex, much less is known
about alterations in dendritic spines, although
Mathieu and Colonnier (1968) demonstrated
that sectioning of parallel fibers produces a loss
of spines along the dendrites of Purkinje cells.
In a significant study Rakic and Sidman (1973a
and b) found that in the mouse mutant "weaver"
the dendritic spines of Purkinje cells develop
even though the parallel fibers are almost completely lacking. In this mutant, Sotelo (1973)
also showed the presence of dendritic spines
and found that they may be contacted by axons
with which they would not normally form synapses. In the staggerer mouse (Sotelo, 1973;
Sotelo and Changeux, 1974), the converse situation obtains, for tertiary dendrites of the Purkinje
cells in this mouse lack spines, so that the parallel
fibers are unable to reach their normal synaptic
targets (see page 68). Finally, Purkinje cells
can be induced to put out an excessive number
of thorns. In rats it is possible to eliminate the
climbing fiber afferents to the Purkinje cells by
giving an intraperitoneal injection of 3-acetyl-
pyridine. This poison selectively and completely
destroys the inferior olivary nucleus, which is
the source of climbing fibers to the cerebellum
(Desclin, 1974; Desclin and Escubi, 1974). In the
cerebella of animals that have survived this treatment for two weeks or more, the thick Purkinje
cell dendrites exhibit a profusion of thorns, some
of them synapsing with parallel fibers but many
of them free of synapses altogether (Sotelo,
Hillman, Zamora, and Llinás, 1975). Evidently
the generation of new thorns is evoked by the
loss of a major afferent fiber system.

Before leaving the subject of dendritic
spines or thorns, we should consider their role
or function. At the outset, it must be stated that
their function is unknown. Clearly, they form
synapses with axon terminals, but contrary to

Figure 3–8.   **A Spiny Branchlet of a Purkinje Cell Dendrite.**

   In this freeze-fractured preparation a spiny branchlet extends obliquely across
the field. The broken stems of several thorns *(arrows)* protrude from the exposed surface of the dendrite, and an intact thorn *(t)* extends into the neuropil on the right. The
stem of another thorn runs into the neuropil above it. Both of these are surrounded
by the neuroglial cytoplasm that ensheathes the Purkinje cell dendritic tree. The A
face of the dendrite is covered with numerous intramembranous particles. Attached
to the shaft of the dendrite is an irregularly shaped fragment of membrane displaying
the characteristic features of the presynaptic B face—a cluster of small papular protuberances in a relatively particle-free area. This is probably the location of a synaptic
junction with a stellate cell axon, an inhibitory synapse.
Cerebellar cortex of adult rat. × 76,000.

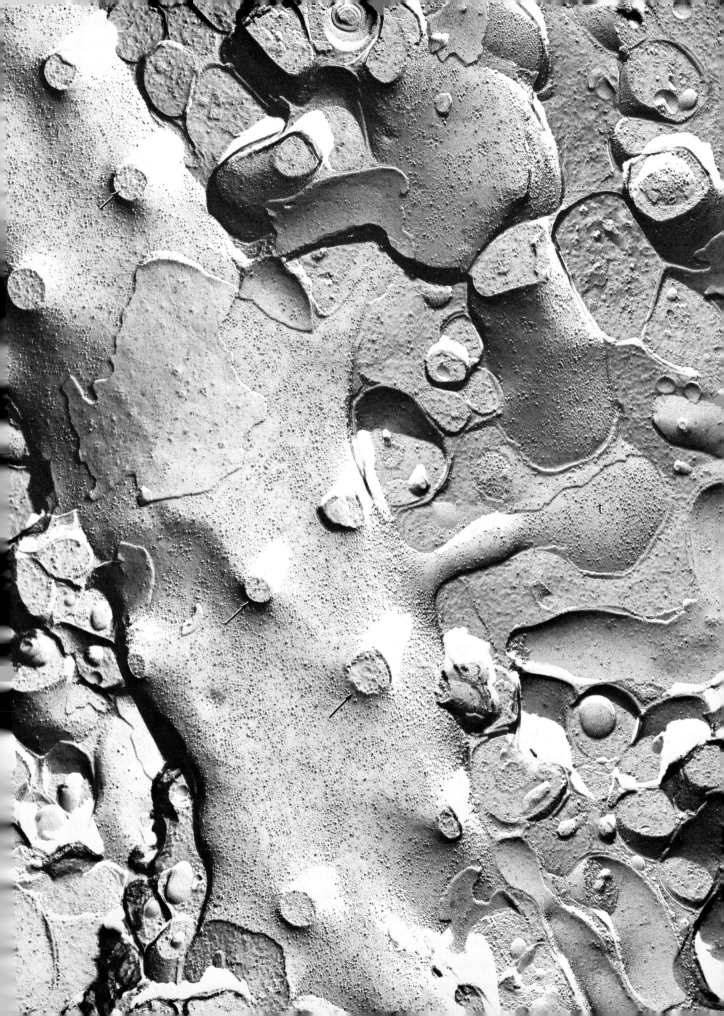

the hypotheses of earlier morphologists, they do not serve primarily to increase the amount of dendritic surface for the reception of axon terminals, for the main shafts of most spiny dendrites are largely free of synapses. One possibility is that they are important in the organization of the neuropil and reach out to synapse with appropriate afferents that are intermingled with many different axons pervading the neuropil (Peters and Kaiserman-Abramof, 1970).

It should be recalled that in the Purkinje cells of the cerebellar cortex the spines are the exclusive locations of excitatory synapses, whereas the shafts of the dendrites are the exclusive sites of inhibitory synapses. In addition, spines may provide postsynaptic surfaces that are effectively isolated from the influence of potential changes in other parts of the neuron (Diamond, Gray, and Yasargil, 1969 and 1970; Llinás and Hillman, 1969; Chan-Palay and Palay, 1970; Palay and Chan-Palay, 1974). According to this hypothesis, the dendritic spine is viewed as a current injection device (Llinás and Hillman, 1969). Upon activation by an appropriate post-synaptic depolarization, it releases a small amount of current into the dendritic shaft. This current is necessarily attenuated by the high longitudinal resistance of the slender stem of the spine. The resultant potential changes spread along the dendrite and summate with those coming from the activation of other spines as well as with those from inhibitory synapses on the shaft. By the same mechanism the resistance of the slender stem protects the postsynaptic surface membrane of the spine from the influence of large alterations in the potential of the dendritic shaft. If this hypothesis is correct in principle, the spine plays an important role in regulating the excitatory input to a nerve cell.

Finally, it should be noted that not all dendritic spines are purely postsynaptic elements, for in the olfactory bulb (Figure 3–7) the spines (so-called gemmules) of the external granule cells contain synaptic vesicles and form reciprocal synapses with the dendritic shafts of mitral cells (see Rall, Shepherd, Reese, and Brightman, 1966).

GROWING TIPS OF DENDRITES

In Golgi preparations Morest (1969a and b) has identified the growing tips of dendrites as enlargements from which one or more filopodia extend. In a fine-structural study of the dendritic growth cones of mitral cells in the neonatal mouse olfactory bulb, Hinds and Hinds (1972) confirmed the presence of these filopodia, each about 0.2 micron in diameter, and demonstrated that they extend from the expanded tips of growing dendrites. The cytoplasm of these dendritic growth cones contains microfilaments, each about 5 nm thick. These fill the enlarged tips and are accompanied by a few mitochondria and cisternae of smooth endoplasmic reticulum, although no microtubules are in evidence.

A similar picture is presented by Vaughn, Henrikson, and Grieshaber (1974), who also comment upon the loose feltwork of filamentous material in the dendritic growth cones. An example of the growth cones in the cervical spinal cord of a 14-day mouse embryo is shown in Figure 3–9 in which it can be seen that axon terminals form synapses (*arrows*) with the growth cones. Vaughn, Henrikson, and Grieshaber propose that the new synapses are formed between axon terminals and the filopodia of dendritic

---

Figure 3–9. **Dendritic Growth Cones.**

A motor neuron dendrite *(Den)* and its growth cone *(GC)* pass between the transversely sectioned axons *(Ax)* of the lateral marginal zone of an embryonic spinal cord. Another dendritic growth cone *(GC₁)* is located in the lower right portion of the micrograph. The growth cones differ from other dendritic profiles in that they contain few microtubules and have varying numbers of smooth-surfaced vesicles *(v)*, vacuoles or cisternae. The growth cone cytoplasm is characterized by a feltwork of fine, filamentous material. Both growth cones in this figure are contacted by developing presynaptic boutons *(arrows)*.
Cervical spinal cord of 14-day mouse embryo. × *11,000.*

Micrograph provided by C. K. Henrikson and J. E. Vaughn.

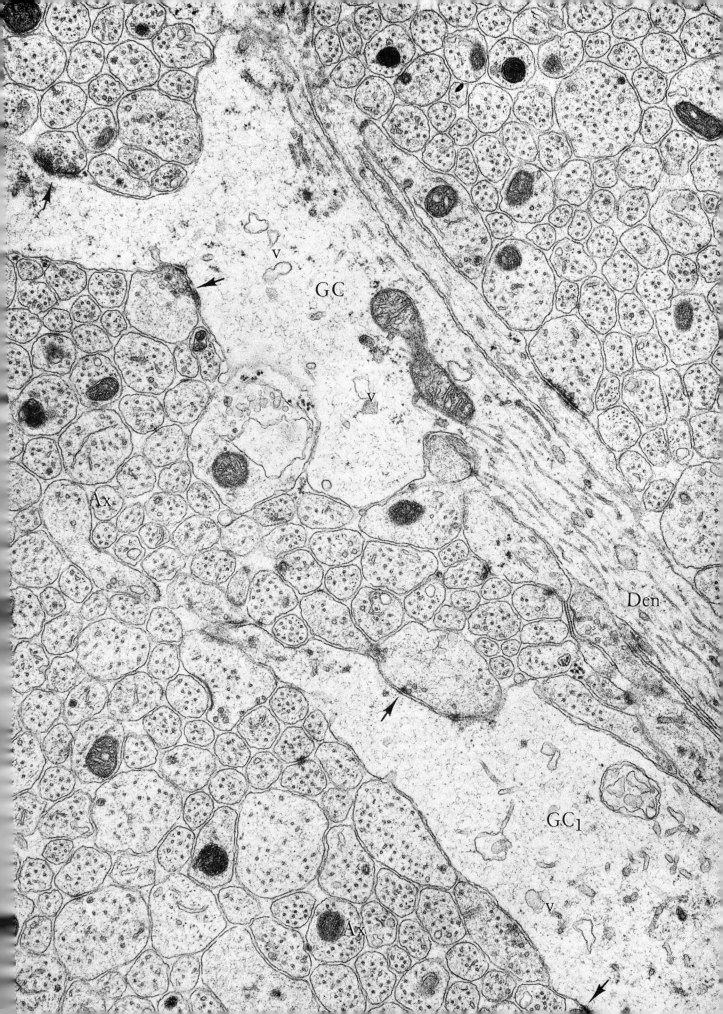

growth cones. When such a synapse has been formed, the involved filopodium expands to form a new growth cone, while the region of the old growth cone acquires the features of a mature dendrite. By this progression the dendrites extend forward and the filopodial synapses come to be positioned upon the dendritic shafts.

From a study of the embryonic chick spinal cord Skoff and Hamburger (1974) conclude that the dendritic growth cones having the form of bulbous enlargements only represent one type. The other type which they encountered had the form of a filopodium of about the same diameter as the dendritic shaft. Skoff and Hamburger (1974) also emphasize the frequency of synapses on dendritic growth cones, and like Vaughn, Henrikson, and Grieshaber (1974) they propose that new synapses are formed with the growth cones. The study of Skoff and Hamburger is useful in that it also emphasizes the differences between dendritic and axonal growth cones. As will be shown in the next chapter, Skoff and Hamburger found that axonal growth cones tend to have a denser cytoplasmic matrix than dendritic growth cones and that they are larger and more irregular structures, with more filopodia. Axonal growth cones also display filopodia, or sheet-like cytoplasmic extensions (Figures 4–10, and 4–11), which dendritic growth cones do not seem to possess.

In the lateral vestibular nucleus of mature rats, Sotelo and Palay (1968) observed that some of the dendrites suddenly enlarge to form varicosities or swellings filled with mitochondria (Figure 3–10). Such varicosities generally vary from 1 to 3 microns in diameter, and in nearly every case the dendritic nature of the swelling has been confirmed by the presence of axon terminals forming synapses upon its surface. The mitochondria of the varicosities are long and slender and either are arranged parallel to the long axis of the dendrite or form gently swirling figures around the long axis. The numbers of mitochondria in such swellings are very large. For example, in one swelling with a cross-sectional area of 12.5 square microns, 134 mitochondrial profiles were present; and in another with an area of 26 square microns, 297 mitochondria were found (Figure 3–10). Glycogen particles are also common in the cytoplasm of these varicosities.

Similar swellings of dendrites have also been encountered in other regions of the nervous system such as the cerebellar cortex, hypothalamus, and superior cervical ganglion. In a more recent electron microscopic study of the central cerebellar nuclei in the cat, Sotelo and Angaut (1973) have found similar formations, which they equate with certain complex dendritic appendages seen in Golgi preparations. Although this equation is apparently in error (see Chan-Palay, 1973c), the appearance of this structure in the cat and in still another nucleus demonstrates that it is not a peculiarity of the rat and suggests that it may be a general phenomenon. Analyses of profiles of these swellings suggest that many of them are the ends of dendrites, and Sotelo and Palay (1968) came to the conclusion that they represent growing dendritic tips. If so, they are quite different from the dendritic growth cones in the developing nervous system that have just been described above. It is possible that they are associated in some way with dendritic growth and remodeling in the terminal parts of the arborization without being themselves the growing tips. They have not yet been noted in developing nervous systems and dendritic growth cones have not been reported in mature nervous systems. The crowding of large numbers of mitochondria into these varicosities remains a puzzling feature, which has not received any explanation.

Figure 3–10.   **A Dendritic Terminal.**

Occupying the center of the field is a large dendritic expansion filled with mitochondria *(mit)* and glycogen granules *(gly)*. Such profiles are abundant in the dorsal part of the lateral vestibular nucleus, and they are interpreted as being the growing tips of dendrites.
Lateral vestibular nucleus from adult rat. × 42,000.

Micrograph by C. Sotelo.

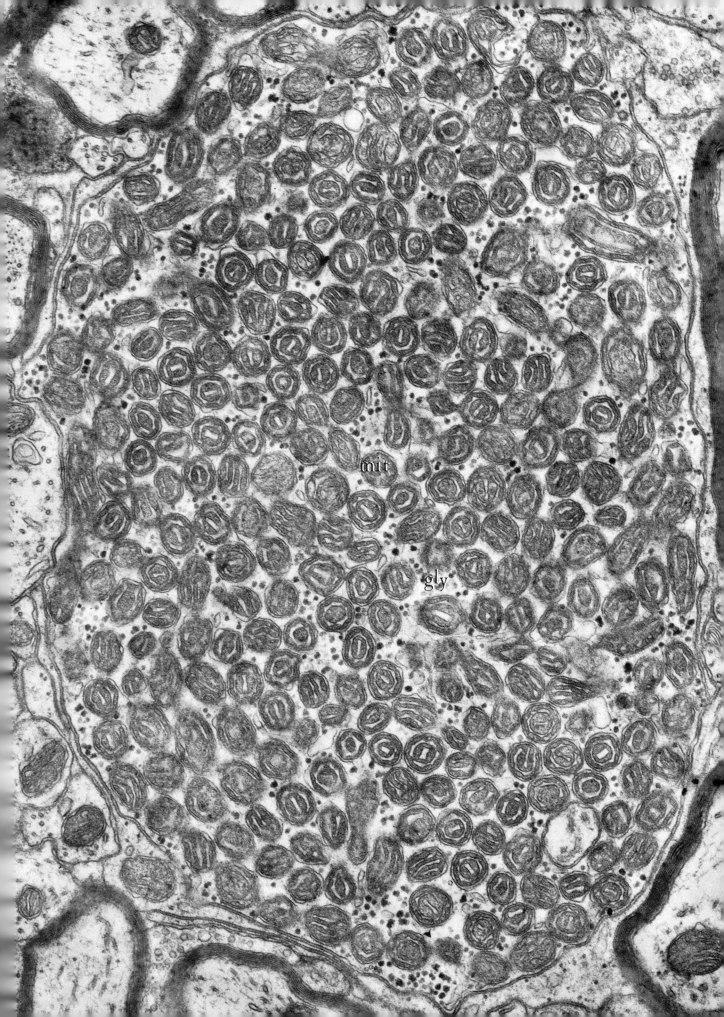

Chapter IV

THE AXON

AXON HILLOCK AND INITIAL AXON SEGMENT

In multipolar neurons the axon hillock is a cone-shaped elevation from which the axon originates. In most histology texts the hillock is described as a region of the perikaryon that is distinguished by its deficiency of Nissl substance or basophilic material. Such a zone is readily apparent in electron micrographs of large neurons, in which the axon hillock has a considerably reduced amount of granular endoplasmic reticulum (Palay, Sotelo, Peters, and Orkand, 1968; Sotelo and Palay, 1968; Conradi, 1969c; Peters, Palay, and Webster, 1970). The organelles predominating in the cytoplasm of this region (Figure 4–1) are free ribosomes and mitochondria and the neurofilaments and microtubules that pass into the axon. The axon hillocks of smaller neurons are less readily identified in light microscope preparations, and the reason for this is apparent in electron micrographs. For example, in the pyramidal neurons

of the rat cerebral cortex (Peters, Proskauer, and Kaiserman-Abramof, 1968) there are no radical differences between the cytoplasm of the axon hillock and the rest of the neuronal cell body. As the axon hillock narrows down into the initial segment there is a gradual diminution in the number of ribosomes (Figure 4–1) but not an abrupt change of the type suggested by classical light microscope descriptions of the axon hillock. A few ribosomes are present in the initial segment, but these usually do not extend much beyond it. The remainder of the axon is generally devoid of ribosomes.

The only other difference between the cytoplasm of the axon hillock and of the neuronal perikaryon is that at the base of the hillock many of the microtubules and neurofilaments change their orientation and funnel into it. As the axon hillock becomes narrower some of the microtubules come together to form fascicles (Figures

---

Figure 4–1. **Axon Hillock and the Initial Axon Segment.**

In the upper part of this picture is part of the perikaryon of a pyramidal neuron. The axon leaves the perikaryon at the axon hillock, and the initial segment begins at the level indicated by the *arrows*. This is the point where the characteristic undercoating, or dense layer (D), appears beneath the axolemma. The initial segment is also characterized by the presence of bundles of microtubules (m).

Although many clusters of ribosomes (r) occur in the axon hillock, they diminish in number (r_1) in the initial segment. The other cytoplasmic components of the initial segment, neurofilaments (nf), mitochondria, and vesicles (v), all pass from the axon hillock into the initial segment without undergoing any distinctive change in their appearance or aggregation. In the cerebral cortex it is common to find axon terminals (At) forming synapses with the initial segment.

Note that the initial segment of this cell is not covered by neuroglial processes, but there is an incomplete layer of dense material (D_1) in the sometimes expanded extracellular space around the initial segment.
Cerebral cortex of adult rat. × 24,000.

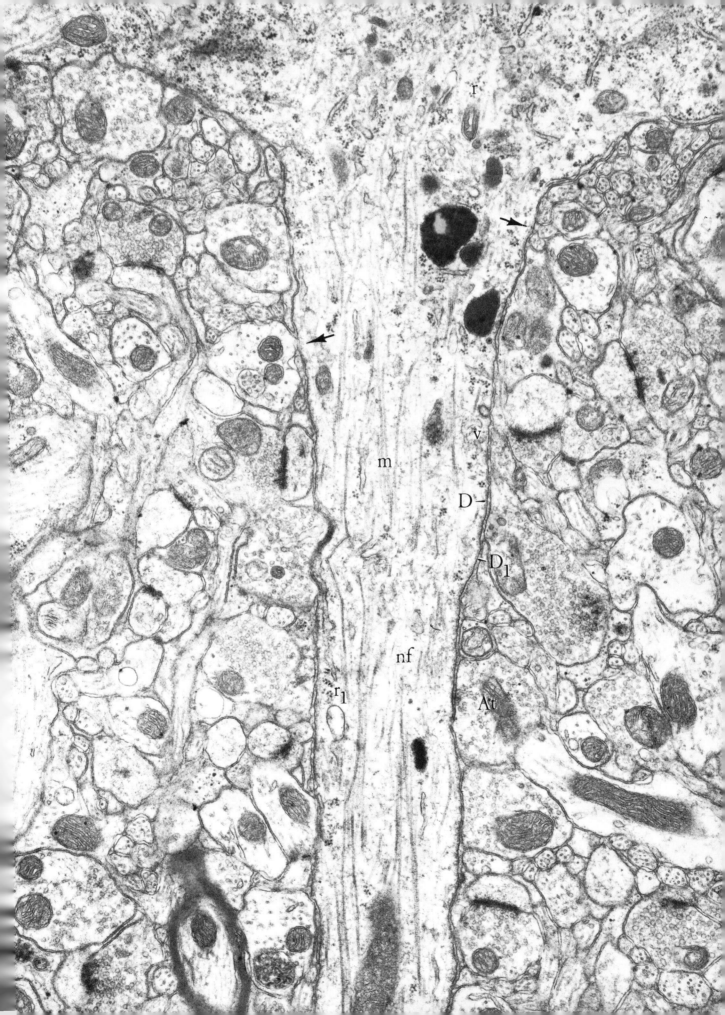

4–1 and 4–2), the existence of which allows cross sections of the hillock to be distinguished from those of large dendrites, in which the microtubules are more homogeneously distributed. These fascicles pass into the initial segment of which they form a very characteristic and diagnostic feature (Figures 4–1 and 4–2). In low power electron micrographs the clusters or fascicles of microtubules appear as dense, elongate structures, lying more or less parallel to the longitudinal axis of the initial segment (see Robertson, Bodenheimer, and Stage, 1963; Kohno, 1964; Palay, 1964; Palay, Sotelo, Peters, and Orkand, 1968; Peters, Proskauer, and Kaiserman-Abramof, 1968; Conradi, 1969c; Westrum, 1970; Mugnaini, 1972). The density of the fascicles apparent in longitudinal sections is in part due to the superimposition of the profiles of microtubules within the section. In transverse sections it can be seen that the microtubules in a fascicle are separated from one another by a distance of about 25 nm (Figure 4–3). Furthermore, the members of a fascicle are connected by cross arms that pass between the microtubules like the rungs of a ladder. To some degree, the number of fascicles of microtubules in the initial segment is proportional to its diameter. They can be numerous in thick initial segments, but the thin initial segments of small neurons may contain only one such fascicle.

In addition to the clusters of microtubules, another characteristic feature of the initial segment is a layer of dense material beneath the plasma membrane (Palay, Sotelo, Peters, and Orkand, 1968). In low power electron micrographs the dense layer makes the plasma membrane appear thickened (Figure 4–1), but at higher resolution it is evident that the dense layer is not in contact with the inner surface of the plasma membrane, but separated from it by a distance of about 6 to 10 nm (Figure 4–3). This undercoating is composed of a somewhat granular material, and although its boundaries are not definite, the thickness of the layer is about 15 to 25 nm. In unosmicated blocks of tissue treated with ethanolic phosphotungstic acid Sloper and

Powell (1973) find the undercoating to have a somewhat dentate appearance. This appearance is explained by the observations of Chan-Palay (1972), who has shown that the undercoating of the initial segment can be resolved into three layers. Directly beneath the axolemma is a layer of granules, each about 7.5 nm wide and separated from its neighbors by an interval of about 7.5 nm in the long axis of the axon and about 9.5 nm in the transverse plane. Beneath the layer of granules is a dense lamina about 7.5 nm thick, and deep to the lamina longitudinal sections show a layer of triangular units or tufts of matted filaments. Each filament in the tufts is about 5 nm thick and branches several times or interweaves rather loosely with other filaments. The base of each tuft is about 55 nm wide and extends 60 to 70 nm toward the center of the axon. Because of the appearance of alternating dense and clear lines passing across the profiles of tangentially grazed initial segments, Chan-Palay (1972) concludes that the tufts represent sections through a continuous ridge that may wind in a tight spiral along the inner face of the dense lamina.

An undercoating similar to that of the initial segment is present at the node of Ranvier of myelinated nerve fibers (see page 220), and in both locations there is also a layer of granular material outside the axolemma (Peters, Proskauer, and Kaiserman-Abramof, 1968; Sloper and Powell, 1973). Since both of these portions of the axon are involved in the generation and propagation of the axon potential, it can be supposed that these membrane coatings are in some way related to that function.

The undercoating of the initial axon segment commences at the site where the axon hillock narrows down to the diameter of the axon (Figure 4–1, *arrows*) and in myelinated fibers it extends as far as the beginning of the myelin sheath (Figure 4–4). This is also the extent of the fascicles of microtubules. In unmyelinated fibers the transition between the initial segment and the remainder of the axon may be defined as the site where the undercoating and the fasci-

Figure 4–2. **The Initial Segment of a Motor Neuron, Longitudinal Section.**

This micrograph displays the features that characterize the axon initial segment: (1) the dense granular layer (*D*) situated beneath the axolemma, (2) the collection of the microtubules (*m*) into fascicles, and (3) the scattered clusters of ribosomes (*r*). Also present in the axoplasm are neurofilaments (*nf*), mitochondria (*mit*), and tubular cisternae and vesicles of the smooth endoplasmic reticulum (*SR*).
Anterior horn of rat spinal cord. × 48,000.

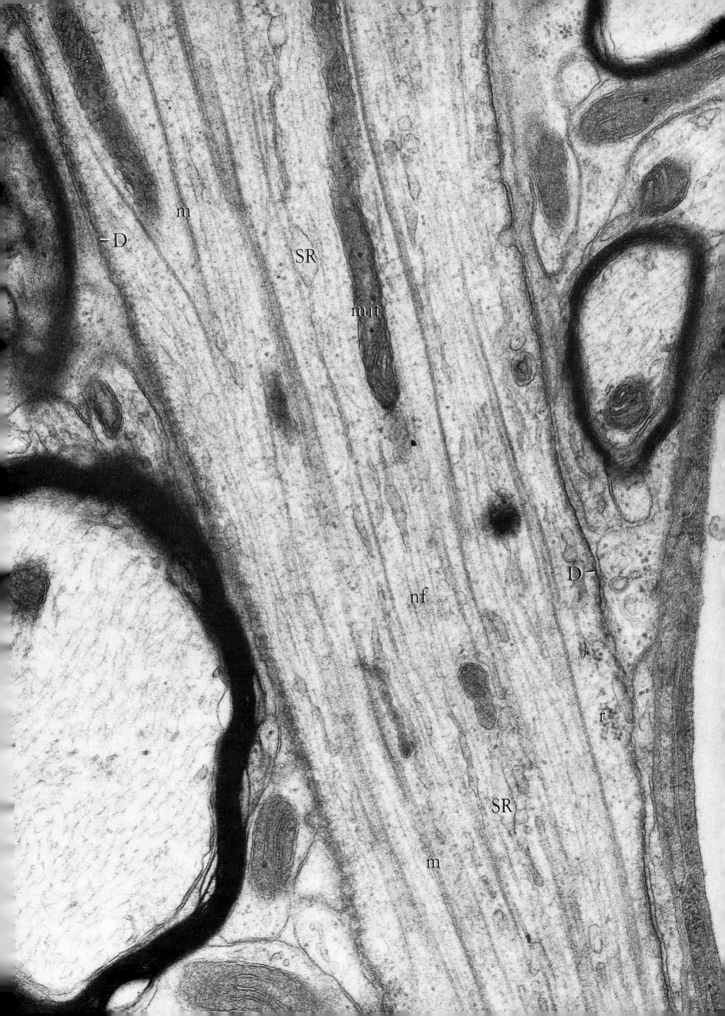

cles of microtubules terminate. The length of the initial segment is very variable. In motor neurons of the cat spinal cord (Conradi, 1969c) it is between 23 and 38 microns long. In pyramidal cells of the monkey cortex (Sloper and Powell, 1973) the initial segments vary in length between 23 and 45 microns, with no correlation between the length and the mean size of the perikarya from which they spring. Saito (1972) gives the length of an initial segment from a dorsal spinocerebellar tract neuron of the cat as 28 microns.

At present, the only observations on the development of the initial axon segment appear to be those by Hinds and Ruffett (1973), who studied the mitral cells of the developing olfactory bulbs of the mouse. Hinds and Ruffett (1973) found that during development the perikarya and processes of mitral cells change from a tangential to a radial orientation and that when the cells are in tangential orientation their axons exhibit no distinctive features. However, in the last five days of prenatal development, most radially oriented mitral cells show distinct microtubules in the proximal portion of the axon, and these are continued into the perikaryal cytoplasm as a parallel bundle that passes to one side of the nucleus. Hinds and Ruffett (1973) suggest that the final position of the axon is determined by this perikaryal bundle of microtubules along which the cell body migrates peripherally. The mature features of the axon initial segment of the mitral cell gradually develop during late embryonic and early postnatal life. First a decrease in the number of ribosomes is noted, and the next characteristic to develop is the fasciculation of the microtubules. Last to appear is the undercoating of the axolemma which begins as dense patches. The difference in the time of appearance of the fascicles of microtubules and of the undercoating lead Hinds and Ruffett (1973) to conclude that these two features are unrelated, and they support the earlier postulate of Palay, Sotelo, Peters, and

Orkand (1968) that the undercoating is concerned with the action potential and the fasciculation of the microtubules with provision of the motive force for protoplasmic streaming or axonal transport (see page 107).

An interesting situation exists when an initial axon segment takes origin from a dendrite (Peters, Proskauer, and Kaiserman-Abramof, 1968); then a fasciculation of the microtubules occurs in the dendrite only in the cytoplasm of that side from which the axon arises. The cytoplasm on the other side of the dendrite displays the normal homogeneous distribution of microtubules.

Both the axon hillock and the initial segment may bear synapses which are symmetrical (Figure 4–1). Where synapses occur along the initial axon segment the undercoating is interrupted beneath the synaptic junction and is replaced by the typical postsynaptic densities (Palay, Sotelo, Peters, and Orkand, 1968; Peters, Proskauer, and Kaiserman-Abramof, 1968). Sloper and Powell (1973) confirmed this description in material stained with ethanolic phosphotungstic acid. In cerebral cortex (Westrum, 1970) the synapses may occur on spines that project from the initial segment. Very like the spines of dendrites, the axonal spines may be either pedunculate or sessile, and the undercoating of the axolemma often ends at the base of the spine. In some spines an organelle similar to that occurring in dendritic spines (pages 81–82) may be present. These organelles, which may also occur in the main shaft of the initial axon segment, where they lie often parallel to the axolemma (Peters, Proskauer, and Kaiserman-Abramof, 1968; Jones and Powell, 1969c), have been termed cisternal organelles. They consist of two or more flattened cisternae separated from each other by intervals about 40 nm wide which contain a granular, dense plate about 20 nm thick, and at higher resolution each plate can be seen to consist of two parallel sheets, 50 nm apart.

None of the above features seem to charac-

Figure 4–3. **The Initial Segment, Transverse Section.**

The initial segments are from a pyramidal neuron of the cerebral cortex (**upper picutre**) and a Purkinje cell of the cerebellar cortex (**lower picture**).

These two initial segments are very similar. The dense undercoating (*D*) beneath the axolemma (*Al*) is about 10 nm thick and is separated from the axolemma by a clear interval. The fasciculation of the microtubules (*m*) is most clearly shown in this plane of section.

The microtubules within each fascicle are regularly spaced and appear to be strung together by thin, dark cross bands (*arrows*). Other components of the axoplasm are mitochondria (*mit*), neurofilaments, and various vesicles.

Upper picture: *Cerebral cortex of rat, pyramidal neuron.* × *100,000.*

Lower picture: *Cerebellar cortex of rat, Purkinje cell.* × *82,000.*

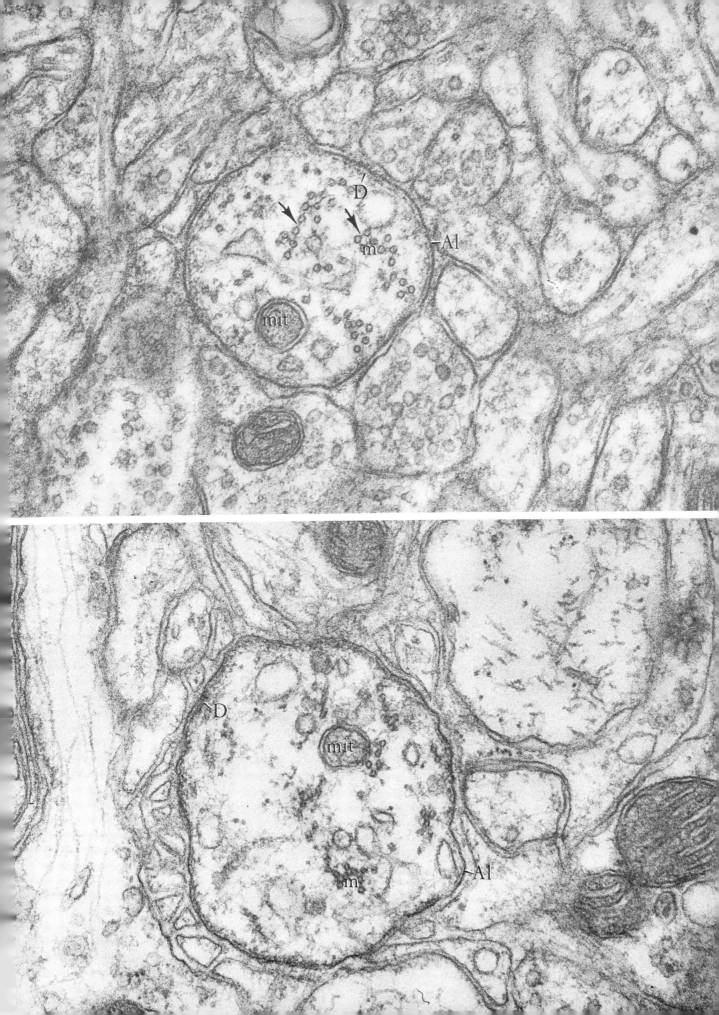

terize the axon arising from the soma of the sensory ganglion cell (Figures 4–5 and 4–6), although it also does not have Nissl bodies extending into it (see Wyburn, 1958; Rosenbluth and Palay, 1961; Rosenbluth, 1962a; Pineda, Maxwell, and Kruger, 1967). Recently Zenker and Högl (1976) have shown that the typical features of the initial segment first appear in the axon of the sensory ganglion cell at some distance from its origin and just before the onset of its myelin sheath. The difference between the initial segments of sensory ganglion cells and those of neurons in the central nervous system may be related to the fact that the initial segment of the ganglion cell is not the site of origin of the action potential. However, Zelená (1971) has found that in some of the dorsal root ganglia, neurons that do not show typical chromatolysis after axotomy contain increased numbers of neurofilaments in their cytoplasm and some fascicles of microtubules in the initial segment. The meaning of this observation is not presently apparent.

It would be interesting to determine where the action potential arises in anaxonal or amacrine cells in the central nervous system. In the olfactory bulb the internal granule cells, which are considered to be anaxonal, have no processes whose proximal portions resemble those of initial axon segments (Hinds, pers. comm.).

THE AXON BEYOND THE INITIAL SEGMENT

Like other portions of the neuron, the axon beyond the initial segment (for example, Figures 4–4, 4–8, 4–9, 6–9, and 6–15) contains mitochondria, microtubules, neurofilaments, agranular endoplasmic reticulum, and multivesicular bodies. However, it is characterized by an absence of two components present elsewhere, namely, the granular endoplasmic reticulum and free ribosomes. This should, however, be qualified by the statement that this is a generalization, for note has been made of the presence of small numbers of free ribosomes in some axons. For example, Jones and Powell (1969b) depict a few free ribosomes at a node of Ranvier in the cat somatosensory cortex, and Zelená (1970 and 1972) has shown them in the myelinated axons from dorsal roots in the rat, but such reports are exceptional. In contrast to large dendrites, large axons contain few microtubules and many neurofilaments, both of which are oriented parallel to the long axis of the process.

In an electron microscope comparison of the number of microtubules in the accessory nerve and one of its more terminal branches in the rat, Zenker and Hohberg (1973) found the number of microtubules per unit of cross-sectional area to be the same in the two parts of the nerve. However, during the course of forming its terminal branches the total cross-sectional area of the accessory nerve increases about 11 times. Thus, there is an indication that while microtubules may extend for long distances, in the accessory nerve at least, microtubules must be added to the axoplasm as the nerve extends away from its stem.

NEUROFILAMENTS AND MICROTUBULES

Neurofilaments are of indefinite length and about 10 nm in diameter (Figure 4–7). With the refined techniques of recent years it can be shown that neurofilaments are not solid structures but tubular, so that in cross section they appear as profiles with dense walls, 3 nm thick, surrounding a clear center (Palay, 1964; Sandborn, 1966; Peters and Vaughn, 1967; Wuerker

Figure 4–4. **The Initial Segment and the Preterminal Axon Compared.**

This plate presents longitudinal sections of two axons.

The axon (*Ax*) in the picture on the **left** is an initial segment entering into its myelin sheath (*my*). This portion of the axon is characterized by both the dense undercoating (*D*) beneath the axolemma and the fascicles of microtubules (*m*) in the axoplasm. The axoplasm contains only a few neurofilaments (*nf*) but many vesicular profiles, the dilated portions of the tubular endoplasmic reticulum.
Cerebral cortex from adult rat. × 30,000.

The axon (*Ax*) in the picture on the **right** is the preterminal portion of an axon emerging from its myelin sheath (*my*). This axon shows neither the dense undercoating beneath the axolemma nor the fascicles of microtubules that characterize the initial segment. Instead, the axoplasm has a central core of neurofilaments (*nf*) and individual microtubules (*m*), which pass through two dilatations containing many synaptic vesicles (*sv*).
Cerebral cortex from adult rat. × 23,000.

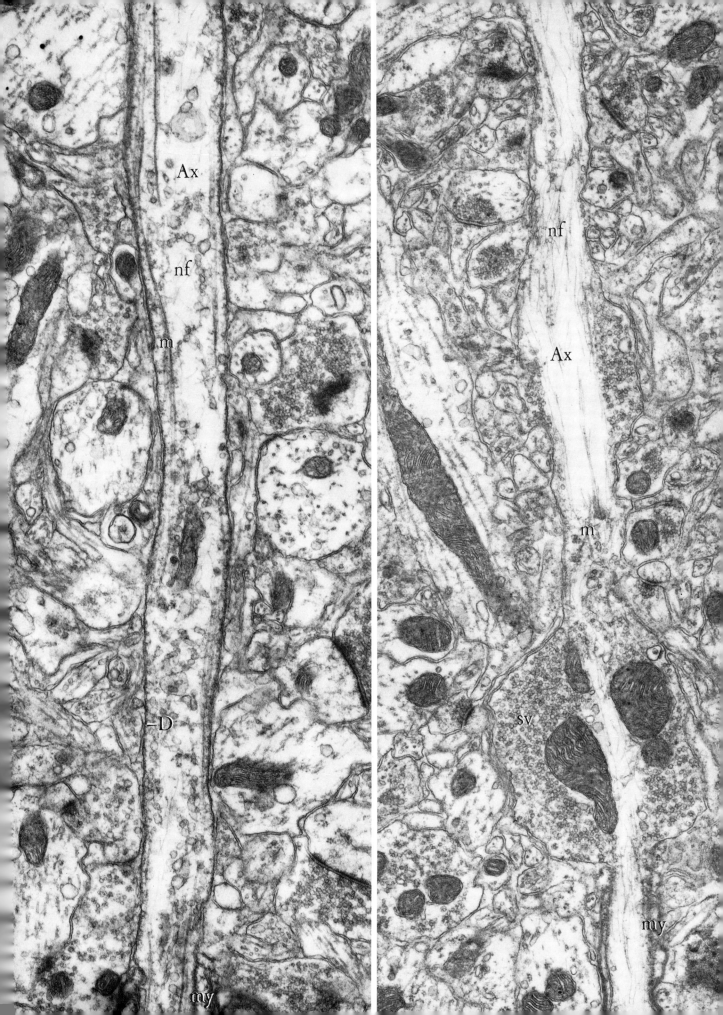

and Palay, 1969; Wuerker, 1970). Consequently, in longitudinal sections the neurofilament appears as two parallel, dark lines separated by a lighter zone (e.g., Metuzals, 1963). Wuerker (1970) believes the wall of each neurofilament to be usually composed of four elements, each about 3.5 nm in diameter, joined together by interconnecting cross bars. These elements appear to be globular subunits from which short, spike-like processes radiate (Wuerker and Palay, 1969). From the work of Schmitt and Davison (1961) on the structure of filaments extracted from the axoplasm of the giant squid, it is supposed that each neurofilament is a helically coiled thread with four or five subunits making up the wall at any one level (see also Kadota and Kadota, 1973a and b. An analysis of preparations of neurofilaments from the axoplasm of squid nerves (Davison and Huneeus, 1970; Huneeus and Davison, 1970) has led to the identification of a single protein subunit named *filarin*. Filarin is an acidic protein with a subunit molecular weight of about 80,000, and this protein is not identical with any of the proteins isolated from microtubules in the same axoplasm. On the other hand, Shelanski (1973) found the neurofilaments from vertebrate brain to be composed of proteins with a molecular weight of about 59,000. Using a similar but more elaborate method, Davison and Winslow (1974) have also extracted a filamentous protein from calf brain axons. The subunits of this protein have a molecular weight between 50,000 and 60,000 (range of three different methods of determining molecular weight), thus confirming the results of Shelanski (1973). This protein is readily distinguishable from tubulin, the subunit of microtubules, by differences in solubility, amino acid composition, and electrophoretic mobility. It is also evident from these studies that the neurofilament protein of mammalian axons differs from the filamentous protein obtained from squid axons. Davison and Winslow (1974) point out that electron micrographs of invertebrate axons fail to show the nicely oriented parallel neurofila-

ments found in the axons of mammals. Instead the axoplasm exhibits randomly oriented fine filaments, interwoven into a cottony meshwork. Such appearances had been attributed to inadequate preservation of the axoplasm, consistent with the disrupted mitochondria and swollen endoplasmic reticulum often displayed by the axons of invertebrates. In the light of these recent chemical studies, it must be considered that perhaps the native state of the filamentous protein in the invertebrates is not represented by fine parallel axial neurofilaments as in the vertebrates. Additional work is necessary in order to ascertain the relationship between the proteins of vertebrate and invertebrate axons and to understand the differing roles that they may play in these two situations.

Microtubules are also tubular structures of indefinite length, but they have a larger diameter (Elfvin, 1961). As seen in transverse sections (Figures 4–3, 4–6, 4–7, and 4–9), microtubules measure 20 to 26 nm across. The dense wall is about 6 nm thick and in the middle of the clear center is a dense dot (see Figure 4–3; Peters and Vaughn, 1967) which seems to represent a thin central filament or a row of granules (Rodríguez-Echandía, Piezzi, and Rodríguez, 1968).

Microtubules were first visualized by Fawcett and Porter (1954) in the shafts of cilia. In neurons they were first encountered by Palay (1956a and 1958b), who did not distinguish them clearly from certain varieties of the agranular endoplasmic reticulum. Since the introduction of glutaraldehyde as a fixative for electron microscopy (Sabatini, Bensch, and Barrnett, 1963) they have been described in a variety of cells (see Slautterback, 1963; Silveira and Porter, 1964; de-Thé, 1964; Sandborn, Szeberenyi, Messier, and Bois, 1965; Sandborn, LeBuis, and Bois, 1966; Fawcett, 1966a; Anderson, Weissman, and Ellis, 1966) and recognized as a universal cytoplasmic component. Because of their great numbers in the axostyles and axopods of protozoans (for example, see McIntosh, Ogata, and Landis, 1973; Tilney, 1971) it is in

---

Figure 4–5.   **Axon Hillock and Initial Segment of a Trigeminal Ganglion Cell.**

The initial segment of the axon (*Ax*) emerges from the axon hillock which is at the upper right. The cytoplasm of the ganglion cell contains cisternae of granular endoplasmic reticulum (*ER*). These do not extend into the axon, although a few clusters of ribosomes (*r*) are present in the axonal cytoplasm. Unlike the initial segments of neurons in the central nervous system, those of ganglion cells do not possess an undercoating beneath the axolemma (*Al*), and the microtubules (*m*) do not form fascicles.

The sheath around the axon is formed by Schwann cell processes (*SC*), which turn around the axon and extend into flattened sheets as they approach the axolemma. Compare with Figure 4–6.

Trigeminal ganglion of adult mouse. × 23,000.

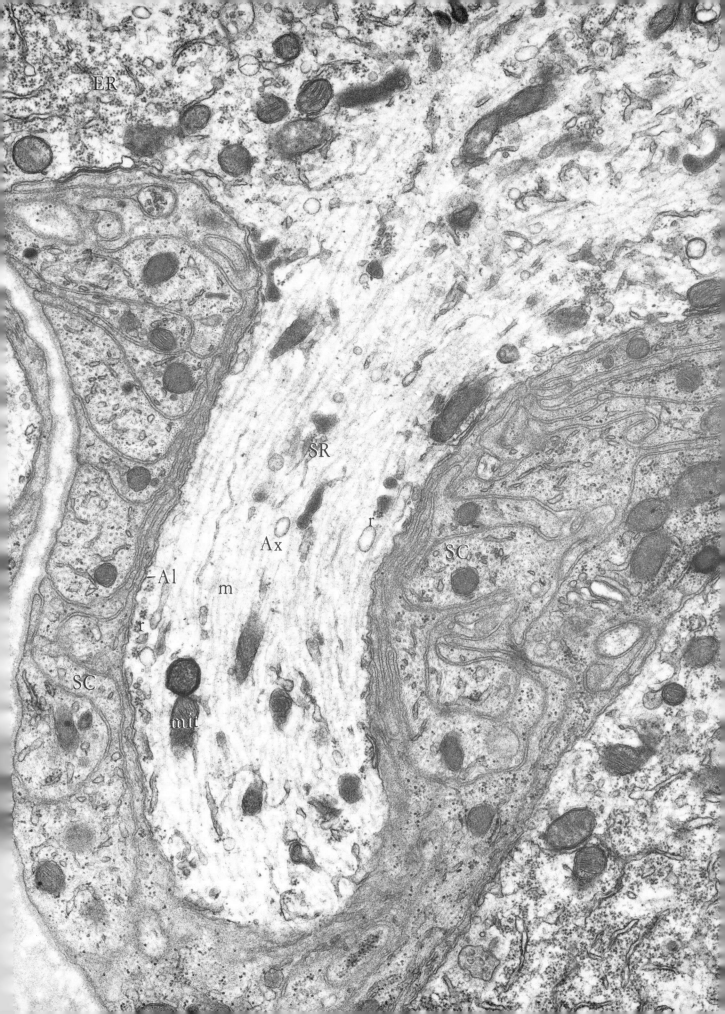

these unicellular organisms that their organization into groups has been most fully studied.

Transverse sections of microtubules from nerve (e.g., Sandborn, 1966; Peters and Vaughn, 1967; Wuerker and Palay, 1969) and other tissues (e.g., Ledbetter and Porter, 1963; Silveira and Porter, 1964; Porter, 1966; Lane and Treherne, 1970; Tilney, 1971) show their walls to be composed of about 13 globular subunits. In a study of photographic reinforcement of profiles of microtubules from nerves by rotation of electron microscope images, Frisch (1969) has found that most microtubules from nerves have 13 subunits in their wall, but a few have 12 or 14. More direct evidence for the validity of accepting 13 as the number of subunits has come from the recent study of Tilney, Bryan, Bush, Fujiwara, Mooseker, Murphy, and Snyder (1973), who fixed microtubules, from seven different sources, in glutaraldehyde in the presence of tannic acid. One source was repolymerized chick brain microtubules. This type of fixation results in an image similar to that obtained by negative staining, and the subunits of the microtubules show very clearly. The subunits have been taken to represent profiles of subfilaments or protofilaments, but until this latter study by Tilney and his colleagues there has been no direct evidence for their existence in microtubules oriented longitudinally in tissue sections. Previous evidence for their existence had, however, come from examination of negatively stained, homogenized preparations from mammalian brain (Kirkpatrick, Hyams, Thomas, and Howley, 1970) and in microtubules that have been mechanically disrupted (Pease, 1963; Grimstone and Klug, 1966; Barnicot, 1966).

Since the centers of microtubules display no electron-dense contents other than the central dot seen in cross sections, it has been suggested that they might be hollow. This concept seems to receive some validity from the observations of Lane and Treherne (1970) who fixed and incubated cockroach ganglia in lanthanum hydroxide. They found the lanthanum to enter the cores of the microtubules. The outer parts of the walls were left unstained, but the lanthanum also stained a zone outside the wall. Lane and Treherne (1970) believe that the lanthanum image does not represent a movement of the substance into the tubules but rather a specific staining of materials already present. The picture obtained with ruthenium red staining is somewhat different (Tani and Ametani, 1970). In cross sections the staining is confined to a layer 3 to 5 nm thick inside the wall, and a central core remains clear. Perhaps this core corresponds to the electron-dense dot in conventional preparations.

Reviews of the present state of knowledge about the chemistry of microtubules have recently been presented by Shelanski and Feit (1972) and Shelanski (1973). From a variety of microtubules a class of closely related acidic proteins, the *tubulins*, have been isolated. When microtubules are disassembled, a dimeric protein with a sedimentation rate of 6S and a molecular weight between 100,000 and 120,000 is isolated. Denaturation of this dimeric protein results in two subunits of approximately equal molecular weights, between 55,000 and 60,000, but differing slightly in their amino acid composition. A variety of plant alkaloids, including colchicine and vinblastine, all of which arrest cell division in metaphase, have been shown to interact with the tubulins, and the binding of colchicine in particular appears to be very specific. In addition, all the microtubular proteins so far isolated have been found to contain guanine nucleotide, which appears to be necessary for the assembly of microtubules from the dimer. The nucleotide is bound as guanosine triphosphate (GTP), in the ratio of 2 moles for each 6S dimer of tubulin. While one GTP molecule exchanges readily with free GTP in the medium, the other is more tightly bound.

Although neurofilaments predominate in large axons, the ratio of neurofilaments to microtubules decreases in smaller axons and the total number of neurofilaments and microtubules together seems to be proportional to the caliber of the axon (Friede and Samorajski, 1970). This may perhaps be due to the relatively uniform spacing between these elongate organelles. As axons branch and become smaller, the neurofilaments become fewer and less prominent, until in thin unmyelinated axons, neurofilaments are rare and generally only microtubules are present. This condition can make the distinction between small axons and small dendrites difficult. Consequently, features in addition to their content of neurofilaments and microtubules must be used to distinguish between the two types of process. The question of the identification of small diameter dendrites and axons will be considered in a later section (see page 116).

The function of neurofilaments is not known. However, Wuerker and Palay (1969) suggest that they may be involved in the movement of substances in the cell. Thus, microcinematography of living cells and their processes shows two-directional streaming in the perikaryon, the streaming being confined to the zones, or "roads" between Nissl bodies. The most prominent element in these roads is the fascicles of neurofilaments. Hence these might contribute to a mechanism whereby substances can be transported from the Nissl bodies, where they are produced, to the neuronal processes where they are consumed (see page 107).

With the recent surge of interest in microtubules a number of functions have been postulated for them: for example, the skeletal support of anisodiametric structures, contraction, cell division, and the intracellular transport of ions, metabolites, and vesicles. Since this literature is expanding so very rapidly, only a few examples will be cited here. The evidence that microtubules may offer skeletal support has come largely from studies on structures such as long extensions, or axopods, protruding from some protozoans. If the microtubules in the elongate processes are made to disappear, through the application of low temperatures or high hydrostatic pressures, for example (see Tilney and Porter, 1967; Tilney, Hiramoto, and Marsland, 1966), the axopods collapse. In the nervous system the microtubules may play a similar supporting role, particularly in the early phases of development when the axons and dendrites are growing out from neurons into a relatively open matrix (e.g., see Hinds, 1972). It is unknown whether the microtubules are necessary for the maintenance of cell shape in the mature brain and spinal cord, in which the elements are packed tightly together, or in the peripheral nervous system, in which they are supported by collagen and reticular fibers. There is no direct evidence for the role that microtubules may play in motility. However, the occurrence of microtubules in cilia, sperm tails, and flagella suggests that they play some role in motility. In cell division it is well known that microtubules form part of the mitotic apparatus and that they represent the classical spindle fibers seen in the light microscope. Colchicine blocking of mitosis in metaphase is thought to be due to the strong binding of colchicine with microtubular proteins and the consequent disassembly of microtubules. For a further discussion of these possible roles for microtubules the reader is referred to the review by Schmitt and Samson (1968). The possible role of microtubules in intracellular transport, as exemplified by axoplasmic flow, will be discussed in a later section of this chapter (see page 108).

It is of interest that in immature animals (Bodian, 1966b; Peters and Vaughn, 1967) nerve fibers contain many microtubules but very few neurofilaments. In the optic nerve of the rat neurofilaments only become common at about five days after birth (Peters and Vaughn, 1967), and they tend to appear first in groups. With increasing maturity the number of groups of neurofilaments in each axon increases, and at the same time the members of the groups become dispersed. Even in the adult optic nerve, where the number of neurofilaments in a large axon is greater than the number of microtubules, the neurofilaments still tend to be aggregated in groups. These observations on the appearance of neurofilaments in axons of the rat optic nerve led Peters and Vaughn (1967) to postulate that neurofilaments may be formed by the breakdown of the walls of microtubules into their component filaments. A possible interconnection between neurofilaments and microtubules was also suggested by the experiments of Wiśniewski, Shelanski, and Terry (1968). They showed that in animals treated with colchicine and other mitotic spindle inhibitors such as vinblastine the neurons initially lose their microtubules while the neurofilaments proliferate. Colchicine produces a similar loss of microtubules and a proliferation of filaments in neurons in tissue culture (Yamada, Spooner, and Wessells, 1971; Daniels, 1973). Some time after the removal of colchicine the process reverses, and neurofilaments are replaced by microtubules. The injection of aluminum salts into the cerebrospinal fluid also leads to a proliferation of fibrillar material, and in the anterior horn the affected neurons display dense tangles of filaments, each about 10 nm in diameter (Terry and Peña, 1965). In the light microscope these masses of filaments resemble the dense tangles seen in Alzheimer's disease (see Terry and Wiśniewski, 1968), although in this disease the aggregations of filamentous material are largely composed of twisted microtubules 22 nm in diameter with constrictions 80 nm apart (Terry, 1963). Since the diameter of a neurofilament is greater than that of one of the component subfilaments in the wall of a microtubule, it is unlikely that a direct transformation between these two elements could occur. If any exchange between them does take place, it must involve a rearrangement of the constituent subunits of the two. The difference in chemical composition between the proteins of neurofilaments and microtubules, of course, rules out any possibility that mere morphological rearrangements could result in the transformation of the one into the other.

Some indication of the form of the subunits

of microtubules may be gained from the work of Rodríguez-Echandía and Piezzi (1968) who subjected the peripheral nerves of toads to cold. They found that after two hours of cooling with cracked ice most of the microtubules of the axoplasm disintegrated into ill-defined aggregations of cotton-like material, similar to the matrix that surrounds the microtubules in normal nerves. If a nerve, either *in vivo* or *in vitro*, was warmed again, the microtubules re-formed. Hence, it appears that low temperatures affect the disaggregation of the subunits in microtubules. Cold treatment did not alter the form of the neurofilaments. It remains to be seen whether the results of these experiments can be generalized to microtubules in other species and in other parts of the nervous system.

In relation to the changes that can be induced by chemicals, mention should be made of the observation by Burton and Fernandez (1973) that treatment of the nerve cord of the crayfish with hyaluronidase induces the formation of large tubular elements in the axoplasm. These elements, which Burton and Fernandez (1973) refer to as macrotubules, are 40 to 50 nm in diameter (about twice the size of microtubules) and have a wall thickness of about 8.5 nm. When they are induced to appear, these elements tend to be randomly oriented in the axoplasm. The macrotubules often occur in groups or pairs in which they are in close approximation to each other. The significance of this observation is presently unknown.

The appearance of fibrils in the cytoplasm of living neurons has been reported many times (e.g., Schultze, 1878; Bozler, 1927; Weiss and Wang, 1936; see Schmitt, 1968), but it is probable that these structures, visible with the light microscope, represent an aggregation of microtubules and neurofilaments (Bullock and Horridge, 1965) or the narrow interspaces (*Plasmastrassen*) between clumps of other organelles. It can also be presumed that neurofilaments and microtubules form the neurofibrils apparent in perikarya and nerve fibers stained with silver. The results of Gray and Guillery (1961), on the other hand, seem to indicate that the neurofilaments are the only components contributing to the appearance of neurofibrils and that microtubules are not argyrophilic. Thus, for example, Gray and Guillery (1966) and Guillery (1967) have shown that in locations where silver stains demonstrate the presence of neurofibrillar rings in nerve terminals, corresponding rings of neurofilaments can be demonstrated with the electron microscope. If only the neurofilaments react with silver to produce neurofibrils, then it would be expected that the intensity of silver staining would correspond to the concentration of neurofilaments in a neuronal process. It is true that axons stain darker than dendrites in silver-stained preparations, but it is important to note that dendrites are stained, even though their cytoplasm contains very few neurofilaments. In a study of this problem, Potter (1971) concluded that neurofibrils may be stained in locations where either neurofilaments or microtubules predominate, depending upon the staining procedure employed, but that the more commonly used recent techniques of silver staining largely depend upon the presence of neurofilaments.

An unusual association between neurofilaments and microtubules is found in the cytoplasm of ganglion cells from the nervus terminalis in some teleost fishes. In these cells there is a round, strongly argyrophilic body which is either as large as or bigger than the nucleus. In the electron microscope, Rossi and Palombi (1969) have shown this body to be composed of swirling bundles of neurofilaments and microtubules. In transverse sections of the bundles it is found that each microtubule is surrounded by 9 or 10 filaments which are equidistant from each other and 3 to 4 nm from the central microtubule.

Figure 4–6.   **The Initial Segment of a Trigeminal Ganglion Cell.**

In the center of the field is the transversely sectioned initial segment of a ganglion cell axon (Ax). Unlike the initial segments of axons from neurons in the central nervous system, initial segments of ganglion cells have no undercoating beneath the axolemma (Al), and the microtubules (m) are homogeneously dispersed. In addition to the microtubules, this initial segment contains mitochondria (mit) and tubular profiles of the smooth endoplasmic reticulum (SR).

Surrounding the axon is a thick satellite sheath composed of circularly arranged Schwann cell processes (SC) containing microtubules (m₁).

The axon lies in an indentation of a ganglion cell (N) which is covered by a sheath of Schwann cell processes (SC₁).

Trigeminal ganglion of adult mouse. × 26,000.

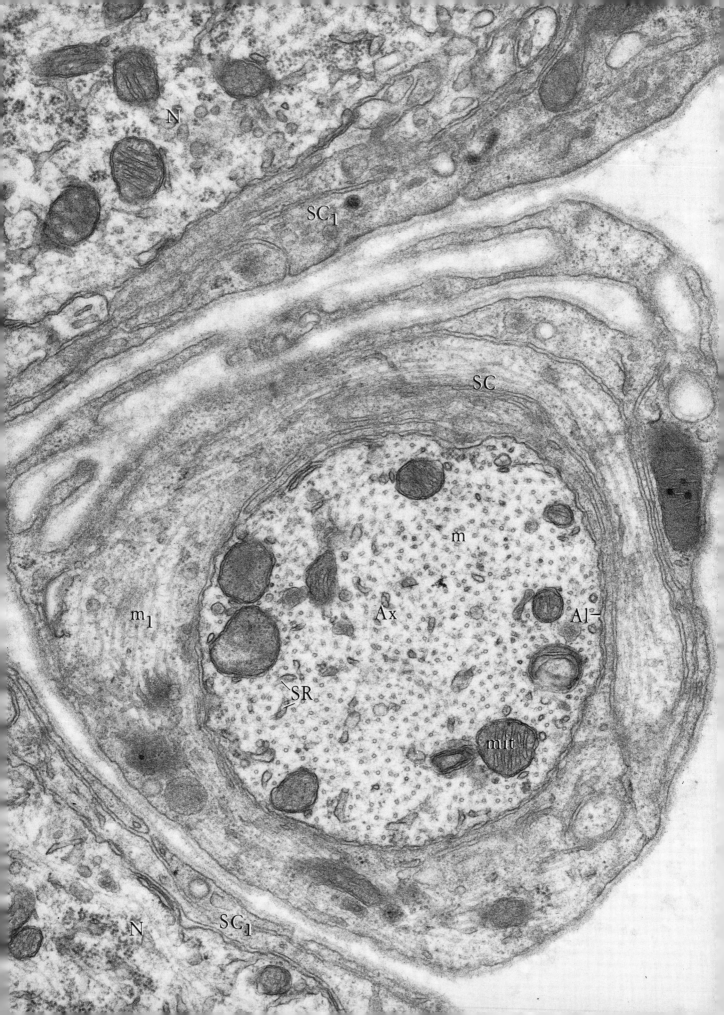

THE ENDOPLASMIC RETICULUM AND MITOCHONDRIA

As mentioned earlier, in the central nervous system the granular endoplasmic reticulum does not extend into the cytoplasm of axons beyond the axon hillock and the first part of the initial segment. However, the agranular endoplasmic reticulum is represented by a few irregular vesicles, tubules, and cisternae that are generally arranged in rows parallel to the length of the axon (see Figures 4–3, 4–5, 6–5, 6–14, and 6–15). These structures lie between the neurofilaments and microtubules, and, as pointed out by Metuzals (1963), the irregularly shaped cisternae are sometimes joined together by narrow constrictions. This suggests that the cisternae may represent a continuous system extending along the length of the axon, although it must still be proved.

An unusual form of the agranular endoplasmic reticulum has been described in the axoplasm of the Purkinje cells of the cerebellum (Andres, 1965b; Morales and Duncan, 1966; Hámori and Szentágothai, 1968) and in axons in the lateral vestibular nucleus of the rat (Sotelo and Palay, 1971). According to the description of Andres (1965b) it consists of a number of parallel and interconnecting tubules whose outer surfaces are covered either by particles 8 to 10 nm in diameter (type A) or by a series of regularly arranged ring-like structures (type B). Sotelo and Palay (1971) make the point that the particles are not ribosomal in nature, and they show that the lumina of the tubules have an acid phosphatase activity. Other altered forms of agranular endoplasmic reticulum shown by Sotelo and Palay (1971) are whorls of concentrically arranged lamellae. These and other proliferations of the agranular endoplasmic reticulum were also found in some axon terminals of the lateral vestibular nucleus. Sotelo and Palay (1971) suggest that these atypical forms of agranular reticulum represent stages in the degeneration of axons and their terminals and reflect a continuing remodeling of synaptic connections that may go on throughout life in the adult animal.

A somewhat different and unusual form of agranular endoplasmic reticulum is also present in the growing olfactory nerve axons. There the cytoplasm has flattened cisternae that are arranged transversely across the axon to form partial septa (Hinds, 1972). Somewhat similar arrangements of agranular endoplasmic reticulum have also been described in crayfish nerve fibers (Peracchia, 1970), fish olfactory nerve axons (Holz and Weber, 1970), axons in the hypothalamus of fish (Follenius, 1970), and axons and dendrites in frog cerebellum (Lieberman, 1971a). In these latter studies the transverse cisternae, which are apparently connected to one another by longitudinal tubules, have been seen to be perforated by small pores through which microtubules pass.

It has been proposed by Sandborn (1966) that the components of the agranular reticulum are connected together by microtubules and that microtubules also serve as interconnections between other organelles of the neuronal cytoplasm. Such continuity is difficult to establish on the basis of sections in which there is a superimposition of the images of organelles and may be illusory. It should be also pointed out that, unlike microtubules, the membrane-limited

---

Figure 4–7. Microtubules, Neurofilaments, and Neuroglial Fibrils.

The **inset at the upper right** shows part of the perikaryon of a protoplasmic astrocyte that contains a large bundle of cytoplasmic fibrils (*f*) located in a recess of the nucleus (*Nuc*). With diameters of 6 to 8 nm, these fibrils are thinner than neurofilaments but, like them, are hollow and when sectioned transversely display a dark wall surrounding a lighter core.
Spinal cord from adult rat. × 211,000.

The remainder of the figure is a transverse section through a dendrite of an anterior horn cell. The cytoplasm contains numerous profiles of the smooth endoplasmic reticulum (*SR*), microtubules (*m*), and neurofilaments (*nf*). Each microtubule has a dense wall formed by globular subunits. In the light centers of some microtubules a dense dot is sometimes seen, but it is not prominent in this field.

The neurofilaments (*nf*), which in this type of dendrite are grouped into fascicles instead of being dispersed, display a light core and a dark wall beset with radiating spokes (*arrows*). Notice that nearly all of the microtubules and neurofilaments appear in transverse section. Their regularity reflects the rigorous parallelism in the arrays of these linear structures.
Spinal cord from adult rat. × 211,000.

Micrographs by R. B. Wuerker.

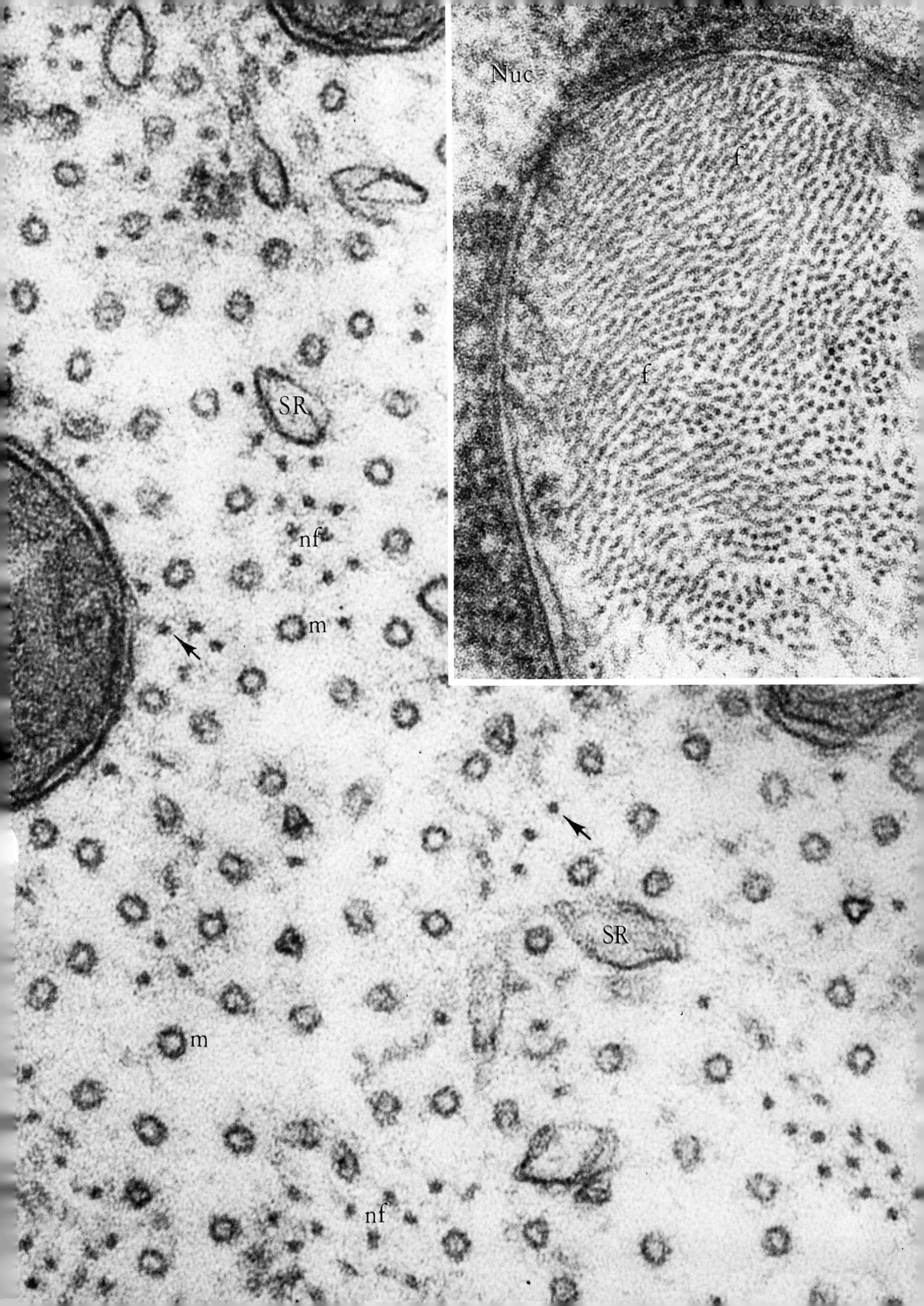
Nuc
f
f
SR
nf
m
SR
m
nf

components of the neuron have walls possessing a trilaminar structure. It is true, however, as mentioned by Sjöstrand (1963a) and Sandborn (1966), that the membranes of mitochondria may also display a globular or micellar structure (also see Frisch, 1969), so that they resemble the walls of microtubules as seen in transverse section. The contrast between the walls of the microtubules and those of the membranous organelles is perhaps best illustrated by the observations of Gray (1964). In potassium permanganate–fixed material he has shown that, although the walls of such components as the endoplasmic reticulum have a trilaminar appearance, the microtubules are not even clearly preserved.

The mitochondria of the axon are thin and often several microns long (e.g., see Vaughan and Peters, 1973). They are oriented parallel to the length of the axon, branch infrequently, and may have longitudinally arranged cristae (Figures 4–1, 4–2, and 4–5). Other than this, they show no unusual features. Much shorter mitochondria also exist in the axon, especially in the terminal boutons (Figures 5–2 and 5–3) and in boutons en passant (Figure 4–4). In such sites the mitochondria are associated with accumulations of synaptic vesicles.

THE AXONAL MEMBRANE

In electron micrographs, the plasma membrane of the axon (axolemma) resembles the plasma membrane limiting other parts of the cell. Namely, it is 7 to 8 nm thick and has the form of two dense lines, or leaflets, separated by an intervening lighter zone. In material fixed with osmic acid, either directly or after primary fixation in aldehydes, the plasma membrane appears asymmetrical because the outer leaflet is less dense than the one adjacent to the axoplasm (see Figures 6–5, 6–9, and 6–16).

Since the axon is actively involved in ionic exchange during the passage of an impulse down the axon, a question arises as to whether the membrane undergoes any detectable change during excitation (see Cohen, 1973). Optically detectable changes that can be presumably attributed to changes in the axolemma do occur during excitation (see Keynes, 1970). Thus, the birefringence of the squid axon increases during the passage of the action potential, and the intensity of the optical change closely follows changes in the membrane potential (Cohen, Keynes, and Hille, 1968). It has also been reported that living

nerves stained with certain fluorescent dyes exhibit a small increase in fluorescence during the passage of an impulse (see Tasaki, Carnay, Sandlin, and Watanabe, 1969; Cohen, 1973). Keynes (1970) suggests that both of these effects are related to the activity of the membrane of the axon, since it is only in the vicinity of the membrane that the potential gradient is large enough to bring them about.

A change in the axolemma during excitation has also been reported by Peracchia and Robertson (1971) in the crayfish abdominal nerve cord. If during electrical stimulation the axons of the cord are fixed with aldehydes and postfixed with osmic acid, the axolemma, the outer membrane of the mitochondria, and the endoplasmic reticulum all become more electrondense than they are in unstimulated nerves. At the same time the overall thickness of the membrane increases to 12 to 15 nm. Peracchia and Robertson (1971) suggest that the increased density is brought about by an unmasking of the —SH groups in the membrane during stimulation. In testing this idea they found that treating control specimens with disulfide reducing agents brought about the same effect as stimulation, whereas blocking the —SH groups prevented the increase in density. No equivalent studies and observations so far appear to have been carried out on the mammalian nervous system.

Modifications of the basic axolemmal structure occur in the following sites:

1. At nodes of Ranvier in both the central and peripheral nervous systems, where a dense layer lies beneath the axolemma in the zone between two adjacent segments of myelin. A similar dense layer undercoats the axolemma of the initial axon segment (see Figures 4–1 to 4–3).

2. In the paranodal region, where the terminal loops of myelin overlie the axolemma in both central and peripheral nerves. In these sites the axolemma and the plasma membrane bounding the terminal loops of the sheath form a junctional complex (see Figures 6–14 and 6–15).

3. At synaptic junctions, where the axon plays the role of either the pre- or postsynaptic component. In chemical synapses, where the axolemma and the plasma membrane of another neuronal component, such as a dendrite, take part in the formation of a synaptic complex, there may be an accumulation of dense material in the cytoplasm adjacent to the axolemma (see Figures 5–3 to 5–6). At electrical synapses the axolemma comes into close apposition with the plasma membrane of the postsynaptic element to form a gap junction (see Figure 5–16).

AXOPLASMIC FLOW

Although suggestions of its existence had been made earlier, the first experimental demonstration of axoplasmic flow was provided by Weiss and Hiscoe (1948; see reviews by Weiss, 1969 and 1970; Schmitt and Samson, 1968; Grafstein, 1969; Lasek, 1970; Davison, 1970; Freide and Seitelberger, 1971; Ochs, 1971; Wuerker and Kirkpatrick, 1972; Lubínska, 1975). In their experiments Weiss and Hiscoe (1948) placed constrictions around axons and showed that the axoplasm and its content of organelles accumulated on the proximal side of the constriction, where it produced an irregular bulge. When the constriction was removed the accumulated material was found to pass down the axon at a somatofugal rate of about 1 mm per day. Components having rates of this order have been termed the slow components of axoplasmic flow (see Weiss, 1969). Later investigations have demonstrated that components in this category have rates in the range of 0.5 to 5.0 mm per day.

Other components of the flow are transported at faster rates, which were only discovered by the use of isotopes. Faster transport takes place at rates in the range of 10 to 2000 mm per day (see Lasek, 1970; Ochs, 1972). Both types of transport are well demonstrated in a large number of experiments in which a tritiated amino acid, e.g., [³H] leucine, is injected into the vicinity of neuronal somata, for example, retinal or dorsal root ganglion cells. This label is incorporated into the proteins of the neuronal soma and subsequently enters the axon. Thereafter it can be traced by either autoradiography or scintillation counting as it passes down the axon to reach the axon terminals. Apparently proteins are transported down the axon in this manner because the axon does not possess the equipment for the synthesis of sufficient protein for its maintenance. As has already been noted (see page 96), the axoplasm is free of ribosomes, although it does contain a small amount of ribonucleic acid. This concept of the manner in which the axon is maintained is largely substantiated by the observation that mammalian axons soon degenerate once they have been severed from the neuronal perikarya, a fact that underlies the use of degeneration methods for studying neuronal projections.

The composition of the material transported by the slow and fast mechanisms appears to be heterogeneous. The whole cytoplasm, however, does not move down the axon, but only selected components; ribosomes, for example, remain in the perikaryon. For the most part, though, the fast component is generally considered to consist of particulate matter such as vesicles, and mitochondria, as well as membrane-bound materials like some proteins, enzymes, catecholamines, and glutamate (see Lasek, 1970; McEwen, Forman and Grafstein, 1971; Sabri and Ochs, 1973). Our knowledge of which substances are transported depends, of coursè, on an ability to test for the presence of those substances. On the whole, however, the substances involved in the fast transport appear to be ones directly necessary for synaptic functions. The slow component, on the other hand, seems to involve high molecular weight and soluble materials such as proteins, and perhaps some particulate elements, but generally it appears to concern materials related to the growth and maintenance of the axon (see Schonbach, Schonbach, and Cuénod, 1973).

The slow-moving materials are constrained in the cytoplasm, for when the slow component of the transport is followed after pulse labelling with an isotope, it is found to move along the axon in a distinct peak of labelling at a rate of about 1 mm per day. The peak, or crest of the label, remains distinct for very long periods and does not diffuse. This suggests that the proteins involved in this slow transport are bound to relatively stationary components of the axoplasm and that they have a long half-life. Weiss (1967) has proposed that the movement of the slow component is brought about by a flow of the cytoplasmic matrix of the axon, while another suggestion (see Schmitt and Samson, 1968) is that the neurofilaments and microtubules are actually part of this slow component. Evidence in support of this latter suggestion comes from two sources. First, the electron autoradiographic studies of Droz (1971) which have indicated that the slow-moving proteins are bound to, or associated with, the microtubules. Second, Grafstein, McEwen, and Shelanski (1970) demonstrated that tritiated colchicine injected into the eyes of goldfish moves down the optic nerve fibers at a slow rate of about 0.5 mm per day. The tritiated colchicine selectively binds with the microtubules and so it is supposed that the slow rate reflects the rate of formation of microtubules (also see McEwen, Forman, and Grafstein, 1971).

Schmitt (1968) has proposed that microtubules are also involved in the fast transport of vesicle-bound components, such as transmitters and neurosecretory products, from the neuronal soma to the nerve terminals. He suggests that the side arms of microtubules become attached to a complementary component on the surface of the vesicles and that the vesicles move along the outsides of the microtubules in much the same way that actin filaments are thought to slide along myosin in muscle. Some backing for this concept seems to be given by the studies of Smith, Järlfors, and Beránek (1970). They studied the axoplasm of the central nervous system of the lamprey and found synaptic vesicles to be generally sparsely distributed throughout the cytoplasm, but arranged in regular arrays associated with microtubules in the vicinity of synapses. Neurofilaments were not associated with vesicles or other components of the cytoplasm in the lamprey. Thus far, similar associations between microtubules and vesicles have not been encountered elsewhere, although Raine, Ghetti, and Shelanski (1971) have noted that microtubules often closely surround mitochondria within some axons. However, this close association is probably unspecific and occurs because the mitochondria have to squeeze between the microtubules as they pass down the axon.

Recent studies have shown that colchicine, a mitotic inhibitor which selectively binds to subunits of microtubules and produces a depolymerization of microtubules and/or prevents their repolymerization into subunits (Shelanski and Taylor, 1967 and 1968), can selectively reduce both fast and slow transport, suggesting that both systems are intimately linked and depend upon the microtubular complex for their integrity (e.g., Kreutzberg, 1969; Karlsson and Sjöstrand, 1969; James, Bray, Morgan, and Austin, 1970; Fernandez, Huneeus, and Davison, 1970). In one of the most careful studies of the effects of drugs on fast transport of radioactive leucine, Edström and Mattsson (1972) studied the effects of colchicine, cycloheximide, and vinblastine sulfate by assessing their differential effects either on the ganglion cell bodies of a frog sciatic nerve preparation or on the nerve itself. They found that cycloheximide almost completely inhibited protein synthesis in the neurons, but treatment of the nerve fibers with the drug had no effect on axoplasmic transport. Contrary to the findings of others, colchicine did not affect transport when placed in nerve fibers, but it did markedly arrest the outflow of proteins along the nerve when the neuronal somata were treated. It did not, however, affect protein synthesis in the ganglion. To explain this result they suggest that colchicine does not cause the breakdown of already formed microtubules, but acts by binding to the microtubular monomer protein, so that the effect on the cell body might be to interfere with the assembly of microtubules. Vinblastine sulfate, whose action is similar to that of colchicine, prevented transport when placed on either the neurons or the nerve.

From these and other studies, then, it can be concluded that microtubules are involved in axoplasmic transport, although the manner of their involvement is unknown.

An example of a contrary view, that microtubules are not the primary structures involved in rapid axoplasmic flow, is given in the study by Byers (1974). Byers examined the effects of colchicine on the transport of tritiated proline along the desheathed vagus nerves of rabbits. She found that normal transport of this substance can continue at the normal rate despite a substantial loss of microtubules. In electron microscopic autoradiographs the silver grains were located over the marginal cytoplasm of the axon, close to the axolemma. Consequently, Byers (1974) suggests that rather than the microtubules the marginal axoplasm, the smooth endoplasmic reticulum, and the axolemma may be the components involved in rapid transport.

Correlative morphological studies of the effects of colchicine on the normal nervous system are those of Hansson and Sjöstrand (1971) and of Echandía, Ramirez and Fernandez (1973), although some of the effects of this drug on anterior horn cells had previously been studied by Wiśniewski, Shelanski, and Terry (1968). Hansson and Sjöstrand (1971) treated rabbits with colchicine which was given either intracister-

Figure 4-8.   **Small Axons in the Molecular Layer of Cerebellum.**

This field consists almost entirely of transversely sectioned axons of granule cells. These axons are termed "parallel fibers" because of their remarkably regular arrangement. This neuropil is unusual in that no neuroglial cell processes intervene between the closely packed axons. Each axon contains a few microtubules (*m*), and some show profiles of smooth endoplasmic reticulum (*SR*). Where mitochondria (*mit*) occur, they almost fill the axon.

Separating the axons from the endothelial cell (*End*) on the left are the neuroglial limiting membrane (*As*) and the basal lamina (*B*) that surround the parenchyma of the brain.

Cerebellum from adult rat. × 62,000.

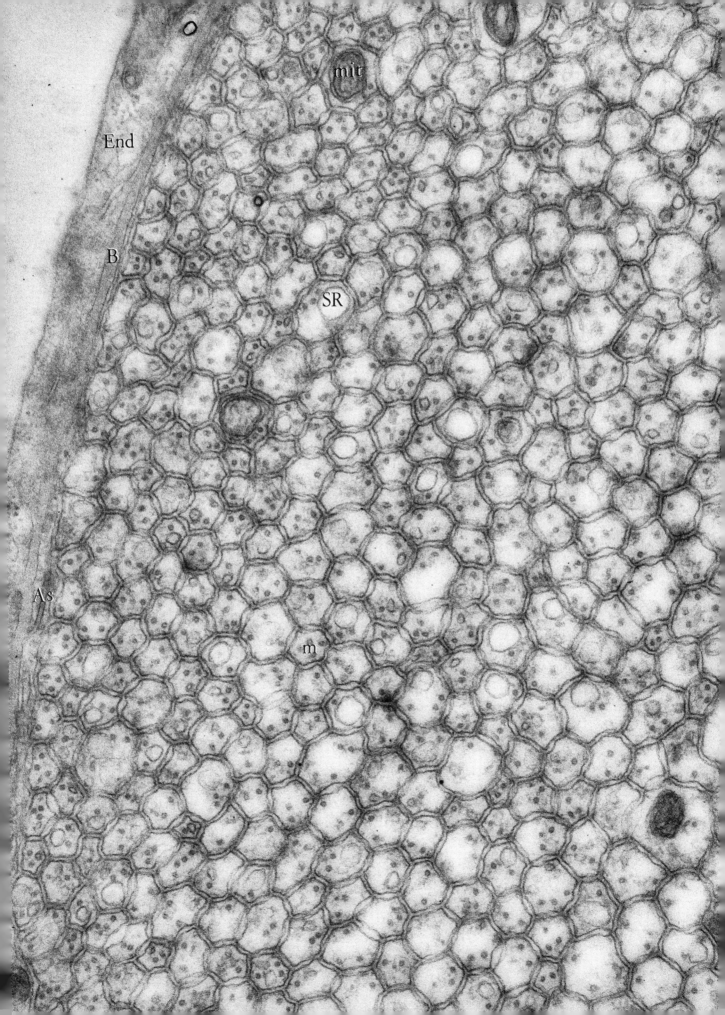

nally or locally to the hypoglossal and vagus nerves through the epineurium. Among the changes observed were a swelling of the hypoglossal neurons and the formation of bundles of 10-nm filaments in the cytoplasm between the Nissl bodies, although there was no obvious change in the number of microtubules. This is somewhat similar to the result obtained by Wiśniewski, Shelanski, and Terry (1968) on anterior horn cells. Vagus neurons did not show an increase in neurofilaments but seemed to increase the number of microtubules. Local treatment of the nerves with colchicine resulted in a blockage of axoplasmic flow, so that proximal to the site of application of the drug the nerve was distended and showed a damming-up of mitochondria, `lysosomes, endoplasmic reticulum, and bundles of 10-nm filaments, in varying proportions. The number of microtubules in the nerve appeared to be maintained in the normal range. The treated and distal portions of the nerves appeared normal in respect of the cytoplasmic constituents.

This observation of the maintenance of the number of microtubules in the nerve is in contrast to the results of Echandía, Ramirez, and Fernandez (1973). They find that injection of colchicine beneath the perineurium of the hypoglossal nerve of the cat leads to a loss of microtubules and an increase in numbers of 10-nm filaments. These filaments seem to form a network in which they are somewhat randomly arranged and joined by interconnecting bridges. Echandía, Ramirez, and Fernandez (1973) find that five days after injection of colchicine the nerves recover and regain their normal features.

How to explain the diverse results obtained by applying colchicine to nerves is not yet apparent. Some diversity may be produced by such factors as the concentration of colchicine used, the method of delivery to the nerve, and differences in the properties of microtubules from different animal phyla.

Vincristine sulfate, which blocks the axoplasmic flow of labelled proteins, produces a loss of microtubules in cultured sympathetic neurons and induces the formation of crystal-

loid structures within the cells and their processes (England, Kadin, and Goldstein, 1973).

At present the effects of cytochalasin-B on axonal transport do not seem to have been established. As will be considered later (see page 116) it has been concluded by Wessells et al. (1971) that cytochalasin-B disrupts microfilamentous networks in the cytoplasm and since well-defined networks of this kind are not obvious in the axon, little effect might be expected. This conclusion seems to be supported by the results of Banks, Mayor, and Mraz (1973) who found that cytochalasin-B does not inhibit the movement of noradrenaline, or dense-cored vesicles, within preparations of autonomic nerves of the cat. They found no marked effects upon the morphology of neurofilaments and microtubules. However, Fernandez and Samson (1973) found the substance to affect both the fast and slow transport of radioactive leucine in the crayfish nerve cord.

The transport of proteins down the axon has been exploited to advantage as a method for studying the projections of neurons (see Cowan, Gottlieb, Hendrickson, Price, and Woolsey, 1972). A radioactive amino acid, usually proline or leucine, is injected around the cell bodies of neurons. The isotope is incorporated into the proteins and transported down the axon to its terminals, where it can be localized by autoradiography at either light or electron microscope levels.

A number of studies have shown that transport of materials in the axon takes place in both directions, although the somatofugal flow is the most obvious one. Somatopetal or retrograde transport along axons is suggested by direct observation of the movements of particles along them (Pomerat, Hendelman, Raiborn, and Massey, 1967), and it can be shown in terms of acetylcholinesterase (AChE) transport, for example. When nerves are transected and the ends of the isolated segments examined for AChE accumulation, the enzyme is found to be present at both ends of an isolated segment (Lubínska and Niemierko, 1971; Ranish and Ochs, 1972).

It has recently been reported that both horse-

Figure 4–9. **Unmyelinated Axons in the Olfactory Bulb.**

This field shows transversely sectioned, unmyelinated axons (*Ax*) in the nerve layer of the olfactory bulb. The cytoplasm of the axons contains microtubules and mitochondria embedded in a cottony matrix. Passing between the axons, and segregating some of them into discrete bundles (*Ax₁*), are irregularly shaped astrocytic processes (*As*).

Rat olfactory bulb. × 30,000.

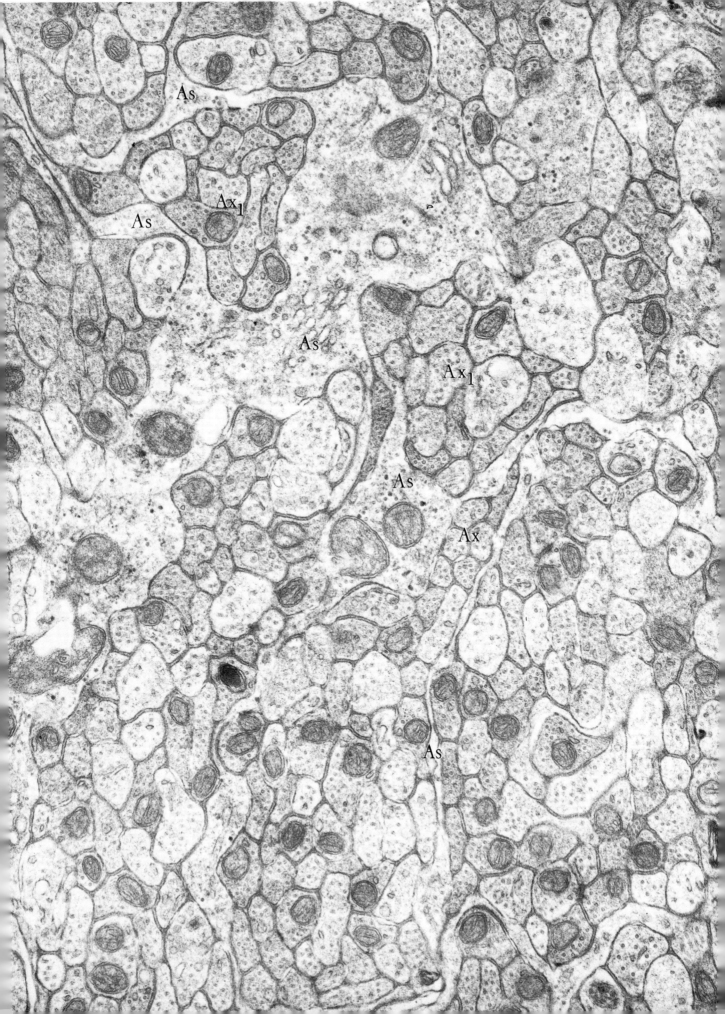

radish peroxidase and a tracer formed by the binding of Evans blue with albumin are transported from an injection site in a muscle to the perikarya of motor neurons innervating that muscle (Kristensson and Olsson, 1971a and 1973). These tracers are taken up by axon terminals, and a similar phenomenon can be demonstrated in the central nervous system where the retrograde transport of horseradish peroxidase may be used as a means of tracing the projections of axons (La Vail and La Vail, 1972 and 1974; La Vail, Winston, and Tish, 1973; Warr, 1973). When the somata and axons of labelled neurons are examined the horseradish peroxidase taken up by the axon terminals is found to be sequestered in numerous vacuoles, small tubules, vesicles, and multivesicular bodies (Kristensson and Olsson, 1971b; La Vail and La

Vail, 1974). No tracer appears free in the cytoplasm, and there seems to be no detectable alteration in the neurons when small amounts of tracer are injected. Although the parameters are not yet clear, this retrograde transport of tracers may vary as a function of age, species, and the system of neurons involved. For example, horseradish peroxidase injected into the tongues of suckling mice appears in almost all the hypoglossal nerve bodies (Kristensson, Olsson, and Sjöstrand, 1971), whereas in older mice only a few neurons become labelled. The same age dependency is also present in the cat (Warr, personal communication), but in adult rabbits uptake of peroxidase, from the tongue at least, occurs with a facility equal to that observed in young animals of other species.

THE AXON GROWTH CONE

Since it is becoming increasingly apparent that the nervous system is a potentially plastic system and not static, some consideration must be given to the form of the ends of growing axons, or axon growth cones. So far these entities have been described only in developing tissue, and the appearance of the growth cones in the light microscope was described many years ago in Golgi-impregnated material (Cajal, 1909), reduced silver preparations (Cajal, 1909), and tissue culture (Harrison, 1910; Pomerat, Hendelman, Raiborn and Massey, 1967). Unequivocal identification of these structures in electron microscopic studies of embryonic material is difficult on the basis of random sections and perhaps the best definitive study of their ultrastructural appearance has been provided by Yamada, Spooner, and Wessells (1971), who examined them in cultures of dorsal root ganglia

from the chick. They examined the growth cones in these cultures with both phase contrast and electron microscopy and so were able to be certain of their identity.

With the phase contrast microscope, Yamada, Spooner, and Wessells (1971) have shown growth cones to be expanded regions at the ends of axons, from which a varying number of continually moving thin processes, filopodia or microspikes, extend (Figure 4–10). In addition, the growth cones have thin membranous structures arising from them, which continually expand and retract. In the electron microscope (Figures 4–10 and 4–11) the cytoplasm of such growth cones is characterized by large amounts of smooth endoplasmic reticulum, vesicles, neurofilaments and a few microtubules as well as a peripheral network of microfilaments, 4 to 6 nm in diameter. The neurofilaments form a core to

Figure 4–10. **Growth Cone from a Sympathetic Neuron in Tissue Culture.**

The **inset** is a phase contrast picture. At the bottom is the highly refractive perikaryon (N) of the neuron and extending from it a fiber (f). This fiber bears the growth cone which displays filopodia (arrows).

The electron micrograph is of the same growth cone; most of the filopodia (arrows) are apparent. The end of the fiber (f) is at the bottom of the picture, and its cytoplasm shows peripheral microtubules (m) that surround a core containing mitochondria (mit) and vesicles (v). As the fiber expands into the growth cone the cytoplasm exhibits closely packed organelles which can be identified as mitochondria (mit_1), many narrow cisternae of the smooth endoplasmic reticulum (SR), vesicles that frequently have dense contents (v_1), and some dense bodies that appear to be myelin figures. Toward the distal border of the growth cone these organelles become less frequent, so that beneath the plasma membrane there is a relatively organelle-free zone in which the matrix seems to be microfilamentous.
Neuron cultured for one day; obtained from one-day-old rat superior cervical ganglion.

Electron micrograph by M. B. Bunge. × 14,000.
Phase contrast photograph by D. Bray. × 1350.

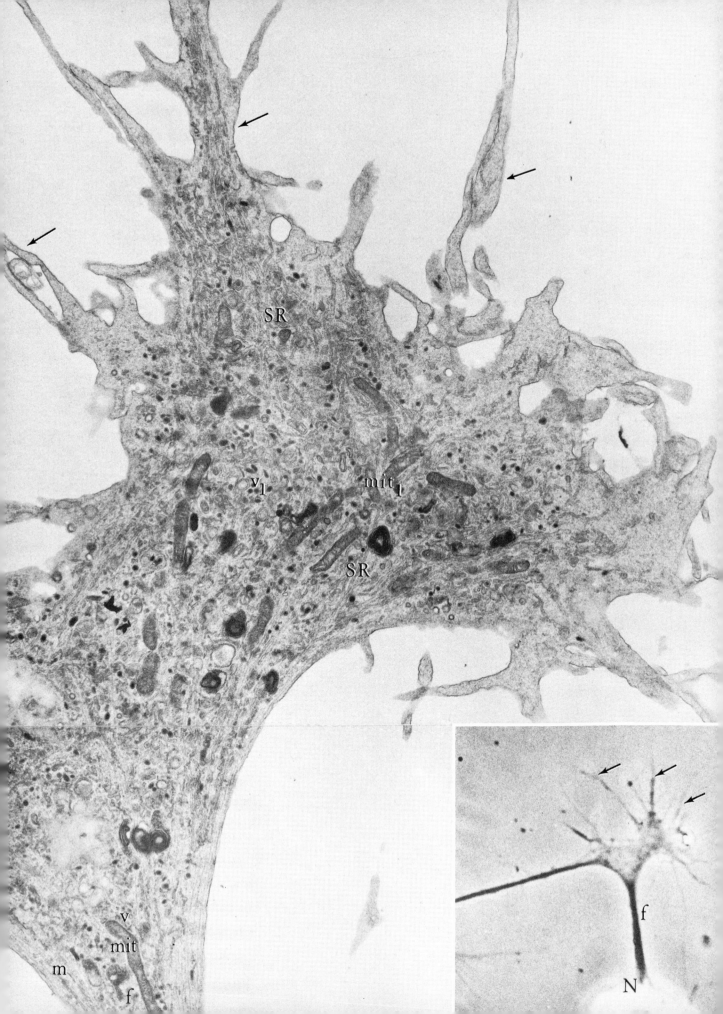

the growth cone, and these are surrounded by interlacing tubules of smooth endoplasmic reticulum through which microtubules penetrate. The microfilaments form a meshwork. They are mainly located beneath the plasma membrane and extend into the filopodia.

Bunge (1973) has found growth cones with a similar form in tissue cultures of sympathetic neurons from the superior cervical ganglion (Figures 4–10 and 4–11). In addition to the disposition of organelles just described she has shown continuity between the surface membrane of the growth cone and the cytoplasmic membranes. Bunge (1973) suggests that these cytoplasmic membranes of the conspicuous smooth endoplasmic reticulum might be involved in the recycling of the surface membrane when the growth cone changes its shape and hence its surface area. A similar recycling of the plasma membrane also seems to occur at axon terminals (see page 122). In an interesting paper accompanying that by Bunge (1973), Bray (1973) showed that two types of motion occur in growth cones at the tips of neuronal processes. Rapid and flame-like extensions and retractions of microspikes were superimposed on a much slower and linear advance of the cone as a whole. This advance was at an almost constant rate of about 40 microns per hour. In almost every case branches were formed by the bifurcation of growth cones that had first broadened. Distances between the cell body and the branching points remained relatively fixed, and the branching angles were smaller for thinner processes. The final growth pattern achieved under these conditions resembled that of dendrites of sympathetic neurons in the animal; axon formation was not observed, but somewhat similar conditions must pertain for the axon.

The description of growth cones given by Yamada, Spooner, and Wessells (1971) and by Bunge (1973) is in good agreement with that given earlier by Tennyson (1970) who examined them in the centrally directed neurites of dorsal

roots in the embryos of rabbits from day 11 to day 12½ of gestation. Tennyson (1970) described some of the cisternae of the smooth endoplasmic reticulum as dilated and suggested that these dilations probably correspond to the pinocytotic vesicles that have been described in cultured preparations. An additional observation was the presence of some clusters of free ribosomes in the cytoplasm of the cones and of their parent axons.

The structure of the growth cones as shown in the three studies cited above differs from that of the entities described as growth cones in studies such as those of developing spinal cord (Bodian, 1966b; Bodian, Melby, and Taylor, 1968) and of developing cerebellum in material taken from intact embryos (Del Cerro and Snider, 1968). These latter authors describe growth cones as bulbs or enlargements, about 0.5 micron in diameter, that contain accumulations of large, clear vesicles which are either rounded or elongate. Kawana, Sandri, and Akert (1971) showed similar structures in the cerebellar cortex, but found filopodia to arise from their enlargements. Tennyson (1970) states that similar bulbous enlargements were present in the posterior fasciculus of the rabbit embryos she examined, at a time when immature synapses were first seen. Whether these bulbous enlargements, which are often poorly preserved and have a tendency to burst during tissue preparation (Peters and Feldman, 1973, unpublished observations), are types of axon growth cones must be held in question at present until more studies of other embryonic tissues have been carried out.

Microfilaments similar to those found in growth cones have been encountered in a large number of other locations such as glial cells in tissue culture (Spooner, Yamada, and Wessells, 1971), dendritic growth cones (Hinds and Hinds, 1972), cultured fibroblasts (Perdue, 1973), pseudopodia of slime molds (Wohlfarth-Bottermann, 1963), and amoebae, (Pollard, Shel-

---

Figure 4–11.   **Growth Cone from a Sympathetic Neuron in Tissue Culture.**

This electron micrograph shows a growth cone with a veil-like ruffled sheet at its distal end as well as a few filopodia (*arrows*). The core of the growth cone shows the same organelles as the one in Figure 4–10. These are mitochondria (*mit*) and dense vesicles (*v*) enmeshed between tubular cisternae of the smooth endoplasmic reticulum (*SR*). The fiber (*f*) connecting the growth cone to the parent neuron passes to the left. It is accompanied by a second fiber (*f₁*), the growth cone of which is at another level. Some of the collagen substrate is seen near the leading edge of the growth cone.

Superior cervical ganglion taken from a one-day-old rat, and cultured for one day.

Micrograph by M. B. Bunge. ×10,000.

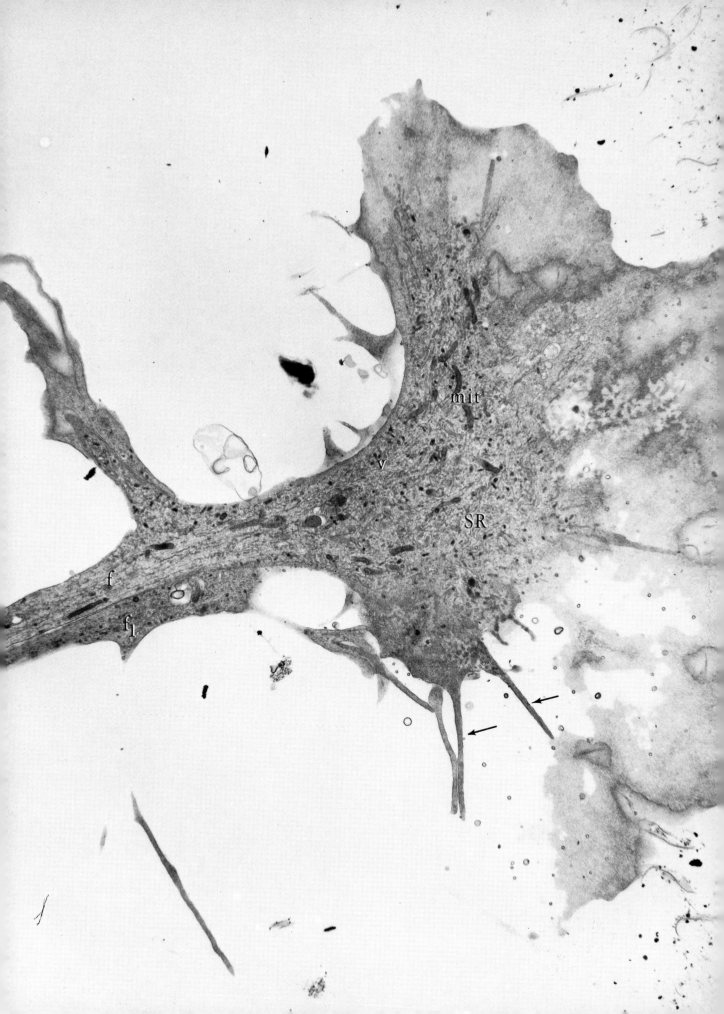

ton, Weihung, and Korn, 1970). It has been suggested that they are contractile in nature and may be involved in such processes as gastrulation (Baker, 1965), neurulation (Baker and Schroeder, 1967; Burnside, 1971), and lens invagination (Wrenn and Wessells, 1969). In cultured glial cells, for example (Spooner, Yamada and Wessells, 1971), microfilaments are present just beneath the plasma membrane of the undulating membrane at the edges of the cells that are migrating in the culture. Application of cytochalasin-B to a glial cell culture (Spooner, Yamada and Wessells, 1971) leads to a rapid cessation of cell migration and at the same time causes a disruption of the microfilamentous network. Other organelles, such as microtubules, are unaffected. Microtubules are, however, affected by colchicine, which does not affect the activity of the undulating membrane, the cell movements or the microfilaments. Cytochalasin-B also causes a rounding up of growth cones in cultured nerve cells (Yamada, Spooner and Wessells, 1971), retraction of filopodia, and a cessation of axon elongation. No organelles other than microfilaments appear to be affected by cytochalasin-B. Hence it seems that the microfilaments are responsible for the movements of the growth cone. Such a function for microfilaments is consistent with the observation by Perdue (1973) that the microfilaments in cultured chick embryo fibroblasts are composed in part of an actin-like protein. Thus fibroblast microfilaments bind rabbit muscle heavy meromyosin and specifically bind antibody directed against isolated actin-like protein.

To return to the microtubules of growing neuronal processes, colchicine inhibits the elongation and retraction of growing processes and disrupts the microtubules, whose place becomes occupied by large numbers of 7 to 10 nm filaments (Yamada, Spooner and Wessells, 1971; Daniels, 1973). Withdrawal of the colchicine from a culture leads to an assembly of microtubules (Daniels, 1973). In addition to apparently providing the skeletal support for the extremely long and thin processes of growing neurons, the microtubules may be responsible for axonal flow or the transport of metabolites from the cell body and into the growing processes (see page 107).

At present the distribution of microfilaments in the mature neurons has not been investigated. They may, however, be responsible for the rather fuzzy material that occurs in dendritic spines (see page 81) and may provide some of the flocculent density present between the microtubules and neurofilaments in axons and dendrites.

With reference to the structure of the plasma membrane of growth cones, Pfenninger and Bunge (1974) have shown that neuronal growth cones in tissue cultures display few intramembranous particles in freeze-fractured preparations. The concentration of particles increases eightfold as the perikaryon is approached. The particles of the growth cone also increase in number as the time in culture is prolonged and the nerve fibers mature. These results suggest that the plasma membrane of the outgrowing nerve fiber, and especially that of the growth cone, is immature and that with maturation more particles are inserted into it.

IDENTIFICATION OF SMALL AXONS AND DENDRITES

As mentioned earlier, the differentiation between small axons and dendrites may present a problem in the interpretation of sections of neuropil, because both types of process contain microtubules but few neurofilaments. Small axons usually have regular contours (Figures 4–8 and 4–9), however, and tend to travel through the neuropil in bundles in which they are arranged parallel to each other, while at sites of either *boutons en passant* or *boutons terminaux* they tend to expand. At such expansions there are increased numbers of synaptic vesicles and mitochondria, even though the typical synaptic densities may not be included in the section. Dendrites, on the other hand, usually have more irregular contours than axons and their surfaces may bear spines or thorns. Furthermore, in most locations dendrites course through the neuropil as individual structures and tend to change direction frequently. Dendrites containing microtubules are almost never as thin as small axons and they usually contain ribosomes in their cytoplasm, although these particles tend to become fewer with increasing distance from the perikaryon.

In view of the recent findings of axo-axonal

and dendro-dendritic synapses (pages 162 and 166), a process cannot be categorically defined as either an axon or a dendrite on the basis of its position in a synapse. It is still true, though, that axo-dendritic synapses are the most common kind to be formed between neuronal processes.

The features outlined above, taken together and considered in the light of the architecture of the region under study, particularly if they are correlated with observations made upon Golgi impregnations, should permit an investigator to differentiate between small axons and dendrites in most instances of doubt.

Chapter V

SYNAPSES

The term "synapse" was first used by Sir Charles Sherrington in 1897 (see Foster and Sherrington, 1897). It was derived from Greek words meaning "to fasten together," and was used to signify a site where the axon terminal of one neuron comes into functional contact with a second neuron. It follows from the neuron doctrine that a synapse is not a site of cytoplasmic confluence between neurons but an interface at which they are functionally related. In the light microscope, synapses are usually revealed by means of silver-staining techniques, but virtually all that these methods show is the profile or silhouette of the expanded end-bulb, or *bouton terminal*, of the preterminal axon attached to the surface of a perikaryon or dendrite. Apart from the mitochondria and, sometimes, neurofibrils, the light microscope shows nothing of the organelles within the *bouton terminal*, and it has remained for the electron microscope to reveal the detailed morphology of synapses. Indeed, it is perhaps in the field of synaptic morphology and organization that electron microscopy has made its greatest contribution to neuroanatomy.

The use of the term "synapse" may be expanded to include not only the functional contacts that occur between two neurons but also those between neurons and effector cells, e.g., muscle cells. Essentially, it is through a study of this latter type of functional contact, the neuromuscular junction, that most of the morphological and functional criteria for the identification of synapses in the nervous system have been derived.

Figure 5–1. **Motor End-plate.**

The **upper picture** is a light microscope picture of a neuromuscular junction. Coming into the field from the right is a myelinated axon (*Ax*). The myelin sheath is lost as the axon branches into its terminals (*At*), which contain the dark profiles of mitochondria. These terminals come into apposition with the muscle fiber below. Surrounding the axon terminals are the nuclei (*Nuc*) of the Schwann cells associated with the nerve ending. The black granules surrounding the nerve terminals are mitochondria (*mit*) in the muscle cell.
Superior oblique muscle of rat. × 2250.

The **lower picture** is an electron micrograph of a motor end-plate similar to that shown above. The terminals (*At*) of the motor nerve fiber contain mitochondria (*mit*) and synaptic vesicles (*sv*) and are separated from the surface of the muscle cell by a wide interval that contains the basal lamina (*B*). In this region the sarcolemma shows junctional folds (*arrows*) and the sarcoplasm is rich in mitochondria (*mit₁*). Covering the axon terminals are two Schwann cells (*SC*).
Superior oblique muscle of two-week-old rat. × 17,000.

Micrographs by J. M. Kerns.

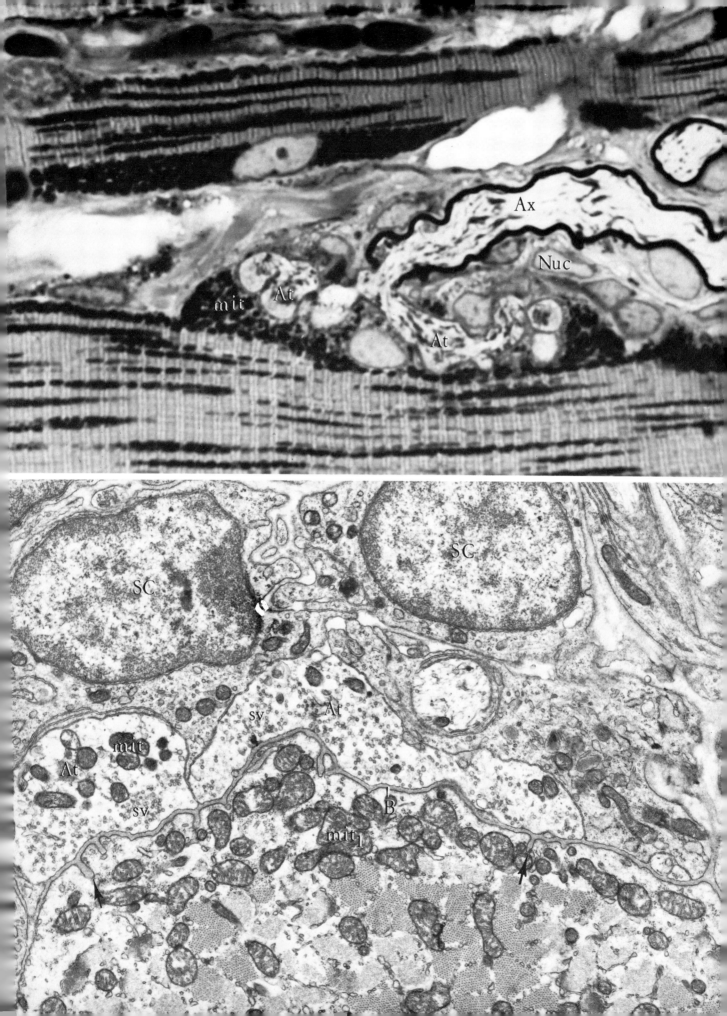

THE NEUROMUSCULAR SYNAPSE

Studies of the vertebrate motor end-plate include those of Robertson (1956 and 1960a), Reger (1958), Birks, Huxley, and Katz (1960), Andersson-Cedergren (1959), Couteaux (1960), Birks (1966), Padykula and Gauthier (1970), McMahan, Spitzer, and Peper (1972), Ceccarelli, Hurlbut, and Mauro (1972 and 1973), Heuser and Reese (1973), and Salpeter, McHenry, and Feng (1974).

At a motor end-plate one of the terminal branches of a motor nerve emerges from its myelin sheath and expands to form terminals which are filled with crowds of synaptic vesicles, 40 to 50 nm in diameter, numerous mitochondria, and tubules of smooth endoplasmic reticulum (Figure 5–1). The nerve terminals (Figure 5–1, *At*) occupy a depression, the synaptic gutter, indenting the surface of the muscle fiber. In this region, the sarcolemma, or muscle plasma membrane, is thrown into folds, the junctional folds (Figures 5–1 and 5–2), which are most elaborate in mammalian end-plates but meager in those of lower vertebrates. At the crests of the folds the sarcolemma is separated from the membrane of the nerve terminal by the synaptic cleft, about 60 nm deep. A single basal lamina (Figures 5–1 and 5–2, *B*) occupies this interval and follows the contours of the sarcolemma, so that it enters and lines the junctional folds. Birks, Huxley, and Katz (1960) described the synaptic vesicles of the nerve terminal as being focused upon special zones of the axonal membrane, where spots of dense material lie on its cytoplasmic face (Figure 5–2, *asterisks*). These spots lie opposite the openings of the junctional folds, and in a recent study of the frog sartorius muscle by Heuser and Reese (1973) these densities have been shown to be the profiles of 100-nm wide bands which are oriented perpendicular to the long axis of the terminal axon. According to their interpretation the motor end-plates may be considered to be formed of a number of "synaptic units," each one being represented by a dense band plus its associated synaptic vesicles. Another set of cytoplasmic densities, but with no associated vesicles, lies within the muscle cell on the crests of the folds of the sarcolemma (Figure 5–2).

The synaptic vesicles in the nerve terminals of the motor end-plate are thought to be packages of neurotransmitter (see Dale, Feldberg, and Vogt, 1936), which are released from the nerve terminals in multimolecular "quanta." In the motor end-plate the neurotransmitter is acetylcholine, and the manner in which this transmitter is released was first indicated by Fatt and Katz (1950). While recording from the subsynaptic region of a skeletal muscle fiber they observed the random appearance of small fluctuations in the resting potential. These fluctuations, or miniature potentials, were always in the direction of depolarization. Subsequent studies by del Castillo and Katz (1954 and 1955) led to the concept that the miniature potentials were due to the release of quanta of transmitter and could be attributed to release of the contents of individual synaptic vesicles. The assumption is that vesicles move toward the synaptic junction and discharge their contents in an all-or-none fashion when they collide with the presynaptic membrane (see Eccles, 1964). It is assumed that the transmitter diffuses across the synaptic cleft and reacts with specific receptor sites on the postsynaptic membrane or sarcolemma to produce a transient increase in the permeability of that membrane to surrounding ions. If such a discharge takes place and the synaptic vesicles coalesce with the plasma membrane of the axon terminal, then there is a problem in explaining the origin of a new supply of synaptic vesicles to replace the ones discharged. Some idea of the amount of membrane involved can be gained from the study of Bittner and Kennedy (1970) on the opener-stretch neuron of the crayfish, which

---

Figure 5–2. **Motor End-plate.**

Passing down the middle of the field is the basal lamina (*B*) which occupies the synaptic cleft separating the plasma membranes of the axon terminal (*At*) and the muscle cell. The axon terminal is crowded with synaptic vesicles (*sv*) that become concentrated at special zones of the axolemma (*). Although no coated vesicles are apparent in the axon terminal, the empty "shells" or "baskets" that form the coats of such vesicles can be seen (*arrowheads*).

While the presynaptic membrane is relatively smooth, the sarcolemma is thrown into junctional folds (*arrows*) lined by the basal lamina (*B*) of the synaptic cleft. At the crests of the folds the cytoplasmic face of the sarcolemma is coated by a dense material.

Rat diaphragm. × 75,000.

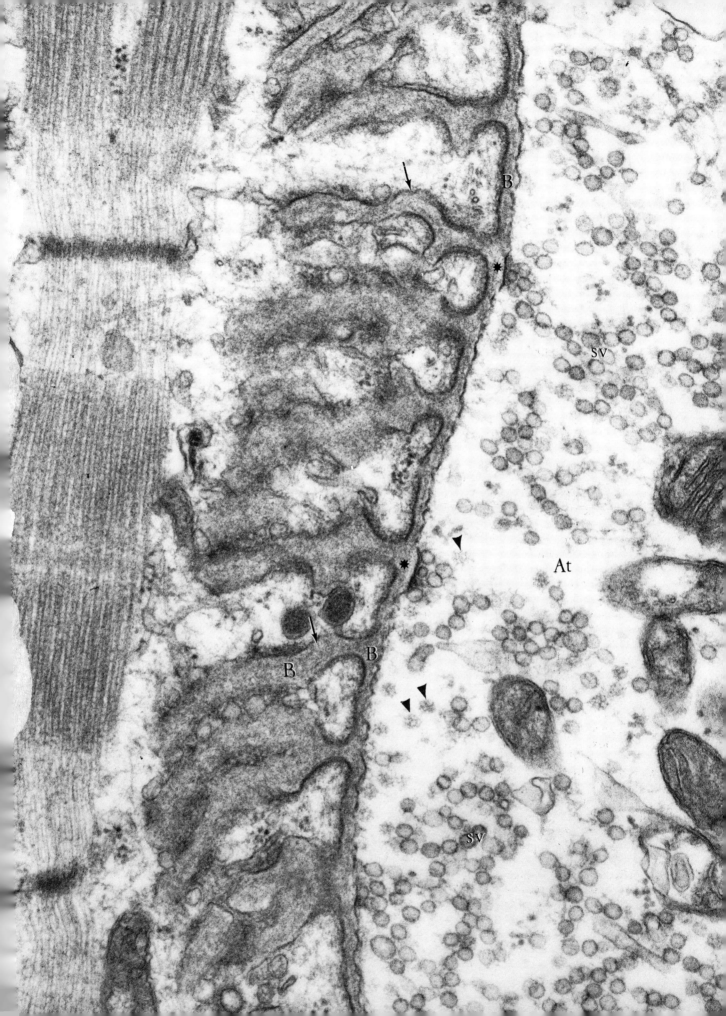

makes about 50 endings upon each of 1200 muscle fibers. In this system Bittner and Kennedy calculated that if the synaptic vesicles are equivalent to quanta of transmitter and the synaptic vesicles fuse with the presynaptic membrane, then the loss of synaptic membrane due to such a fusion would amount to almost 24 square mm of membrane per hour. Their conclusion was that a loss of this magnitude could not be sustained unless the synaptic vesicles are recycled from the presynaptic membrane.

Evidence for such recycling came from the study by Ceccarelli, Hurlbut, and Mauro (1972), who used frog cutaneous pectoris nerve-muscle preparations. They recorded the end-plate potentials and used curare to prevent the muscle twitch. After stimulating at a rate of two stimuli per second for varying intervals the curare was removed, and the specimen was either prepared directly for electron microscopy or treated with black widow spider venom before being prepared for morphological examination. This venom provokes the spontaneous release of an avalanche of several thousand micro end-plate potentials and completely depletes the terminals of their synaptic vesicles (Clark, Hurlbut, and Mauro, 1972) so that it can be used to assess the amount of transmitter left in the nerve terminals. Ceccarelli, Hurlbut, and Mauro (1972) found that about 80 per cent of the transmitter is released from the nerve terminals within about four hours, although the nerve terminals looked normal and still contained many vesicles. After six to eight hours the store of transmitter, and along with it the population of vesicles, was almost completely depleted. At this time the nerve terminals appeared swollen. When horseradish peroxidase was added to the medium bathing the stimulated preparation, it was taken up into many of the synaptic vesicles in the terminals, whereas resting control preparations showed no such uptake. On the basis of these data Ceccarelli, Hurlbut, and Mauro (1972) concluded that during stimulation the vesicles fuse with the axolemma and release their transmitter. In the next phase of the cycle new vesicles derived from the axolemma are returned to the axoplasm. This study was further elaborated upon by Ceccarelli, Hurlbut, and Mauro (1973) in a subsequent publication, in which it was emphasized that the vesicles can re-form both during and after stimulation, and that the re-formed vesicles can store and release transmitter.

These results have been confirmed by Heuser and Reese (1973 and 1974) using iso-lated frog sartorius muscle preparations with their nerves attached. Using higher rates of stimulation they found that after 15 minutes 60 per cent of the synaptic vesicles had disappeared from the nerve endings, an amount that Heuser and Reese (1973) calculate to be equivalent to 3 × 10⁵ synaptic vesicles. Concomitant with the depletion of synaptic vesicles they found numerous cisternae to appear inside the nerve terminals, as shown previously by Heuser and Miledi (1971) and by Korneliussen (1972a). Calculations by Heuser and Reese (1973) indicate that the loss of synaptic vesicle membrane is equal to the amount of membrane incorporated into these cisternae plus an amount by which the plasma membrane of the axon terminal increases, since it becomes irregular as a result of the stimulation. On the basis of a series of elegant experiments using horseradish peroxidase as a marker, Heuser and Reese (1973) concluded that the following sequence of events takes place upon stimulation of a nerve terminal. Synaptic vesicles discharge their contents of transmitter by coalescing with the plasma membrane of the nerve terminal at the regions where the densities occur. The synaptic vesicle membrane thus becomes an integral part of the axolemma. Then equal amounts of membrane are recovered from the axolemma by the formation of coated vesicles. These endocytotic coated vesicles frequently occur in locations where Schwann cell processes occur in the synaptic cleft. They lose their coatings as they coalesce and form the cisternae from which the supply of synaptic vesicles is repleted.

In another approach to the junctional morphology at the frog neuromuscular junction Heuser, Reese, and Landis (1974) examined freeze-fractured preparations. They found that the A face of a fractured nerve terminal possesses a series of transverse ridges on its surface, the ridges being bordered by rows of relatively large particles. From their locations it is apparent that these ridges correspond to the electron-dense bands which have synaptic vesicles clustered along them in sectioned material. In freeze-fractured preparations of resting nerve terminals there were no signs of the synaptic vesicles opening onto the surface, but in stimulated material, especially that fixed in dilute formaldehyde solutions while the stimulation was in progress, the ridges were paralleled on either side by a row of small dimples, which appear to represent sites where synaptic vesicles are attached to the axolemma. Because of the variety of sizes and shapes of these dimples at "vesicle sites," Heuser, Reese, and Landis assume that they represent synaptic vesicles in various stages of discharge. Stimulated axon terminals also showed dimples in the axolemma at points some distance away from the synaptic ridges. These accessory dimples, which frequently occurred above Schwann cell processes in the synaptic cleft, appear to represent the coated vesicles, which have been shown to undergo endocytosis in sectioned material.

The A face of the freeze-fractured sarcolemma exhibits clusters of large particles on the crests of the sarcolemmal folds, where sections show the cytoplasmic densities to be located. Clustered around the large particles (8 to 12 nm in diameter) are assemblies of smaller particles (6 to 7 nm in diameter). Similar large and small particle assemblies also occur in the sarcolemma of rat diaphragm motor end-plates (Rash, Ellisman, and Staehelin, 1973; Rash and Ellisman, 1974). These observations on the appearance of freeze-fractured motor end-plates are substantiated by the results of Peper, Dreyer, Sandri, Akert, and Moor (1974).

At the vertebrate motor end-plate the bursting of synaptic vesicles leads to the deposition of their content of acetylcholine (ACh) in the synaptic cleft. This transmitter then excites or depolarizes the postsynaptic muscle cell through the binding of the ACh with specific receptor sites. The concentration of ACh in the synaptic cleft remains high for only a brief period for it is soon removed. Most of the ACh is removed through hydrolysis by acetylcholinesterase (AChE), although some of it is lost from the synaptic cleft by diffusion. The importance of the rapid removal of the ACh is clearly demonstrated by experiments in which AChE is inhibited by enzyme poisons like eserine or edrophonium (Tensilon) (e.g., see Katz, 1966). In the presence of such inhibitors repeated stimulation produces an accumulation of ACh. The ACh receptors on the sarcolemma become desensitized and neuromuscular transmission fails. A large proportion of the choline produced by the breakdown of the ACh by its esterase seems to be taken up by the axon terminal, which reuses the choline to resynthesize ACh and recharge the synaptic vesicles.

A number of studies indicate that calcium ions are required for the release of ACh at the neuromuscular junction (Katz and Miledi, 1965; Krnjevic, 1974). Recently Politoff, Rose, and Pappas (1974) have shown that when frog neuromuscular preparations are fixed in the presence of high concentrations of calcium, dense parti-

cles appear in the synaptic vesicles, the postsynaptic membrane, mitochondria, and the triads of the sarcolemma. Since such particles are not present in tissue fixed in calcium-free solutions, it is presumed that they are calcium deposits. The particles related to the synaptic vesicles are attached to, or form part of, the vesicle membrane, and each vesicle has one, and rarely two, particles. Thus the vesicles may be polarized, and it may be conjectured that the region of the vesicle displaying the particle has to come into contact with the presynaptic membrane before the vesicle can burst and release its transmitter. Bohan, Boyne, Guth, Narayan, and Williams (1973) found dense particles in synaptic vesicles isolated from electroplaques. Hillman and Llinás (1974) have shown them attached to the axolemma in the vicinity of synapses formed by squid giant axons. Hillman and Llinás used high energy dispersive x-ray analysis to demonstrate the presence of calcium and phosphorus in these particles. Oschman, Hall, Peters, and Wall (1974) presented almost identical results, independently confirming that the dense deposits in the membrane contain calcium and phosphorus.

Gray and Paula-Barbosa (1974) have also shown dense particles attached to synaptic vesicles in tissue fixed in aldehyde mixtures buffered to pH 2 or 4 and postfixed in osmium. Whether these particles represent the calcium deposits or some other entity in the vesicle wall is not yet apparent.

Histochemical techniques for the demonstration of AChE show that the electron-dense product of the reaction is located in the synaptic cleft, where it is mainly associated with the outer surface of the sarcolemma (e.g., see Couteaux, 1955; Lentz, 1969; Salpeter, McHenry, and Feng, 1974; Rash and Ellisman, 1974). The positions of the receptor sites for ACh are much less apparent, although it is presumed that these sites must also be located on the surface of the postsynaptic membrane. One of the most useful chemicals for the study of the receptors has been a group of protein toxins obtained from the venom of some snakes. One of these toxins is α-bungarotoxin which binds to the postsynaptic membranes of skeletal muscle and electroplaques. The binding is such that the response of the cells to ACh is blocked. Using α-bungarotoxin labelled with radioactive iodine, Fambrough and Hartzell (1972) found that at rat diaphragm end-plates there are about 10^7 receptor sites per end-plate, or 13×10^3 sites per square micron. In comparison in an electron microscope autoradiographic study of the mouse diaphragm motor end-plate with tritiated α-bungarotoxin, Porter, Barnard, and Chiu (1973) arrived at a value of about 8×10^3 sites per square micron. This latter article contains a useful table summarizing the data derived from a number of investigations and shows that in both motor end-plates and electroplaques the values obtained for the number of receptor sites per square micron range between about 1×10^4 and 3×10^4.

Entities which may correspond to the receptor sites have been described by Rosenbluth (1973 and 1974) at the myoneural junctions of the body musculature of the leech and at the motor end-plates of tadpoles. In the leech Rosenbluth (1973) has described discrete and concave, 7 nm patches of the postsynaptic muscle membrane, from which projections arise and extend about 20 nm toward the axon terminal. The projections are arranged in hexagonal arrays and have a spacing of about 15 nm. In amphibia (Rosenbluth, 1974) somewhat similar dense patches are located in the outer leaflet of the postsynaptic membrane where it faces the axon terminal, but the patches do not extend into the junctional folds. The patches in amphibia are 6 to 12 nm in diameter and are less regularly spaced than in the leech, for they are spaced at intervals between 10 and 15 nm. In both cases the concentration of the projections is about 10^4 per square micron, which agrees closely with the concentration of receptor sites obtained by the autoradiographic labelling techniques.

INTERNEURONAL CHEMICAL SYNAPSES

Some of the features displayed by motor end-plates are also displayed by interneuronal chemical synapses, that is, synapses in the central and peripheral nervous system which make use of chemical transmitters. Indeed, it was largely on the basis of their similarity to motor end-plates that interneuronal chemical synapses were first recognized in the earlier electron microscopic studies of the nervous system (e.g., Palade and Palay, 1954; De Robertis and Bennett, 1954 and 1955; De Robertis, 1956a and 1958; Wyckoff and Young, 1956; Palay, 1956b and 1958b). Like the neuromuscular junction each interneuronal chemical synapse consists of a *presynaptic element* containing synaptic vesicles and an apposed *postsynaptic element* from which it is separated by a *synaptic cleft*, 20 to 30 nm wide. The pre- and postsynaptic membranes display densities on their cytoplasmic faces, and these specialized membranes together with the synaptic cleft are defined as the *synaptic junction* (see Figures 5–3 to 5–8).

There are, however, certain differences between the neuromuscular junctions of striated muscle and the interneuronal synapses of the central nervous system:

1. In the central nervous system the synaptic junctions occur between cells that are derived from the same germinal layers, whereas the components of the neuromuscular junctions originate from two different germinal layers.

2. The synaptic cleft is narrower in the central nervous system than in the neuromuscular junction.

3. No distinct basal lamina is present surrounding neurons in the central nervous system, although the glycocalyx enclosing them usually extends into the synaptic cleft and often condenses into a dense line running down the middle of the cleft.

4. At the neuromuscular junction the appositional zone is less specialized and more extensive than at central nervous system synapses. Thus, although the presynaptic membrane of the

---

Figure 5–3.   Axon Terminal Emerging from the Myelin Sheath.

In this picture an axon (*Ax*) emerges from its myelin sheath to form a terminal (*At*) containing synaptic vesicles (*sv*) and two mitochondria (*mit*). This terminal synapses with a large dendrite (*Den*) of an anterior horn cell. At the synaptic junction the plasma membranes of the dendrite and the terminal lie parallel to each other, and three specialized areas are visible. Two of these areas are synaptic complexes (*arrows*), for they have synaptic vesicles closely associated with them. The third (*triangle*) is a *punctum adhaerens* and probably has a purely adhesive function; its densities are disposed symmetrically on either side and no synaptic vesicles are intimately related with this area.
Spinal cord from adult rat. ×48,000.

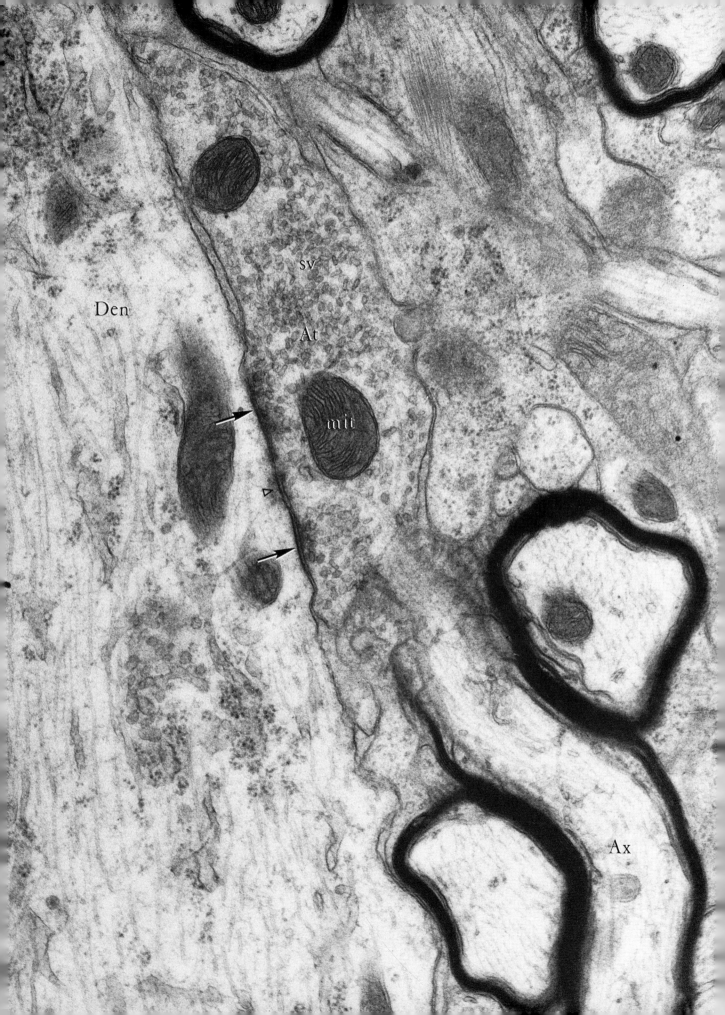

neuromuscular junction has focal aggregations of dense material, as in the central nervous system, this material does not seem to be matched by consistently well-defined postsynaptic aggregations.

Some of the features exhibited by the junctional zones between pre- and postsynaptic membranes of the central nervous system are also shown by the *zonulae adhaerentes* (Farquhar and Palade, 1963) between cells in other epithelia. First, the plasma membrane on one or both sides of the synapse is furnished with tufts of fine cytoplasmic filaments that insert into the cytoplasmic densities. Second, the synaptic cleft may be occupied by vague filamentous material that forms a thin, dark plate midway between the apposed membranes. Third, the pre- and postsynaptic membranes are adherent, for when nervous tissue is prepared by homogenization and differential centrifugation, the isolated axon terminals frequently bear attached fragments of the postsynaptic membrane. The essential difference between the appearance of a zonula adhaerens and a synaptic junction is that the synapse is polarized (Figures 5–3 to 5–7). Thus, the cytoplasmic densities attached to the junctional membranes are usually disposed asymmetrically; the dense filamentous material is usually more conspicuous on the postsynaptic side of the junction, where it is called "the subsynaptic web" (De Robertis, Pellegrino de Iraldi, Rodriguez de Lores Arnaiz, and Salganicoff, 1961; De Robertis, 1962).

Junctional zones with a symmetrical disposition of dense material similar to the zonulae adhaerentes are widely distributed throughout the central nervous system. Such junctions have been found between all components of the tissue, both neuronal and neuroglial. Although one of the components taking part in the formation of such an adhesion may, in some instances, contain synaptic vesicles, the vesicles are never closely associated with these symmetrical junctions (see Figures 5–3 and 5–4). Most commonly, neither of the components contains vesicles. Consequently, such junctions are considered to be purely adhesive and not concerned with the transmission of impulses. The form of these junctions closely resembles the *zonula adhaerens*, for in addition to the symmetrical densities, which have fluffy patches of filaments passing into them, a plate of dense material sometimes bisects the intercellular space between the apposed plasma membranes. These adhesions are confined, however, to small spots. Consequently, in keeping with the Latin nomenclature introduced by Farquhar and Palade (1963), we shall refer to them as *puncta adhaerentia* (see page 6). From the above account it should be clear that, unlike the simple adherent junctions, synapses have a polarized or asymmetrical structure.

In sections of central chemical synapses the dense material may be limited to small areas (Figures 5–3 and 5–4), or may extend for the entire length of the junction (Figure 5–5). When synaptic vesicles are associated with these dense areas, then the whole assemblage of vesicles plus junctional density is referred to as a "synaptic complex" (Palay, 1958b). As at the motor end-plate (Figures 5–1 and 5–2) the aggregation of vesicles in the synaptic complexes suggests that they may represent sites for the extrusion of the chemical transmitter into the synaptic cleft so that it can act upon the postsynaptic membrane. For this reason, Couteaux (1961) has termed the assemblages of synaptic vesicles and dense material the "active zones" of the synaptic junction.

Concentrations of synaptic vesicles occur near the synaptic junction, where the pre- and postsynaptic membranes are separated by a gap

---

Figure 5–4. **Axo-Dendritic Synapses, Anterior Horn.**

Upper picture. In this field are two axon terminals (At_1 and At_2) synapsing with a large dendrite (*Den*). Both terminals contain a mixture of spherical and ellipsoidal synaptic vesicles. At the synaptic junction formed by terminal At_1 two dense patches are present. The second axon (At_2) displays a well-defined synaptic complex (*arrow*). Note that these axon terminals are surrounded by astroglial sheets (*As*). *Spinal cord from adult rat.* × 46,000.

Lower picture. Synapsing with the dendrite (*Den*) is a large axon terminal (*At*) containing spherical synaptic vesicles together with many mitochondria. At the junction between the pre- and postsynaptic membranes there are four dense patches associated with a widening of the intercellular gap. Three of these patches (*arrows*) represent synaptic complexes, for the dense material is asymmetrically disposed and there is an accumulation of synaptic vesicles. Note the dense, fibrillar material beneath the dense layer next to the postsynaptic membrane. The fourth, smaller dense patch (*triangle*) is a *punctum adhaerens*. *Spinal cord from adult rat.* × 46,000.

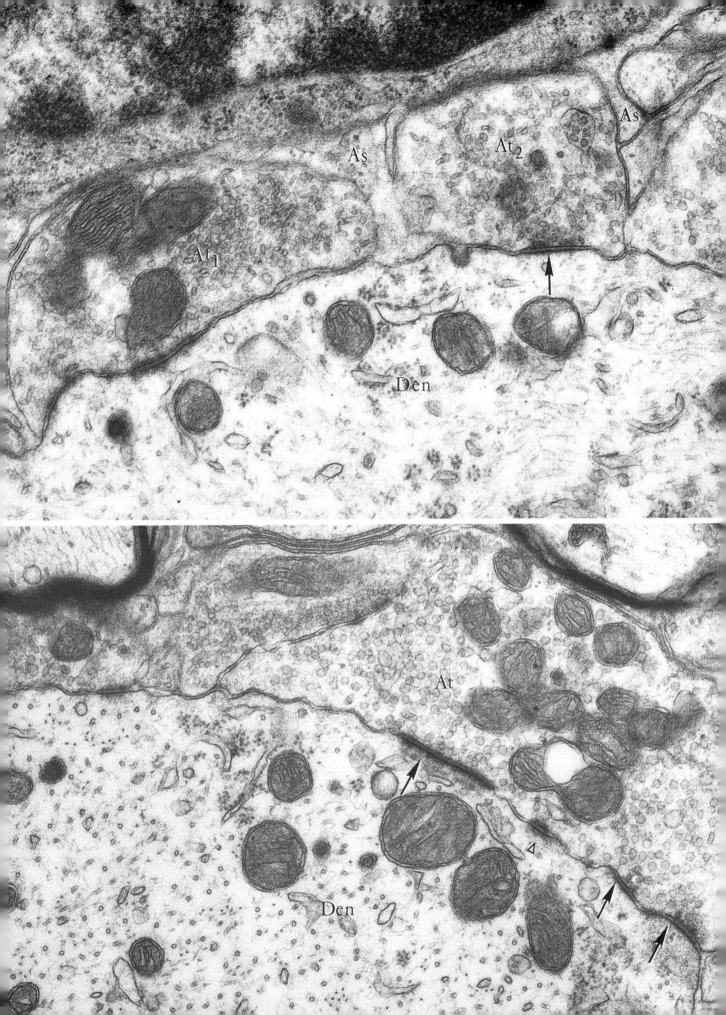

of 20 to 30 nm. The vesicles aggregate particularly near the regions of the junction where there is an accumulation of dense material in the adjacent cytoplasm. In the type of synapse described here (Figures 5–3 and 5–4), the dense material is usually sparse. It may be symmetrical in distribution or somewhat more prominent on the presynaptic side. Also, the density is often discontinuous and forms several patches. Puncta adhaerentia are commonly interspersed with the synaptic complexes. These also appear as dense patches, but they are thicker and more symmetrical than those of the synaptic complexes. The *puncta* (Figures 5–3, 5–4, and 5–9, *triangles*) have no synaptic vesicles immediately associated with them.

There is now a good deal of evidence to indicate that the vesicles of the presynaptic terminals contain the chemicals, e.g., acetylcholine or catecholamines, by which transmission across the synaptic junction is effected (see Whittaker, 1965; De Robertis, 1966 and 1967). Further, as at neuromuscular junctions the synaptic vesicles are considered to represent quanta of transmitter substance, which during quiescence are released a few at a time and produce the miniature end-plate potentials. When an impulse arrives at a synapse, they are released in larger numbers and effect transmission (see Katz, 1966).

The chemical synapse is by far the most common type of synapse in the central nervous system of mammals. In addition, however, there is another type, the "electrical synapse." Such synapses are rare in mammals, but common both in lower vertebrates (see Figure 5–16) and invertebrates. At electrical synapses physiological studies indicate that a chemical transmitter is not released. Their most outstanding morphological feature is the gap junction, which provides close apposition between specialized patches in the pre- and postsynaptic membranes. The gap junction allows current to pass directly between adjacent cells, and since a

chemical transmitter is not involved, the synaptic delay is shorter than that associated with chemical transmission (see Bennett, 1972a and b).

Lastly, some examples have been found of synapses which display a series of different types of specialized junctions along the synaptic interface (see Figure 5–19). Some of the junctions are of the gap type, and others show the characteristics of chemical synapses. These types of association between pre- and postsynaptic membranes are considered to represent mixed areas of both chemical and electrical transmission, and accordingly have been designated as "mixed synapses."

The different styles of synapses will now be described in detail. Reviews of the fine structure of chemical synapses in the nervous system have been given by De Robertis (1959), Hager (1961), Whittaker and Gray (1962), Couteaux (1961 and 1963), Eccles (1964), Robertson (1965), Gray (1966), Gray and Guillery (1966), Pappas (1966), Palay (1967), Sotelo (1971a), Bodian (1972), and Pappas and Waxman (1972). An extensive and valuable review of the physiology and chemistry of chemical transmission has recently been published by Krnjevic (1974). Pfenninger (1973) has published a comprehensive survey of the cytochemistry of the synapse, with special emphasis on the several membranes thought to be involved in transmission.

In most cases the presynaptic element in a chemical synapse is an axon terminal, an enlargement or expansion of the axon that contains synaptic vesicles and mitochondria. Such axon terminals can occur either at the tips of axons, when they are termed *boutons terminaux*, or along the lengths of axons, when they are referred to as *boutons en passant*. Boutons terminaux are formed at the ends of both myelinated and unmyelinated axons. Myelinated axons either lose their myelin sheath just before the terminal expansion (Figure 5–3), or arborize into unmyelinated preterminal branches with expan-

---

Figure 5–5. **Axospinous Synapses, Cerebral Cortex.**

In the lower half of the field is a transversely sectioned dendrite (*Den*) with a short and stubby spine (*sp*). An axon terminal (*At*) with round, clear vesicles is forming an asymmetrical synaptic junction (*s*) with the spine. Two other well-oriented asymmetrical synaptic junctions (s_1 and s_2) between axon terminals (At_1 and At_2) and dendritic spines (sp_1 and sp_2) are also present, and one of these spines (sp_2) contains a spine apparatus (*sa*). Less well oriented asymmetrical axospinous synapses (s_3 and s_4) can be recognized by the presence of the postsynaptic density, as can a synapse (s_5) which has been sectioned parallel to the plane of the synaptic junction.
Rat visual cortex. × 70,000.

Micrograph by J. Saldanha.

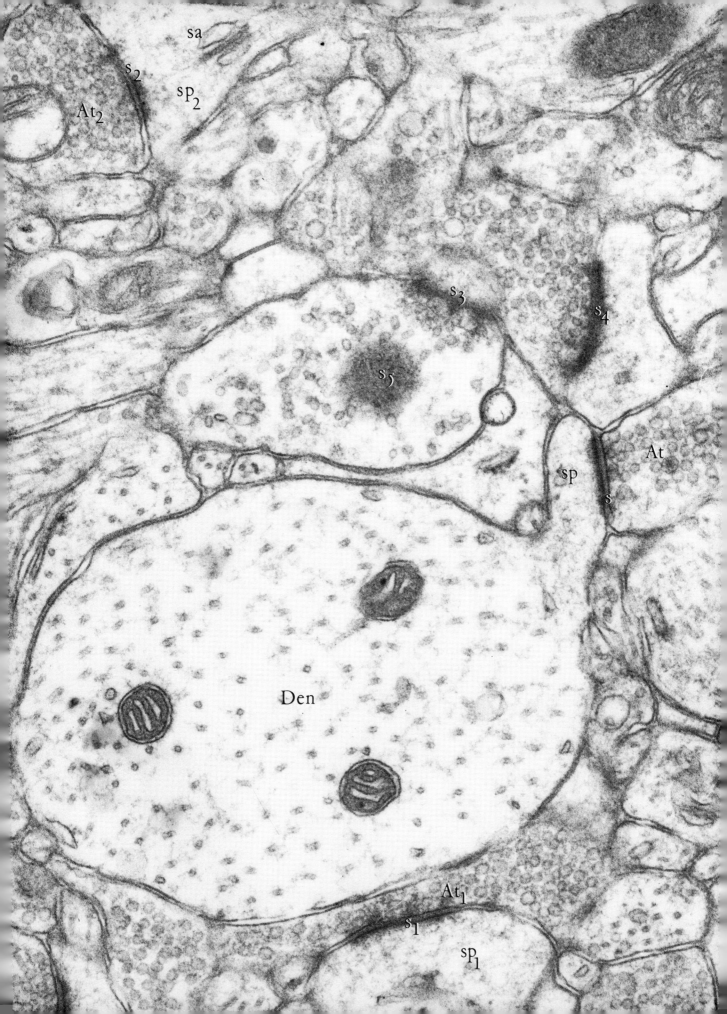

sions at their ends. *Boutons en passant* can occur in the course of unmyelinated axons (Figure 4–4) or at the nodes of Ranvier of myelinated axons (Figure 3–4).

Since an axon terminal can form a synapse with any part of the surface of another neuron, synapses in which an axon forms the presynaptic component may be designated as being

axo-dendritic (Figures 5–3 to 5–7 and 5–9),
axo-somatic (Figures 5–13 and 5–14), or
axo-axonal (Figure 5–15).

In recent years, however, it has become evident that the presynaptic component of a synapse need not necessarily be an axon terminal. Thus, there are now examples of synapses that occur between two dendrites (*dendro-dendritic*; Figures 3–7 and 5–16), between the perikarya of two neurons (*somato-somatic*), and between perikarya and dendrites (*somato-dendritic*). The identification of these structures as chemical synapses is based essentially on the fact that they resemble chemical synapses involving an axon. Specifically, the apposed plasma membranes of the two neuronal components lie parallel to each other but separated by a cleft, there is an associated density in the adjacent cytoplasm, and one of the components contains a concentration of synaptic vesicles close to the junctional specialization.

Morphologically, perhaps the least complex type of synapse is the one formed by an axon terminal and either the perikaryon of a neuron or a large dendritic trunk. This type of synapse is shown in Figure 5–3, which depicts a myelinated axon leaving its sheath and forming a terminal expansion attached to a large dendrite. Another example is depicted in Figure 5–4, in which a number of axo-dendritic synapses are shown. The structure of this type of synapse has been described in many different areas of the central nervous system (e.g., Gray, 1959 and 1961a; Palay, 1958b and 1967; De Lorenzo, 1961; Hamlyn, 1962; van der Loos, 1964; Peters and Palay, 1966; Mori, 1966). In such synapses the postsynaptic element is readily identifiable as either a neuronal perikaryon or a large dendrite. The presynaptic element is less readily identified unless it is seen to emerge from a myelin sheath (Figure 5–3) or to be an expansion of a clearly recognizable unmyelinated axon. Frequently though, continuity with known axons cannot be established in electron micrographs of thin sections. Then, the presynaptic component appears as an isolated oval profile flattened against the postsynaptic surface and containing large numbers of synaptic vesicles and a few mitochondria.

THE SYNAPTIC JUNCTION

The *synaptic junction* consists of the pre- and postsynaptic membranes, the densities associated with their cytoplasmic faces, and the synaptic cleft between them. An attempt to classify synapses on the basis of the form of the junction was first made by Gray (1959). He suggested that in the cerebral cortex there are two kinds of junctions: type 1 and type 2 (also see Whittaker and Gray, 1962). Type 2 junctions, which have just been described, were said to

Figure 5–6. **Asymmetrical Synapses, Cerebral Cortex.**

The **upper picture** shows two asymmetrical synapses (s_1 and s_2) between two axon terminals (At_1 and At_2) and the smooth dendrite (*Den*) of a stellate cell. At the synaptic junctions the pre- and postsynaptic membranes are separated by a cleft that contains intercellular material, and the postsynaptic membrane has a prominent coating of dense material on its cytoplasmic face.
Rat auditory cortex. × 100,000.

The **lower picture** displays a number of asymmetrical synapses formed between axon terminals and dendritic spines. One of the axon terminals (At_1) forms a synaptic junction with a single spine (sp_1), while to the right is an axon terminal (At_2) forming synapses with two spines (sp_2). On the left is a large axon terminal (At_3) synapsing with a large spine (sp_3). These two large profiles appear to form two synaptic junctions (*arrows*), but reconstructions have shown that such images are usually produced by the plane of section passing across a simple ring-like synaptic junction. Other synaptic junctions (s_1 and s_2) are more obliquely sectioned, and one junction (s_3) has been sectioned parallel to the plane of the participating membranes so that the postsynaptic density has the form of a disc.

Note the astrocytic covering (*As*) of the synapse between At_3 and sp_3.
Rat visual cortex. × 50,000.

Micrograph by J. Saldanha.

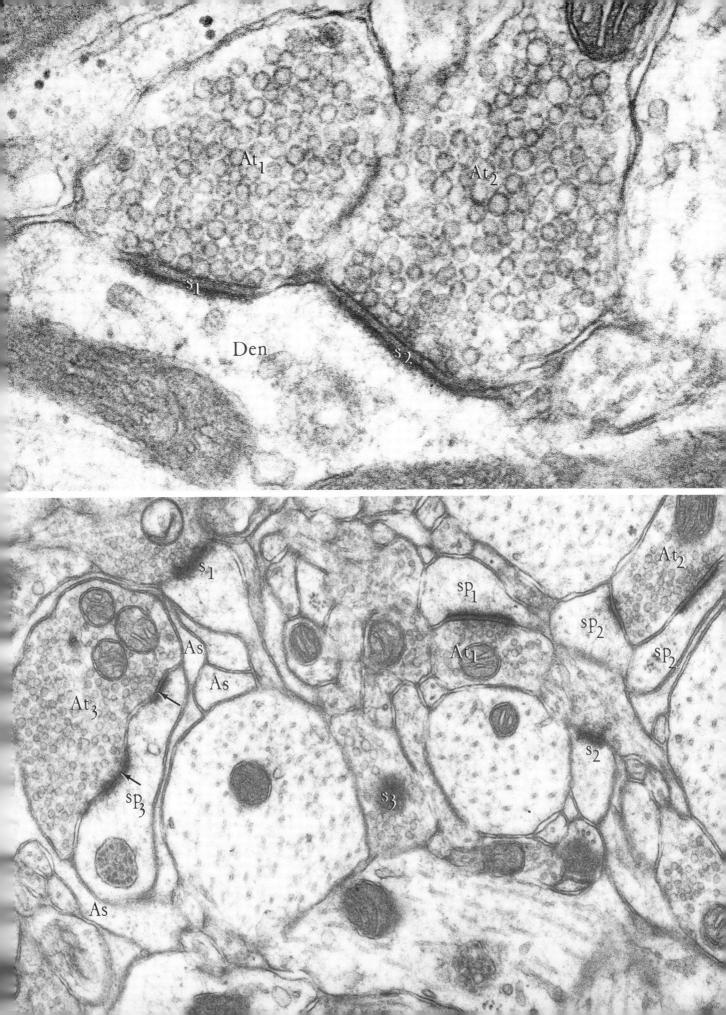

occur on both the dendritic trunks and perikarya of neurons (Figures 5–3, 5–4, and 5–9); the synaptic cleft is about 20 nm wide, and the dense regions of the junction are short and thin. Type 1 junctions, which occur on dendritic spines and on the shafts of the smaller dendritic branches, have a wider synaptic cleft, about 30 nm, that contains a plaque of dense extracellular material (Figures 5–5 to 5–7). In this type of synapse the junction may be extensive and there is a pronounced accumulation of dense material on the cytoplasmic face of the postsynaptic membrane which gives the type 1 junction a marked asymmetry.

Gray and Guillery (1966) have pointed out, however, that this classification is too rigid to apply to all synapses, for forms intermediate between types 1 and 2 occur in subcortical structures. In a later evaluation of the synapses of the cerebral cortex Colonnier (1968) came to the conclusion that the type 1 and the type 2 synapses represent the extremes of a morphological continuum, and he chose to refer to them as *symmetrical* and *asymmetrical* synapses. This is the nomenclature which will be adopted here, although the implication that these are the only morphological forms of synapses is clearly not intended. The terms are nevertheless useful, since they bring definite images to mind. No satisfactory expressions for the intermediate forms have yet been proposed.

In retrospect, it is also apparent that the disposition of the two types of synapse described by Gray (1959) pertains only to the pyramidal cells in the cerebral cortex. Thus, stellate neurons have both asymmetrical and symmetrical synapses on their perikarya, which in addition bear intermediate forms of synapse. These intermediate forms have a wide synaptic cleft with a long and straight junctional zone lacking a prominent postsynaptic density (Peters, 1971). Similar intermediate synapses are also present in the spinal cord (see Figure 5–4) and in the cerebellum (Palay and Chan-Palay, 1974).

Another example of an intermediate form of synapse is one described by Walberg (1964) in the inferior olive. This axo-dendritic synapse has a pronounced postsynaptic density that is not markedly thicker than the presynaptic density, and the synaptic cleft is rather narrow.

To anticipate what is to follow, it may be mentioned that in addition to the width of the synaptic cleft and the prominence of the postsynaptic density, asymmetrical and symmetrical synapses differ in the dimensions of the presynaptic grid and in the character of the synaptic vesicles in the presynaptic component (e.g., Figures 5–13 and 5–14). Consequently, the differences between these two types of synapses are more secure now than when they were first described.

The Presynaptic Grid

Gray (1963) has shown that when pieces of central nervous tissues are stained with phosphotungstic acid before they are embedded, both symmetrical and asymmetrical synapses exhibit a hexagonal array of dense particles attached to the cytoplasmic face of the presynaptic membrane. These particles are also occasionally visible in material stained with lead and uranyl salts (Figure 5–14, *arrows*). They are about 60 nm in diameter, with a center-to-center spacing of around 100 nm. The array of particles is readily shown in sections passing parallel to the plane of the synaptic junction. The particles are limited to those areas of the synaptic junction where vesicles aggregate, the so-called synaptic complexes.

The particles are also a prominent feature of the synaptic complex if the method of Bloom and Aghajanian (1966 and 1968c) is used to stain material. This method is essentially similar to that employed by Gray (1963) but omits the osmication of the material, so that ethanolic phosphotungstic acid is the only electron-dense staining chemical. Consequently, membrane-bound organelles such as mitochondria and synaptic vesicles are not visible. Since the synapses

---

Figure 5–7. **Purkinje Cell Dendrite.**

Extending down the middle of the field is the spiny branchlet of a Purkinje cell dendrite, whose cytoplasm contains mitochondria (*mit*) and cisternae of the smooth endoplasmic reticulum (*SR*). Two thorns (*t₁* and *t₂*) emerge from this dendrite, and passing down through the stalk of each thorn and into its bulb is a thin tubular extension of the smooth endoplasmic reticulum (*arrow*). Other thorns (*t*) in the surrounding neuropil appear as isolated profiles. The dendritic thorns form asymmetrical synapses with the axon terminals (*At*) of parallel fibers (*Ax*), and sometimes an axon terminal (*At₁* and *At₂*) may synapse with two thorns.

Passing between the neuronal elements in this field are the processes of Golgi epithelial cells (*As*).

Cerebellum of adult rat. × 19,000.

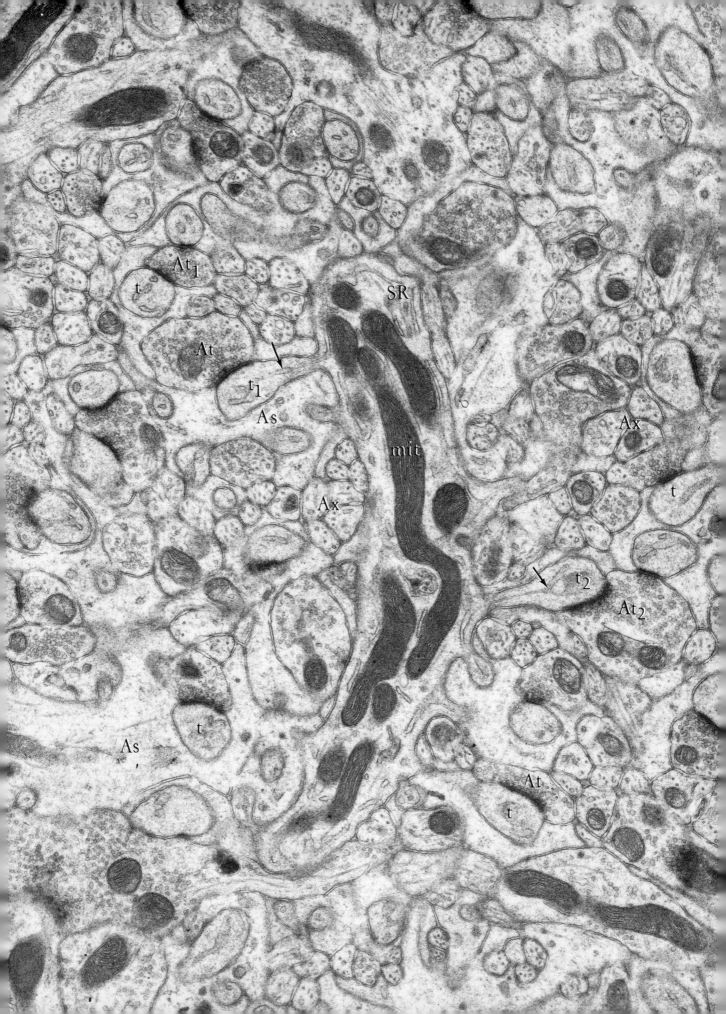

show up clearly and in isolation, Bloom and Aghajanian (1968c) and Lauder and Bloom (1975) have employed this stain for displaying and counting synapses during development. Bloom and Aghajanian (1968c) considered that since the ethanolic phosphotungstic acid selectively "stains" basic amino acids such as arginine, lysine, and histidine at low pH values, the presynaptic particles should be rich in these amino acids (see Bloom, 1972). Using this type of stain, Bloom (1972) describes the presence of one to ten particles or aggregates on the cytoplasmic face of a sectioned presynaptic membrane and states that each particle is 30 to 50 nm wide and separated from neighboring particles by an interval of 20 to 50 nm. In synapses viewed *en face*, that is, sectioned parallel to the synaptic cleft, the approximately hexagonal array described by Gray (1963) is apparent.

With this method the postsynaptic density appears as a dense band, or sheet, 10 to 25 nm wide, lining the cytoplasmic face of the postsynaptic membrane, and sometimes this shows thin wisps of material extending into the cytoplasm of the postsynaptic element. The method also displays a dense line in the middle of the synaptic cleft.

The most complete study of the structure of the presynaptic densities has been made by Akert and his colleagues (Pfenninger, Sandri,

Akert, and Engster, 1969; Akert and Pfenninger, 1969; Akert, Moor, Pfenninger, and Sandri, 1969; Akert, Pfenninger, Sandri, and Moor, 1972). Using small blocks of aldehyde-perfused tissue impregnated with bismuth iodide and poststained with uranyl and lead salts, these workers have explored the structure of the presynaptic grid. The grid consists of the dense particles described above arranged in a regular hexagonal or triagonal array in which they are evenly spaced in the plane of the presynaptic membrane. The particles project into the cytoplasm of the presynaptic element and are joined by filamentous cross bridges. As shown diagrammatically in Figure 5–8, the synaptic vesicles are located between the dense projections and in effect occupy the open spaces in the grid, so that each projection is surrounded by six vesicles. Akert and his colleagues refer to the whole assemblage of synaptic vesicles and dense projections as the "presynaptic vesicular grid." They point out that because of the hexagonal arrangement of the spaces around each dense projection, sections passing perpendicular to the presynaptic membrane may produce different images, depending on their orientation with respect to the grid. Thus, if the synaptic vesicles are seen to alternate regularly with the projections, as would be produced by a section passing through plane A in Figure 5–8, then a section 90

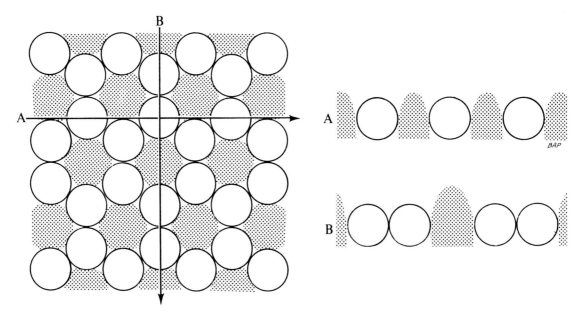

Figure 5–8.   **Presynaptic Grid.**

The left side of this diagram shows the *en face* view of the presynaptic grid in which the synaptic vesicles, represented as circles, lie between the dense projections (*stippled*). Sections passing perpendicular to this grid will produce different images depending upon their orientation. Thus, as shown on the right, a section passing in plane A will produce an image in which synaptic vesicles and densities alternate. Sections passing in plane B will produce images in which two contiguous synaptic vesicles alternate with each projection.

degrees to this plane would display two contiguous vesicles alternating with each projection. This second pattern is shown by the arrow B in Figure 5–8, and is depicted in B on the right. Gray (1966) has proposed that the dense projections may act as guides to ensure that the vesicles reach definite topographical loci at the synaptic junction. Akert, Pfenninger, Sandri, and Moor (1972) support this notion and raise the question of whether the number of spaces in the grid occupied by vesicles can be used to determine the state of activity of a synapse.

In freeze-etched preparations Akert, Pfenninger, Sandri, and Moor (1972) find small circular depressions on the A face of the presynaptic membrane. The spacing of these depressions which they term "synaptopores" seems to correspond to that of the holes in the presynaptic grid. Hence they raise the question as to whether these depressions, which in effect project into the cytoplasm of the presynaptic element, may be sites of attachment for synaptic vesicles. This point will be considered further when the appearance of freeze-fractured preparations of synaptic junctions is discussed under Freeze Fracturing (page 142).

During the development of synapses (Aghajanian and Bloom, 1967; Bloom, 1972) the dense projections appear to grow from small flattened patches, so that interconnected peaks are first apparent. Later the peaks separate into the densely stained, rounded and discrete projections of the mature form.

As mentioned, dense material also occurs at motor end-plates on striated muscle (Akert, Moor, Pfenninger, and Sandri, 1969; Heuser and Reese, 1973). In this case presynaptic material apparently forms strips opposite the mouths of the junctional folds indenting the surface of the muscle cell (see Figure 5–2).

The Synaptic Cleft

The synaptic cleft between the pre- and postsynaptic membranes is 20 to 30 nm wide and is not a free space, for it contains material binding these two membranes together. Thus, in preparations of synaptosomes, which are presynaptic terminals detached from their axons (see Gray and Whittaker, 1962; Whittaker, 1972), the postsynaptic membrane often remains attached to the presynaptic terminal. In fact this adhesion is the basis for a method for separating postsynaptic membranes in bulk from whole brains.

A dense, or intermediate plaque of intercellular material is often seen within the synaptic cleft (Figure 5–6) and this is usually more prominent in asymmetrical than in symmetrical synapses. A series of filaments appears to bridge the cleft. Van der Loos (1963 and 1964) and De Robertis (1962) consider that these filaments contribute to the intercellular plaque, some of them extending across the entire width of the cleft and others occupying only its postsynaptic portion (also see Cotman and Taylor, 1972). Van der Loos (1964) remarks that what appear to be filaments could represent small vertically oriented platelets.

The intercellular plaque shows up more frequently in material stained in the block with ethanolic phosphotungstic acid (Bloom, 1972), and in such material it is 5 to 10 nm thick. In their bismuth iodide–impregnated blocks, Akert and Pfenninger have shown two dense layers each about 6 nm thick in the synaptic cleft, separated from each other by a lighter zone 2 to 3 nm wide. The dense layers lie against the pre- and postsynaptic membranes, and in effect, they occupy the spaces on each side of the intercellular plaque. Consequently, the image is the reverse of that perceived in conventionally prepared material. At the edges of the synaptic cleft, the dense layers diverge and follow the surfaces of the pre- and postsynaptic components.

In a study of the chemical constituents of the synaptic cleft, Pfenninger (1971a and b) examined the effects of various solutions and enzymes on the appearance of the cleft in material primarily fixed with glutaraldehyde, osmicated, and then either stained with lead and uranyl salts or impregnated by the bismuth iodide technique. Used prior to fixation, enzymes such as trypsin and peptidase opened up the synaptic cleft, whereas they had no effect on material previously fixed with glutaraldehyde. There appear to be two components in the synaptic cleft, one being mainly acidic, uranyl positive and trypsin-labile, and the other being trypsin-resistant, with basic groups which react with bismuth iodide. Papain, pepsin, and pronase, on the other hand, produced a complete loss of material stainable by any method, so that the synaptic cleft appeared empty. Pfenninger (1971b) concluded that the synaptic cleft contains proteins, both acidic and basic, and that the cleft material may maintain the attachment between the pre- and postsynaptic membranes through a form of polyionic binding.

Although Pfenninger (1971b) was unable to split the pre- and postsynaptic components apart by exposure of unfixed tissue to solutions containing low concentrations of calcium ions, chelators, or sucrose, salt solutions of 2 molar concentration did lead to a dissociation of the synaptic components. In many cases thin strands, or filaments, seemed to extend across the synaptic cleft. These filaments were extremely thin, and Pfenninger (1971b) believes them to represent uncoiled macromolecules. He suggests that clumped together, the macromolecules may give rise to the thicker filaments described as crossing the synaptic cleft by van der Loos (1963 and 1964), De Robertis (1962), and Gray (1966).

It should be mentioned that trypsin prevents uranyl salts from staining the pre- and postsynaptic densities but does not prevent staining with bismuth iodide. Consequently, the cytoplasmic dense material seems to be like that in the synaptic cleft.

As shown by the use of silver methenamine (Rambourg and Leblond, 1967), which is regarded as a relatively specific technique for the detection of glycoprotein, extracellular spaces throughout the central nervous system contain glycoprotein, although it appears to be most concentrated in the synaptic clefts. Similarly, ruthenium red, which is considered to be a marker for mucopolysaccharides, is concentrated in the synaptic clefts (Bondareff, 1967). Tani and Ametani (1971) state that if the ruthenium red does not become too concentrated, the substance binding the dye can be seen to be arranged in a system of striations bridging the cleft.

Hence the synaptic clefts contain both proteins and mucopolysaccharides as does the glycocalyx on the surface of almost all cells. The presence of the intercellular plaque, however, and the differential effects of enzymes on the cleft material show that the substances are not homogeneously distributed in the cleft. Nor do the substances completely fill it, for it is open to penetration by lanthanum and horseradish peroxidase, like other extracellular spaces in the central nervous system (Brightman, 1967).

Furthermore, mention should be made of the possible presence of sialic acid in the cleft. This substance is present in quite large amounts in synaptosome fractions and is involved in sialoglycolipids and sialoglycoprotein, which appear to be important in synaptic transmission. These substances are able to bind transmitter molecules (Wesemann, Henkel, and Marx, 1971). Bondareff and Sjöstrand (1969) treated synaptosomes with neuraminidase, which releases sialic acid, and showed a decrease in the staining density of both the pre- and postsynaptic components, as well as the synaptic cleft material. Consequently, Bondareff and Sjöstrand (1969) suggest that at least some of the sialic acid occupies the cleft. Sialic acid also appears to be contained in the membrane of synaptic vesicles and other membranous components isolated from nerve terminals, as recently demonstrated by Marx, Graf, and Wesemann (1973).

Although definite evidence is lacking, it may be speculated that the synaptic cleft material has a specific composition and plays a role in intercellular recognition. If this is so, then the cleft substance would be important in the formation of synapses at specific sites on the surfaces of neurons. Additionally, if the molecules are filaments disposed across the intercellular cleft, as the results of Pfenninger (1971b) and others suggest, the substance could ensure a rapid movement of transmitter from the pre- to the postsynaptic membrane and interfere with diffusion away from the synapse.

Postsynaptic Densities

The characteristic morphological feature of the postsynaptic membrane is the accumulation of dense material on its cytoplasmic face. In con-

Figure 5–9. **An Axo-Dendritic Synapse, Anterior Horn.**

The sides of the picture are occupied by large dendrites (Den_1 and Den_2) of anterior horn cells, and in the interval between them are five terminals (At_1 to At_5). Each terminal contains synaptic vesicles (*sv*) and mitochondria (*mit*). The large terminal (At_1) synapses with both dendrites, and where the synaptic complexes (*arrows*) occur there is a slight widening of the gap between the pre- and postsynaptic membranes. At these synaptic complexes, vesicles are accumulated and the density is most prominent beneath the postsynaptic membrane. A *punctum adhaerens (triangle)* is also present at the synaptic junction on the left. This *punctum* has symmetrical densities and no clearly associated vesicles.

One of the other axon terminals (At_2) also synapses with the dendrite on the right, but the remaining terminals do not form obvious synaptic junctions. The suggestive densities marked by an asterisk (✱) near terminal At_4 cannot be interpreted because of the oblique plane of section.
Spinal cord from adult rat. $\times 44,000$.

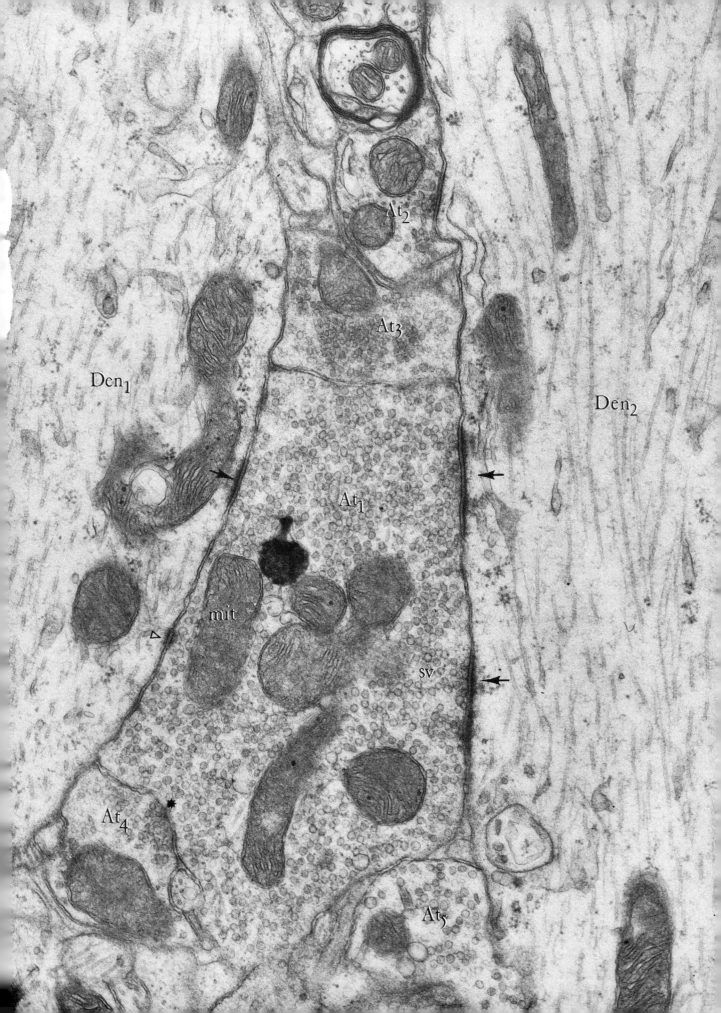

ventionally prepared tissues this postsynaptic density is more prominent than that of the presynaptic membrane, but morphologically it is much less complex. The postsynaptic density (Figures 5–5 and 5–6) is a relatively even sheet of somewhat granular material which seems to have filaments embedded in it, and as pointed out above, the accumulation of material is thicker and more prominent at asymmetrical than at symmetrical synapses. Filaments are sometimes apparent extending from the postsynaptic density, and these have been termed the postsynaptic web (De Robertis, Pellegrino de Iraldi, Rodriguez de Lores Arnaiz, and Salganicoff, 1961).

Reference to Figure 5–5 and the lower part of Figure 5–6 shows that at the smaller asymmetrical junctions the postsynaptic density has the form of a complete disc when viewed *en face* (Figures 5–5, s_5, and 5–6, s_3) or when reconstructed from serial sections (Peters and Kaiserman-Abramof, 1969). At larger junctions, however, the disc may be perforated and at the largest junctions, there may be two or three perforations. Thus, although only one postsynaptic density is usually present at an asymmetrical synapse, when a junction is viewed in sections passing perpendicular to the plane of the synaptic membranes, the existence of the perforations can result in images which show two or more, seemingly discontinuous, postsynaptic densities (Figure 5–6, *arrows*; Peters and Kaiserman-Abramof, 1969).

In symmetrical synapses the postsynaptic densities are disposed in a number of small, discrete patches (Figures 5–3, 5–4, and 5–9, *arrows*). The number of patches is variable and increases with the size of the synaptic interface. Interspersed with the densities of the synaptic complexes are *puncta adhaerentia* (Figures 5–3, 5–4, 5–9, and 5–13, *triangles*). These are usually smaller than the densities of the synaptic com-

plexes and as has been mentioned above, they seem to be purely adhesive structures and not sites for synaptic transmission.

A somewhat different type of postsynaptic density has been described by Sotelo (1971a) in the cerebellum of pleurodeles. This consists of a spherical cytoplasmic dense zone, which is formed of small vesicles, each about 10 nm in diameter, apparently embedded in a rather dense matrix, giving the whole structure an alveolate appearance.

In the habenular and interpeduncular nuclei, Milhaud and Pappas (1966a) described subsynaptic, or postjunctional, dense bodies beneath the postsynaptic density. These small dense bodies, each about 20 to 25 nm in diameter, are arranged in a hexagonal array to form a plate situated about 50 nm below the postsynaptic density. Each dense body consists of material resembling that of the postsynaptic density. Postsynaptic dense bodies occur at axo-somatic and axo-dendritic synapses, and Milhaud and Pappas (1966a) estimate that they were present in about one-third of the synapses they examined. When a spine is surrounded by synapses a single row of bodies forms a central axis to the spine. Such an assemblage has been termed a "crest synapse" by Akert, Pfenninger, and Sandri (1967) who studied them in the subfornical organ of the cat. Postjunctional dense bodies also occur in the lateral vestibular nucleus and cerebellar granular layer of the cat and rat (Milhaud and Pappas, 1966a and b; Palay and Chan-Palay, 1974; Jones, 1973) and in the lateral nucleus of the rat cerebellum (Chan-Palay, 1973g), as well as in the oculomotor nucleus of the chameleon, cat, and monkey (Waxman and Pappas, 1970), the pineal body of the ferret (David, Herbert, and Wright, 1973), and the trochlear nucleus of the cat (Bak and Choi, 1974). They are occasionally found in the superior colliculus of the rat (Lund, 1969). Like the

---

Figure 5–10. **The Synaptic Junction Between an Axon and a Dendritic Thorn.**

Near the center of the field of this freeze-fractured preparation an axonal varicosity (*At*) makes contact with a dendritic thorn (*t*). The varicosity, shown as a cross-fracture of the axoplasm, contains round synaptic vesicles (*sv*) and a mitochondrion (*mit*). The presynaptic face of the varicosity curves inward to match the dome-like configuration of the thorn, and the synaptic cleft is represented by the widened interspace between the two. The thorn is represented only by the B face of its plasmalemma, which displays an accumulation of membrane particles in the postsynaptic location, characteristic of excitatory synaptic junctions. A cross-fractured sheet of astroglial cytoplasm (*As*) encapsulates this synaptic pair.
Parallel fiber and Purkinje cell dendritic thorn in the molecular layer of the cerebellar cortex, adult rat. × 106,000.

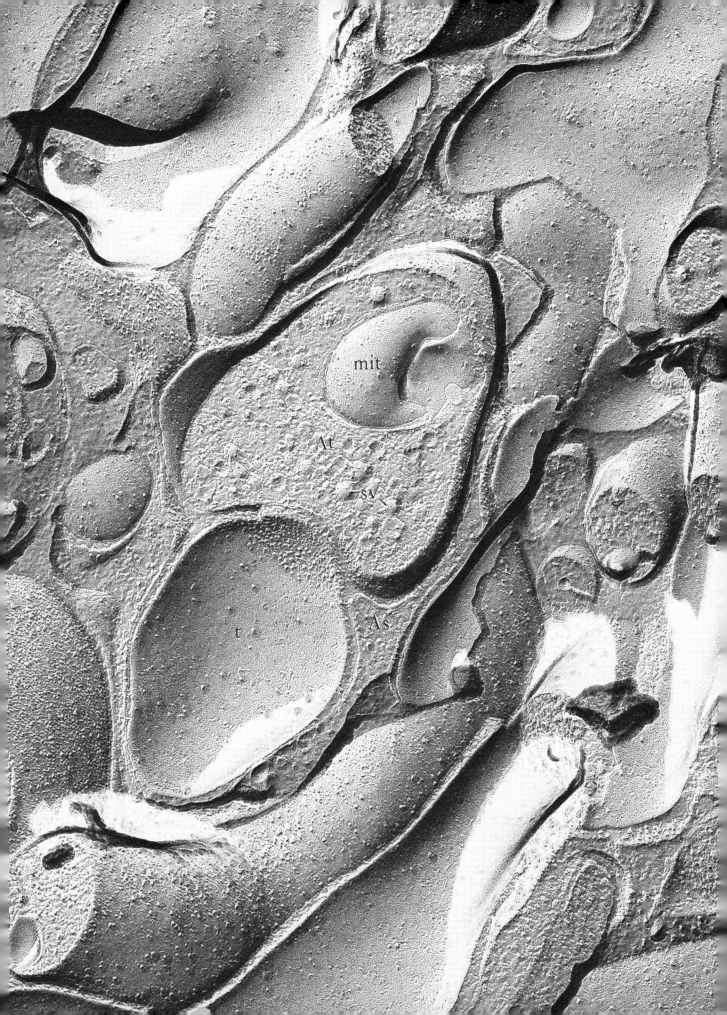

postsynaptic density, these subsynaptic dense bodies impregnate strongly with bismuth iodide (Akert, Moor, Pfenninger, and Sandri, 1969).

Taxi (1961 and 1964) has described a subsynaptic bar in the autonomic ganglia of amphibia. This structure (Figure 5–13, *arrowhead*) consists of one or two dense plaques, each about 40 nm thick, separated from each other by a distance of about 40 nm. In appearance the dense plaques resemble the postsynaptic density. Each plaque is slightly shorter than the one above it, so that in sections the whole apparatus, including the postsynaptic density, appears to have a triangular shape. It is of interest that the uppermost bar is separated from the postsynaptic density by about the same distance as are subsynaptic bodies and that sometimes the bars are discontinuous (Sotelo, 1968). Hence, the subsynaptic dense bodies and the bars are probably variations of the same structure. The possible relation between these structures and nematosomes is considered by Grillo (1970) and Le Beux (1972a).

The function of these subsynaptic structures is unknown, but if frog sympathetic ganglia are denervated (Sotelo, 1968) so that almost all the axon terminals disappear from the neuronal surface, the subsynaptic bars remain unchanged. A similar persistence of the subsynaptic dense bodies is reported by Lund (1969). Postsynaptic densities also persist for long periods after degeneration of axon terminals, and consequently the existence of the postsynaptic dense material appears to be relatively independent of the presence of presynaptic terminals, although the material almost certainly disappears eventually after loss of the presynaptic element.

Since the postsynaptic membrane receives presynaptic terminals over only part of its surface, it is a mosaic, and it can be assumed that those areas involved in the formation of synapses are also sites for the reception of neurotransmitters discharged by the presynaptic elements. Although densities whose concentration is consistent with the number of receptor sites have been described at neuromuscular junctions (Rosenbluth, 1973 and 1974), efforts to determine the locations of the receptors at interneuronal synapses have not been fruitful. The only difference between the interneuronal receptive areas and the remainder of the postsynaptic membrane is the presence of postsynaptic dense material. Attempts to localize receptor sites chemically are hampered by the difficulty of separating the postsynaptic from the presynaptic membrane, and the reader is referred to a discussion edited by Bloom, Iversen, and Schmitt (1970) for a further consideration of receptor sites.

Since the postsynaptic densities usually disappear when presynaptic elements are caused to degenerate following experimental lesions, it has been generally assumed that the existence of the postsynaptic density is dependent upon the presence of the presynaptic element. The study by Rakic and Sidman (1973a and b) of the cerebellum of the weaver mouse mutant indicates that the situation may be more complex. In this mutant almost all the granule cells die in the proliferation zone near the outer surface of the cerebellum. Hence, parallel fibers are almost completely lacking. Nevertheless, the spines of the Purkinje cell dendrites still develop, and each one displays a postsynaptic density. In this instance, then, the postsynaptic density is not dependent for its existence upon the presence of a presynaptic component, and this suggests that the dependence is only established after a synapse has been formed.

Figure 5–11. **The Presynaptic Membrane, A Face.**

A broad cross fracture of a mossy fiber terminal (*At*) occupies most of the field. Round synaptic vesicles (*sv*) are dispersed throughout this terminal along with a few mitochondria (*mit*) and occasional tubules of the endoplasmic reticulum (*SR*). The A face of the plasmalemma (*AlA*) of this terminal displays the usual large population of membrane particles. There are, however, clearings among them, in which arrays of small, round depressions or craters (*arrows*) appear. These depressions mark the mouths of synaptic vesicles, attached within the terminal to the plasmalemma and apparently opening onto its surface. A *double-headed arrow* in the right lower corner of the picture indicates a synaptic vesicle that is at the point of discharging onto the surface. The B (*AlB*) face of the plasmalemma presents the complementary appearance as is shown near the bottom of the picture. Here two fragments of the B face display the typical smooth surface from which small papules project, corresponding to the round depressions in the A face. The postsynaptic member of this synapse is shown as several cross-fractured dendrites (*Den*), containing mitochondria (*mit*) and cisternae of the endoplasmic reticulum (*SR*).

Mossy fiber rosette and granule cell dendrites composing a glomerulus in the granular layer of the cerebellar cortex, adult rat. × 88,000.

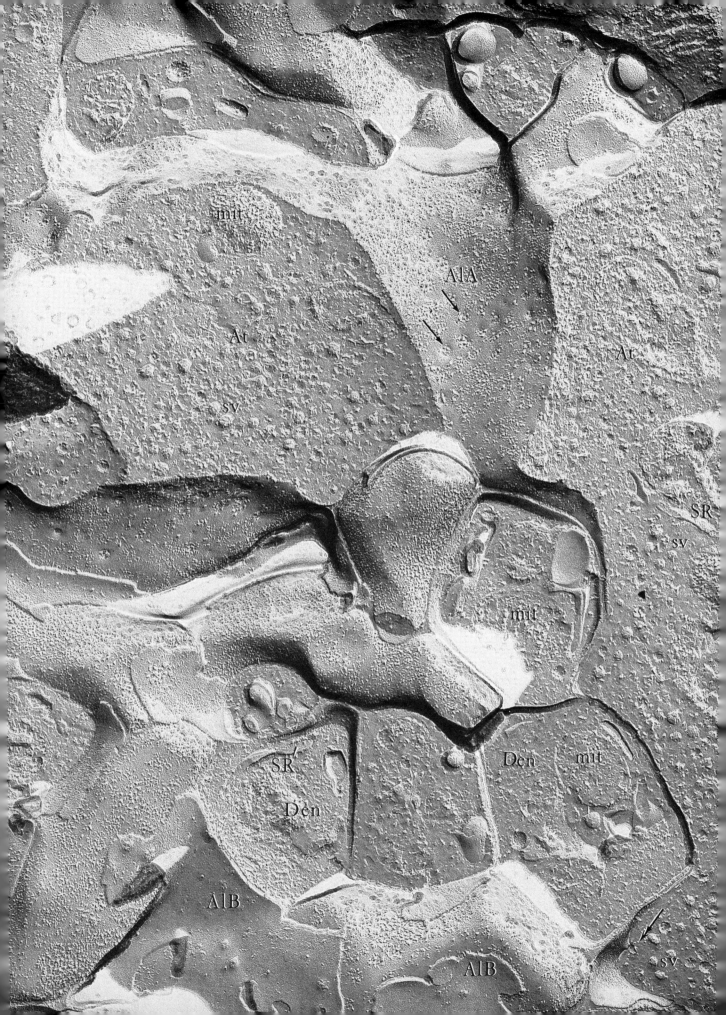

Sotelo (1973) has made the same observation in the weaver mouse mutant, and in addition has shown that some of these spines are contacted by axons with which they would not form synapses under normal conditions. Another mouse mutant, the staggerer mouse, is characterized by abnormal Purkinje cells lacking tertiary spine branchlets, so that the parallel fibers are unable to reach their usual presynaptic targets. In this mutant Sotelo (1973) has shown that a few of the axon terminals of the parallel fibers have a normal presynaptic morphology, although the axon faces a neuroglial process.

Gentschev and Sotelo (1973) also found unusual conditions to exist in the anterior ventral cochlear nucleus of the rat. In this nucleus primary deafferentation can lead to two different events. Some of the denervated postsynaptic sites are reoccupied not by collateral sprouting of axon terminals undamaged by the deafferentation but by nearby axon terminals that seem to move and so occupy the postsynaptic density. Other denervated postsynaptic sites become totally engulfed by the postsynaptic cytoplasm and eventually disappear.

Although the studies are still in their infancy, Cotman, Banker, Churchill, and Taylor (1974) have succeeded in isolating a subcellular fraction which is rich in postsynaptic densities. Analysis (Banker, Churchill, and Cotman, 1974) shows that this fraction contains 90 per cent protein in which two polypeptides predominate.

Freeze Fracturing

A number of investigators have examined the freeze-etched appearance of synapses in the central nervous system (Akert, Pfenninger, Sandri, and Moor, 1972; Pfenninger, Akert, Moor, and Sandri, 1972; Palay and Chan-Palay, 1974; Landis and Reese, 1974b; Landis, Reese, and Raviola, 1974), and basically their results are in agreement with one another. Hence their conclusions will be presented in a general fashion rather than in a chronological sequence.

At asymmetrical synapses a characteristic structure is seen in the postsynaptic membrane which shows a striking aggregation of particles, each 8 to 11 nm in diameter, attached to the B face, or external half of the membrane (Figure 5–10). This aggregation is matched by an array of pits in the complementary A face, or cytoplasmic leaflet of the same postsynaptic membrane. The presynaptic membrane of an asymmetrical synapse shows no similar specialization with respect to the particle distribution. There is some increase in number of particles, but basically it resembles the fracture surfaces of plasma membranes not involved in synapse formation. That is, the particles preferentially split with the A face. The A face of the presynaptic membrane is marked, however, by a series of small indentations (Figure 5–11, *arrows*) that are mirrored by protuberances on the B face (Figure 5–12, *arrows*). These protuberances often show a dimple or crater on their tops. Their form has been analyzed by Pfenninger, Akert, Moor, and Sandri (1972) who conclude that the protuberances represent sites of vesicle attachment rather than openings where synaptic vesicles are emptying into the synaptic cleft.

It should be mentioned that these vesicle attachment sites are more prominent in unanesthetized than in anesthetized animals (Streit, Akert, Sandri, Livingston, and Moor, 1972). In the lamprey spinal cord Pfenninger and Rovainen (1974) have found the number of sites to be increased also in tissue which has been incubated in solutions of high potassium content in the presence of calcium ions. It should be noted that, as pointed out earlier, the presence of calcium in the fixing solution also allows particles containing this cation to be seen at one site on the membrane of a synaptic vesicle (Politoff, Rose, and Pappas, 1974). Pfenninger and

Figure 5–12.   **The Presynaptic Membrane, B Face.**

Most of the field of this freeze-fractured preparation is occupied by a large mossy fiber terminal. The cross-fractured axoplasm (*At*) to the right and left of the figure contains many synaptic vesicles (*sv*) and mitochondria (*mit*). Large expanses of the B face (*AlB*) of the presynaptic plasmalemma are exposed by the fracture plane. As is usual, the B face is relatively free of membrane particles except on the summits of small papular projections (*arrows*), which correspond to the attachment sites of synaptic vesicles within the terminal. The ridge-like elevations in the contours of the B face are produced by granule cell dendrites passing beneath it. Several of these dendrites (*Den*) can be seen in the lower part of the picture.
Mossy fiber rosette and granule cell dendrites in the granular layer of the cerebellar cortex, adult rat. × 94,000.

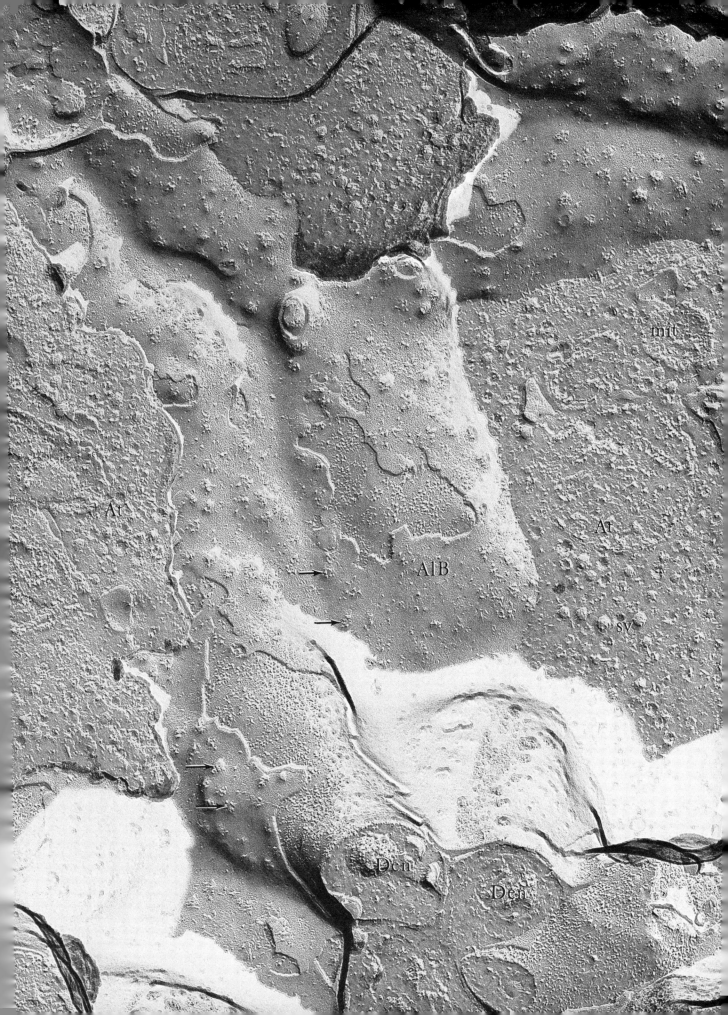

Rovainen (1974) found that electrical stimulation increases the number of vesicle attachment sites above control values.

As will be discussed later, there is good evidence that in some locations asymmetrical synapses are excitatory. One example is the asymmetrical synapse of the reciprocal pair of synapses in the olfactory bulb between the mitral cell dendrites and the gemmules of granule cells, and other examples occur in the cerebellum (Figures 5–10 to 5–12). These same two portions of the central nervous system also have well-defined symmetrical synapses, which are inhibitory. Making use of this knowledge of the location of symmetrical synapses, Landis and Reese (1974b) examined them in freeze-fractured preparations of the olfactory bulb, and Palay and Chan-Palay (1974) and Landis, Reese, and Raviola (1974) examined them in preparations of the cerebellar cortex. These studies both showed that unlike the asymmetrical synapses, the postsynaptic membranes of symmetrical synapses show no well-marked internal specializations. Again, however, the presynaptic membrane does show the presence of vesicle attachment sites. Thus, there is a difference in the distribution of particles in the postsynaptic membranes of symmetrical and asymmetrical synapses, but the significance of this difference is not yet apparent.

In anticipation of what is to be presented in the next section of this chapter, it may be stated that Palay and Chan-Palay (1974) and Landis, Reese, and Raviola (1974) also encountered some puncta adhaerentia in their studies of the cerebellum. These nonsynaptic junctions are each characterized by small circular patches of aggregated particles symmetrically disposed on the B faces of the participating membranes. The locations of these particle aggregates are marked by complementary groups of pits on the A faces of the fractured membranes.

NONSYNAPTIC JUNCTIONS BETWEEN NEURONS

As pointed out earlier, not all the junctional complexes between neurons and their processes have accumulations of synaptic vesicles associated with them. When synaptic vesicles are absent and a cleft is maintained between the apposed plasma membranes, then the junctional complex is considered to be purely adhesive and not a functional site for synaptic transmission. Such structures are termed *puncta adhaerentia* (see page 6).

Puncta adhaerentia occur widely throughout the central nervous system and are most prominent between adjacent astrocytes. As far as neuronal processes are concerned, they have been recorded between the following:

1. *Neighboring dendrites* (see Gray, 1961b; Palay, 1961b; Peters and Palay, 1966; Pappas, Cohen, and Purpura, 1966)
2. *Dendrites and axons* (see Hamlyn, 1962; Peters and Palay, 1966)
3. *Dendrites and somata* (see Gray and Guillery, 1966; Pappas, Cohen, and Purpura, 1966)
4. *Adjacent somata* (see Shofer, Pappas, and Purpura, 1964)
5. *Axon terminals and initial segments of axons* (see Westrum, 1966; Palay, Sotelo, Peters, and Orkand, 1968; Peters, Proskauer, and Kaiserman-Abramof, 1968)
6. *Neuronal processes and astrocytes* (Sotelo, 1971a)
7. *Axon membranes and their surrounding sheaths*

Although puncta adhaerentia are considered to be simple points of attachment, it is not uncommon for them to occur at interneuronal interfaces characterized by symmetrical synaptic junctions as well (Figures 5–3, 5–4, 5–9, and 5–13, *triangles*). Thus Hamlyn (1962) showed puncta in the hippocampus of the rabbit between the terminals of mossy fibers and dendrites at the bases of dendritic spines projecting into them.

Gray and Guillery (1966) have demonstrated puncta in the spinal cord of cat, and they seem to be common at synaptic junctions in the spinal cord of the rat (Figures 5–3, 5–4, and 5–9). A similar intermingling of synaptic complexes and puncta also occurs at the junctional interfaces between large axon terminals and dendrites in the lateral geniculate body of the cat (Figure 11–4; Peters and Palay, 1966) and in the lateral vestibular nucleus of the rat (Figure 5–19; Sotelo and Palay, 1968).

Interesting forms of puncta adhaerentia appear in the synaptic glomeruli of the lateral geniculate body of the cat (e.g., Peters and Palay, 1966; Guillery, 1967). The glomeruli are closely packed groups of axons and dendrites dispersed in the neuropil of laminae A and A_1. Between the plasma membranes of adjacent dendrites the puncta often occur in a series. They are symmetrical structures with many filaments inserted into thick dense plaques on the cytoplasmic aspects of the membranes. When one of the processes contributing to the adhesion is an axon, then a somewhat different appearance obtains. Now the punctum is asymmetrical. The asymmetry occurs because, although the dendritic side of the junction has many filaments associated with it, the axonal side is devoid of filaments and the plaque of dense material beneath the axonal plasma membrane is thin. Similar forms of puncta also appear in the glomeruli in the lateral geniculate body of the monkey (Colonnier and Guillery, 1964) and in the midthalamic nuclei of the cat (Pappas, Cohen, and Purpura, 1966; Pappas, 1966).

SYNAPTIC VESICLES WITH CLEAR CENTERS

Shapes and Sizes of Vesicles

The most commonly occurring synaptic vesicles are 40 to 50 nm in diameter. They have clear centers or agranular contents, and with few exceptions (e.g., Fukami, 1969) in tissues fixed primarily with osmic acid or potassium permanganate, they are roughly spherical. Such vesicles are found in nerve terminals at neuromuscular junctions (Figure 5–2), in some sympathetic nerve endings and throughout the central nervous system (e.g., Figures 5–3 to 5–9). At present it is not absolutely certain that these vesicles contain transmitter substances since no histochemical techniques have yet been devised that allow direct visualization of such chemicals in electron micrographs. There is, however, strong circumstantial evidence, based upon studies of fractions from homogenates of brain tissue, which indicates that at least some of these clear vesicles contain acetylcholine (see De Robertis, Rodriguez de Lores Arnaiz, Salganicoff, Pellegrino de Iraldi, and Zieher, 1963; Whittaker, 1965, 1969, and 1972; Whittaker, Michaelson, and Kirkland, 1964; De Robertis, 1967; Whittaker and Zimmerman, 1974).

While it is generally assumed that acetylcholine is the transmitter associated with agranular vesicles, especially in the motor end-plates, it is becoming apparent that nerve terminals containing such vesicles may have other transmitters in them. For example, in experiments using tritiated γ-aminobutyric acid ([³H]GABA), which is known to be an important inhibitory transmitter in the central nervous system, Iversen and Bloom (1972) found it to be localized in nerve terminals with agranular vesicles. In homogenates these nerve terminals constituted 13 per cent of those from the cerebellum and 42 per cent of those from the hippocampus and showed no unusual features. Tritiated glycine, which is another inhibitory chemical, was taken up by a different set of boutons in homogenates used by Iversen and Bloom (1972). Matus and Dennison (1971) found tritiated glycine to be associated with boutons containing flattened agranular vesicles in studies using slices of spinal cord. On the other hand, in the rat retina, tritiated GABA was associated with Müller fibers, which are cytoplasmic processes of astrocytes (Neal and Iversen, 1972).

In the past few years, attention has been drawn to variations in both the size and shape of clear vesicles (see Figures 5–4, 5–13 and 5–14). For example, Lenn and Reese (1966) have shown that some terminals in the ventral cochlear nucleus contain clear vesicles with a mean diameter of 40 nm, whereas others have vesicles of 45 nm. Lenn and Reese (1966) interpreted these measurements to indicate that the nerve endings with the smaller vesicles are associated with inhibitory afferent terminals (also see McDonald and Rasmussen, 1971). Somewhat similar conclusions have been reached by Larramendi, Fickenscher, and Lemkey-Johnston (1967), who measured the sizes of synaptic vesicles in axon terminals in the cerebellum. The axon terminals they assume to be excitatory contain larger vesicles than those considered to be inhibitory in function. Moreover, these investigators find that vesicles become smaller with age. In the cerebellum of the Syrian hamster, on the other hand, Duncan, Morales, and Benignus (1970) found differences in the sizes of synaptic vesicles in four different locations, but they were not able to correlate these size differences with the form of the synaptic junction or with the neuronal components taking part in the synapses.

The results of these studies may be equated with those of Akert, Pfenninger, Sandri, and Moor (1972), who examined freeze-etched nerve endings in the spinal cord of the monkey and cat both in aldehyde-fixed material and in unfixed tissue. They also find two populations of spherical vesicles in the nerve terminals. One has a mean size of 39 nm and the other 48 nm. From the dimensions of the presynaptic grids present in the terminals (see page 132), Akert, Pfenninger, Sandri, and Moor (1972) conclude that the larger vesicles are present in the axon terminals forming asymmetrical synapses and the smaller vesicles in the terminals forming symmetrical (type 2) synapses.

Although primary fixation with osmic acid produces essentially round vesicles, the expanded use of aldehydes for primary fixation has brought to light vesicles variously described as elongate, flattened, or ellipsoidal (see Figures 5–13 and 5–14) in different areas of the central nervous system (e.g., Walberg, 1965a; Uchizono, 1965 and 1973; Bodian, 1966a and b; Lund and Westrum, 1966; Gray, 1969b; Price and Powell, 1970a; Chan-Palay, 1973f; Palay and Chan-Palay, 1974). These elongate vesicles are usually described as being about 20 nm wide and 50 nm long, although the extent of elongation depends largely upon the type of axon terminal being examined and the osmolarity of the fixative employed. Thus, Bodian (1970a and 1975) has shown that in the monkey spinal cord there are terminals (S bulbs) which contain spherical vesicles with a resistance to flattening or elongation and other terminals (F bulbs) that flatten readily after aldehyde perfusion followed by osmication. In addition, there are other axon terminals (L and R bulbs) which show an intermediate sensitivity to flattening, for while such vesicles do not usually flatten and are rather irregularly rounded, they can be induced to flatten if tissue is washed in an appropriate buffer before osmication.

More recently, Valdivia (1971) carried out a systematic study of the effect of different parameters upon the shapes of clear synaptic vesicles in the axon terminals of the cerebellum of the rat. In effect, he found that when aldehydes are used as primary fixatives, there are three forms of vesicles: small round vesicles less than 40 nm in diameter, large round vesicles with diameters of 40 to 50 nm, and flat vesicles measuring 50 to 60 nm by 25 nm (see Figure 5–14). While different types of axon terminals showed distinctive vesicle populations in terms of these three forms, the proportion of each form present basically depended upon the osmolarity of the fixative. Valdivia (1971) also found that the concentration of aldehydes and the length of fixation and dehydration have no effect on vesicle shape. However, if the osmolarity of the buffer solution containing the aldehydes used for fixation, or that of the solution used to wash the specimens before osmication, is increased, the formation of flattened vesicles is favored. Thus, axon terminals such as those of the parallel fibers (Figure 5–7) and mossy fibers have a predominant population of rounded vesicles and few flattened vesicles under any conditions. In contrast, the terminals of the basket cell axons and of the Golgi cell axons in the glomeruli contain significant numbers of flattened vesicles, and the number is increased by increasing the osmolarity of the buffer or of the washing solution.

A similar result was obtained by Korneliussen (1972b) in a study of the synaptic vesicles in the motor end-plates of the rat diaphragm. In standard preparations fewer than 10 per cent of the vesicles are elongate, the remainder being spherical. But the proportion of flattened vesicles can be increased to as much as 50 per cent by increasing the molarity of the buffer solution containing the aldehydes used for fixation, or by increasing the molarity of the solution used for washing tissue prior to osmication. Hence the vesicles are osmotically sensitive and change shape both during and after fixation with aldehydes. The reason for this is that aldehydes do not stabilize membranes (see Bone and Denton, 1971). However, fixation in osmic acid renders them no longer sensitive.

Differences in the size and shape of synaptic vesicles and their response to either osmic acid or aldehyde fixation are also emphasized by Nakajima (1974), who studied the synaptic terminals on the Mauthner cell of the goldfish. Nakajima's article should be consulted for details of the distribution of the various types of terminals on the Mauthner cells, since only a

---

Figure 5–13. **Axo-Somatic Synapses.**

In the bottom right of the picture is part of the perikaryon of a neuron which forms synapses with three axon terminals (*At₁* to *At₃*). One of these terminals (*At₂*) contains spherical synaptic vesicles (*sv*), while the lower terminal (*At₁*) contains predominantly ellipsoidal synaptic vesicles (*sv₁*). The synaptic complexes (*arrows*) formed between the plasma membranes of the perikaryon and the axon terminals are symmetrical. At other locations the lower axon terminal (*At₁*) is involved in the formation of a punctum adhaerens (*triangle*), and the middle terminal (*At₂*) has a junction (*arrowhead*) that appears to have no synaptic vesicles associated with it but shows an asymmetrical density beneath which is a dense plaque resembling a subsynaptic bar.

These axon terminals are enclosed by astrocytic processes (*AsP*).

Ventral cochlear nucleus of adult rat. × 60,000.

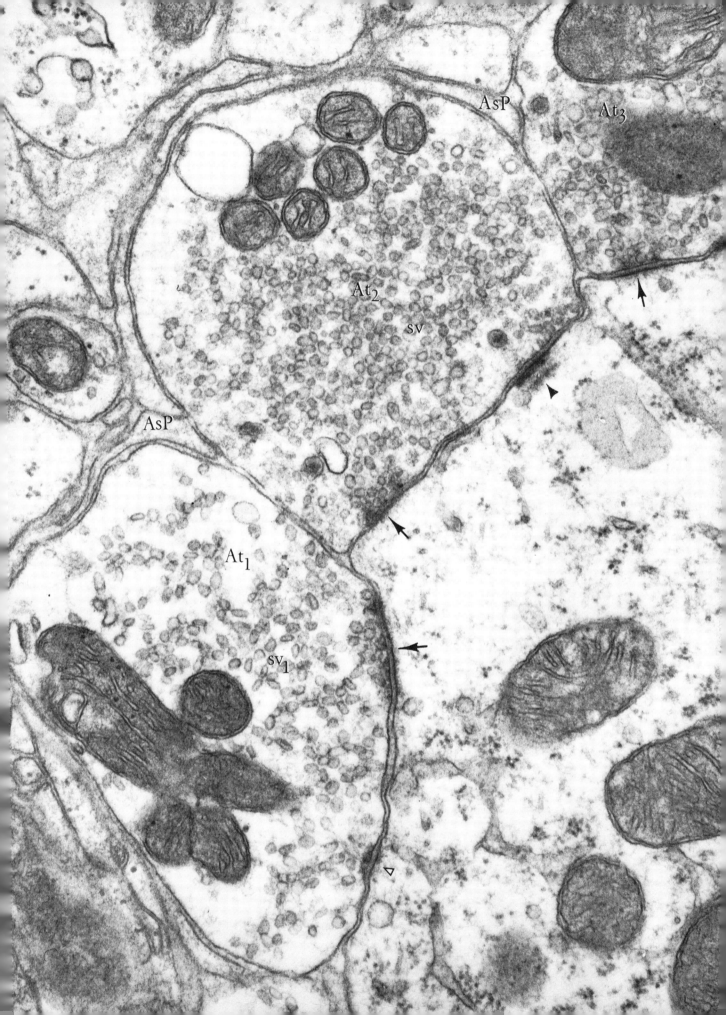

summary will be presented here. Some terminals, such as the club endings issuing from myelinated axons, have large spherical vesicles, 46 to 48 nm in diameter, whose shape and size are not altered by the fixative. Much smaller vesicles occur in other terminals. These vesicles are 40 nm in diameter in osmic acid–fixed material. They are spherical but become elongate after aldehyde fixation. A third type of vesicle is seen in the spiral fiber endings on the initial segment of the Mauthner cell. This medium-sized vesicle is 42 nm in diameter and remains spherical in all fixatives. In contrast, the vesicles in the unmyelinated club endings are also 42 nm in diameter and spherical in osmic acid–fixed material, but they become elongate after aldehyde fixation.

Dennison (1971) stereoscopically examined the clear synaptic vesicles in the goldfish spinal cord and in the rat olfactory bulb. The tissue was perfused with solutions containing a mixture of formaldehyde and glutaraldehyde, and after a brief wash it was postfixed in osmic acid. Some of the tissue was impregnated with zinc iodide–osmic acid according to the method of Kawana, Akert, and Sandri (1969) to render the vesicles opaque. In boutons of the goldfish spinal cord, Dennison (1971) found that in addition to the round or spherical vesicles, there are both cylindrical and disc-shaped vesicles. In the rat olfactory bulb, however, she found no cylindrical vesicles but only those which were spherical and disc-shaped.

It is surprising that synaptic vesicles do not simply swell or shrink in aldehyde solutions of different tonicities, and that some assume discoidal or cylindrical shapes when the tonicity of the solution is increased. This may mean that the surface area of the vesicle membrane cannot alter, even though the contents of the vesicles change in volume. However, no data are available for this calculation, and even if this assumption is correct, it does not explain why some vesicles form discs and others cylinders.

It is interesting that in freeze-fractured material, whether previously fixed in aldehydes or unfixed, synaptic vesicles in all types of nerve terminals prove to be spherical (Akert, Pfenninger, Sandri, and Moor, 1972; Palay and Chan-Palay, 1974; Landis and Reese, 1974b; see Figures 5–10 to 5–12). This observation suggests that primary osmic acid fixation preserves the native shape of the vesicles whereas initial fixation in aldehydes permits subsequent alterations in their shapes. However, the change in shape is not caused by the aldehydes but, as Valdivia

(1971), Korneliussen (1972b) and others have shown, is influenced by the osmolarity of the salt solution in which the fixative is dissolved, or the buffer used for washing the tissue afterward. The altered shape is then stabilized by the subsequent stage of postfixation in osmium tetroxide. The nonspherical shape of the vesicles after these fixatives is, then, an artifact of the method of preparation. But since only vesicles of certain presynaptic terminals are affected, the change must depend upon some specific property of these nerve endings. The consistency of this change permits the neurocytologist to use the shape of the vesicles in differentiating among synaptic terminals of different origins.

Other factors affecting the form of vesicles have been reported. Thus, Akert, Cuénod, and Moor (1971) showed that synaptic vesicles enlarge during the initial phases of Wallerian degeneration in the tectum of the pigeon. Similar results have also been reported for degenerating axons terminals in the caudate nucleus of the rat (Kawana, Akert, and Bruppacher, 1971), spinal trigeminal nucleus of the cat (Westrum, 1973), and lateral geniculate nucleus of the cat and monkey (Lloret and Saavedra, 1975). In the latter study, it has been shown that the vesicles increase their volumes by as much as 280 per cent. Whether this enlargement is a common and reliable indication of early degeneration has yet to be established.

The reasons for this swelling have not been elucidated, but most likely it can be attributed to nonspecific permeability changes in the membrane of the nerve ending which make the contents of the ending more hypotonic.

In another study of the retinotectal system of the pigeon, Cuénod, Sandri, and Akert (1972) reported that intraocular injection of colchicine induced the appearance of enlarged synaptic vesicles, two or three times larger than normal, in the optic terminals in the tectum.

Correlation Between Vesicle Shape and Function of Chemical Synapses

Eccles and his coworkers have attempted to correlate the types 1 and 2 synaptic junctions of Gray (1959) with different functions (Andersen, Eccles, and Voorhoeve, 1963; Eccles, 1964; Andersen and Eccles, 1965). Their early results suggested that type 1 (asymmetrical) junctions are excitatory and type 2 (symmetrical) junctions are inhibitory. As discussed in the previous section, other studies have shown that the axon terminals forming these two types of junction also differ in respect of the shapes of the synaptic vesicles. For the most part, after aldehyde fixation, the presynaptic components of asymmetrical synapses contain only round vesicles (see Figures 5–5 to 5–7) and those of symmetrical synapses contain some elongate or flattened vesicles (see Figures 5–4, 5–13, and 5–15) (e.g., Uchizono, 1965; Bodian, 1966a; Lund and Westrum, 1966; Walberg, 1966b; Valdivia, 1971). This correlation prompted speculation that the shapes of the synaptic vesicles could be used as a better guide to the functions of synapses than the form of the junction. Thus it was proposed that axon terminals containing round vesicles are excitatory and those containing elongate vesicles are inhibitory. Uchizono (1965, 1967, 1968, 1969), in particular, produced evidence in favor of this concept. He noted that terminals in the cerebellar cortex containing round vesicles synapse on the dendritic spines of Purkinje cells (Figure 5–7), whereas terminals containing elongate vesicles synapse upon the perikarya. He correlated his results with the evidence derived from physiological studies of the cerebellar cortex (Andersen, Eccles, and Voorhoeve, 1963) which showed that the fibers ending on the Purkinje cell spines are excitatory, while the endings around the cell bodies of the Purkinje cells are inhibitory. Uchizono (1967) also showed that inhibitory components in the stretch receptors of the crayfish muscle have elongate vesicles. Other arguments in favor of this concept have been put forward by Bodian (1966a). He found that in the developing neuropil of the monkey spinal cord, synaptic bulbs with round vesicles appear initially, when the first reflexes can be elicited, and presynaptic terminals with elongate vesicles only occur later, when inhibitory inputs develop (also see Bodian, 1970b). Gray (1969a and b) also considers that his studies on the distribution of flattened and rounded vesicles support the concept.

Although acceptance of this hypothesis correlating the form of synapses with excitatory and inhibitory functions is very tempting, the final evidence in favor of it must come from morphological studies of neuronal systems in which the necessary physiological evidence is available. The number of such systems presently available is rather limited. Strongly suggestive evidence is certainly forthcoming from studies of the cerebellar cortex, in which, for example, the climbing fibers are known to be excitatory. Larramendi and Victor (1967) were the first to recognize the terminals of climbing fibers (in the mouse),

which they showed to be full of spherical synaptic vesicles. This conclusion has been confirmed in a number of forms, including fish (Kaiserman-Abramof and Palay, 1969), frog (Sotelo, 1969), rat (Chan-Palay and Palay, 1970; Palay and Chan-Palay, 1974), and cat (Mugnaini, 1972; Sotelo, 1971a). As all these authors, among others, have shown, the climbing fibers synapse with thorns projecting from the large Purkinje cell dendrites with which they effect Gray's type 1 synaptic junctions, thus providing corroboration for the correlations suggested by Uchizono.

In a recent study of the hippocampus and the dentate gyrus of the rat and cat, Gottlieb and Cowan (1972) correlated the appearance of presynaptic terminals containing either flattened or rounded vesicles with the physiologically known properties of these regions. They found that most of the terminals on the pyramidal cell somata where there is a focus of postsynaptic inhibition contain flattened vesicles. Conversely, in regions containing the terminations of the extrinsic, commissural, and long association pathways which are excitatory, virtually all of the presynaptic terminals contain rounded vesicles. These authors point out, however, that terminals containing rounded vesicles also form axo-somatic synapses, but those with flattened vesicles predominate. Also Gottlieb and Cowan (1972) find that some terminals containing round vesicles form axo-somatic synapses which are symmetrical. Gottlieb and Cowan (1972) concluded that their study supports the correlation of vesicle shape with function, at least in the hippocampal formation.

Additional support for the concept seems to come from a study by Matus and Dennison (1971). Since glycine is thought to be an inhibitory transmitter at some synapses in the spinal cord (see Curtis, 1969; Hebb, 1970; Krnjevic, 1974), these authors soaked pieces of the lumbosacral spinal cord of rats in tritiated glycine. In electron microscopic autoradiographs, there was an accumulation of grains repeatedly associated with terminals containing flattened vesicles. Although not all terminals containing flat vesicles had grains associated with them, no grains above background frequency were ever present over boutons with round vesicles.

It is unfortunate that an acetylcholine reaction has not been devised and used in a similar fashion to show what kinds of boutons contain this transmitter. That there is no correlation between vesicle shape and acetylcholinesterase activity is shown in a study of the cochlear nucleus by McDonald and Rasmussen (1971). They found that some terminals containing round and others containing flattened vesicles have the enzyme reaction product covering their limiting membranes.

Problems associated with the correlation of presynaptic terminals containing flattened vesicles with inhibition and those containing rounded vesicles with excitation are as follows:

In the cuneate nucleus, Walberg (1966a) found that axons belonging to the pyramidal tract, which is excitatory, contain elongate vesicles. Some elongate vesicles are also present in motor end-plates of the rat diaphragm. These synapses are excitatory, and as pointed out earlier, the proportion of elongate vesicles can be altered by adjusting the molarity of the fixing solution (Korneliussen, 1972).

Although the specific localization of the inhibitory transmitter γ-aminobutyric acid (GABA) in tissue sections is difficult, McLaughlin, Wood, Saito, Barber, Vaughn, Roberts, and Wu (1974) have developed a promising antibody technique. In a study of the cerebellum they have shown that this transmitter is present in basket cell endings and in Golgi cell endings in the glomeruli. In conventional preparations, however, the basket cell endings have mainly rounded synaptic vesicles intermixed with only a few that are flattened, while the Golgi cell terminals in the glomeruli have mainly flattened vesicles.

One of the obvious corollaries of the basic hypothesis is that the difference in shape of vesicles corresponds to a difference in the kind of transmitter they contain. What this means when applied to axon terminals which contain both spherical and elongate vesicles, or disc-shaped as opposed to cylindrical vesicles, is far from obvious at present. For if the shapes of vesicles can be correlated with postsynaptic excitation or inhibition, then terminals with a mixture of vesicles could presumably exercise both functions and release two kinds of transmitter substance. Also, the existence of cylindrical and disc-shaped vesicles must lead to the assumption that elongate vesicles with these two different shapes contain different inhibitory transmitters. It is conceivable, of course, that the appearance of a mixture of vesicle shapes in a presynaptic terminal could be the result of a graded response to a fixative (Bodian, 1972; Valdivia, 1971; Korneliussen, 1972b). Even on the basis of this possibility, however, it would still be necessary to show inhibitory transmitters in vesicles that tend to elongate and excitatory transmitters in those that tend to maintain a spherical shape. Additionally, it must be assumed that the postsynaptic effects of a given transmitter are always the same, but it is clear from neurophysiology that the response elicited by presynaptic stimulation is a complex result of the interaction between the transmitter and the postsynaptic cell. Indeed, the same transmitter may induce different results in different locations. For example, acetylcholine is excitatory in sympathetic ganglia and inhibitory at the postganglionic terminations in the heart.

There is the problem of synapses which are intermediate, not only in the form of the vesicles, but in the form of the synaptic junction. And added to this is the rare finding that two different synaptic interfaces formed by the same presynaptic terminal may have different features, one being asymmetrical and the other symmetrical (Palay, 1967; Mugnaini, 1970; Sotelo, 1971a). In addition, as Kane (1974) has recently shown, ablation of the cochlea in the cat brings about degeneration of both boutons which contain spherical vesicles and form asymmetrical synaptic junctions, and boutons which contain pleomorphic populations of vesicles and form symmetrical synaptic junctions. In the cochlear nucleus this author claims that a single axon can apparently form both of these bouton types, and so on the basis of the hypothesis relating structure of synapses to their function, the implication would be that the same axon might form both excitatory and inhibitory axon terminals.

Consequently, while attempts to correlate synaptic function with either the morphology of the synaptic vesicles or the form of the synaptic junction must be pursued, at present it is premature to draw general conclusions. It is hoped that morphological features of synapses will one day allow statements about function to be made, but many more carefully correlated studies must be carried out before this goal can be attained.

Morphological Aspects of the Dynamics of Synaptic Activity

As pointed out in the discussion of the motor end-plate, there is a good deal of evidence to support the idea that synaptic vesicles recycle at the motor nerve endings, but for interneuronal synapses the events that take place during synaptic activity are less well documented. However, as early as 1957 De Robertis and Vaz Ferreira noted that stimulation of the splanchnic nerve of the rabbit at a rate of 100 stimuli per second led to an increase in the number of synaptic vesicles in axon terminals in the adrenal medulla. A decrease in their number only occurred at higher rates of stimulation. On the other hand Perri, Sacchi, Raviola, and Raviola (1972) recently showed that in the superior cervical ganglion stimulation of the preganglionic fibers for 3½ hours leads to a reduction in the numbers of agranular vesicles in the nerve endings. Furthermore, although the synaptic vesicles are initially distributed evenly throughout the nerve endings, the loss caused by prolonged stimulation is most prominent in those parts of the endings that are most distant from the synaptic junction. They take this to suggest that there is a movement of vesicles toward the presynaptic membrane during synaptic activity. A loss of vesicles during stimulation of terminals in the superior cervical ganglion has also been reported by Birks (1974) and by Pysh and Wiley (1974). Birks (1974) reported a loss of as much as 46 per cent of the vesicles after stimulation at 1 or 4 stimuli per second for 20 minutes. Pysh and Wiley (1974) found similar amounts of vesicle depletion and noted that the plasma membranes of the axon terminals expanded in such a manner that the profiles of the normally bulbous terminals became crescent-shaped and seemed to wrap around the postsynaptic dendrites. After a period of rest the stimulated terminals once again assumed their bulbous shapes, and their synaptic vesicles increased in number. Thus Pysh and Wiley (1974) assume that those observations support the concept that release of acetylcholine is associated with exocytosis of synaptic vesicles whose membranes become incorporated into the presynaptic membrane, in a fashion similar to that postulated for nerve terminals at motor end-plates.

On the other hand, Birks (1974) considers that since he did not find a depletion in the amount of acetylcholine in terminals despite a loss of vesicles at stimulation, his results cannot be readily accounted for on the basis of the vesicle theory of transmitter storage and release. Thus, he concluded that while the acetylcholine may be stored in the vesicles during rest, more than half of the transmitter is set free into the cytoplasm under conditions of maintained activity.

This view raises the point that despite the attractiveness of the theory that attempts to correlate synaptic vesicles with quanta of transmitter substance, there is no indication of how the transmitter gets into the vesicles and becomes concentrated. Using synaptosomes and synaptic vesicles prepared from the cerebral cortex, Marchbanks (1969) differentiates between two pools of acetylcholine. One pool is in the cytoplasm and can be released by osmotic shock, and the other is related to the synaptic vesicles. Synthesis of acetylcholine appears to take place first, or more rapidly, in the cytoplasmic rather than the vesicular compartment, and this more recently formed acetylcholine is the first to be released upon stimulation. These findings would consequently argue against the synaptic vesicles being equivalent to quanta. On the contrary, they would indicate that acetylcholine in the vesicles is only a reserve pool and that it is the cytoplasmic pool which is released during synaptic activity. Recently Marchbanks (1975) has thoroughly and critically reviewed the evidence concerning the vesicle hypothesis. Since this evidence is far from being unequivocally in support of the hypothesis, Marchbanks reiterated his suggestion that synaptic vesicles play an indirect role in transmitter release, that they constitute some kind of reserve store from which the extravesicular pool of transmitter is replenished.

Many examples of the fusion of synaptic vesicles with the presynaptic membrane have been recorded in transmission electron microscope studies, and more recently they have been shown in freeze-etched material (e.g., Nickel and Potter, 1970; Heuser, Reese, and Landis, 1974; Figure 5–11). In addition, the presence of coated vesicles has been recorded, not only at the presynaptic membrane, but also at postsynaptic surfaces and at locations where no synapses are present. Such vesicles have been shown to take up markers like saccharated iron oxide (e.g., Waxman and Pappas, 1969) and ferritin (Rosenbluth and Wissig, 1964; Brightman, 1965b; Birks, Mackey, and Weldon, 1972) which ultimately become sequestered into multivesicular bodies (Rosenbluth and Wissig, 1964; Birks, Mackey, and Weldon, 1972).

In our discussion of the motor end-plate, it was pointed out that Heuser and Reese (1973) propose that synaptic membrane is taken up as coated vesicles to be used again in the ultimate formation of new synaptic vesicles. The first demonstration of coated vesicles in axon terminals at interneuronal synapses was given by Gray (1961b, 1963, and 1966) who used phosphotungstic acid as a block stain for his material. At that time Gray referred to the coated vesicles as *complex vesicles* and described them as synaptic vesicles surrounded by an outer shell of smaller vesicles. Andres (1964) also noticed such vesicles and referred to them as "pinocytotic vesicles with spiky fringes." Somewhat later, Westrum (1965) suggested that synaptic vesicles are derived from the complex vesicles, and this view has been supported by Kanaseki and Kadota (1969) who examined sections of brain fractions after both normal and negative staining. Kaneseki and Kadota have shown that the complex vesicles are enclosed in a shell, or basket, composed of hexagonal and pentagonal subunits. They therefore termed these entities "vesicles in a basket." They propose that these structures are identical to the "complex" (Gray, 1961b), "dense-rimmed" (Brightman and Palay, 1963; Brightman, 1962), "alveolate" (Palay, 1963b), and coated vesicles described by other investigators. Kanaseki and Kadota (1969) further propose that these structures are formed at the neuronal membrane, then move away from it, lose their shell, and become synaptic vesicles. They support this suggestion by demonstrating the existence of empty as well as fragmented shells (see also Kadota and Kadota, 1973a and b).

Using the same method of preparation as Kanaseki and Kadota (1969), namely fixation in 4 per cent unbuffered osmic acid followed by 12 per cent glutaraldehyde, Gray and Willis (1970) studied a variety of tissues and interpreted the profiles encountered in axon terminals as forming a sequence. They came to the conclusion that synaptic vesicles are produced by liberation from complex vesicles, which themselves take origin from the surface membranes of presynaptic boutons. Gray and Willis (1970) show the presence of pieces of shell and further postulate that some of the fragments which remain adherent to the walls of the liberated vesicles become incorporated into the dense projections of the presynaptic membrane as the vesicles discharge. Somewhat related to this concept is that of Altman (1971). He suggests that coated vesicles are budded off from the Golgi apparatus during development and migrate to the neuronal membrane with which they become fused and provide the synaptic densities at sites where early interneuronal attachments are formed.

In another study, Gray and Pease (1971) examined the retinal receptor-bipolar synapses in the guinea pig eye. In this instance the authors found evidence for the formation of synaptic vesicles at the presynaptic membrane lying around the presynaptic ribbon. No complex vesicles are found around the ribbon in the cytoplasm, however, and Gray and Pease (1971) suggest that the ribbon acts as a guide in directing vesicles to the rather narrow strip of active zone at the presynaptic membrane. For a consideration of whether the shell, or coat, of coated vesicles is "real" or an "artifact," reference should be made to a recent discussion by Gray (1972).

In these latter studies there is no record of synaptic vesicles taking origin from agranular cisternae, as proposed by Heuser and Reese (1973), but evidence for synaptic vesicles pinching off from the agranular endoplasmic reticulum has been noted by a number of investigators, including Palay (1958b), Robertson (1960a), Birks (1966), Düring (1967), Lovas (1971), Stelzner (1971), and Korneliussen (1972a).

Finally, mention may be made of a miscellaneous group of studies that have shown alterations of axon terminals in different phases of synaptic activity. In a study of the effects of stimulation on the primary auditory cortex of cats, Fehér, Joó, and Halász (1972) found that after 45 minutes of stimulation by clicks, the largest axon terminals forming asymmetrical synapses in layers 4 and 5 of the auditory cortex show a decrease in their content of synaptic vesicles, whereas some smaller terminals show either an increase or a decrease. In anesthetized cats any loss of vesicles was less apparent. Since these authors did not know which axon terminals were from the specific thalamocortical pathway, they were obliged to measure a random sample of terminals. They assume, though, that those showing a reduction of vesicles are the thalamocortical terminals.

Another interesting study is that of Cragg (1969), who examined the rod-bipolar synapses in newborn rats. The receptor terminals showed a small, but statistically significant increase in size during prolonged exposure to darkness, and the synaptic vesicles dispersed, although apparently they did not alter in number. Earlier, Mountford (1963) could find no effects on either the size or concentration of synaptic vesicles at the receptor-bipolar synapses of the retinas of guinea pigs exposed to intense light as opposed to those left in darkness for long periods. Lund and Lund (1972) have also shown that the ratio between different morphological types of synapses in the superior colliculus of the rat is altered in young postnatal animals deprived of light.

GRANULAR VESICLES

A slightly larger vesicle (40 to 60 nm) containing a dense granule, 15 to 25 nm in diameter, is encountered in the axon terminals of autonomic fibers (see Grillo and Palay, 1962; Grillo, 1966; Bloom and Barrnett, 1966; Bloom and Giarman, 1968; Hökfelt, 1968; Tranzer, Thoenen, Snipes, and Richards, 1969; Bloom, 1970; Geffen and Livett, 1971), in the intestine, vas deferens (Richardson, 1962; Tranzer, Thoenen, Snipes, and Richards, 1969), and pineal body (De Robertis and Pellegrino de Iraldi, 1961; Bak, Hassler, and Kim, 1969). The dense granule is usually spherical, but it may be rod-shaped about 13 by 34 nm. Synaptic vesicles of this type have become associated with catecholamines and especially norepinephrine (noradrenalin), because they occur in sites where adrenergic nerve fibers are known to be present. Evidence for this concept comes from a variety of sources. For example, small granular vesicles are common in the nerves of the dilator muscle of the albino rabbit iris, which is innervated predominantly by adrenergic nerves, whereas only small agranular synaptic vesicles are present in the cholinergic nerves to the sphincter muscle (Richardson, 1964). By use of electron microscopic autoradiography Wolfe, Potter, Richardson, and Axelrod (1962) demonstrated that tritiated norepinephrine is concentrated in those nerve endings of the pineal body that contain granular vesicles. This type of labelling has been confirmed by a number of authors including Budd and Salpeter (1969), who also pointed out that the distribution of dense-cored vesicles and of the labelled norepinephrine do not coincide perfectly.

Other evidence is presented by De Robertis and Pellegrino de Iraldi (1961), who showed that after a single dose of reserpine, the granular contents rapidly disappear from vesicles of the pineal body, an observation which has been repeatedly confirmed. A similar depletion is caused by oxypertine (Bak, Hassler, and Kim, 1969). In other studies combining electron microscopy, microfluorescence, and biochemical observations Van Orden, Bloom, Barrnett, and Giarman (1966) and Van Orden, Bensch, and Giarman (1967) also showed a good correlation between the number of small, granule-containing vesicles and the quantity of catecholamines in adrenergic nerve fibers under experimental conditions of depletion and forced uptake of exogenous norepinephrine.

Hence, at the present, the weight of evidence indicates that the small granular vesicles are storage vesicles for catecholamines. However, in nearly all electron microscopic preparations of adrenergic nerve endings there is a varying proportion of electron-lucent vesicles.

The proportion present depends upon the type of fixative used. Thus, Tranzer, Thoenen, Snipes, and Richards (1969) show that fixation in osmic acid alone produces more clear vesicles than fixation in aldehydes followed by osmic acid. Moreover, these authors conclude that all vesicles in adrenergic nerve terminals are capable of taking up and storing norepinephrine, since preincubation of tissues in solutions containing norepinephrine increases the proportion of vesicles containing granules. In fact some of the norepinephrine probably diffuses out during fixation, as indicated by the use of exogenously administered "false" transmitters, such as alpha-methylnorepinephrine, 5-hydroxydopamine, and 5-hydroxytryptamine. These compounds become insoluble and electron-dense when tissues are fixed in glutaraldehyde followed by osmic acid. If they are used to replace norepinephrine, a large percentage of the vesicles in adrenergic nerve endings contain quite opaque granules (e.g., see Bondareff, 1966; Eccleston, Thoa, and Axelrod, 1969; Taxi and Droz, 1966; Tranzer, Thoenen, Snipes, and Richards, 1969; Chiba, 1973). According to the results of Chiba (1973) in the vas deferens of the mouse, however, about 10 per cent of the vesicles still retain clear centers.

Until recently these small granular synaptic vesicles were found only in the endings of autonomic nerves in the peripheral nervous system and were not seen in the central nervous system (Fuxe, Hökfelt, Nilsson, and Reinius, 1966; Palay, 1967). Instead there was only a larger diameter granule-containing vesicle, with a mean diameter of 80 to 90 nm, with a dense spherical core of about 50 nm (Figure 5–15). Small numbers of such larger dense-cored vesicles occur in endings throughout the central nervous system (see Figure 5–13). Some authors have associated these larger granular vesicles with biogenic amines (e.g., Pellegrino de Iraldi, Farini Duggan, and De Robertis, 1963; Aghajanian and Bloom, 1966; De Robertis, 1967), ignoring the great difference in size between them and the accepted catecholamine-containing granules, as well as the discrepancy between the numbers of the larger granules and the regional concentration of biogenic amines (Fuxe, Hökfelt, and Nilsson, 1965; Fuxe, Hökfelt, Nilsson, and Reinius, 1966). The confusion arising from these different points of view has engendered considerable discussion (see for example, Kety and Samson, 1967). The problem has been partially clarified, however, by Hökfelt (1967a and b and 1968), who discovered that when central nervous tissue is fixed in potassium permanganate, small, dense granules appear in the synaptic vesicles in regions of the brain known to have a high amine content such as the outer layer of the median eminence. This very important observation resolves the question concerning the localization of the catecholamines in the nerve terminals of the central nervous system and brings the results of electron microscopy into line with the results of histochemistry and pharmacology. As yet though, no autoradiographic studies have been performed that give confirmation that the permanganate-preserved vesicles are catecholamine-containing, for potassium permanganate either is ineffective in retaining tritiated norepinephrine in sections or oxidizes the labelled norepinephrine (see Descarries and Droz, 1970; Bloom and Giarman, 1968; Bloom, 1970).

Use of potassium permanganate fixation does not contribute to our understanding of the larger dense-centered vesicles, and it revives another problem that seems to have been ignored. This problem is the significance of the clear-centered vesicles, which had been equated with acetylcholine. Obviously, clear-centered vesicles can no longer be considered as a homogeneous population, for Hökfelt's observations and those of others concerned with the effects of fixation on small granular vesicles suggest that these vesicles can release their charge of transmitter with loss of the granules but without loss of the limiting membrane. The present evidence in favor of this concept is reviewed by Bloom, Iversen, and Schmitt (1970) and by Geffen and Livett (1971). In summary, the evidence to date indicates that in addition to catecholamines, the small granular vesicles contain some adenosine triphosphate, the enzyme dopamine β-hydroxylase, and considerable amounts of soluble proteins collectively known as chromogranins. These appear to be released from the granular vesicles by exocytosis, so that the vesicle wall, or membrane, is left intact and returned to the cytoplasm to accumulate and store more transmitter.

The larger dense-centered vesicle is usually between 80 and 150 nm in diameter and contains a dense spherical core about 50 to 70 nm across. The core may appear either fibrillar or granular. These larger vesicles are numerous in the presynaptic terminals of autonomic ganglia, making up about 5 per cent of the vesicle population, and in the neuromuscular endings of smooth muscle (Richardson, 1962 and 1964; Grillo and Palay, 1962; Elfvin, 1963). Small numbers of them also occur in some of the terminals in various parts of the central nervous system (e.g., Chan-Palay, 1973g), where they are often in the company of clear synaptic vesicles (Figure 5–15); they are usually located away from the synaptic junction. They even occur in the cholinergic motor terminals of skeletal muscle.

The role of these larger granular vesicles has been studied in recent years, but it is still enigmatic. Their contents are difficult to analyze. Since they stain with ethanolic phosphotungstic acid, at least part of their opacity may be due to a proteinaceous matrix (Bloom and Aghajanian, 1968a and b). There is some suggestion that the larger granular vesicles may constitute a mixed population. In comparison to the contents of the small granular vesicles the larger ones are relatively resistant to depletion by reserpine (e.g., Tranzer, Thoenen, Snipes, and Richards, 1969; Bloom and Barrnett, 1966; Hökfelt, 1966), and so far as can be determined by electron autoradiographic studies using labelled norepinephrine, the larger granular vesicles are not obviously associated with this transmitter (Descarries and Droz, 1970; Sotelo, 1971b). On the other hand, in boutons that store catecholamines the content of the larger granular vesicles increases in density after loading with 5-hydroxydopamine, which is a false transmitter (Tranzer, Thoenen, Snipes, and Richards, 1969; Chiba, 1973). This indicates that the large vesicles, like the small ones, are capable of concentrating 5-hydroxydopamine and therefore may normally store catecholamines, but larger vesicles in boutons presumed to be cholinergic because of their predominant content of clear vesicles do not show a similar increase in density.

In a study of the substantia nigra and area postrema of the rat, Sotelo (1971b) noted some labelling of axon terminals from which granular vesicles were absent. He also noticed a high phosphatase activity of the larger granular vesicles in the region of the Golgi apparatus, and raised the question of whether these granular vesicles might be considered as primary lysosomes.

NEUROSECRETORY VESICLES

In mammals the prototype of a neurosecretory system is represented by the supraoptic and paraventricular nuclei, the supraopticohypophysial tract, and the neurohypophysis. The perikarya, axons, and terminals of this system contain characteristic vesicles, which are 120 to 150 nm in diameter and which enclose large, dense droplets that almost completely fill them (Palay, 1957; Bargmann, 1966; Ishii, Thomas, and Nakamura, 1973; Krisch, 1974). A great deal of experimental evidence suggests that these characteristic droplets contain the hormones (vasopressin and oxytocin) produced by the supraoptic and paraventricular nuclei. They are depleted along with the hormones by such stimuli as dehydration and suckling (for references, see Bargmann, 1966; Sloper, 1966; Krisch, 1974). Furthermore, isolated neurosecretory granules from the neurohypophyses of mammals and fishes contain high concentrations of the hormones (Weinstein, Malamed, and Sachs, 1961; Barer, Heller, and Lederis, 1963; Sachs, 1963). Consequently, these droplets have been termed elementary neurosecretory granules. These granules are not of a constant size; Krisch (1974), for example, has found that granules of the supraoptic nucleus are larger than those of the paraventricular nucleus, and that the granules of the supraoptic nucleus are made distinctly smaller as a result of dehydration. In another study, Ishii, Thomas, and Nakamura (1973) measured the granules in the pars nervosa of the rat and concluded that the axons can be classified into five groups which contain granules with median sizes of 143, 155, 167, 180, and 193 nm.

There are two hypotheses put forward to account for the manner in which the hormones are secreted from the granular vesicles. One is that the hormones diffuse out through the vesicular membranes into the axoplasm and from there pass through the axolemma into the surrounding extracellular space. The second is that the contents of the granular vesicles are discharged into the extracellular space by exocytosis as the vesicle fuses with the axolemma. A study of freeze-fractured neurosecretory endings by Dreifuss, Akert, Sandri, and Moor (1973) favors the latter postulate. Those authors observed several large depressions, or pits, 40 to 80 nm in diameter, on the A faces of fractured membranes surrounding the axon terminals, which had been stimulated to secrete by soaking the tissue in either potassium or lanthanum chloride.

It is interesting that the terminals in the neurohypophysis also contain small clear vesicles. These vesicles have diameters of about 50 nm and resemble those in synaptic endings elsewhere. Their role in this situation is unknown, but they may be residual vesicles left after discharge of the granular contents.

The terminals containing neurosecretory granules display another very important and identifying characteristic; they abut upon a perivascular space, not against another neuron or effector cell. Therefore, they can be considered as nerve endings that innervate nothing, although Krisch (1974) has shown puncta adhaerentia between neurosecretory axons and pituicytes. Their secretory product is released into the perivascular space, is transported somehow into the lumen of the vessel, and is carried in the blood to the appropriate organs whose activity it modifies. Neurosecretory systems of this kind have been recognized in almost all vertebrates and invertebrates. Although the secretory droplets vary in size and chemical properties, the principle of gland-like morphology and free nerve endings has been repeatedly confirmed in a wide variety of animals (Hofer, 1968).

In mammals, as in other animals, there is another example of a neurosecretory system in the same region of the brain. This second example, which has come to light in recent years, consists of the tuberal nuclei, especially the arcuate nucleus, and the median eminence (see Weindl, 1973). Here nerve fibers presumably originating from the arcuate nucleus in the floor of the third ventricle course into the median eminence, where they terminate in the external layer. The terminals form palisades around the capillaries of the primary hypophysial portal plexus. The relationship of the terminals to the perivascular space and its limiting basal lamina is exactly the same as it is in the supraopticohypophysial neurosecretory system. The granule-containing vesicles in these endings are, however, smaller. Two types of vesicle have been described: small, clear vesicles resembling typical synaptic vesicles, and larger ones about 120 to 150 nm in diameter containing a dense central droplet (Rinne, 1966; Kobayashi, Kobayashi, Yamamoto, and Kaibara, 1967). This larger vesicle corresponds in size to the enigmatic vesicle described in an earlier paragraph as occurring sporadically in nerve terminals of all types. In this sytem, however, it is common, and each ending is likely to have at least two or three, and most of them have many more. Furthermore, as mentioned above, when the median eminence is fixed in potassium permanganate, the small, clear vesicles in some terminals prove to contain minute dense granules resembling those found in adrenergic terminals (Hökfelt, 1967a and b). These terminals may be involved in regulating the secretion of hormones from the tuberohypophysial fiber system into the portal circulation. Although this median eminence system does not contain the special granules characteristic of the classic supraopticohypophysial system, morphologically it satisfies the criteria for a neurosecretory system and must be accepted as such. Consequently, the terminology currently in use for the vesicles will have to be revised when more is known about their chemistry and functions. The median eminence system is thought to be involved in the elaboration and control of various releasing factors regulating the activity of the adenohypophysis. Hökfelt's studies suggesting that at least some of the fibers are simply adrenergic introduce new and interesting complications, although the secretion of pituitary regulating factors also seems to be influenced by a system of nonadrenergic neurons (Ganong, 1972).

The term neurosecretion was invented to designate a special class of neurons that had gland-like properties—producing secretory granules and innervating nothing. Although it is now possible, by slight changes in the original concept, to assimilate all nerve cells into this class, there is still considerable virtue in retaining the original meaning of the term, at least until a systematic revision of the terminology applied to terminals, their enclosed vesicles, and synapses can be achieved.

OTHER PRESYNAPTIC ORGANELLES

Mitochondria are often encountered in the terminal boutons of axons (Figures 5–2 to 5–4, 5–9, 5–11, 5–13, 5–14, and 5–19). Although their role in the terminal has not been specified, it seems reasonable to suggest that the mitochondria might be concerned with the provision of the energy necessary for synaptic transmission. Energy is required for the maintenance of the sodium pump, for restoring the integrity of the surface membrane, and for sustaining enzymatic reactions in connection, perhaps, with the synthesis of the transmitter and the construction of the synaptic vesicles. In fact, the maintenance of synaptic vesicles and synaptic activity appears to depend upon an adequate oxygen supply and respiratory activity. Thus Webster and Ames (1965) have shown that if retinas are incubated for only three minutes in solutions lacking oxygen and glucose, there is a generalized swelling of mitochondria and a loss of synaptic vesicles in the presynaptic portions of rod-bipolar synapses. This change is correlated with abolition of a response to light when recordings are made from the attached optic nerve. The effects are reversible if the anoxia lasts less than 20 minutes. Also in a recent study, Vaughn and

Grieshaber (1972) have made the interesting observation that the glycogen content of boutons is much greater in perinatal rats than in adults, while conversely the mitochondria occupy a proportionally greater volume of boutons as animals mature. They relate these data to the progressive addition of aerobic pathways to anaerobic ones during development and to the fact that the time when most glycogen is present is the time when animals can tolerate long periods of anoxia.

Mitochondria are also capable of concentrating cations from their surrounding medium, and their role in maintaining the ionic balance in the presynaptic axoplasm was suggested long ago (Palay, 1956a and b). In particular, their capacity to take up calcium, even against a large concentration gradient, has attracted considerable attention (Lehninger, 1967 and 1968). The activity of these ion uptake mechanisms is coupled to the oxidative phosphorylation and electron transport functions of mitochondria. Recently experimental evidence has been brought forward which supports a more specific role for mitochondria in the release of transmitters from nerve terminals. Working with the frog neuromuscular junction, Alnaes and Rahamimoff (1975) have demonstrated that interference with the calcium uptake mechanism of mitochondria, by inhibiting either oxidative phosphorylation or the electron transport chain, increases the frequency of spontaneous miniature end-plate potentials and also increases the amount of transmitter released by a nerve impulse. Since immersion in a calcium-free medium had the same enhancing effect, these authors suggested that the presynaptic intracellular free calcium, close to the presynaptic membrane, is the important factor regulating spontaneous release of transmitter (Katz and Miledi, 1965 and 1967a and b). Ruthenium red, which inhibits calcium uptake by mitochondria, also increased the spontaneous release of transmitter from the nerve ending, but with decreased quantal content. On the basis of these experiments, Alnaes and Rahamimoff proposed that the presynaptic mitochondria help to regulate the release of transmitter from nerve terminals by participating in the regulation of intracellular free calcium.

However, it should be pointed out that mitochondria are not a constant feature of presynaptic terminals. Thus, although they are commonly present in the larger boutons (e.g., Figures 5–3 and 5–4) (Palay, 1958b) they are frequently absent from smaller ones (e.g., Figures 5–5 to 5–7) (Gray, 1959). This distribution of mitochondria may be construed to indicate that they play no special role in synaptic transmission. They may reach the axon terminals merely as a result of centrifugal axonal flow (see Weiss and Pillai, 1965) and collect in axon terminals large enough to accommodate them. However, it should not be forgotten that the mitochondria do not occupy stable positions within the cell. They are probably in constant migration, as is shown by studies of living cells and nerve fibers in culture.

Neurofilaments and *microtubules*, which are common constituents of axonal cytoplasm, also continue into preterminal axons (Figures 5–3 and 11–4). In *boutons en passant* these organelles merely form the axis of the enlargement and do not enter the lateral protuberances, which are filled with mitochondria and synaptic vesicles. When the terminal has only a unilateral protuberance, the microtubules and neurofilaments pass to one side, away from the synaptic zone. Reference must again be made to the observations of Smith, Järlfors, and Beránek (1970), who showed synaptic vesicles to be arranged in regular arrays with respect to microtubules in the central nervous system of the lamprey. Although such an association between microtubules and vesicles has not yet been encountered elsewhere, this observation suggests the possibility that microtubules may act to guide or transport synaptic vesicles within the axon.

In most preparations the axonal microtubules seem to end short of the terminal enlargement, or *bouton terminal*. Gray (1975 and 1976) has recently shown that by using a special fixation procedure microtubules can be demonstrated in nerve terminals of rat and frog brain. He examined fragments of brain that had been teased apart in a solution of bovine serum albumin before fixation in the succession of solutions recommended by Kanaseki and Kadota (1969): unbuffered osmium tetroxide, glutaraldehyde, and uranyl acetate. In sections of these fragments Gray found that microtubules not only occurred in the usual places, including axons and dendrites, but also could be traced right down into the synaptic terminals, in which they were closely associated with synaptic vesicles. Westrum and Gray (1976) also noted microtubules in presynaptic terminals, sometimes attaching close to the inner surface of the axonal plasmalemma. Immunohistochemical investigation, however, has not yet demonstrated the presence of tubulin in the presynaptic terminal (Matus, Walters, and Mughal, 1975). On the contrary, in synapses both *in situ* and in synaptosome fractions tubulin appears to be confined entirely to the postsynaptic density (Walters and Matus, 1975; Matus, Walters, and Mughal, 1975). The appraisal of Gray's recent findings must therefore await further exploration.

Like microtubules, neurofilaments also usually fail to enter into the boutons terminaux, but Gray and Guillery (1961 and 1966) and Gray (1964) have shown that in the cat, for example, the boutons may contain loops of neurofilaments. In the rat such loops have not been observed, although most axon terminals contain a few neurofilaments. Their number seems to depend upon the size of the terminal. For example, in the large nerve endings of the lateral vestibular nucleus and lateral geniculate nucleus (Figure 11–4), neurofilaments may be prominent, while they are generally absent from the smaller axon terminals of the cerebral cortex (Figures 5–5 and 5–6).

Gray and Guillery (1961 and 1966) have suggested that only boutons containing loops of neurofilaments are visible in light microscopic preparations stained by the Bielschowsky and similar silver methods. Conversely, they attribute the failure of this method to stain boutons in certain parts of the central nervous sytem—for example, the cerebral cortex—to a lack of neurofilaments. It is of interest that during experimental degeneration some boutons become filled with neurofilaments. This stage of neurofibrillary degeneration precedes the final granular disintegration of the boutons (for references, see Gray and Guillery, 1966).

Little information is available about the morphology of axon terminals in neurological disorders. In tissue taken from the vicinity of senile plaques from patients with Alzheimer's presenile dementia, Gonatas and Gambetti (1970) found many enlarged axon terminals. These terminals contained lamellated dense bodies, or tubular and vesicular components. Large axon terminals containing branching tubular and vesicular profiles were also encountered by Gonatas (1967) in biopsy material from a patient with severe psychomotor retardation, and by Gonatas and Goldensohn (1965) in a patient with generalized convulsions, mental retardation, and cortical blindness.

Other components of the cytoplasm in presynaptic axon terminals may be coated vesicles, *multivesicular bodies*, smooth endoplasmic reticulum, and as indicated earlier, *glycogen*.

Presynaptic ribbons were first described in the presynaptic regions of rods and cones of the vertebrate retina by Sjöstrand (1958). A similar structure also occurs in the inner plexiform layer of the retina (Kidd, 1962; Dowling and Boycott, 1966; Raviola and Raviola, 1967; Dowling, 1968) and in pinealocytes of a wide range of vertebrates (see Wolfe, 1965; Collin, 1971). Other locations of presynaptic ribbons are at the synapses of hair cells of the guinea pig cochlea (Smith and Sjöstrand, 1961a and b), at electroreceptors (Wachtel and Szamier, 1966), and in lateral line hair cells of fishes (Hama, 1965). The presynaptic ribbon is a dense, rod-like structure lying near and perpendicular to the presynaptic junction. Synaptic vesicles are usually clustered around it, and it has been suggested that it acts as a guide to direct vesicles to the presynaptic membrane (Bunt, 1971; Gray and Pease, 1971). According to Bunt (1971), who has studied the effects of various digestive enzymes on presynaptic ribbons, they are composed, at least in part, of a protein or polypeptide rich in aromatic amino acids, and they do not contain appreciable amounts of nucleic acids. Szamier (1974) has also shown that presynaptic ribbons are digested by pronase or protease, although no other components of the synapses are affected by this treatment.

Structures resembling synaptic ribbons have also been encountered in the presynaptic terminals of the squid giant synapse (Martin and Miledi, 1975). In the squid the structure consists of thin rectangular lamellae surrounded by vesicles.

OTHER POSTSYNAPTIC ORGANELLES

The *spine apparatus* is the best known of the specialized postsynaptic structures (Gray, 1959; Gray and Guillery, 1963b and 1966). First described in the dendritic spines of the cerebral cortex (Figures 5–5, *sa*, and 11–3), the spine apparatus usually appears as two or more profiles of flattened sacs, or cisternae separated from each other by plaques of dense material, which at high resolution can be seen to be composed of pairs of parallel sheets. Although serial reconstruction of these structures is difficult because of their small size, it would appear that the profiles of the sacs are part of a single complex cisterna, and that this cisterna is in continuity, through a small tubular extension in the neck of the spine, with the smooth endoplasmic reticulum of the dendritic trunk (Peters and Kaiserman-Abramof, 1969). The appearance of the spine apparatuses is highly variable. Sometimes the sacs are distended, and at other times they are collapsed so that their walls are more or less apposed.

So far, the spine apparatus has been described in all parts of the cerebral cortex, including the hippocampus (Hamlyn, 1962; Westrum and Blackstad, 1962), and Pappas and Waxman (1972) also record its presence in the caudate nucleus. Spine apparatuses do not appear to

occur frequently in subcortical portions of the central nervous system, however, although Colonnier and Guillery (1964) observed structures resembling spine apparatuses in the lateral geniculate nucleus of the monkey, and Sotelo (1971a) encountered them in the spines of the tertiary branches of Purkinje cells in one out of five cats he studied. A simple form of the spine apparatus also occurs in the lateral horn of the spinal cord (Gray and Guillery, 1966).

An organelle resembling the dendritic spine apparatus occurs in the axon initial segments of cortical pyramidal cells. Westrum (1970) described them in the spines protruding from initial segments, and similar organelles are also encountered lying free in the shaft of this part of the axon (Peters, Proskauer, and Kaiserman-Abramof, 1968; Jones and Powell, 1969a). In such extraspinous locations these structures are called *cisternal organelles*. They consist of two or more flattened cisternae separated by granular dense plates, 20 nm thick, which at high resolution can be resolved into two parallel plates, 5 nm apart. Cisternal organelles have also been encountered in the shafts of dendrites in the cerebral cortex (Gray and Guillery, 1966; Kaiserman-Abramof and Peters, 1972; Jones and Powell, 1969b). They resemble those in the initial axon segment, but in dendrites they are surrounded by free polysomes.

Contrary to our experience, Schultz and Karlsson (1966) have concluded that the occurrence of spine apparatuses in the cerebral cortex is dependent on the type of fixation used. Thus, they state that primary fixation by dripping on, or immersion in, osmium tetroxide produces more spine apparatuses than primary fixation in aldehydes. Hence they conclude that the spine apparatuses may be a fixation artifact. If so, they are complex, and their precursors have not been defined.

Virtually nothing is known of the development of the spine apparatus, although Gray (1963) records that they originate at about 16 days after birth in the rat occipital cortex, and Pappas and Waxman (1972) state that they appear in tissue cultures at the time when synapses develop. The function of these organelles is totally unknown. The suggestion that they may be implicated in memory has been voiced many times, but without any substantiation.

Even in spines that do not contain a spine apparatus, there are tubules or cisternae of smooth endoplasmic reticulum, as for example, in the spines of the Purkinje cells of the cerebellum (Kaiserman-Abramof and Palay, 1969; Palay and Chan-Palay, 1974; Figure 5–7) and the perikaryal spines of the stellate cells in the rat cerebral cortex. Since the flattened sacs of the spine apparatus in the cerebral cortex can occasionally be observed in direct confluence with the cisternae or tubules of the smooth endoplasmic reticulum, the spine apparatus is probably a local specialization of this ubiquitous membranous system which permeates all parts of the neuron.

The postsynaptic density plus the bands and granules that may lie beneath it are, together with the spine apparatus, the only specialized postsynaptic organelles so far observed. The specific relations of other organelles to the postsynaptic membrane are less certain. However, Rosenbluth (1962b) reported that subsurface cisternae are sometimes present beneath synaptic junctions and suggested that the proximity of these organelles to the postsynaptic membrane may be fortuitous. In most cases this is probably true, but in the synapses formed by the efferent nerves of the acousticolateralis system subsurface cisternae are consistently present (Engström, 1958; Hama, 1965 and 1969; Jande, 1966; Sjöstrand, 1961; Wersall, Flock, and Lundquist, 1965). Also, subsurface cisternae appear to occur consistently beneath certain synapses of the oculomotor nucleus (Pappas and Waxman, 1972).

Gray (1963) has reported that mitochondria often lie adjacent to the postsynaptic thickening in the spinal cord, and Bodian (1964 and 1972) has drawn attention to the fact that it is not uncommon to find Nissl bodies lying beneath aggregates of certain large synaptic bulbs terminating on anterior horn cells in the monkey.

SYNAPTIC RELATIONS

As stated in the introduction to this chapter on chemical synapses, a wide variety of synaptic relations is possible between neurons. Not all possible relations exist in any one part of the central nervous system, and indeed, it is usual to find one or two forms of synapse predominating in a given nucleus or portion of the brain and spinal cord. In the following section, we shall survey some of them. All combinations between different parts of neurons have now been recorded. The existence of dendro-axonic and somato-axonic synapses must bring about radical changes in our thoughts about the function of connections between neurons. Such synapses could alter the input into a system and could have very complex regulatory effects, as indeed they have been assumed to do in the places

where somato-axonic synapses occur; namely, the carotid body and the cardiac ganglion. Even the discovery of dendro-dendritic synapses, whose individual effects should be minor, placed a strain upon accepted concepts of neuronal functioning.

Axo-Dendritic Synapses

These are by far the most common synapses encountered in the neuropil. They may occur on the shafts of dendrites (Figures 5–3, 5–4, and 5–6) or on the appendages protruding from them (Figures 5–5 to 5–7). The identification of such synapses is usually not difficult, since in most instances the dendritic nature of the postsynaptic component can be established on the basis of its content of relatively evenly spaced microtubules, rosettes of free ribosomes, and profiles of granular endoplasmic reticulum, although the latter tends to become more sparse as a dendrite extends further away from the neuronal perikaryon.

Axo-dendritic synapses can be either asymmetrical (Figures 5–5 and 5–6) or symmetrical (Figures 5–3, 5–4, and 5–9). On dendrites lacking spines or thorns, the distribution of synapses along the shafts may vary considerably. For example, there is a relatively tight packing on the dendrites of the stellate cells of the cerebral cortex (Figure 5–6, *upper picture*), of cells in the basal ganglia, and of anterior horn cells in the spinal cord (Figure 5–4). At the other extreme synapses are absent along the dendrites of granule cells in the cerebellar cortex which receive axonal terminals only at their ends.

On dendrites bearing spines, like those of pyramidal cells in the cerebral cortex and the hippocampus, and like the Purkinje cells in the cerebellum, these protrusions are the main receptive sites for axon terminals (Figures 5–5 and 5–7).

Axo-Somatic Synapses

Differences in the density of axo-somatic synapses (Figures 5–13 and 11–2) on the perikarya of various neurons in the central nervous system can be appreciated even in silver-stained preparations examined with the light microscope, and in recent years the electron microscope has been used to obtain some values of the percentage of perikaryal surface covered by synapses. Thus, Blackstad and Dahl (1961) calculate that 15 per cent of the perikaryal surface of granule cells in the fascia dentata of the rat is covered by axon terminals, and Lemkey-Johnston and Larramendi (1968a and b) estimate a 15.2 per cent coverage of basket cell perikarya and 4.5 per cent coverage of stellate cell perikarya in the cerebellum of the mouse. The perikarya of Betz cells in the cat have 23 per cent coverage (Kaiserman-Abramof and Peters, 1972). In the lateral geniculate nucleus of the rat, Karlsson (1966c) gives values of 5 and 15 per cent for two individual neurons. All these values are much lower than the 47 per cent coverage determined by Conradi (1969b) for the somata of neurons in the lumbosacral spinal cord of the cat. Other neurons, such as the granule cells of the cerebellar cortex (see Palay and Chan-Palay, 1974), have no axo-somatic synapses. Hence the variation in the amount of the perikaryal surface covered by synapses is very large and the extent of the coverage is characteristic for each cell type.

Kaiserman-Abramof and Peters (1972) calculate that there are about 13 boutons per 100 square microns of Betz cell perikaryal surface in the cat and about 870 boutons on an entire perikaryon. This is lower than the values of 17 and 22 boutons per 100 square microns calculated by Conradi (1969b) for two dendrites of motor neurons in the lumbosacral spinal cord of the cat and higher than the figures of 133 and 83 boutons that Karlsson (1966c) found on the perikarya of two neurons in the lateral geniculate nucleus of the rat.

For a comparison with these values, some reference can be made to calculations of the total numbers of synapses on average neurons. These values are obtained by dividing the total number of synapses in a given volume of tissue by the total number of neurons it contains, regardless of neuronal type. On this basis, Cragg (1967) has calculated the total number of synapses on average neurons in the motor cerebral cortex of the mouse and cat to be 13,000 and 60,000, respectively. Consequently, it must be concluded that the perikaryon is not the principal site of synaptic input to nerve cells.

Axo-somatic synapses may be either asymmetrical or symmetrical, although on most perikarya symmetrical synapses seem to predominate (Figure 5–13). There is great variation, however, for while the pyramidal cells of the cerebral cortex apparently form only symmetrical synapses, some of the stellate cells in the same cortex form both symmetrical and asymmetrical synapses (Colonnier, 1968; Jones and Powell, 1970a) in addition to those with an intermediate morphology (Peters, 1971). In the spinal cord of the monkey, on the other hand, Bodian (1966a, 1970a, and 1972) recognizes five different forms of synapses on the anterior horn cells, and rather similar types have been described by Conradi (1969a) in the cat. These synapses differ in the shape of the synaptic vesicles they contain after primary fixation with aldehydes and in the relative concentration of agranular and granular vesicles, as well as in the form of the synaptic junctions and their related organelles. A complex situation also exists in the nucleus dorsalis of the cat (Saito, 1974), in which the large cells have a variety of axon terminals on their somata.

In addition to these variations in the diversity of form of axo-somatic synapses and the numbers per unit area of perikaryal surface, there are also differences in the extent to which the perikarya are covered by thin sheets of astrocytic processes. Thus, the perikarya of Purkinje cells (Figure 11–2), anterior horn cells, and neurons of the substantia gelatinosa are completely covered by a sheath of astrocytic processes that is only penetrated by synapsing axon terminals. In contrast, the perikarya of pyramidal cells in the cerebral cortex (Figures 2–1 and 2–3) and granule cells in the cerebellar cortex are free of such a covering, and hence are directly adjacent to other neuronal components in their vicinity (see page 248).

Figure 5–14.   **A Variety of Synapses.**

Occupying the center of the field is a large spine or protrusion from the perikaryon of a neuron, and surrounding this structure is a variety of axon terminals. Two of the terminals (At_1 and At_2) contain small, spherical synaptic vesicles, while the spherical vesicles in two other terminals (At_3 and At_4) are somewhat larger. The other axon terminals (At_5 to At_9) contain some elongate synaptic vesicles. The synaptic junctions in which these various axon terminals participate all seem to be symmetrical. The junction formed by At_5 is noteworthy because of the regular array of presynaptic densities (*arrows*). At the other synaptic junctions, only one or two of these densities (*arrows*) are apparent.
Ventral cochlear nucleus of adult rat. × 44,000.

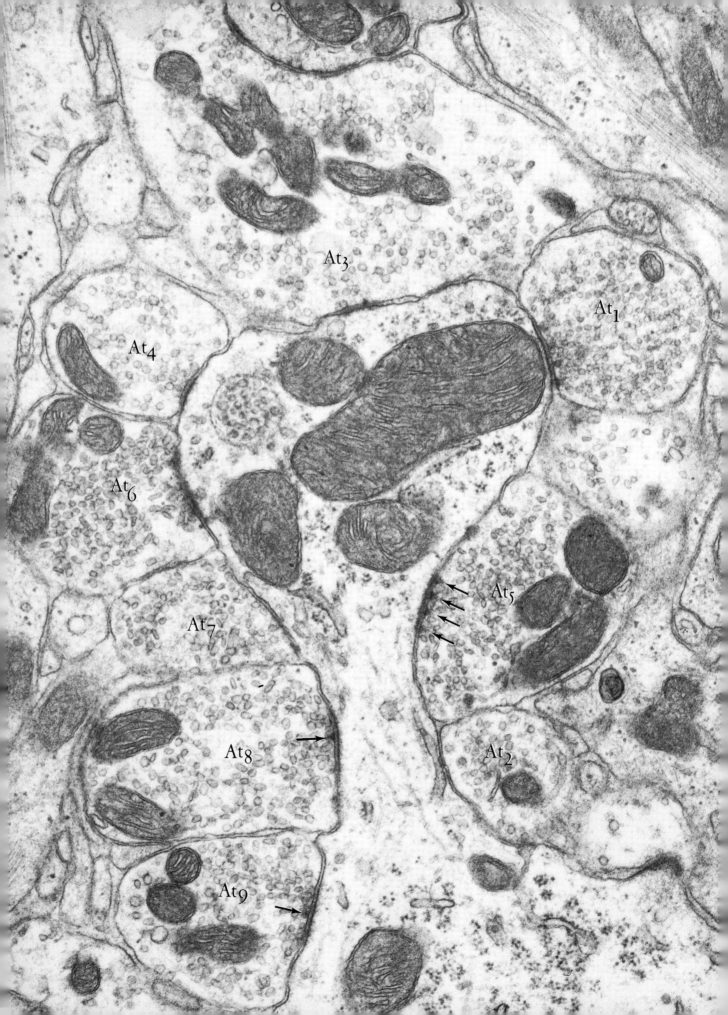

Axo-Axonal Synapses

The acceptance of a synapse as axo-axonal depends upon two criteria: (1) the identification of *both* components as axons and (2) the close association of synaptic vesicles with at least one side of the junction. It is the first of these criteria that is crucial in the recognition of an axo-axonal synapse, and so in all the examples collected until now, the postsynaptic component has been either (1) a typical axon initial segment (Figures 5–15, upper picture, and 4–1) or (2) an axon terminal with synaptic vesicles clustered against a second synaptic interface on a recognizable dendrite or perikaryon. In this latter it is assumed, of course, that dendro-dendritic and dendro-somatic synapses are sufficiently rare for the intermediate component of such a serial synapse not to be a preterminal or terminal dendrite. On the basis of such an assumption, Peters and Palay (1966), for example, reported the existence of axo-axonal synapses in the glomeruli of the dorsal nucleus of the lateral geniculate body of the cat. However, a more recent study by Famiglietti and Peters (1972) has thrown doubt upon the original interpretation of this situation; as shown in Figure 5–18, a vesicle-containing terminal of an optic nerve fiber (As_1) synapses upon a second vesicle-containing terminal (Den_2), which in turn synapses upon a dendritic thorn (Den_1). In this more recent study it has been determined that the second vesicle-containing profile of the series (Den_2), which is postsynaptic to the terminals of axons of the optic nerve, is the dendritic terminal of an intrinsic neuron. Hence the synapse between the two vesicle-containing elements is axo-dendritic (also see Figure 11–4). A similar conclusion was also reached by Lieberman and Webster (1972) after their investigation of the dorsal lateral geniculate nucleus of the rat. Hence the second

criterion for the identification of an axo-axonal synapse proved to be insufficient in this case. Consequently, one must be very cautious in its application.

Axo-axonal synapses defined on the basis of the presence of synaptic vesicles in both components have been identified in a number of different areas of the central nervous system. These include the spinal cord of the rat and cat (Gray, 1962 and 1963), the lumbosacral substantia gelatinosa of the cat (Ralston, 1965), the posterior column nuclei of the rat (Valverde, 1966), the main sensory nucleus of the trigeminal nerve (Gobel and Dubner, 1969), the nucleus dorsalis of the cat (Saito, 1974), the oculomotor nucleus of the cat and monkey (Waxman and Pappas, 1970), the gracile (Rustioni and Sotelo, 1974) and cuneate nuclei of the cat (Walberg, 1965b), and the lateral geniculate nucleus of the cat (Szentágothai, Hámori, and Tömböl, 1966) and monkey (Colonnier and Guillery, 1964), as well as other nuclei of the thalamus (Pappas, Cohen, and Purpura, 1966; Jones and Powell, 1969a; Morest, 1970). Axo-axonal synapses have also been recognized in the inner plexiform layer of the retina by Kidd (1962).

In all these situations, where both neuronal profiles contain synaptic vesicles, the profile with vesicles accumulated close to the synaptic junction is designated the presynaptic component. Synaptic vesicles in the postsynaptic component do not concentrate close to the axo-axonal interface; instead, they are related to the second interface in the series, i.e., the junction between this terminal and either a dendrite or a perikaryon. This arrangement, consisting of an axo-axonal synapse superimposed upon an axon terminal that itself participates in an axo-dendritic or axo-somatic synapse, could be the structural basis for one type of presynaptic inhibition (see Eccles, 1961; Katz, 1966). Indeed, in most

---

Figure 5–15. **Axo-Axonal Synapse and Dense-Cored Vesicles.**

The **upper picture** shows an axo-axonal synapse between an axon initial segment (Ax) and an axon terminal (At). The initial segment is characterized by the presence of fascicles of microtubules (m) and a typical dense undercoating (D). The undercoating is less prominent at the synaptic junction (*arrow*) which has a symmetrical form. In the axon terminal (At) some of the synaptic vesicles tend to be elongate. The form of this axo-axonal synaptic junction should be compared with that of the asymmetrical junction between the dendritic spine (sp) and its axon terminal (At_1) on the right.
Rat cerebral cortex. × 90,000.

The **lower picture** shows two axon terminals (At_1 and At_2) synapsing with a dendrite (Den). One of the axon terminals (At_2) contains only agranular, or clear, vesicles, but the other (At_1) also has granular vesicles. These granular vesicles have dark cores and are 75 to 95 nm in diameter.
Dentate nucleus of monkey. × 90,000.

Micrograph by V. Chan-Palay.

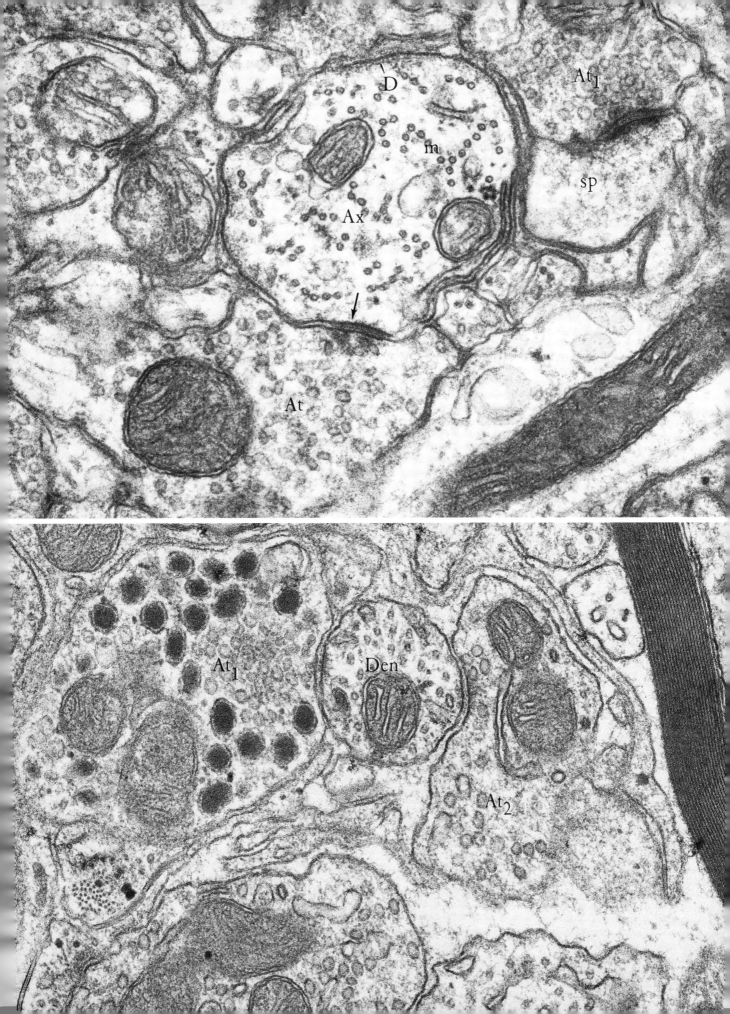

of the areas in which this type of axo-axonal synapse has been found, there is also some corroborative physiological evidence for the existence of presynaptic inhibition.

The other form of axo-axonal synapse that has been encountered in electron microscopic investigations is one in which an axon terminal synapses with the initial segment of an axon (Figure 5–15, upper picture). If the postsynaptic process is not directly continuous with the perikaryon of a neuron at the axon hillock, the initial segment can still be identified by means of the characteristics described in Chapter IV. In brief, these are the undercoating beneath the plasma membrane and the bundles of microtubules within the axoplasm (see Figures 4–1 to 4–3). Axo-axonal synapses involving the axon initial segment as the postsynaptic element have been found in, among other locations, the cerebellar cortex (Palay, 1964; Palay and Chan-Palay, 1974), cerebral cortex (Westrum, 1966; Peters, Proskauer, and Kaiserman-Abramof, 1968), and the lateral vestibular nucleus (Sotelo and Palay, 1970). The presynaptic boutons forming these synapses show no unusual features. At the synaptic junction, which is of the symmetrical type, the vesicles in the axonal terminal show some elongation. Immediately beneath the synaptic complexes the characteristic undercoating of the initial segment gives way to the postsynaptic density (Figure 5–15). The function of these synapses upon the initial axon segments is unknown. In theory their location is very suitable for the exertion of an inhibitory effect upon the initiation of an action potential. It is, however, equally possible, by assuming slight differences in the physiological properties of the postsynaptic membrane, to consider that their location is strategic for inducing an action potential in the initial segment.

It should be noted that in the olfactory bulb, the initial axon segment of the mitral cell may form reciprocal synapses with another element (Price and Powell, 1970b; Willey, 1973). In this case the junction at which the initial axon segment is postsynaptic is symmetrical in form and the junction at which it is presynaptic is asymmetrical.

Two examples have been described of a different form of axo-axonal relationship that functions as a synapse. One is the pinceau around the initial axon segment of the Purkinje neuron of the cerebellum (Palay, 1964; 1967; Palay and Chan-Palay, 1974; Hámori and Szentágothai, 1965; Gobel, 1971; Mugnaini, 1972), and the other is the axon cap around the Mauthner cell

axon of the goldfish (Robertson, Bodenheimer, and Stage, 1963; Kohno, 1970; Nakajima, 1974). In each situation the afferent axons terminate in numerous branching twigs that are filled with small vesicles and surround the initial segment of the axon without forming typical synapses with it. Physiological evidence shows that both of these axo-axonal synapses are inhibitory in function (Furukawa and Furshpan, 1963; Andersen, Eccles, and Voorhoeve, 1963; Eccles, Llinás, and Sasaki, 1966a). The inhibitory influence seems to be produced by a gross alteration in the ionic environment surrounding the postsynaptic membrane, rather than the action of a chemical transmitter.

Since in these two examples no typical junctions were thought to be present between the afferent axons and the initial segments, the question arises as to whether their relation is truly synaptic. Physiologically, it must be synaptic, for the activity of the afferent fibers definitely affects the functional state of the second neuron. If the relation is regarded as a true synapse, however, then it becomes more difficult to define the essential morphological criteria for the identification of synapses.

Recent studies of both the Mauthner cell axon cap and the pinceau around the Purkinje axon have somewhat clarified this problem. Since the latter instance is simpler and better understood, it will be considered first. The most complete description is given by Palay and Chan-Palay (1974). The pinceau consists of a plexus of branching terminal axon collaterals intertwined around the initial segment of the Purkinje cell axon. The axon collaterals originate from a variable number of basket cells, each of which may contribute branches to the pinceaux on several Purkinje cells. The larger branches descend vertically below the Purkinje cell body, and their branches clasp the initial segment like long fingers, forming a kind of palisade around the periphery of the pinceau. In transverse sections the formation appears as a whorl of branching axonal profiles arranged around the Purkinje cell initial segment. The large axons give off robust branches and these subdivide into smaller terminal twigs with blunted tips. Some of the smaller branches contain groups of round and elliptical synaptic vesicles, and the terminal twigs are crowded with them. All these processes in the axonal plexus are bound together by occasional specialized intercellular formations which have been tentatively identified as septate junctions (Gobel, 1971; Sotelo and Llinás, 1972; Palay and Chan-Palay, 1974). At these junctions the adjacent axonal surface membranes become strictly parallel, and the interspace is crossed by discs about 8 nm thick and regularly spaced with a center-to-center distance of about 20 nm. It is these discs that give the junctions their name, for they appear as septa crossing the intercellular space. Viewed *en face* the discs form a honeycomb pattern. Since these junctions have not yet been examined in freeze-fractured preparations, their identification with apparently similar septate junctions in invertebrates must be provisional. But it is worth recalling that in invertebrates septate junctions have been thought to be the sites of electrical coupling between cells (e.g., Lowenstein and Kanno, 1964; Satir and Gilula, 1970). This correlation of structure and function is uncertain, however, since gap junctions have also been found at the same interfaces in invertebrates. If, on further critical analysis, the interaxonal junctions in the pinceau prove to be septate junctions, then it will be important to find out whether the axons are indeed electrically coupled, for no gap junctions have yet been found among them.

The vast majority of the axonal branches in the pinceau terminate freely at some distance from the initial segment of the Purkinje cell axon. In fact, this axon is itself almost completely ensheathed in ribbons of neuroglial cytoplasm. The pinceau can be considered, therefore, as a good example of the synapse *à distance*, an interneuronal junction in which the two members of the synapse fail to come into apposition and remain at a discreet distance. This description of the pinceau was presented in some early electron microscopic analyses of its architecture (Palay, 1964 and 1967; Peters, Palay, and Webster, 1970). At that time direct axo-axonal synapses between basket cell axons and the initial segment of the Purkinje cell axon had been seen only rarely. Hámori and Szentágothai (1965), however, presented a drawing of the pinceau in the cat indicating that in this animal, at least, true Gray's type 2 synapses covered the initial segment of the Purkinje cell axon. This claim has not been substantiated by later studies of this species (Mugnaini, 1972; Sotelo and Llinás, 1972). Nevertheless, examination of a large collection of electron micrographs through the pinceau indicates that in the rat there is regularly a small number of true chemical synaptic junctions (perhaps one or two) between basket cell axon terminals and the Purkinje cell axon initial segment, especially at the border between its first and second thirds (Palay

and Chan-Palay, 1974). Thus, the pinceau included not only a voluminous synapse *à distance*, but also a few precisely placed axo-axonal synaptic junctions of a more conventional type. These terminals contain pleomorphic synaptic vesicles and the symmetrical densities characteristic of Gray's type 2 junctions.

The situation is little better understood concerning the axonal cap of the Mauthner cell. Here the morphological arrangement is far less clear and the physiological studies also leave much detail unexplored. The most comprehensive description is that given by Nakajima (1974). The axonal cap is a highly complicated neuropil surrounding the initial segment and the axon hillock of the Mauthner cell. It consists of fine unmyelinated fibers and their terminals, which form a spiral plexus around the Mauthner cell axon initial segment. They contain clear, round synaptic vesicles. Although some of these axons terminate on the initial segment of the Mauthner cell axon, they also appear to synapse with each other by way of symmetrically placed clusters of round vesicles and membrane densities (first described by Kohno, 1970). Thus the central core bears some resemblance to the pinceau around the Purkinje cell axon. However, the peripheral part of the axonal cap is much more complex. This part is traversed by thin dendrites, which extend from the axon hillock and are covered by small terminal boutons containing flattened synaptic vesicles. There are also many fine unmyelinated axons which originate either from the spiral fibers in the central core of the axonal cap or from large myelinated fibers that are found in the peripheral part of the axonal cap. The former terminate on the axon hillock as small to medium-sized boutons containing round synaptic vesicles, and some of them form mixed synapses with gap junctions like those found in the central core. The fibers originating from large myelinated axons end as unmyelinated club endings on the edges of the axon hillock, and they form only chemical synaptic junctions containing flattened synaptic vesicles. The whole axonal cap is enclosed by neuroglial cells (probably astrocytes), which send delicate processes centrally through the neuropil to surround the initial segment except where terminals are attached. Thus there is a morphological basis in this complex synaptic field for a variety of synaptic mechanisms, both chemical and electrical.

Furukawa and Furshpan (1963) provided evidence that activation of the afferent fibers in the axonal cap produces a brief electrical inhibition of the Mauthner cell followed by a longer-lasting chemically mediated inhibition. These two effects could be produced by the same terminals with mixed synaptic junctions. However, the morphological arrangement is now seen to be so complicated that it would justify a re-examination of the electrophysiology of this synaptic formation. Nakajima's paper (1974) discusses some of the problems posed by the new electron microscopic findings.

Dendro-Dendritic Synapses

Previously it was generally assumed that dendrites could not occupy presynaptic positions, but this assumption was shown to be invalid as a result of the study by Rall, Shepherd, Reese, and Brightman (1966). They produced physiological evidence that the granule and mitral cell dendrites of the olfactory bulb are in synaptic contact, and their morphological studies showed the presence of synapses between the gemmules of the granule cell dendrites and the smoother-surfaced mitral cell dendrites. Apart from the fact that both components are dendrites (see Figure 3–7), some of the synapses are also unusual in that separate and *reciprocal synapses* with opposite polarities occur side by side at the same junctional interface. As in other situations, the direction of transmission is determined by the location of the synaptic vesicles. The side of the junction at which they are clustered is said to be presynaptic. As can be seen in Figure 5–16, the mitral-to-granule cell synapses have a prominent density only on the postsynaptic side of the junction; therefore these synapses are asymmetrical. The granule-to-mitral cell synapses differ from this in having a narrower synaptic cleft and symmetrical densities. These findings have been confirmed by Andres (1965a), Price (1968), and Price and Powell (1970a). It is of interest that on the basis of the physiological evidence, Rall, Shepherd, Reese, and Brightman (1966) postulate that the mitral-to-granule cell synapses are excitatory and the granule-to-mitral cell synapses are inhibitory (see also Rall and Shepherd, 1968; Reese and Shepherd, 1972).

As is well known from Golgi preparations, the granule cells of the olfactory bulb have both peripherally and centrally directed dendrites but no axon. Like the granule cells, the amacrine cells of the retina lack axons, and their dendrites form reciprocal synapses with the central processes of bipolar cells (Dowling and Boycott, 1966; Dowling, 1968). Although the central process of a bipolar cell conducts away from the perikaryon, and so is usually considered to be an axon, Reese and Shepherd (1972) raise the question of whether, on the basis of its morphology and its short length, this process should be regarded as a dendrite. If this concept is accepted, and it does not appear to be necessary, then the synapses between amacrine cells and bipolar cells would also be regarded as dendro-dendritic.

Other reciprocal dendro-dendritic synapses have been observed in the olfactory bulb glomeruli between the dendrites of periglomerular cells and of mitral cells. Again the two oppositely directed synapses differ in their morphology (Hinds, 1970). Pinching (1970) has also shown reciprocal synapses between dendrites of mitral cells and periglomerular cells and between tufted cells and periglomerular cells. In these examples from the olfactory glomeruli both neurons participating in the reciprocal synapse

---

Figure 5–16. **Dendro-Dendritic and Electrical Synapses.**

Upper picture. In the lower half of the field is the secondary dendrite (*Den*) of a mitral cell. This dendrite synapses with a gemmule (*gem*) protruding from a granule cell dendrite. At the synaptic junction between these two dendritic components are two synaptic complexes with opposite polarities, as indicated by *arrows*. Where the direction of transmission, as judged by the grouping of the synaptic vesicles, is from the mitral dendrite to the gemmule, a dense filamentous material (*f*) underlies the postsynaptic membrane. Where the direction is from the gemmule to the mitral cell dendrites, the polarity is not marked by a postsynaptic density.
Olfactory bulb from rat. × 62,000.

Micrograph by T. S. Reese and M. W. Brightman.

Lower picture. In the center of the field is a gap junction forming an electrical synapse between a mossy fiber (*At*) and a granule cell dendrite (*Den*). The separation between the *pre-* and *post*synaptic membranes is about 3 nm. At each end of the gap junction the membranes diverge from each other to form punctate junctions (*triangles*). Within the mossy fiber terminal are synaptic vesicles. (*sv*).
Cerebellum of viper (Vipera aspis). × 230,000.

Micrograph by C. Sotelo.

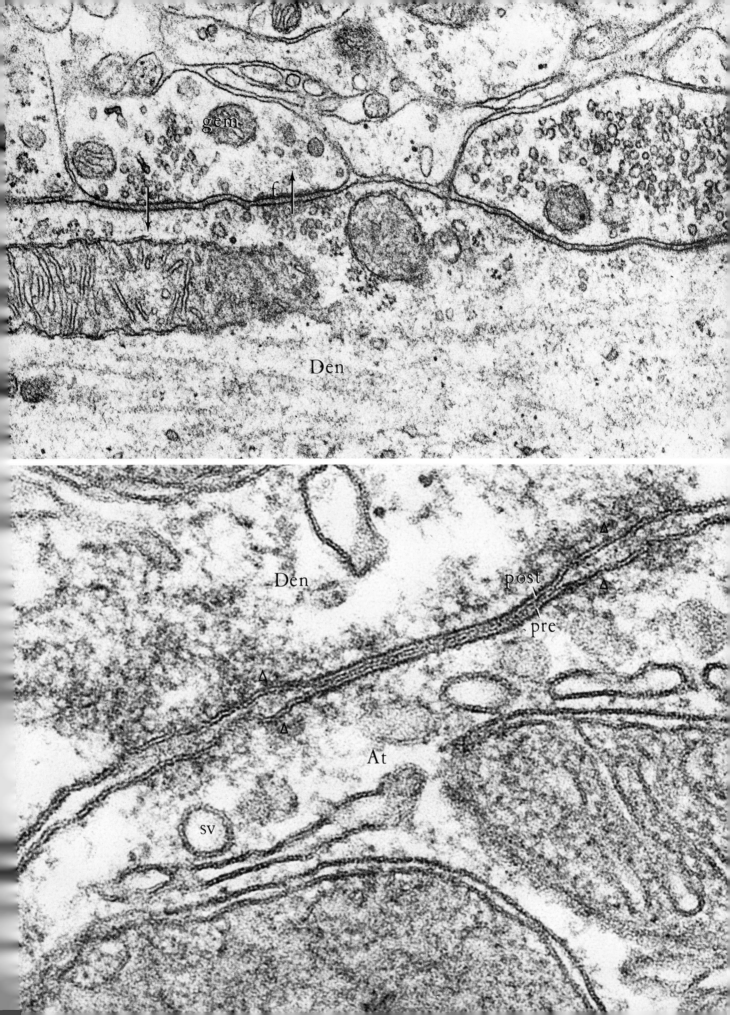

have axons, and the same appears true of the ventrobasal nucleus of the thalamus in the monkey (Harding, 1971) and in the nonglomerular neuropil of the dorsal nucleus of the lateral geniculate body in the cat (Famiglietti, 1970), monkey (LeVay, 1971), and rat (Lieberman and Webster, 1972). In the thalamic examples, however, except for the differences in their polarities, both synapses appear to have a similar morphology.

Other locations in which dendro-dendritic synapses have been recorded, in these cases single and unpaired synapses, are the superior colliculus of the rat (Lund, 1969), cat (Sterling, 1970), and monkey (Lund, 1972); the dorsal horn of the spinal cord (Ralston, 1968); the ventrobasal thalamic nuclei of the cat (Ralston and Herman, 1969; Ralston, 1971) and monkey (Wong, 1970; Harding, 1971); the dorsal nucleus of the lateral geniculate body of the rat (Rafols and Valverde, 1973; Lieberman, 1973) and cat, in both the glomeruli (Famiglietti and Peters, 1972; see Figure 5–18) and the nonglomerular neuropil (Famiglietti, 1970; Wong, 1970; Wong-Riley, 1972; LeVay, 1971); the medial geniculate body of the cat (Morest, 1970 and 1971); and the suprachiasmatic nucleus of the rat hypothalamus (Güldner and Wolff, 1974).

In most of these cases, the studies have been strongly supported by Golgi-impregnated material to show the form of the neuronal processes. In the electron micrographs the identification of the presynaptic component as a dendrite is based upon the presence of ribosomes and sometimes profiles of granular endoplasmic reticulum in the cytoplasm; it is very rare to find ribosomes in axons (see page 90), except in the initial segment, which has a very characteristic morphology (see page 92). In some cases, however, continuity of the presynaptic process with the cell soma has been illustrated and the identification of the process as a dendrite thereby firmly established (e.g., Lund, 1969; Harding, 1971; LeVay, 1971). It should be noted that in nearly all the examples concerning areas outside the olfactory bulb and retina, the accumulation of vesicles at the synapse is very small and not conspicuous.

Somato-Dendritic, Dendro-Somatic, Somato-Axonic, and Somato-Somatic Synapses

Using the accepted criteria for the identification of a chemical synapse, Sétáló and Székely (1967) described somato-dendritic synapses in the optic tectum of the frog. Although they were unable to determine the origin of the dendritic component of the synapse, they considered the presynaptic neuron to be a stellate cell. At the junction the plasma membranes of the two components lie parallel to each other, and the associated density is most conspicuous in the cytoplasm of the dendrite. One or two synaptic complexes may be present at the same junction. Among the synaptic vesicles in the perikaryon there may be one or two which are granular. Clearly, these junctions fulfill all the morphological criteria used for the identification of a chemical synapse. An interesting feature pointed out by Sétáló and Székely (1967) is that these somato-dendritic synapses are often located close to axo-somatic synapses involving the same neuronal perikaryon. Whether this close association between the two types of synapses has a physiological significance is unknown.

Somato-dendritic synapses have also recently been described by Lieberman (1973) in the rat lateral geniculate nucleus. In this nucleus are small cells which, in addition to having dendrites that are presynaptic, have presynaptic perikarya. The perikarya have focal accumulations of elongate vesicles associated with prominent presynaptic densities or projections, and at these points the perikarya are presynaptic to elements described as dendrites. Blunt or stalked appendages may also arise from the perikarya or main dendrites of these small neurons and enter into the synaptic glomeruli that are present in the nucleus.

In addition to the dendro-dendritic synapses already described in the glomeruli of the olfactory bulb, Pinching (1970) has also reported dendro-somatic and somato-somatic synapses. At these junctions the periglomerular cell is presynaptic to the dendrites of mitral cells and to the somata of tufted cells, respectively. Also in the olfactory bulb, Sotelo (1971a) showed reciprocal synapses between the perikarya of mitral cells and the gemmules of granule cells, and Fisher (1972) described somato-somatic synapses in the cat retina in which the perikarya of amacrine cells are presynaptic to those of bipolar cells.

An example of a somato-somatic synapse outside the central nervous system has been described by Matthews and Nash (1970) in the superior cervical ganglion. The participants in the synapse are a small granule-containing cell, which is presynaptic, and the perikarya of principal neurons. In this example some of the vesicles in the granule-containing cells are dense-cored. The somata of these small cells are also presynaptic to other neuronal components which are not perikarya (Matthews and Raisman, 1969).

What may be a somato-somatic synapse has been described in the pineal body of the rat (Arstila and Hopsu, 1964; Hopsu and Arstila, 1965). This junction has small vesicles accumulated close to a site where the plasma membranes of two adjacent perikarya are apposed and lie parallel to each other. The apposed membranes have no visible density associated with them, but between the vesicles are ribbons that closely resemble presynaptic ribbons. In some instances vesicles lie on both sides of the apposed plasma membranes.

Somato-Axonic Synapses

Interesting forms of synaptic relations have also been described in the cardiac ganglion of both the turtle (Yamauchi, Fujimaki, and Yokota, 1975) and rat (Yamauchi, Yokota, and Fujimaki, 1975) and in the rat carotid body (McDonald and Mitchell, 1975). In the cardiac ganglion there are reciprocal synapses between the postganglionic cholinergic axons and granule-containing adrenergic interneurons. At the junction polarized from the cholinergic to the adrenergic element, clear vesicles are concentrated near the presynaptic membrane of the axon terminal, while at the adrenergic to cholinergic synapse the granular vesicles accumulate near the membrane of the granule-containing cell. Similar reciprocal relations exist in the rat carotid body between clear vesicle–containing axon terminals and the granular vesicle–containing glomus cells. The axon terminals in the carotid body are from two sources, the afferent glossopharyngeal axons and the afferent preganglionic sympathetic axons. McDonald and Mitchell (1975) regard the glomus cells as interneurons and comparable with the amacrine cells of the retina and granule cells of the olfactory bulb. If this is so, then the rat carotid body and the turtle cardiac ganglion provide us with examples of somato-axonic synapses.

Dendro-Axonic Synapses

The only suggestion of the existence of dendro-axonic synapses comes from studies of the olfactory bulb. Although no description is given, Pinching and Powell (1971b) indicate that the dendrites of periglomerular cells may be presynaptic to the initial segments of axons from short-axoned (stellate) cells. In another study Willey (1973) described synapses between the initial segments of mitral cell axons and profiles containing synaptic vesicles. The synapses between these two elements are reciprocal and are morphologically unusual because of the presynaptic role of the initial axon segment. Although the element synapsing with the initial segment of the mitral cell is not identified, it is assumed that it is dendritic.

It should be emphasized that in neither of these two examples has the origin of the vesicle-containing profile synapsing with the initial segment been firmly established, so that the existence of dendro-axonic synapses is still equivocal.

Synaptic Glomeruli

A glomerulus is a globular tangle of nerve cell processes reminiscent, in shape and intricacy, of the knots of capillaries that are found in the renal cortex. In the nervous system the name was first applied to complicated ball-like formations of neuropil that are visible to the naked eye or with slight magnification in the superficial layers of the olfactory bulb (see following discussion). Held (1897) used the term to designate certain rounded cell-free areas in the granular layer of the cerebellar cortex within which the rosettes of mossy fibers articulate with the dendrites of granule cells. Each mossy fiber is presynaptic to many granule cell dendrites (Figure 5–17). In this type of glomerulus the large mossy ending, which is filled with many synaptic vesicles and mitochondria disposed around a core of neurofilaments and microtubules, occupies a central position and is surrounded by numerous granule cell dendrites (Figure 5–17, *Den*), which indent its surface (Gray, 1961b; Palay, 1961b and 1964; Mugnaini, 1972; Palay and Chan-Palay, 1974). Occupying a more peripheral position in the glomerulus are the axons of Golgi cells (Figure 5–17, *At*). In contrast to the generally spherical synaptic vesicles of the mossy fiber, in aldehyde-fixed preparations the Golgi cell axons have more flattened vesicles (see Szentágothai, 1970; Mugnaini, 1972; Palay and Chan-Palay, 1974). The Golgi cell axons also synapse upon the granule cell dendrites. Bordering the whole glomerulus and partially separating it from the neuronal elements of the surrounding neuropil are a few astrocytic processes (Figure 5–17).

The glomeruli in the olfactory bulb are more complex (see Shepherd, 1974). Within these glomeruli the terminals of olfactory axons synapse with the dendritic tufts of the principal neurons of the olfactory bulb, the mitral and tufted cells (Andres, 1970; Reese and Brightman, 1970), as well as with the dendrites of the intrinsic periglomerular neurons. These synapses are of the asymmetrical variety. It has been established that numerous synapses also occur between the mitral and periglomerular cell dendrites within a glomerulus (Pinching and Powell, 1971b; White, 1972). The mitral-to-periglomerular cell synapses are asymmetrical, while the periglomerular cell-to-mitral cell synapses are symmetrical and these dendro-dendritic synapses may be either reciprocal, when they are side by side, or serial, when they are separated by a greater distance. Synapses may also be present between two periglomerular cells; and at the outsides of the glomeruli, axon terminals from periglomerular cells may synapse with the larger mitral cell dendrites. The components of a glomerulus are at least partially enclosed by astrocytic sheets.

The meaning of the term "glomerulus" has more recently been expanded to encompass other intimately related groups of neuronal processes which were not recognizable at the level of the light microscope. Although the definition is rather loose, a glomerulus may now be defined as a complicated synaptic field consisting of a more or less discrete globular cluster of intricately intertwined neuronal processes. Structures fitting this definition occur in the lateral geniculate nucleus (Szentágothai, 1963; Colonnier and Guillery, 1964; Szentágothai, Hámori, and Tömböl, 1966; Peters and Palay, 1966; Guillery, 1969; Guillery and Colonnier, 1970; LeVay, 1971; Famiglietti and Peters, 1972; Lie-

berman and Webster, 1972 and 1974; Lieberman, 1974a) and other nuclei of the thalamus (Pappas, Cohen, and Purpura, 1966; Pappas, 1966; Jones and Powell, 1969a; Hajdu, Somogyi, and Tömböl, 1974; Špaček and Lieberman, 1974); in the substantia gelatinosa of the spinal cord (Ralston, 1965; Réthelyi and Szentágothai, 1969) and descending trigeminal nucleus (Gobel, 1974); in the main sensory trigeminal nucleus (Gobel and Dubner, 1969), the inferior olive (Sotelo, Llinás, and Baker, 1974), and the olfactory bulb (Pinching and Powell, 1971a; White, 1972).

The synaptic glomeruli of the dorsal laminae of the dorsal lateral geniculate nucleus in the cat (Guillery, 1969; Szentágothai, 1970; Famiglietti and Peters, 1972; Figure 5–18), mouse (Rafols and Valverde, 1973), rat (McMahan, 1967; Lieberman and Webster, 1972), and monkey (Guillery and Colonnier, 1970; LeVay, 1971) are much more complex than those in the cerebellum and are not yet fully understood. As in the cerebellum (Figure 5–17) a predominating axon terminal (Figure 5–18, Ax_1), which originates from an optic nerve fiber, occupies the central position in the glomerulus. As shown in Figure 5–18, surrounding it, in postsynaptic positions, are both vesicle-filled profiles (Den_2) and the dendritic spines (Den_1) of the thalamocortical relay cells. In early studies (e.g., Peters and Palay, 1966) the vesicle-filled terminals around the central axon were mistakenly identified as axons, and hence the synapses formed between them and the central axon were considered to be axo-axonal. However, in recent studies on the cat (Famiglietti and Peters, 1972), rat (Lieberman and Webster, 1972), and monkey (LeVay, 1971), it was suggested that these vesicle-filled profiles (Figure 5–18, Den_2) are actually dendritic in origin. Thus, the central axon must be considered as being presynaptic in the axo-dendritic synapses it forms with both the vesicle-filled peripheral terminals and the dendritic thorns of

Figure 5–17.   **The Glomerulus, Cerebellar Cortex.**

In this complex structure the presynaptic component is a large axon terminal (the mossy fiber) which sweeps down the middle of the field. It has a light core occupied by neurofilaments and microtubules, which are surrounded by numerous mitochondria. The contour of the terminal is very irregular with many protuberances, which are filled with synaptic vesicles. The postsynaptic component consists of the small terminals of granule cell dendrites (*Den*), which are let into recesses in the surface of the axon terminal and its protuberances to form synapses (*s*). Each dendritic terminal is typically fitted with a single mitochondria. Also participating in the glomerulus are the terminals of Golgi axons (*At*). Although not apparent in this micrograph, these Golgi axons also synapse with the dendrites of the granule cells.
Granular layer in cerebellar cortex of adult rat. × 22,000.

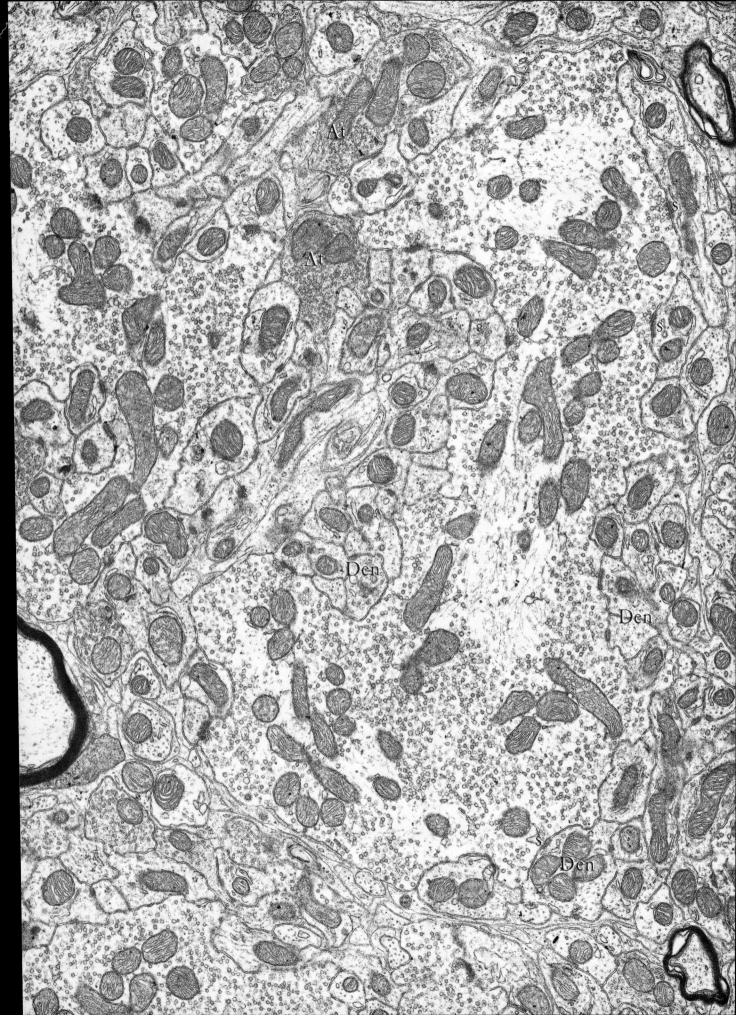

the relay neurons. In addition these thorns have also proved to be postsynaptic to the same vesicle-filled peripheral terminals (Figure 5–18, *arrows*). Most of these vesicle-filled profiles (Figure 5–18, Den_2) seem to be derived from dendrites of the Golgi type II cells of this thalamic nucleus, but the glomeruli also seem to contain axon terminals (Figure 5–18, Ax_2) of the same Golgi type II cells, as well as terminals of corticogeniculate fibers. Since there is still debate about the exact origins of the components of these glomeruli, reference should be made to the original accounts for a fuller discussion of the intricacies of this structure. Besides the synaptic junctions, rather complex puncta adhaerentia also occur between the plasma membranes of adjacent components in this glomerulus.

In the medial geniculate nucleus of the thalamus (Jones and Powell, 1969a; Morest, 1970), the structure of the glomeruli seems, in many respects, to be very much like that of the lateral geniculate nucleus. One difference, however, is that the central element of the medial geniculate glomerulus is a dendritic protrusion, or thorn. A similar situation also seems to occur in the pulvinar (Majorossy, Réthelyi, and Szentágothai, 1965; Szentágothai, 1970; Hajdu, Somogyi, and Tömböl, 1974). In both cases one of the vesicle-filled profiles is presynaptic to the other and to the dendritic protrusion, while the second vesicle-filled process is presynaptic only to the dendritic protrusion.

Three components are also present in the glomeruli of the somatosensory nucleus of the thalamus of the rat (Špaček and Lieberman, 1974). One of these is a dendritic protrusion that is embedded in a large axonal terminal, derived from the fibers of the medial lemniscus, which makes extensive synaptic contacts with dendritic protrusions. The lemniscal terminals have round vesicles. The other component is a small terminal with flattened vesicles and this is also presynaptic to the dendritic component. However, there are apparently no synapses between

the vesicle-containing terminals, although both vesicle-containing terminals are presynaptic to the dendrite.

In the substantia gelatinosa of the spinal cord (Ralston, 1965; Réthelyi and Szentágothai, 1969), a large axon terminal occupies the center of the glomerulus, and its surface is indented by vesicle-filled profiles and by the spines of dendrites. The large central axon terminals originate from the pyramid-shaped neurons of the dorsal horn. They are presynaptic to both the vesicle-filled peripheral terminals and to the dendritic processes, which probably belong to intrinsic neurons of the substantia gelatinosa. At the same time, the peripheral axons, which are in part derived from the axons of the primary sensory neurons (Szentágothai, 1970), are also presynaptic to the dendritic processes. This synaptic field lacks a conspicuous astrocytic covering.

According to the recent study of Gobel (1974) the synaptic glomeruli in the substantia gelatinosa (nucleus caudalis or descending nucleus) of the cat spinal trigeminal nucleus are more complex than those in the lower spinal cord. Thus, Gobel described a large central axon derived from a trigeminal nucleus neuron that is surrounded by dendritic shafts, two kinds of dendritic spines, and small axon terminals. The central axon is presynaptic to each of the dendritic components, the most common of which is a dendritic spine with no synaptic vesicles in its cytoplasm. This type of spine also articulates with the second type of dendritic spine, which has synaptic vesicles in its cytoplasm, as well as with vesicle-containing dendritic shafts and with the small axon terminals. These small axon terminals, which are derived from neurons contained within the substantia gelatinosa, are also presynaptic to the central axon, and consequently Gobel suggests that these interneurons are inhibitory in function.

In the main sensory nucleus of the trigeminal nerve of the cat (Gobel and Dubner, 1969), the synaptic glomeruli again have a cen-

---

Figure 5–18. **The Glomerulus, Lateral Geniculate Nucleus.**

This large synaptic glomerulus contains a number of different neuronal components. The most prominent one is the large central axon (Ax_1) which is an optic nerve terminal. This synapses *(arrow)* upon both bulbous dendritic profiles (Den_1) of the geniculocortical relay cells and vesicle-filled dendritic terminals (Den_2). The vesicle-filled dendritic terminals also synapse *(arrowhead)* on the dendrites (Den_1) of the geniculocortical cells. A fourth type of profile (Ax_2) with some flatter synaptic vesicles is also present in the glomerulus.

Note that the glomerulus is surrounded by sheet-like astrocytic processes (As).
Dorsal nucleus of lateral geniculate body, cat. × 40,000.

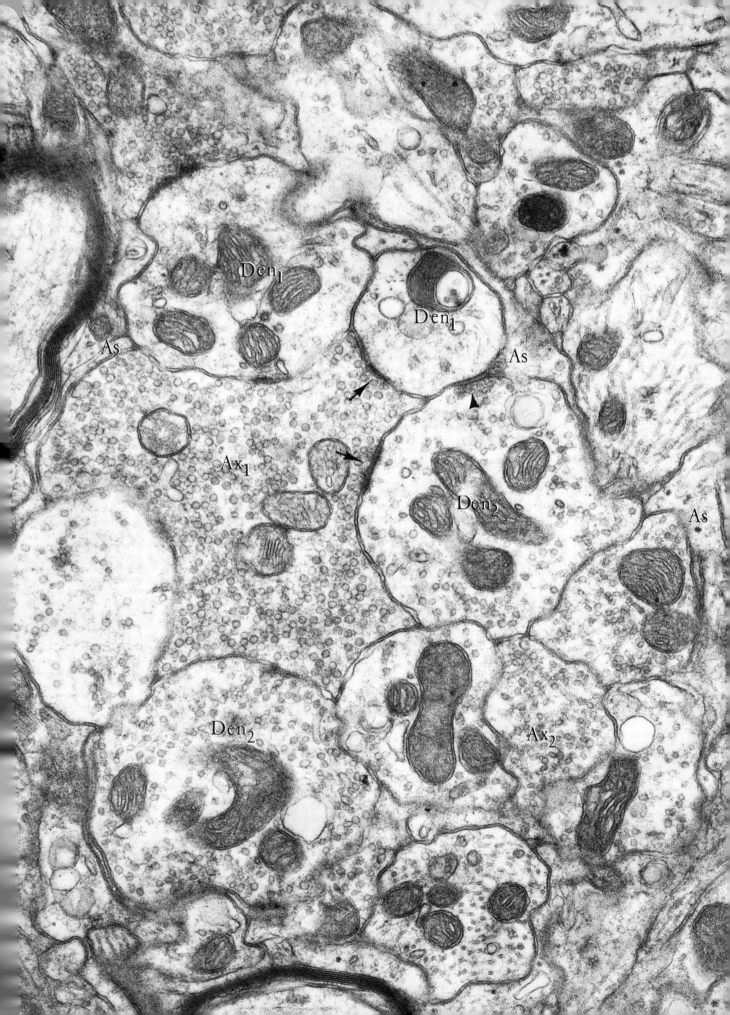

tral axon, but one derived from the primary trigeminal afferent fibers. The central axon is surrounded by smaller, vesicle-filled boutons and dendritic processes. The central axon and peripheral boutons both synapse upon the dendritic component and, judging from the distribution of synaptic vesicles, Gobel and Dubner suggest that the peripheral axons are presynaptic to the central ones.

Although no complete generalizations are possible, it seems that in these glomeruli there is a common pattern of organization in that at least three principal components are involved in the structure. Two of them are vesicle-containing components and the other is a dendritic component with no vesicles. In most thalamic glomeruli the large central axon carrying the primary sensory information is presynaptic to the other two components, while the dendritic processes of the relay cell are postsynaptic to both vesicle-containing components, the smaller of which is probably derived in each case from an interneuron, or Golgi type II cell. In the somatosensory nuclei of the rat thalamus the situation is simpler, for although both vesicle-containing components are presynaptic to the dendritic component lacking vesicles, there are no synapses between the vesicle-containing components. In contrast, in the substantia gelatinosa and in the main sensory nucleus of the trigeminal nerve the primary afferent axons from the sensory ganglion cells are postsynaptic to the other vesicle-filled component, even though the primary sensory axon occupies a central position in the glomeruli of the main sensory trigeminal nucleus and trigeminal substantia gelatinosa and a peripheral position in the glomeruli of the spinal substantia gelatinosa.

ELECTRICAL SYNAPSES

As the techniques for intracellular recording developed, it became evident that electrotonic transmission occurs between neurons at a number of sites, both in invertebrates and in vertebrates. The first electrical synapse to be examined morphologically was the giant motor synapse of the crayfish (Robertson, 1953, 1955a, and 1964; Hama, 1961). This was also the first synapse at which electrical one-way transmission was clearly demonstrated (Furshpan and Potter, 1959; Furshpan, 1964). Since then, electrotonic transmission has been demonstrated in a number of fishes, particularly by Bennett and Pappas and their coworkers who have carried out extensive correlative studies of the morphology and physiological properties of such synapses.

It is now evident that where electrotonic transmission occurs between two neurons their plasma membranes come close together (see Bennett, 1974). As seen in Figure 5–16 (lower figure) a gap of about 2 nm is maintained between them, and so in sections taken perpendicular to the junction, an apparently seven-layered structure appears. It consists of four dense lines, two from each of the plasma membranes (*pre* and *post*), alternating with three lighter lines. Hence these are *gap junctions* and not zonulae occludentes, in which the space between apposed membranes is obliterated. At the present time there is no reason to believe that zonulae occludentes couple cells electrotonically. Consequently, the morphology of electrical synapses differs significantly from that of chemical synapses at which there is a cleft of about 20 nm. Furthermore, the electrical synapses are generally symmetrical and display little or none of the dense material associated with the cytoplasmic faces of plasma membranes involved in chemical synapses.

Since the early studies of the crayfish giant motor synapse, the electromotor neurons of mormyrid fish have been studied (Bennett, Aljure, Nakajima, and Pappas, 1963) as well as the club endings on Mauthner cells in the goldfish (Robertson, Bodenheimer, and Stage, 1963; Nakajima, 1974). The occurrence of gap junctions has also been correlated with physiological studies of electrotonic coupling in a number of other sites.

In fish (see Pappas and Waxman, 1972), axo-dendritic and axo-somatic electrical synapses have been described in locations such as the spinal electromotor nucleus of the electric eel (Pappas and Bennett, 1966; Mezler, Pappas, and Bennett, 1972 and 1974), swimbladder neurons of the toadfish (Pappas and Bennett, 1966), spinal and medullary electromotor nuclei of mormyrid fishes (Bennett, Pappas, Aljure, and Nakajima, 1967), giant electromotor neurons of the electric catfish (Bennett, Nakajima, and Pappas, 1967b), medullary pacemaker and relay nuclei of gymnotid fish (Bennett, Pappas, Giménez, and Nakajima, 1967), and the cerebellar cortex of mormyrid fish (Kaiserman-Abramof and Palay, 1969) and gymnotid fish (Sotelo and Llinás, 1972). Dendro-dendritic electrotonic junctions have been observed in gymnotid medullary electromotor nuclei (Bennett, Pappas, Giménez, and Nakajima, 1967) and in mormyrid mĕdullary electromotor nuclei (Bennett, Pappas, Aljure, and Nakajima, 1967), which also have dendro-somatic and somato-somatic synapses. In addition there are axo-axonal contacts, and these have been described in supramedullary neurons of several species of teleosts (Bennett, Nakajima, and Pappas, 1967a).

In amphibia there is morphological evidence for electrical synapses between axons and dendrites in the spinal cord of the frog (Charlton and Gray, 1965 and 1966), in which electrotonic transmission has been recorded (Grinnell and Miledi, 1965; Grinnell, 1966). In birds similar synapses have been described in the tangential nucleus (Hinojosa and Robertson, 1967), and in the ciliary ganglion of the chicken (Brightman and Reese, 1969).

In mammals interneuronal gap junctions have been recorded at only a few sites. These are the lateral vestibular nucleus (Sotelo and Palay, 1970), the inferior olive (Sotelo, Llinás, and Baker, 1974), possibly the mesencephalic trigeminal nucleus (Hinrichsen and Larramendi, 1968 and 1970), the bipolar-ganglion cell junction of the primate retina (Dowling and Boycott, 1966), between photoreceptor cells in the monkey and rabbit retina (Raviola and Gilula, 1973), between cone bipolar cells and amacrine cells in the cat retina (Kolb and Famiglietti, 1974), and between dendrites of the primate cortex (Sloper, 1972). Of these, electrotonic transmission has been recorded in the mesencephalic trigeminal nucleus (Baker and Llinás, 1970), and there is some evidence for such coupling at the bipolar-ganglion cell junction (Ogden 1966) and in the inferior olive (Llinás, Baker, and Sotelo, 1974). In addition, Sotelo and Llinás (1972) have described the presence of gap junctions in the molecular layer of the cerebellum of the cat and rat. Here they occur between neuronal perikarya and dendrites, between neuronal perikarya, and between dendrites.

To return to the form of the gap junctions involved in electrotonic coupling, Robertson (1963) was the first to show a highly differentiated structure that seemed to exist in the gap. Obliquely sectioned junctions displayed delicate cross striations that were about 8 to 9 nm

apart so that a regular ladder-like pattern occurred along the extent of the contact. Sections passing in the plane of the junction displayed an array of closely packed, hexagonal subunits, the walls of which corresponded to the ladder-like striations in more normally oriented planes of section. These appearances were confirmed by studies on electrical synapses in other fishes (Bennett, Nakajima, and Pappas, 1967a; Pappas and Bennett, 1966). Peracchia (1973a) showed a similar appearance between the ends of segments of the lateral giant fibers in the crayfish. Each subunit has a dense dot in its center, and this pattern is clearly shown in isolated synaptic discs from the goldfish nervous system (Zampighi and Robertson, 1973).

When the first descriptions of electrical synapses were presented, gap junctions had not been differentiated from tight junctions (zonulae occludentes). The distinction between these two types of junctions was made clear when dense tracers were introduced into the extracellular space (Revel and Karnovsky, 1967). By applying this technique to the Mauthner cell synapses, Brightman and Reese (1969) not only confirmed the earlier observation of Robertson, Bodenheimer, and Stage (1963) but also showed that the apposed plasma membranes are separated by a gap of about 2 nm which can be penetrated by lanthanum salts. The lanthanum delineated a lamina of honeycombed subunits corresponding to that described by Robertson (1963). Since the lanthanum filled the intercellular spaces it appeared as though the subunits occupied the narrow intercellular gap of the junction. It was not known, however, whether the subunits actually lay in the junction or were matching bulges from the apposed plasma membranes.

The structure of the gap junction was clarified by the application of freeze-fracturing techniques (Chalcroft and Bullivant, 1970; McNutt and Weinstein, 1970; Goodenough and Revel, 1970; Goodenough and Gilula, 1974). These studies show a system of globular particles within the membrane. The particles are arranged in closely packed hexagonal array and are approximately 8 nm in diameter and about 9.5 nm from center to center. Hence their size corresponds to that of the hexagonal subunits delineated by lanthanum. The particles contained within the apposed plasma membranes and shown by freeze fracturing are in exact register so that the rounded elevations produced by the particles of one membrane exactly match those of its facing partner. The penetration of lanthanum between these matched elevations produces the hexagonal subunit patterns seen in sectioned material.

In a study of the known electrical junctions between segments of the lateral giant fibers of the crayfish, Peracchia (1973a and b) has described two patterns of globular subunits after immersion of the tissue in lanthanum. One pattern displays a hexagonal array of globules which are closely packed and have a center-to-center spacing of about 20 nm. The other, less regular pattern of subunits, has a center-to-center spacing of about 13 nm. This result is supported by studies of freeze-fractured preparations (Peracchia, 1973b). In these preparations, the A face directed toward the gap between the two membranes forming the gap junction displays pits 6 to 10 nm in diameter, arranged in a hexagonal pattern with center-to-center spacing of about 20 nm, which corresponds to the larger pattern observed in the lanthanum preparations. A few of the pits are occupied by globules about 12.5 nm wide. Globules of a similar size are more frequent on the B, or internal, face of the outer leaflet, where they commonly are spaced by about 20 nm, but occasionally by about 12.5 nm like the finer pattern of globular subunits in the lanthanum preparations.

It should be noted that in these preparations the preferential retention of the globules on the B face is the converse of their behavior in mammalian gap junctions, in which they are most prominently retained with the A face. Gap junctions with these characteristics may be typical of arthropods since similar features are also displayed by insect gap junctions after freeze fracturing.

In the center of the top surface of each globule in the freeze-fractured preparations Peracchia (1973b) noted a central depression with a diameter of about 2.5 nm, which is matched by an elevation at the bottom of each pit. Peracchia suggests that these 2.5 nm entities, which are arranged perpendicular to the plane of the plasma membranes forming the junction, are the equivalents of the 2.5 nm dense dots seen in the centers of the hexagonally packed subunits after lanthanum staining of gap junctions. Because of their form he proposes that they represent the ends of channels which cross the electrotonic junctions (see also Pappas, Asada, and Bennett, 1971).

Evidence for the existence of such small channels is provided by introducing a fluorescent dye, Procion yellow, into one of the coupled septate axons of the crayfish. After intro-

duction, the dye appears in the next axon on the other side of the junction (Payton, Bennett, and Pappas, 1969). When introduced extracellularly, no such passage of dye occurs. Fluorescein (Pappas and Bennett, 1966), sucrose (Bennett and Dunham, 1970), small ions, neutral red (Bennett, Dunham, and Pappas, 1967), micro-peroxidase of molecular weight 1800 (Reese, Bennett, and Feder, 1971), and cobalt ions (Politoff, Pappas, and Bennett, 1974) also pass between coupled cells. In view of such evidence for the passage of small molecules and ions between cells that are connected by gap junctions, Simionescu, Simionescu, and Palade (1975) recommend that these junctions should be called *maculae communicantes* in order to distinguish them from the zonulae occludentes.

Apart from the gap junctions between plasma membranes at electrical synapses, Bennett and Pappas and their coworkers found that adherent junctions occur at the same interfaces (Figure 5–16, *triangles*). The presynaptic element may also contain clear vesicles (*sv*) of the same size range as those associated with chemical synapses, but these are usually less numerous than at most chemical synapses and apparently do not cluster in the vicinity of the adherent junctions. Pappas and Bennett (1966) conclude that no functional significance can be ascribed to these vesicles, since although they occur in the catfish (Bennett, Nakajima, and Pappas, 1967b) and the gymnotids (Bennett, Pappas, Giménez, and Nakajima, 1967), there is no electrophysiological evidence for chemical transmission.

In the lamprey, however, in which the Müller cell axons form synapses which display both gap junctions and chemical junctions at the same interface, Rovainen (1974b) has shown that composite bursts of excitatory postsynaptic potentials are produced by excitation of the Müller fibers. He attributes these composite excitatory postsynaptic potentials to the existence of the two types of junction at the same interface. Rovainen suggests that the failure to detect chemical transmission at the synapses in electric fish, like those studied by Bennett and Pappas and their coworkers, can probably be attributed to the fact that the small chemical components are masked by the massive, and more extensive, electrical junctions.

These junctions, at which definite electrical and chemical synapses occur at the same interface, are termed "mixed synapses" (Figure 5–19), and more examples of such synapses will be presented in the next section.

From this discussion, then, it is apparent that, unlike a chemical synapse, an electrical synapse does not function through the action of a chemical transmitter. Instead the gap junction of the electrical synapse offers a low-resistance pathway between the cells. The close approximation of the pre- and postsynaptic membrane and the probable existence of intramembranous channels, matched and in register, through which ions can pass, minimize the current leakage across the junction and maximize the flow of current into the postsynaptic component. In addition, since a chemical transmitter does not have to be mobilized, electrical synapses show less delay than chemical synapses. It seems that unlike chemical synapses, whose direction of transmission is determined by the disposition of the transmitter, electrical synapses may transmit in both directions, although the direction of the transmission is usually determined by the interrelations of the neurons in the pathway. For a further consideration of the comparison between the properties of electrical and chemical synapses reference should be made to the excellent discussions by Bennett (1972a and b).

Gap junctions between adjacent plasma membranes also occur elsewhere in the central nervous system, notably between astrocytes (see Chapter VII), and here again they provide low resistance pathways (see Kuffler and Nicholls, 1966). They may also exist between adjacent oligodendrocytes (Sotelo and Angaut, 1973).

MIXED SYNAPSES

Mixed synapses occur at interfaces where there is evidence, either physiological or morphological, for the existence of both chemical and electrical transmission (Figure 5–19).

One structure in which there is physiological evidence of both types of transmission is the ciliary ganglion of the chick. Martin and Pilar (1963a and b) found that, in addition to displaying chemical transmission, the synapses of the ciliary ganglion of three- to five-day-old chicks also exhibit electrotonic coupling. Furthermore, the amount of electrotonic coupling apparently increases with age, at least until four weeks of age.

Electron microscope studies of this ganglion (De Lorenzo, 1960; Hess, 1965) have shown that it possesses some very interesting features. First, the perikarya, together with the presynaptic terminals seated upon them, are ensheathed by lamellae of both loose and compact myelin. Second, in the newly hatched chick each ganglion cell rests in a cup formed by a calyciform axon terminal. Third, in later development the calyciform ending appears to break up into small boutons. Thus, in a six-month-old chicken calyces appear upon only about half of the neurons, and by one to two years of age the transformation is so complete that only small boutons exist.

In a study of these synapses Hess (1965) failed to find sites of close apposition between the plasma membranes of the afferent nerve fibers and the ganglion cells. He postulated that the electrotonic coupling demonstrated by Martin and Pilar could be accounted for by the presence of the myelin lamellae that surround the preterminal axon, the calyciform terminal, and the ganglion cell. In effect, this myelin sheath encloses the synapse within an internode so that the impulses could pass by saltatory conduction from the preterminal axon to the axon exiting from the ganglion cell. He also suggested that the increase in electrical transmission that occurs with maturation is due to the increase in thickness of the myelin sheath surrounding each ganglion cell and hence the progressively more effective insulation. The possibility of saltatory conduction was also mentioned by Martin and Pilar (1964).

Takahashi and Hama (1965), on the contrary, found areas of close apposition at the interface between the plasma membranes of the calyciform axon terminal and the ganglion cell. They pointed out, however, that these appositions occur so rarely that it is uncertain whether they can play any effective role in electrotonic transmission. Much more common at the same interface are *puncta adhaerentia* and synaptic junctions with associated vesicles. De Lorenzo (1966) also observed areas of close apposition between the pre- and postsynaptic membranes, particularly in the region of the axon hillock of the ganglion cell. Brightman and Reese (1969) confirmed these observations and once again showed that the areas of close apposition are further examples of typical gap junctions.

At present it must be concluded that, although chemical synapses and gap junctions have both been observed in the chick ciliary ganglion, there is still some uncertainty about whether the latter structures entirely account for the electrotonic transmission. The role played by the myelin sheaths surrounding the neurons has not yet been elucidated (see also, Bennett, Pappas, Giménez, and Nakajima, 1967). In a recent detailed account of the ciliary ganglion in the adult chicken Cantino and Mugnaini (1975) showed that gap junctions between the pre- and postsynaptic membranes are small but not uncommon. They calculated that gap junctions occupy about 0.17 per cent of the appositional area between the axonal terminals and the ganglion cell, whereas conventional chemical synaptic junctions occupy about 9 per cent. On the basis of the number of gap junction particles (counted in freeze-fractured material) and theoretical estimates of the electrical resistance through a single intercellular channel in these particles, they concluded that the gap junctions, despite their size and number, are sufficient to account for the electrotonic coupling between the preganglionic fibers and the ganglion cells.

Another example of a mixed synapse has been reported by Sotelo and Palay (1970) in the lateral vestibular nucleus of the rat (Figure 5–19). In this nucleus there are large terminal boutons that make synaptic contacts with the giant Deiters neurons. The terminals are about 10 to 12 microns long and 2 to 4 microns deep and generally arise from the afferent axons immediately beyond the termination of their myelin sheaths. As displayed in Figure 5–19, at the interface between the pre- and postsynaptic membranes three types of junctional specialization occur: (1) synaptic complexes that are asymmetrical and have the characteristics of chemical synapses (*arrows*); (2) symmetrical complexes with the characteristics of *puncta adhaerentia* (*triangles*); and (3) complexes in which the pre- and postsynaptic membranes are closely apposed, as at the electrical synapses described above (*asterisk*). In possessing these three types

of complex, the synapses on the Deiters neurons resemble the calyciform synapses in the ciliary ganglion of the chick. The synapses of the club endings upon the Mauthner cell of the goldfish probably have the same form (Robertson, Bodenheimer, and Stage, 1963; Brightman and Reese, 1969; Nakajima, 1974).

Sotelo and Llinás (1972) have recently described mixed synapses between mossy fiber endings and the dendrites of granule cells in the cerebellum of gymnotid fish and frogs. Where vesicles accumulate, the synaptic complexes are asymmetrical, and the gap junctions of the synaptic interface are only about 0.08 to 2.0 microns long. In this instance, as in the lateral vestibular nucleus of the rat, the surface area of the synaptic junction occupied by the chemical synaptic complexes is much greater than that involved in gap junctions. In the cerebellum, the difference factor is two to six times.

As pointed out above, mixed synapses also occur in fish. Apart from those involving the Mauthner cell (Robertson, Bodenheimer, and Stage, 1963), they have been encountered in the ventral horn of the spinal cord in the goldfish and tench (Gray, 1969b), the electromotor neurons of the catfish (Bennett, Nakajima, and Pappas, 1967b), the electromotor relay nucleus of gymnotid fish (Bennett, Pappas, Giménez, and Nakajima, 1967), the teleost oculomotor nucleus (Waxman, Kriebel, Bennett, and Pappas, 1968; Pappas and Waxman, 1972) and the tangential nucleus of the goldfish (Hinojosa, 1973). The mixed synapses between the Müller axons and unidentified dendrites in the spinal cord of the sea lamprey (Rovainen, 1974a and b) have already been mentioned in the previous section. A review of published pictures and descriptions indicates that most of the synapses described in vertebrates as electrotonic synapses are actually only parts of mixed synapses in which the chemical component for some reason failed to receive equal emphasis.

Figure 5–19. **A Mixed Synapse.**

Occupying the center of the field is a large axon terminal containing many synaptic vesicles (*sv*) and mitochondria (*mit*). This terminal forms a mixed synapse with the perikaryon of a Deiters neuron. At the synaptic junction complexes of three types occur: (1) Complexes in which there is close apposition between the pre- and postsynaptic membranes (✱). These are considered as probable electrical synapses. (2) Complexes at which there is a cleft between the pre- and postsynaptic membranes and a prominent postsynaptic accumulation of dense material (*arrow*). Although not shown here, such junctions usually have synaptic vesicles associated with them so that they have the form of typical chemical synapses. (3) Complexes at which there is a space between the pre- and postsynaptic membranes and symmetrically disposed dense material (*triangles*). These are typical *puncta adhaerentia* and do not have associated synaptic vesicles.
Lateral vestibular nucleus of rat. × 41,000.

Micrograph by C. Sotelo.

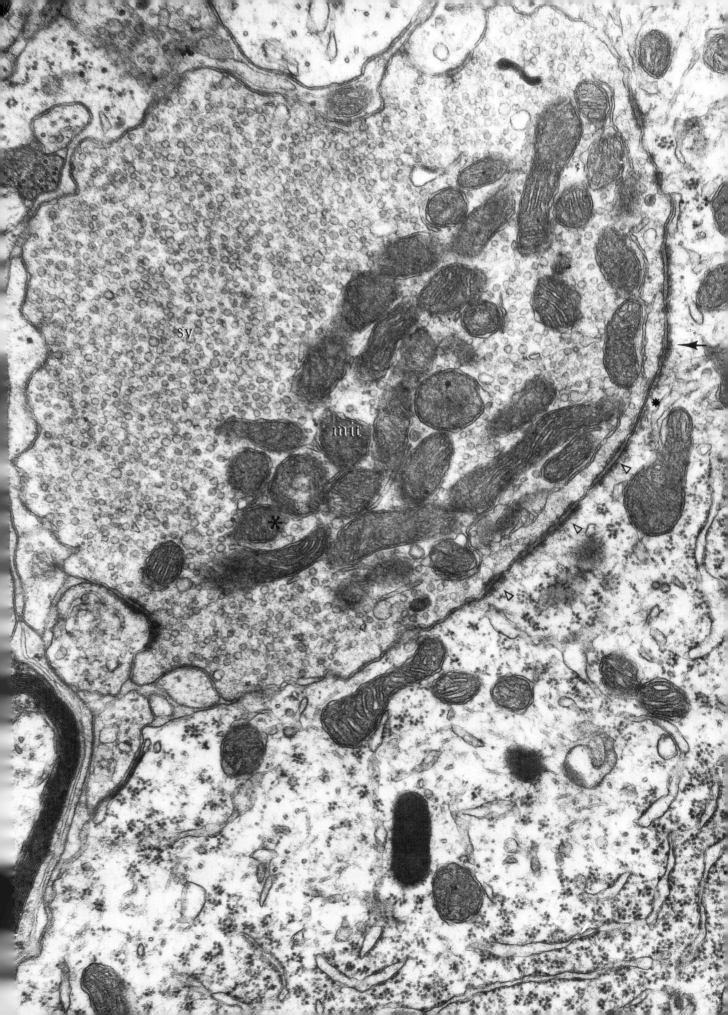

The existence of mixed synapses—that is, the coexistence of chemical synaptic junctions and adjacent gap junctions on the same intercellular surface—raises the question of what possible functions could be served by having both types of transmission occurring at the same interface. It might be assumed that when an impulse invades a presynaptic terminal it would immediately cross the gap junction to depolarize the postsynaptic member of the synapse, thus apparently short-circuiting the mechanisms of chemical transmission and rendering it useless. But this is not necessarily the case. Under natural conditions the effect of the leak across the gap junction may be only a brief, local change in postsynaptic membrane potential, since the postsynaptic component in these synapses usually has a large volume in relation to that of the nerve ending. Thus the effect of transmission through the gap junction may be to prepare the postsynaptic membrane for the receipt of the slower chemical transmission, ensuring that the membrane potential is close to threshold and that it will respond to each impulse transmitted. Another possible function may be displayed if the gap junction transmits in only one direction and has a functional polarity opposite that of the chemical synapse. Then the electrical transmission would follow the postsynaptic potential evoked by chemical transmission and would flow in the opposite direction, that is, into the nerve terminal, where it could augment or depress the efficiency of synaptic discharges according to its timing. Such speculations suggest that the device of placing both chemical and electrical mechanisms for transmission at the same interface provides for very subtle interactions between two neural elements. It is surprising that these possibilities have not attracted more interest among neurophysiologists.

"SYNAPSES" INVOLVING NEUROGLIAL CELLS

In the past year there have been two descriptions of entities which appear to be "axo-glial synapses." These entities meet the morphological criteria for synapses on the basis that a vesicle-containing profile forms a specialized junction with another structure. In these cases the second component has been identified as a neuroglial cell.

Thus, in the developing mouse spinal cord Henrikson and Vaughn (1974) have found that vesicle-containing axon terminals form synapse-like junctions with the processes of radial glial cells. These junctions show a marked similarity to axo-dendritic synapses which are also present in the spinal cord at the same time. However, the existence of these junctions is quite brief. There are none at the tenth day of gestation, a few at the eleventh and twelfth days, many at the thirteenth and fourteenth days, and none again at the fifteenth and sixteenth days of gestation. Based upon these observations Henrikson and Vaughn (1974) suggest that these axo-glial unions may reflect errors in development and that they disappear because there are no specific requirements in the system to sustain their maintenance.

In the general cortex of the turtle, however, axon terminals forming junctions with perikarya of ependymal cells are present in the adult. Ebner and Colonnier (1975) are not able to come to any conclusion about the function of these junctions which they refer to as neuro-ependymal contacts. They suggest that the junctions may, in the light of Henrikson and Vaughn's conclusions, indicate that the turtle brain is continuously growing, or alternatively that the junctions allow for some form of neuronal control over ependymal cell function.

At present insufficient data are available to draw any conclusions about the nature and function of these axo-glial junctions. However, it is important that their existence should be documented at this time.

Chapter VI

THE CELLULAR SHEATHS
OF NEURONS

In the peripheral nervous system both axons and cell bodies of neurons are surrounded by sheaths. The cells encapsulating neuronal cell bodies are usually referred to as satellite cells, and those surrounding axons as Schwann cells. However, these two cells have essentially the same morphology and function, and in addition both are derived from the neural crest, so that there is little reason to consider them as different types. Nevertheless, for the purposes of description the terms "satellite cells" and "Schwann cells" are useful, and they will be retained here.

Sometimes the sheath formed by these cells is basically simple in form. For example, the satellite cells of most of the peripheral neurons are arranged to form a single layer around the enclosed neuron (Figures 6–1 and 6–2). In the nerve a row of cells, now termed Schwann cells, extends along a group of axons, each axon lying in a separate longitudinal invagination of the ensheathing cell. Nerve cell bodies and axons enclosed in such a simple manner are said to be unmyelinated (Figure 6–3). More complex sheaths—myelin sheaths—can also be formed by Schwann and satellite cells (Figure 6–5). In the myelinated nerve fiber a single axon is enclosed by a series of Schwann cells arranged along its length. Each Schwann cell in the series wraps the axon within a spiralled sheet of plasma membrane that constitutes the myelin. The length of myelin formed by each Schwann cell is termed an internodal segment, and the region where two adjacent Schwann cells abut, and the

myelin is interrupted, is referred to as a node of Ranvier (see Frontispiece). At a node no myelin covers the axon, so that in a light microscope preparation stained for myelin the node appears as a discontinuity in the sheath. The elongated nuclei of the Schwann cells forming the myelin internodes are located at the midpoint of the extent of each cell (Frontispiece). At such a site the Schwann cell nucleus and the organelles surrounding it form a bulge. The satellite cells surrounding certain ganglion cells of the peripheral nervous system are also capable of forming myelin sheaths. However, except within the ganglion of the eighth nerve, myelinated cell bodies are relatively uncommon in mammals.

In the central nervous system axons can also be myelinated, and the cells forming their sheaths are the oligodendrocytes, which in white matter tend to be arranged in rows parallel to the nerve fibers (Frontispiece). The myelin-forming cells are located some distance away from the sheaths they form, but as in peripheral nerves a spiralled sheet of membrane forms the myelin which is similarly produced in internodal lengths separated from each other by nodes of Ranvier. In contrast to the peripheral nervous system, however, only the myelinated axons are ensheathed. Other axons passing through the neuropil, or contained in tracts of white matter, are essentially bare and lie directly adjacent to other neuronal and neuroglial components. So far as we are aware, no neuronal perikarya of the mammalian central nervous system are systematically surrounded by myelin sheaths, but they may be surrounded by a sheath composed of astrocytes and their processes. The extent of this covering is variable, however, for while the perikarya of such neurons as anterior horn cells, Purkinje cells, and neurons of the lateral vestibular nucleus have a complete covering of astroglial processes that is only interrupted where the neuron forms synapses with axon terminals, other neurons, such as the majority of those in the cerebral cortex, lack a definite covering. The astroglial sheaths will not be described in the present chapter but will be considered in the chapter dealing with neuroglial cells (see page 242).

Of interest is the recent finding that dendrites in the olfactory bulb of the Rhesus monkey (Pinching, 1971) and cat (Willey, 1973) may be myelinated. But this seems to be a rather unusual situation, for no myelinated dendrites have yet been described in other parts of the central nervous system.

Another anomaly that may be referred to is the presence of amyelinated axons in the spinal and cranial nerve roots of dystrophic mouse mutants (Biscoe, Caddy, Pallot, Pehrson, and Stirling, 1974; Stirling, 1975a). The term "amyelinated" is used because the majority of the axons in the proximal portions of the roots of these mutants are completely without Schwann cell investments, although they are ensheathed close to the central nervous system, as well as more distally. Where sheaths are lacking the axons are closely packed together with nothing between them. It is of interest that myelin formation can be induced experimentally in these regions by crushing the roots (Stirling, 1975b). Both proximal and distal to the injury site, Schwann cells increase in number, surround regenerating axons, and then form myelin sheaths.

THE SHEATHS OF UNMYELINATED GANGLION CELLS

As mentioned above, the perikarya of most neurons in the peripheral nervous system are completely invested by simple sheaths composed of a single layer of satellite cells (Figures 6–1 and 6–2). In light microscopic preparations of spinal and cranial nerve ganglia the nuclei of the satellite cells appear to be bean- or crescent-shaped. They are surrounded by a basophilic cytoplasm that extends from the perinuclear region as thin stellate processes to cover the neuronal surface. In general terms, the thickness of the capsule and the number of satellite cells comprising it are proportional to the size of the enclosed neuron. The quantitative aspects of this relationship have been investigated by Pannese and his collaborators (Pannese, 1960; Pannese, Bianchi, Calligaris, Ventura, and Weibel, 1972). In a light microscopic study, Pannese

(1960) showed that in both newborn and adult mammals, the number of satellite cells forming the capsule of a neuron is proportional to the surface area of the neuron and that this ratio is relatively constant, regardless of neuronal size. He further estimates that throughout development each satellite cell covers approximately 400 square microns of perikaryal surface. Finally, in a recent electron microscopic study (Pannese, Bianchi, Calligaris, Ventura, and Weibel, 1972), it was found that the volume of the satellite sheath is directly proportional to both the volume of the neuronal cell body and its surface area.

Most commonly, the nuclei of the satellite cells sit upon flattened portions of the neuronal surface (Figures 6–1 and 6–2). The chromatin is more concentrated than that of the nucleus of

---

Figure 6–1. **The Sheath Surrounding a Dorsal Root Ganglion Cell.**

The nerve cell on the left is separated from the darker satellite cell by a cleft of about 20 nm. Part of the satellite cell nucleus (*Nuc*) projects into the upper part of the field, and in the perinuclear cytoplasm are cisternae of the Golgi apparatus (*G*) and the granular endoplasmic reticulum (*ER*), mitochondria (*mit*), free ribosomes (*r*) and a few microtubules (*m*). Outside the satellite cell is a basal lamina (*B*), and beyond that are collagen fibrils. Note the invaginations (*arrows*) of the neuron indenting the satellite cell.
Dorsal root ganglion of adult rat. × 35,000.

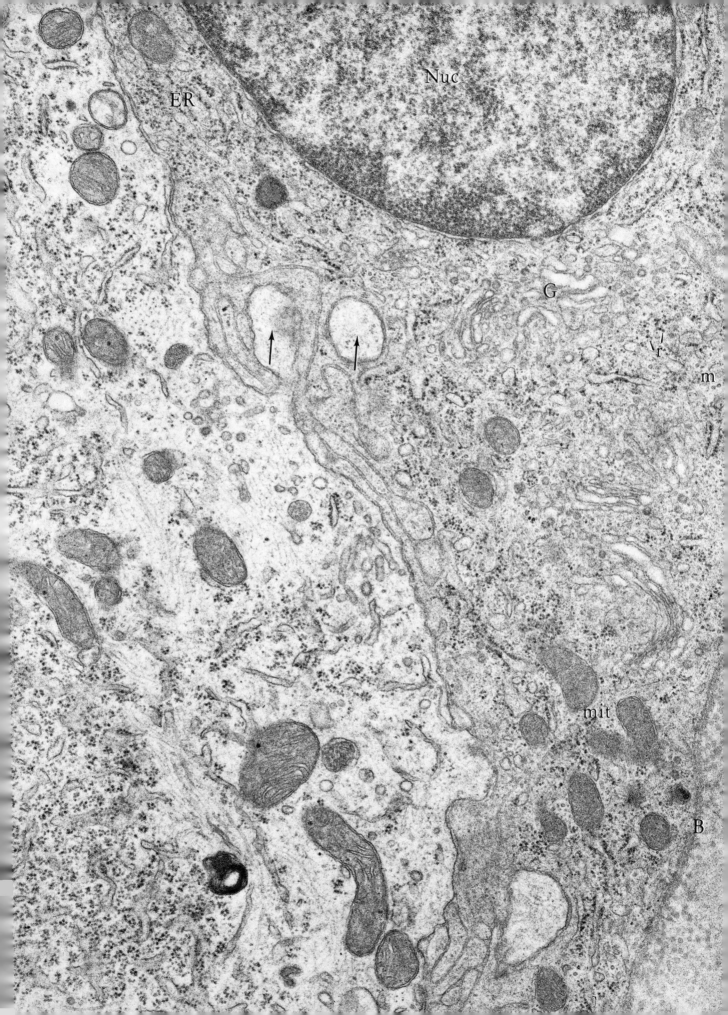

the enclosed neuron (Hess, 1955; Cérvos-Navarro, 1960; Bunge, Bunge, Peterson, and Murray, 1967; Pineda, Maxwell, and Kruger, 1967). Also, the chromatin is homogeneously dispersed, being clumped, if at all, only peripherally and near the center (Figures 6–1 and 6–2), where one or more nucleoli may occur. As in other cells, the nuclear envelope of the satellite cell consists of two layers and is interrupted by nuclear pores. Ribosomes frequently stud the cytoplasmic surface of the nuclear envelope (Figure 6–2) as well as the outer surfaces of the membranes of the endoplasmic reticulum, which in the perinuclear zones of the cells forms distinct parallel cisternae. As shown in Figures 6–1 and 6–2, the Golgi apparatus and many rounded mitochondria are also prominent in the perinuclear zone. The mitochondria are usually shorter and narrower than those in the enclosed neurons. In this case, the intramitochondrial granules are about as prevalent in the neurons as in the satellite cells. Peroxisomes (Figure 6–2) are often closely associated with mitochondria and profiles of endoplasmic reticulum. These cytoplasmic bodies are about 0.2 micron in diameter, are membrane-bound, and have a moderately dense heterogeneous matrix that contains catalase and several oxidative enzymes (Citkowitz and Holtzman, 1973; Arnold and Holtzman, 1975).

Other organelles in the satellite cell cytoplasm (Figure 6–1) include microtubules and filaments. These elongated structures course irregularly through the perinuclear cytoplasm, but in the more attenuated portions of the satellite cells they follow the cell contours and so lie more or less parallel to the surface of the neuron. The cytoplasm of the satellite cell contains lysosomes and multivesicular bodies in addition to glycogen granules and clusters of free ribosomes. The ectodermal origin of these cells is suggested by the cilia that project from the satellite cells surrounding autonomic ganglion cells and from the Schwann cells ensheathing unmyelinated axons (Grillo and Palay, 1963).

Relatively few organelles occur farther away from the perinuclear zone, where the cytoplasm of the satellite cells becomes attenuated to form thin sheet-like processes (Figure 6–2) which extend out toward those of neighboring cells. Where such processes meet they remain separated by a distance of about 20 nm. Sometimes the apposed processes form a simple abutment, but especially in the capsules of the larger neurons, many complex junctional areas occur in which the processes of adjacent satellite cells overlap and interdigitate (Figure 6–1).

An interval of about 20 nm also separates the satellite cells of the capsule from the outer surface of the enclosed neuron. The contours of this interface are irregular, and it is common to find neuronal processes of various sizes projecting into the satellite cells (Figures 6–1 and 6–2). A few of these projections extend through almost the entire thickness of the satellite cell. As shown by Rosenbluth (1963), the dimensions and appearance of the small projections depend somewhat upon the type of fixative that has been used.

Covering the outer surface of the satellite cell sheath is a fluffy basal lamina (Rosenbluth and Palay, 1961; Thomas, 1963). As shown in Figures 6–1 and 6–2, this lamina is confined to the outer surface of the capsule; it does not enter into the 20-nm clefts between adjacent satellite cells.

The sheath of satellite cells extends along the axon as it leaves the neuronal perikaryon. As there is no break in the continuity of the sheath, the same cell may be found covering part of the perikaryon and the beginning of the axon as well (Figures 4–5 and 4–6). Such instances emphasize the artificiality of the distinction between the capsule cells around the peikaryon and the Schwann cells around the axon. In small dorsal root ganglion cells the initial part of the

---

Figure 6–2. **The Sheath Surrounding a Trigeminal Ganglion Cell.**

The cytoplasm of the ganglion cells *(N)* is lighter than that of the ensheathing satellite cell, which occupies the center of the field. The nucleus *(Nuc)* of the satellite cell has a homogeneous karyoplasm and the outer membrane of the nuclear envelope is studded with ribosomes *(r)*. Above the nucleus is the Golgi apparatus *(G)* and other organelles in the cytoplasm are mitochondria *(mit)*, cisternae of the granular endoplasmic reticulum *(ER)*, ribosomes *(r₁)*, and peroxisomes *(p)*. The interface between the satellite cell and its neuron has irregular contours, and the plasma membranes of the two cells are separated by a space about 20 nm deep.

At the bottom of the field the basal lamina *(B)* on the outside of the satellite cell is visible.

Mouse trigeminal ganglion. × 34,000.

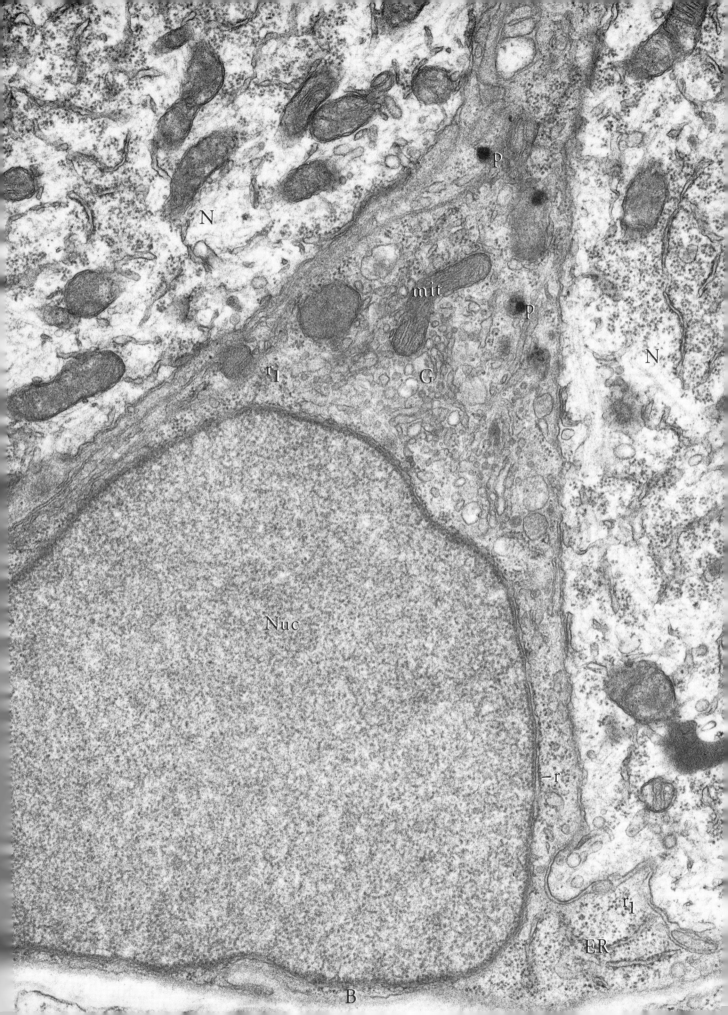

axon is relatively short and straight (see Frontispiece). It is ensheathed by the overlapping processes of a few satellite cells that are separated from each other by a 20-nm gap (Figures 4–5 and 4–6). The initial portion of the axon of a large neuron is longer and more tortuous than that of a smaller neuron (Dogiel, 1908; Cajal, 1909–1911; Pineda, Maxwell, and Kruger, 1967).

Frequently, the initial part of the axon coils about the perikaryon (see Dogiel, 1908), forming a kind of glomerulus, before dichotomizing into its central and peripheral divisions (Frontispiece). The part of the axon coiling around the perikaryon is covered by a thick and complex sheath. On emergence from this sheath, if the axon is to be myelinated, it first acquires a short internode of thin myelin (Spencer, Raine, and Wiśniewski, 1973). Subsequent internodes may be longer and have thicker myelin sheaths until the site is reached where the axon bifurcates.

Elsewhere in the peripheral nervous system there are several important variations in the surface relationships between neurons and their satellite cells (see Hess, 1965; De Lemos and Pick, 1966; Dixon, 1966). In autonomic ganglia the satellite cell sheath may be incomplete, leaving the surface of the ganglion cell exposed directly to the basal lamina for variable distances, and in these same ganglia preterminal and other nerve processes may be enfolded into the satellite cells (see De Lemos and Pick, 1966). Some of these latter processes are projections from the perikaryon of the sympathetic neurons, and sometimes these are regarded as dendrites, for they form synapses with preganglionic axon terminals. Another deviation from the pattern of the dorsal root ganglion is produced in these ganglia by the multiple origin of the axon. A number of short adjacent processes leave the perikaryon and unite to form a single axon trunk. The satellite cells collect around these processes and thicken the capsule in the region of the separate axon hillocks. Focal thickenings of the neuronal capsule also occur where complex arrays of satellite cell processes surround the synaptic endings of the preganglionic fibers.

A consideration of the myelin sheaths formed around some peripheral neuronal cell bodies, in particular those of the eighth nerve ganglion, will be left until the structure of the myelin sheaths of peripheral nerve fibers has been described.

THE SHEATHS OF UNMYELINATED NERVE FIBERS

The structure of unmyelinated nerve fibers was first shown in electron microscope preparations by Gasser (1952 and 1955). Individual axons, which are generally less than 1 micron in diameter, indent the surface of the Schwann cell and become embedded in separate troughs (Figures 6–3 and 6–4). Each Schwann cell can ensheath many axons in this manner. For example, Elfvin (1958) records that in the splenic nerve of the cat there are generally from 5 to 15 unmyelinated axons ensheathed by a single cell, and Dixon (1963) commonly finds 7 to 21 per cell in the trigeminal ganglion fibers of the rat (Figure 6–3). A single Schwann cell, however, does not ensheath a group of axons for their entire length, for the sheath is formed by a chain of Schwann cells, the axons being passed on from cell to cell. In teased preparations of the rat sural nerve and cervical sympathetic trunk, the spacing of Schwann cell nuclei along the same bundle of unmyelinated axons varies greatly, from 20 to about 300 microns, although the mean distance is

---

Figure 6–3.   **Unmyelinated Axons, Adult Peripheral Nerve.**

In the center of the field is the nucleus (*Nuc*) of a Schwann cell, which ensheathes many transversely sectioned unmyelinated axons. The boundary of the Schwann cell is difficult to establish in some places, but it can be generally determined by following the basal lamina (*B*). Some of the axons (*Ax₁*) are embedded in separate pockets of the Schwann cell, others (*Ax₂*) share a pocket, and some axons (*Ax₃*) seem to be shared by this and adjacent Schwann cells. The cytoplasm of the axons contains mitochondria (*mit*), microtubules (*m*), and neurofilaments (*nf*). *Mouse trigeminal nerve.* × 35,000.

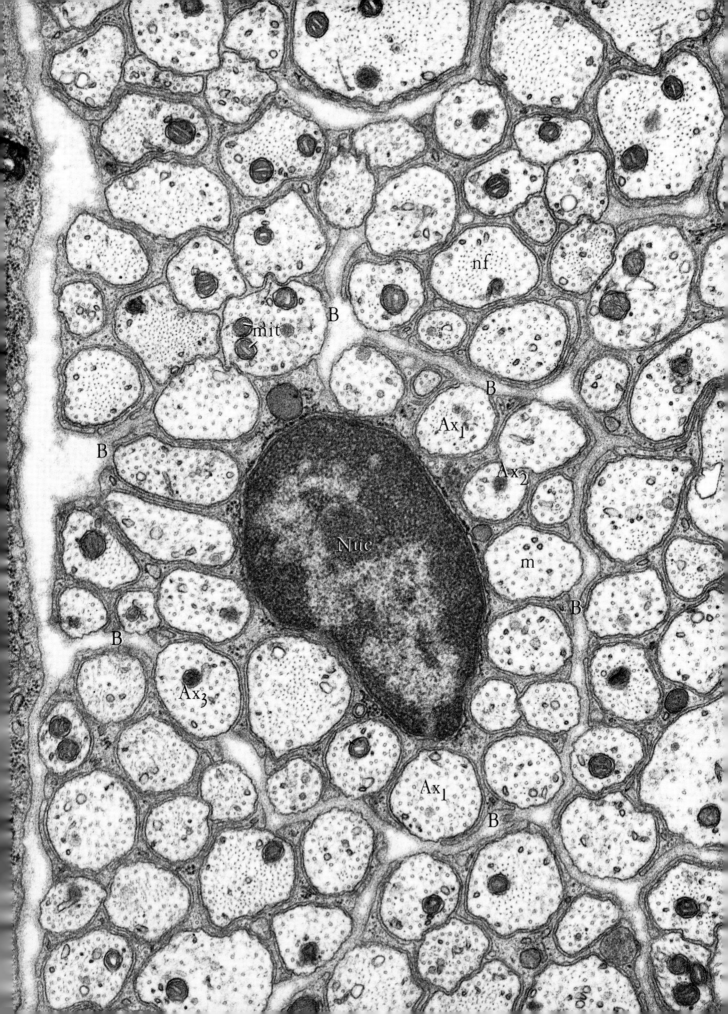

about 100 microns (Peyronnard, Aguayo, and Bray, 1973), while in the human sural nerve the lengths of Schwann cells estimated from the frequency of profiles of their nuclei in cross sections of the nerve is 200 to 500 microns (Carlsen, Knappeis, and Behse, 1974). Where adjacent cells of the series come together, a certain amount of interdigitation and overlap occurs between them, so that a cytoplasmic extension of one cell may sometimes accompany an axon for some distance into the territory of the next cell in the series (see Figure 6–4, Ax_3).

The nucleus of each Schwann cell in the series is usually located midway along the extent of the cell (Figures 6–3 and 6–4), and at this site the nucleus and the organelles in the perinuclear cytoplasm produce a bulge in the sheath. As in the satellite cells forming the capsules of peripheral nerve cell bodies, most of the granular endoplasmic reticulum lies within the perinuclear regions, and it is here that the Golgi apparatus is usually found. Other organelles occurring in the cytoplasm of the Schwann cells are microtubules, filaments, mitochondria, and occasional lysosomes. Consequently, apart from the difference in overall shape, the Schwann cells and satellite cells are almost identical in appearance. However, in Schwann cells surrounding adrenergic axons in bovine splenic nerves, there also are giant mitochondria that are 1.5 to 2.5 microns in diameter and up to 4 microns in length (Thureson-Klein, 1972).

This form of ensheathment, in which a number of individual, unmyelinated axons are enclosed by the same Schwann cell, has been described in the peripheral nerves of several species, for example, the cat (Gasser, 1955; Elfvin, 1963), the rat (Dixon, 1963; Gamble, 1964), and man (Gamble and Eames, 1964). In all species the extent of envelopment provided by a Schwann cell varies from axon to axon. In the simplest situation the unmyelinated nerve fiber is only partially embedded, so that in transverse sections of the nerve the enveloping lips of the Schwann cell remain open. This leaves a small portion of the axonal plasma membrane covered only by the basal lamina (Figure 6–4, Ax_2). More commonly, the enveloping lips of the Schwann cell come together so that their apposed plasma membranes run parallel to each other, separated by a cleft 12 nm wide. This pair of apposed membranes has been called the "mesaxon," a name that alludes to the similarity between this structure and the mesentery suspending the intestine. The length of the mesaxon is variable. Sometimes it is short and straight, but often it may be long and either contorted or loosely coiled around the enclosed axon (Figure 6–4).

Gamble and Eames (1964) have shown that in human peripheral nerves bundles of collagen fibrils are sometimes enclosed by Schwann cells in the same manner as axons.

In the autonomic nerve plexuses a somewhat different relationship exists between unmyelinated nerve fibers and Schwann cells. Although some axons are individually enclosed, it is also common for groups of axons to be enclosed within the same trough of the Schwann cell (see Richardson, 1960; Ross, 1964). As such axons approach their terminations, they gradually lose the Schwann cell investment and become naked (e.g., Richardson, 1960; Simpson and Devine, 1966).

A somewhat similar situation also occurs in the olfactory nerves (Gasser, 1956; De Lorenzo, 1957; Andres, 1966). Here the small axons are arranged in separate bundles, each bundle having its own mesaxon. The mesaxons of several bundles may be confluent, so that they have a branched appearance in transverse sections of the nerve.

Unmyelinated axons of the central nervous

Figure 6–4. Unmyelinated Axons, Adult Peripheral Nerve.

Above the center of the field is a myelinated axon *(Ax₁)* sectioned transversely through the paranodal region. Sections through the paranodal region can be identified by the close apposition between the plasma membranes of the axon and of the inside of the sheath. Another characteristic is the rather thick layer of cytoplasm between the axon and the myelin lamellae, which terminate on the outside of the sheath as the external mesaxon *(mes)*.

The other axons in the field are unmyelinated, and a number of them are separately embedded within each Schwann cell. Although most axons are completely surrounded by their Schwann cell, others *(e.g., Ax₂)* are only partially enclosed. In such cases part of the axon is covered only by the basal lamina *(B)* that surrounds the Schwann cell *(SC)*. Another unmyelinated axon *(Ax₃)*, although apparently embedded within this Schwann cell, is surrounded by a completely separate process, which is probably an extension of the next Schwann cell in the series. Note the microtubular and neurofilamentous components of the axons.

Between the Schwann cells is the collagen *(Col)* of the endoneurium.

Sciatic nerve from adult rat. × 48,000.

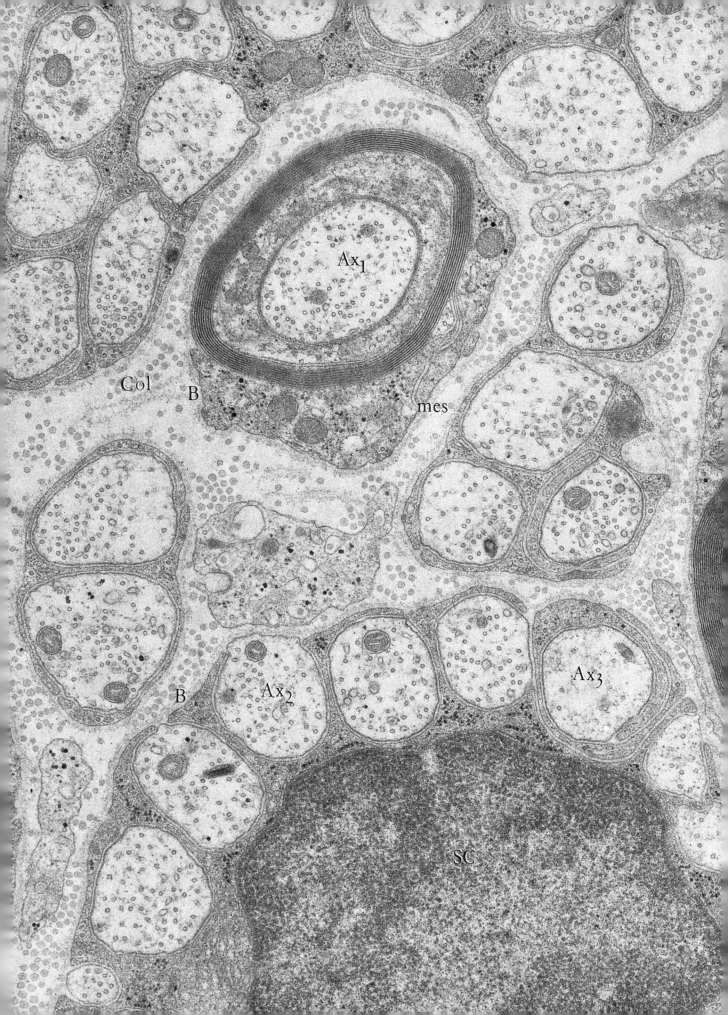

system generally lack individual sheaths (Figures 4–8 and 4–9). In white matter they may be intermixed with myelinated axons. Where unmyelinated axons predominate, as in the hypothalamus or Lissauer's tract, they may be segregated into groups by sheets or trabeculae of astroglial processes. As they enter the neuropil the unmyelinated axons can form small bundles which may be associated with neuroglial processes to a variable degree (Figure 4–9). At their terminals, however, an astroglial process frequently covers an axon terminal and overlies the contiguous portion of the postsynaptic component, so that in effect such a synapse is isolated from the adjacent neuronal components of the neuropil.

THE SHEATHS OF MYELINATED FIBERS

In light microscope preparations stained for either fat or neurokeratin, myelin sheaths appear as tubes surrounding the axons, and at regular intervals along their length the sheaths are interrupted. These interruptions are the nodes of Ranvier (see Frontispiece). The segments of myelin between consecutive nodes of Ranvier are the internodes. In a given peripheral nerve (Duncan, 1934; Schmitt and Bear, 1939; Young, 1945; Williams and Wendell-Smith, 1971) or a tract of the central nervous system (Bernstein, 1966), the greater the diameter of the enclosed axon, the thicker the myelin sheath. The ratio between these two parameters remains relatively constant over a wide range of nerve fiber diameters. However, the ratio between axon diameter and fiber diameter—that is, the diameter measured across the outside of the sheath—is different in the peripheral and central nervous systems. For mature peripheral nerves in the rat, Williams and Wendell-Smith (1971) calculate the ratio to be about 0.6, with lower values for fibers of smaller diameter. However, in the central nervous system the value is higher, and in the pyramidal tract, for example, the ratio is about 0.75 (Bernstein, 1966), which reflects the fact that for axons of similar diameter, peripheral sheaths are thicker than central sheaths.

The lengths of internodes of myelinated fibers also increase in proportion to axon or fiber diameter (Hiscoe, 1947; Hess and Young, 1949; McDonald and Ohlrich, 1971; Schlaepfer and Myers, 1973), and as a rough estimate, the length of the internode is between 100 and 200 times the diameter of the fiber. In some teleost fishes the lengths of the internodes are proportionally much shorter (see Waxman, 1972). The lengths of the internodes change throughout life, however, and they vary from fiber to fiber in the mature animal. The main developmental factors (see Thomas and Young, 1949; Hess and Young, 1952; Thomas, 1955 and 1956; Cragg and Thomas, 1957) which determine the lengths of internodes along mature nerve fibers are the following:

1. A maturing axon acquires its full complement of sheath-forming cells (i.e., Schwann cells and oligodendrocytes) once it has reached its end-organ, for example, a muscle fiber or the skin.

2. Myelination occurs when the axon attains a diameter of 1 to 2 microns.

3. Any subsequent increase in the length of the axon after myelin has formed involves only an increase in the length of the existing internodes, and not the addition of more internodes. Consequently, since the linear growth of the lower limb is greater than that, say, of the head, the sciatic nerve fibers have longer internodes than the facial nerve fibers, even when fibers of the same diameter are compared.

4. In any particular nerve or tract, the axons destined to have the largest diameters in the adult are the first to myelinate. Consequently they have longer internodes than small axons which acquire their myelin sheaths somewhat later in development. It is worthwhile to point out, however, that the internodal lengths along a single nerve fiber are not uniform. Thus, there is a decrease in the length of internodes near the termination of nerve fibers (Whitear, 1952; Quilliam and Sato, 1955). In addition, some short irregular internodes may exist along nerve fibers. In young animals these short internodes may spontaneously degenerate, leaving denuded lengths of axons that are then covered by growth of the adjacent internodes. In mature animals (Lascelles and Thomas, 1966; Lubínska, 1958; and 1961) short internodes probably arise through a restitution of myelin following a local neuritis which resulted in the destruction of existing myelin and the formation of new lengths

of myelin thereafter. Such local "demyelinization" also occurs in the peripheral nerves of the young cat (Berthold, 1973b).

The myelin sheath is an example of an orderly lipoprotein system, and x-ray diffraction studies have shown that in the fresh state it contains about 40 per cent water. Protein and phospholipids each account for about one-third of the dry weight, and glycolipid and sterols, especially cholesterol, each make up about one-sixth of the dry weight. The composition of myelin appears to differ, however, between species and there are differences in the composition of central and peripheral myelin. On the whole, peripheral myelin is generally richer in phospholipid and has less glycolipid. Also, peripheral myelin sphingolipids, which are long-chain fatty acids, make up less than 2 per cent of the total fatty acids, while in central myelin they account for 5 to 20 per cent of the total. Myelin proteins differ in the central and peripheral nervous systems; both contain basic proteins that are antigenic. The other major protein in the central nervous system is proteolipid, and there are small amounts of glycoprotein and other high-molecular-weight proteins. In contrast, the major protein constituent of peripheral myelin is a glycoprotein, and there is little, if any, proteolipid (see Davison, 1970; Mokrasch, Bear, and Schmitt, 1971; Norton, 1972; Quarles, Everly, and Brady, 1973; Everly, Brady, and Quarles, 1973). Because of the orderly array of molecules, correlation has been possible between the results obtained by physical techniques and electron microscopy, and a great deal of the progress made in understanding plasma membranes can be traced to these correlations. It is perhaps due to the high degree of correlation that confidence was first expressed in the images obtained by electron microscopy of tissue sections.

Only a summary of the findings obtained from polarized light and x-ray diffraction studies of peripheral nerve will be given here. Fuller accounts are contained in reviews by Picken (1960), Finean (1961), Robertson (1961), Sjöstrand (1963b), Caspar and Kirschner (1971), and Levine (1972). The polarized light studies indicate the myelin sheath to be composed of concentric layers in which protein and lipid alternate. The lipid molecules are radially oriented in their layers, and the protein molecules are arranged tangentially. X-ray diffraction studies show that myelin is composed of a fundamental, radially arranged repeating unit. In fresh peripheral myelin this unit has a spacing of 17 to 18.5 nm

(Schmitt, Bear, and Palmer, 1941). This information, in conjunction with other data, has led to the conclusion that the repeating unit is composed of two subunits, each consisting of a bimolecular leaflet of lipid sandwiched between monolayers of proteins. It is now known that each one of these subunits corresponds to a single layer of plasma membrane derived from the myelin-forming cell. In effect, then, the radially repeating unit of 17.5 to 18.5 nm observed in x-ray diffraction patterns of fresh myelin can be attributed to two thicknesses of plasma membrane. This repeating unit is considerably larger than the one of 11.5 to 13.0 nm first obtained by measuring the thickness of myelin lamellae in electron micrographs of peripheral nerve fibers fixed primarily in osmic acid fixatives, and the difference can be attributed to a substantial shrinkage that takes place during the preparation of the tissue (Fernández-Morán and Finean, 1957; Finean, 1958 and 1960). Primary fixation with aldehydes gives a slightly larger periodicity to the myelin lamellae (13 to 14 nm), and stabilization of the cholesterol of the myelin with digitonin results in a periodicity of similar dimensions to that found by x-ray diffraction of fresh myelin (Napolitano and Scallen, 1969), as does the use of polymerized glutaraldehyde-urea as the embedding medium, rather than the conventionally used epoxy resins (Peterson and Pease, 1972; Pease, 1973).

INTERNODAL PERIPHERAL MYELIN

The first electron microscope studies of peripheral myelin were undertaken by Sjöstrand (1950) and Fernández-Morán (1950a). Using homogenized preparations, they were able to demonstrate the layered structure that had been predicted earlier by polarization optics and x-ray diffraction. When sectioning techniques had been evolved for the preparation of electron microscope specimens, a number of papers were published in which the existence of lamellae was shown more clearly (Fernández-Morán, 1950b; Rozsa, Morgan, Szent-Györgyi, and Wyckoff, 1950; Hartmann, 1951). In later studies carried out at high resolution (Sjöstrand, 1953; Fernández-Morán, 1954), it soon became apparent that myelin had a concentrically laminated structure in which lamellae repeat radially at a period of about 12 nm (Figure 6–5).

The concentric lamellae of the internodal myelin sheath are derived from the plasma membrane of the myelin-forming Schwann cells of the peripheral nervous system. In transverse sections of internodes Schwann cell cytoplasm is usually present as complete layers on both the inside and the outside of the myelin. The elongated Schwann cell nucleus is present in the outer layer of cytoplasm, generally located halfway along the internode, and the plasma membrane bounding the outer layer of cytoplasm is covered by a basal lamina (Figure 6–5). As pointed out above, the myelin itself is composed of a series of regularly repeating lamellae that are in reality the turns of a spirally wrapped pair of plasma membranes. The spiral terminates on the outer side of the sheath at the external mesaxon (Figure 6–5, *mes*) and on the inner side of the sheath at the internal mesaxon (Figure 6–5, *mes*). At the mesaxons, two areas of the Schwann cell plasma membrane come together so that their outer faces are apposed and as a consequence of this apposition, the intraperiod line (Figure 6–5, *IL*) of the myelin is formed. In the sheath this rather light and somewhat irregular line alternates with the more prominent major dense line (Figure 6–5, *DL*), which is produced by the apposition of the cytoplasmic or inner faces of the same pair of plasma membranes.

In sections of aldehyde-fixed material embedded in epoxy resins (Figure 6–5) the major dense line is about 3.5 nm wide and the less prominent intraperiod line has a width of about 5.5 nm. In earlier studies both lines were thought to be single, but recent high resolution examination of myelin (Revel and Hamilton, 1969; Napolitano and Scallen, 1969; Peters and Vaughn, 1970; Peterson and Pease, 1972) has shown the apparently single line to be composed of two thinner lines separated by an interval of about 2 nm. Peterson and Pease (1972) have termed this interval the intraperiod gap and Revel and Hamilton (1969) have shown the gap to be open to penetration by colloidal lanthanum which enters through the mesaxon.

Hall and Williams (1971) have noted a similar penetration by lanthanum nitrate, but could not get ferritin to enter the gap. It is perhaps surprising that these tracers enter the intraperiod gap, since Peters and Vaughn (1970) and Schnapp and Mugnaini (1975) have shown the presence of small tight junctions in sectioned material. These tight junctions are also evident in freeze-etched material (Schnapp and Mugnaini, 1975; Mugnaini and Schnapp, 1974) as longitudinal strands, or occasionally as rows of particles, that are displayed on the A face of the Schwann cell membrane at the outer mesaxon (Figure 6–17) and complemented by furrows on the B face (Figure 6–17). However, these tight junctions seem to be of the leaky variety and open only to small molecules. Thus, while lanthanum enters into the intraperiod gap, larger molecules such as ferritin (Hall and Williams, 1971), horseradish peroxidase (Hirano, Becker, and Zimmerman, 1969), and ruthenium red do not enter it.

To complete the picture about tight junctions in the myelin sheath, it may be mentioned at this point that Schnapp and Mugnaini (1975) have also found longitudinally extending tight junctions at the inner mesaxon, and in central myelin at the inner and outer ends of the intraperiod gap. Tight junctions are also present at Schmidt-Lanterman clefts and between the membranes bounding the cytoplasmic pockets at paranodes in the central and peripheral nervous systems. These are circumferential junctions (see Figures 6–18, *arrows*, and 6–17, *arrows*).

On the basis of their studies of glutaraldehyde-fixed material embedded in glutaraldehyde-urea polymers, Peterson and Pease (1972) consider the intraperiod gap to contain a highly hydrated carbohydrate gel (the glycocalyx) probably derived from the basal lamina surrounding the outer surface of the Schwann cell. It is clear, however, that the intraperiod gap is not the

---

Figure 6–5. **Myelinated Axon, Adult Peripheral Nerve.**

The transversely sectioned axon (*Ax*) is surrounded by a myelin sheath composed of lamellae formed from the spiralled plasma membrane of a Schwann cell. In the myelin sheath the alternating major dense lines (*DL*) and intraperiod lines (*IL*) are visible. The spiral of the lamellae starts on the inside of the sheath at the internal mesaxon (*mes_i*) where the outer faces of the plasma membrane of the Schwann cell come together to form an intraperiod line, and ends on the outside of the sheath at the outer mesaxon (*mes_o*). The major dense line is formed by apposition of the cytoplasmic faces of this membrane.

Surrounding the myelin is a thin rim of Schwann cell cytoplasm (*SC*). Outside the Schwann cell is a basal lamina (*B*) and beyond this the collagen fibers (*Col*) of the endoneurium.

Adult rat sciatic nerve. × 100,000.

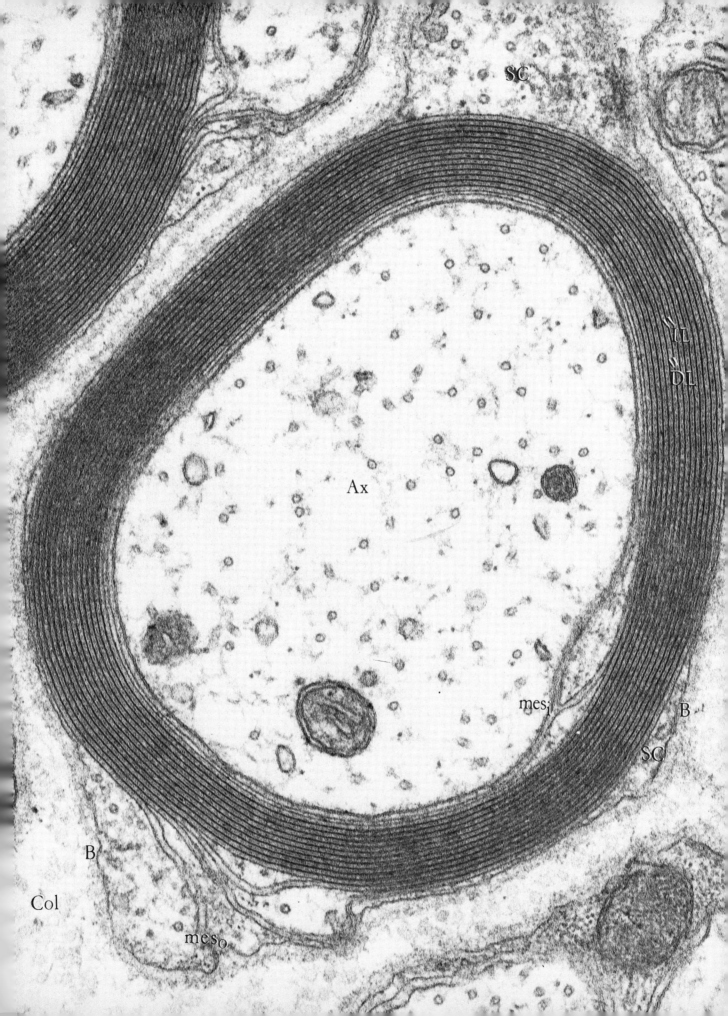

equivalent of a gap junction of the type which occurs between cardiac muscle or epithelial cells (Revel and Karnovsky, 1967) or at electrical synapses (see page 174), since the intraperiod gap (see Figures 6–17 and 6–18) does not display the hexagonal subunits or freeze-cleavage particles that are characteristic of gap junctions. Also, soaking myelinated axons in hypotonic salt solutions dilates the intraperiod gap, as shown by Robertson (1958b), and gap junctions do not dilate under similar conditions.

In addition to an intraperiod gap of about 2.5 nm, when exposed briefly to osmic acid vapor the preparations of Peterson and Pease (1972) showed a gap in the middle of the major dense line, which in their preparations has a width of 5.5 nm. This is thicker than the 3.5-nm wide line of conventionally prepared material.

The interpretation of the electron microscope image is that the major dense and intraperiod lines are where the cytoplasmic and outer leaflets of the apposed surfaces of the Schwann cell membrane forming the myelin sheath are located, and that the lines represent either the protein layers or the lipoprotein interfaces of the plasma membrane. On this basis, the intervening and more lucent zones would represent the sites of the bimolecular leaflets of lipid (see Engström and Finean, 1958; Finean, 1961; Robertson, 1961 and 1966; Sjöstrand, 1963b; Davison, 1968). This conclusion is supported by the study of Napolitano, LeBaron, and Scaletti (1967), who have shown that the periodic lamellar structure of myelin is retained after as much as 98 per cent of the lipid is extracted from the sheath.

Clearly, the plasma membrane of the Schwann cell forming the myelin is not symmetrical in structure, as shown by the difference in appearance of the major dense and intraperiod lines. Peterson and Pease (1972) suggest that some of the differences between the staining properties of the two lines may be attributable to the incorporation of glycoproteins, usually present at the cell surface, into the entity visualized as the intraperiod line. The analysis by Caspar and Kirschner (1971) indicates that one cause of the asymmetry of the myelin structure is the disposition of the cholesterol in the component myelin-forming membrane. They assume the cholesterol to be more concentrated on the external than on the internal side of the lipid bilayer.

THE FORMATION OF THE PERIPHERAL MYELIN SHEATH

Much of our understanding of the structure of peripheral myelin comes from studies of myelin sheath formation. The process was first analyzed in the electron microscope by Geren (1954), who studied the formation of myelin in the peripheral nerves of chick embryos. Her studies have been expanded by a number of later ones that now allow a detailed account of the process to be given.

During the development of a peripheral nerve a pioneer axon extends from a neuron and advances along its path of growth by means of an amoeboid growth cone (see Speidel, 1964; Webster, 1975; page 112). Soon, other axons follow the pioneer and these are closely followed by the Schwann cells, which are derived from the neural crest. Subsequent studies of the distal ends of tadpole nerve fibers growing *in vivo* (Webster and Billings, 1972; Billings-Gagliardi, Webster, and O'Connell, 1974) characterize migratory patterns of Schwann cells and their early association with axons. While moving sporadically at rates of up to 115 microns per day, Schwann cells are ovoid, have several long processes ending in blunt expansions, but lack a basal lamina. They may migrate rapidly for minutes or hours and then remain stationary; movement occurs by process extension, displacement of cytoplasm, and retraction of trailing processes. As Schwann cells associate with and spread along axons, they become spindle-shaped and acquire a basal lamina. In these

Figure 6–6. **Developing Schwann Cell Sheaths.**

At this stage of development most of the smallest axons (*Ax*) are still grouped into bundles, which are enclosed by a common Schwann cell sheath. The sheath is formed by the processes of a number of Schwann cells (*SC*) enclosed within the same basal lamina (*B*). A few of these Schwann cell processes are also involved with individually segregated axons (*Ax₁*), and in one instance (*Ax₂*) an axon has its own Schwann cell sheath. One Schwann cell (*SC₁*) in this field is undergoing mitosis. *Sciatic nerve of newborn rat.* × *21,000.*

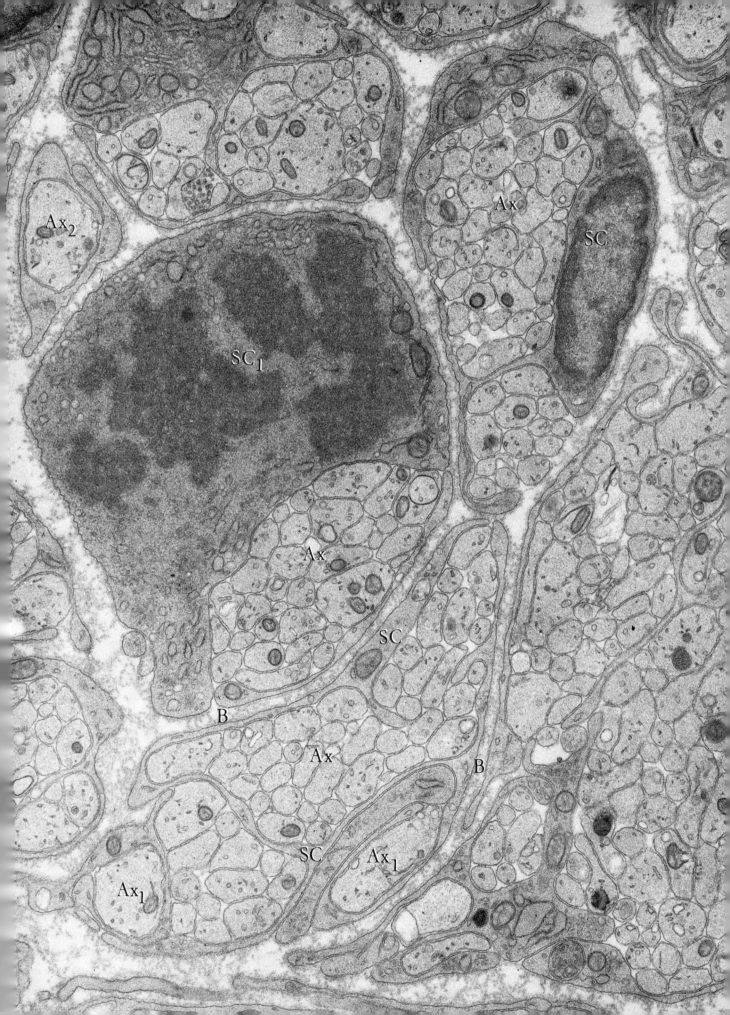

small fiber bundles, the processes of Schwann cells do not form a complete sheath around the entire bundle of growing axons. Some of the axons are either partially or completely enveloped, but the relationships change rapidly and are more complex than Speidel's studies indicated. Further proximally, however, where the maturation of the nerve is more advanced and the migratory Schwann cells have increased their number by mitotic division (Figure 6–6, SC_1), the Schwann cells do form a complete layer on the outside of the fiber bundle, thereby separating them from the surrounding tissues (Peters and Muir, 1959; Peters, 1961a; Gamble and Breathnach, 1965; Gamble, 1966; Peters and Vaughn, 1970; Ochoa, 1971). Schwann cells also start to invade between the axons. In human peripheral nerves, this invasion commences at about 11 weeks of intrauterine life (Cravioto, 1965; Gamble, 1966).

Initially, the invading Schwann cells send out processes that incompletely surround groups of axons, and as the number of Schwann cells increases, families of them, to use the term coined by Webster, Martin, and O'Connell (1973), become associated with groups of axons (Figure 6–6). Such families of Schwann cells are defined by possessing a common basal lamina. Their processes subdivide the axons into groups. Within these groups, some of the larger axons become individually segregated from their fellows (Figure 6–6, Ax_1) and migrate toward the periphery of the group (Webster, Martin, and O'Connell, 1973). Indeed, this stage of the process of nerve maturation seems to be entirely devoted to the sorting out and isolation of individual axons. Early in the process some Schwann cells may initially enclose one or two groups of small axons in addition to one or two individually segregated axons; and conversely, groups of axons may be enclosed by processes derived from more than one Schwann cell (Figure 6–6).

As maturation continues, some Schwann cells become concerned with only a single axon, and these are usually the axons of larger diameter (Figure 6–6, Ax_2 and Figure 6–7, Ax_1). Obviously, such a one-to-one relationship can only be brought about by a substantial increase in the number of Schwann cells. Much of this increase is accomplished by mitosis (Figure 6–6, SC_1). Martin and Webster (1973) have shown that during prophase the Schwann cells retract the sheet-like processes in which they originally enclosed groups of axons. Thus they become spindle-shaped and highly simplified. The axis of the mitosis is parallel to the long axis of the Schwann cell and of the axons, so that after division is complete the daughter cells are arranged in series along the length of the nerve fiber. Next, each daughter cell extends a slender cytoplasmic process from the vicinity of the nucleus and so reasserts the primitive spindle shape. Now by sending out a new set of sheet-like processes, it once again participates in the formation of the developing sheath.

The acquisition of a length of a single axon by a single Schwann cell seems to be the condition that must exist before myelination can commence. Since this process is taking place all along the axon in its peripheral course, an axon destined to become myelinated acquires its particular string of Schwann cells.

Such an axon becomes isolated in a furrow along the surface of the elongated Schwann cell. The furrow then deepens, and its edges, or lips, come together to form a mesaxon (Figure 6–9, *mes*), which resembles the mesaxon of unmyelinated peripheral nerve fibers in the mature animal (see Figure 6–4). At this stage an axon destined to myelinate is about 1 micron in diameter (Matthews, 1968; Friede and Samorajski, 1968; Webster, 1971), and although axons below this size do not appear to stimulate myelin formation, axons that myelinate later in development seem to be rather larger (Fraher, 1972). This size limit seems to be characteristic of the peripheral nervous system, but not of the central

---

Figure 6–7. **Developing Schwann Cell Sheaths, Later Stage.**

Although some of the axons (*Ax*) are still in bundles, others have become individually separated. The majority of these separated axons (Ax_1) have just been enclosed by Schwann cell processes whose lips come together to form a simple mesaxon (*mes*). Two axons (Ax_2 and Ax_3) enclosed by Schwann cells (*SC*) have sheaths at a later stage of development in which the mesaxon has elongated into a loose spiral, and in the spiral around Ax_3 the plasma membrane of the mesaxon has become partially apposed to form the beginning of the intraperiod line. Another axon (Ax_4) has a more mature sheath in which the cytoplasm has disappeared from between the turns of the mesaxon so that compact myelin has formed.
Newborn rat sciatic nerve. $\times$ *21,000.*

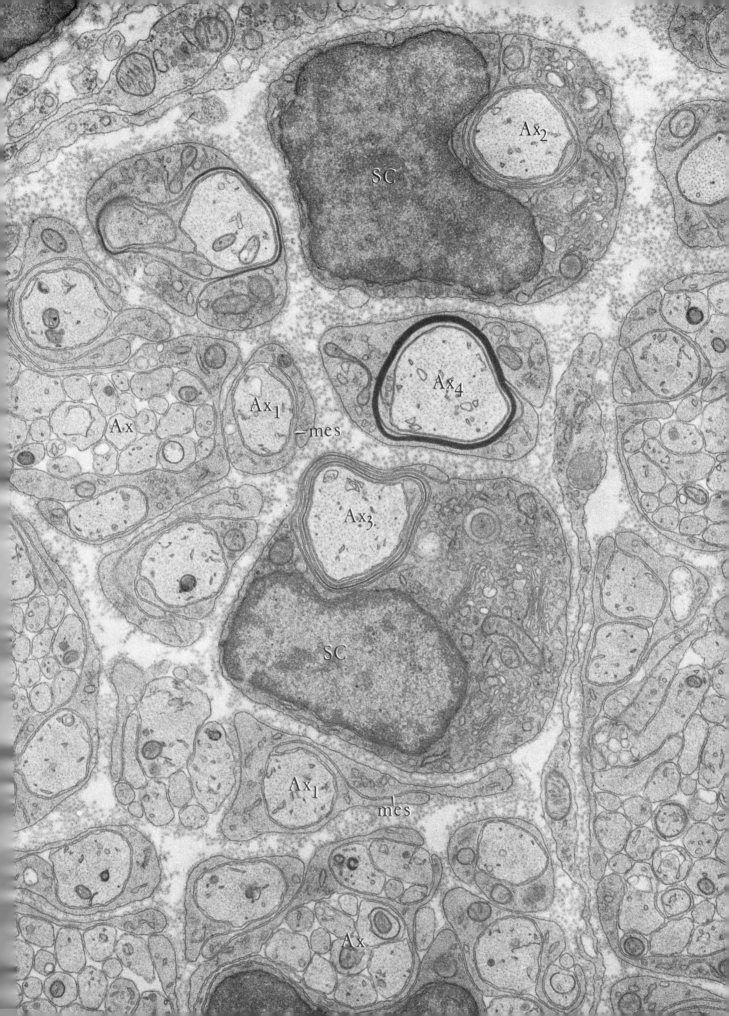

nervous system, in which axons considerably smaller in diameter are found to become myelinated.

At this stage the outer faces of the Schwann cell plasma membrane which come together to form the mesaxon are separated by a gap of about 12 to 14 nm, and only at the outer end of the mesaxon do the membrane surfaces come closer together where they form a tight junction. Next, the mesaxon begins to elongate in a spiral manner around the enclosed axon (Figure 6–9, Ax_2 and Ax_3). Initially the elongation of the mesaxon may not lead to the formation of a simple spiral, but to a tortuous mesaxon that is looped or turns back upon itself (e.g., see Peters and Vaughn, 1970; Webster, 1971). Furthermore, the elongation does not occur at the same rate along the length of an internode, which can be defined as the extent of the territory of a single Schwann cell. The number of turns of the mesaxon is usually greater in the paranuclear regions than at the ends of the Schwann cell where the nodes of Ranvier will form. And even the direction taken by the spiralling mesaxon, either clockwise or counterclockwise, may vary within the same internode (Webster, 1971).

Further elongation of the mesaxon leads to the formation of a more regular spiral. When three to four complete turns are present, the cytoplasm between them is lost and compact myelin begins to form (Figure 6–9, Ax_4). During growth of the compact sheath, the relative amount and distribution of cytoplasm between the layers changes (Webster, 1971). Initially, when there are three to six spiral turns, there are relatively large, longitudinal strips of cytoplasm containing organelles which separate the layers on the side of the fiber where the external mesaxon is located. As the number of turns increases further, the relative size of these strips decreases; they become discontinuous and then disappear. Growth of the compact sheath continues and the only cytoplasm that persists is

contained in a series of small helical pockets, the Schmidt-Lanterman clefts. During this latter phase, the rate of compact myelin sheath growth appears to be relatively constant (Friede and Samorajski, 1968; Fraher, 1972). Similar observations are reported by Williams and Wendell-Smith (1971) who calculate that in the largest sheaths of rabbit sural and gastrocnemius nerves, about 1×10^5 square microns of myelin lamellae are formed per day.

The mechanism of myelin formation and its initial growth rate will be discussed after the formation of central myelin sheaths has been considered.

The compaction of the turns of the mesaxon has two effects. Loss of cytoplasm from between the turns brings the cytoplasmic faces of the plasma membrane forming the mesaxon into opposition to produce the *major dense line*. Simultaneously, the 12- to 14-nm gap in the mesaxon closes to only 2 to 2.5 nm so that the *intraperiod line* forms.

With the addition of further turns to the spiral, compaction of the lamellae becomes more complete, and cytoplasm is now lost from throughout the sheath. It is retained consistently only on the inside and the outside of the myelin (Figure 6–9, Ax_4). The cytoplasmic layer on the inside of the myelin is usually quite thin, but on the outside it is much thicker, and it is here that the elongate Schwann cell nucleus resides. In this more mature sheath in which the spiral of the initial mesaxon has formed compact myelin, only the inner and outer ends of the spiral remain free, and these are referred to as the inner and outer mesaxons, respectively (Figure 6–5). These structures were first defined by Robertson (1955b). As would be expected from the form of the original mesaxon, each end of the spiral terminates at the surface of the Schwann cell. There the two areas of the component plasma membrane diverge from each other and spread over the surfaces of the inner and

---

Figure 6–8. **Diagrammatic Representation of the Formation of Peripheral Myelin Sheaths.**

Early in development (**A**) a Schwann cell contains both bundles of small axons and individual axons. Through an increase in the number of Schwann cells by mitosis, each Schwann cell becomes concerned with only one axon (**B**), which is enclosed in a trough indenting the surface of the Schwann cell. At this time the lips of the enveloping process come together to form a mesaxon (**C**). The lips of the enveloping process then extend so that the mesaxon begins to elongate and the more extensive apposition of the external faces of the enveloping and spiralling process leads to the beginning of the intraperiod line (**D**). Next cytoplasm begins to be lost from the spiralling process and the major dense line results (**E**). As the sheath becomes more mature, the number of turns of the spiralling process increases and the lamellae of the sheath become more compact (**F**).

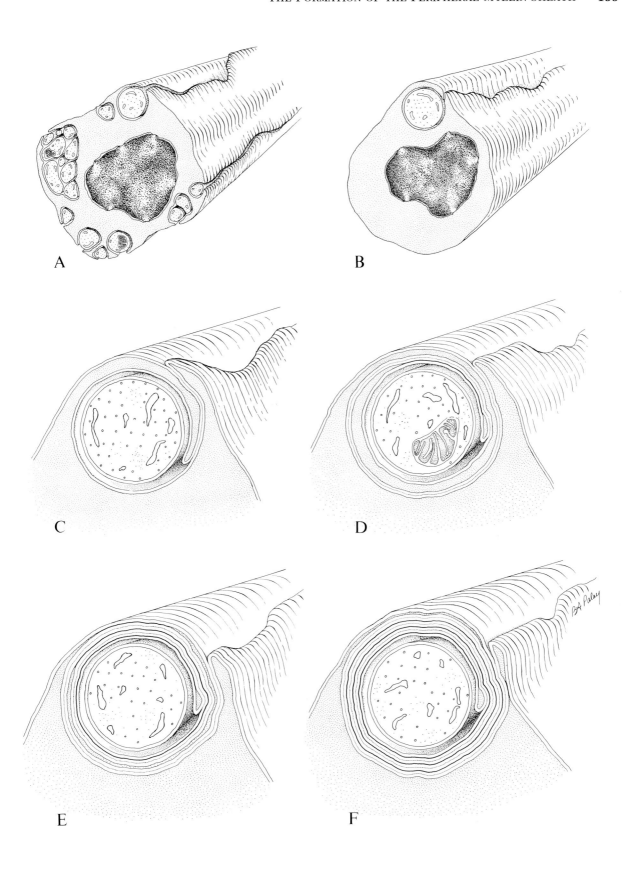

outer layers of Schwann cell cytoplasm. These stages in myelin formation are shown diagrammatically in Figure 6–8.

INTERNODAL CENTRAL MYELIN

Because of the difficulties, which still exist, in producing adequate fixation, the structure of myelin sheaths of the central nervous system was less readily analyzed than that of the peripheral nerves. The first suggestion that central myelin had a spiral structure (Figure 6–9) appears to have come from Fernández-Morán and Finean (1957). However, adequate support in favor of this concept did not appear until three years later, when both Maturana (1960) and Peters (1960a) demonstrated the existence of a spiral in the sheaths of amphibian optic nerve fibers. Their studies showed the presence of both major dense and intraperiod lines (Figure 6–9, *DL* and *IL*) and of an internal mesaxon (Figure 6–9, *mes*). Further, it became evident that the only essential structural difference between peripheral and central myelin sheaths is in the amount of cytoplasm on the outside of the sheath. In central myelin the cytoplasm on the outside of the sheath does not form a complete layer around the myelin but is confined to a narrow longitudinal ridge extending for the length of the internode. In transverse sections this ridge appears as a small tongue process (Figure 6–9, T_1–T_3) or outer loop (Bunge, Bunge, and Ris, 1961).

Theoretically, the central sheath may be considered as resembling a peripheral myelin sheath in which the outer layer of cytoplasm has for the most part been squeezed out so that it forms a narrow ribbon instead of a complete tube on the outside of the myelin. Generally, the outer ridge of cytoplasm, or the so-called outer tongue process, occupies only between 5 and 20 per cent of the outer circumference of the mature sheath (Figure 6–9, T_1–T_3). But in developing sheaths, where the ridge of cytoplasm tends to be more extensive than in the mature animal, a few examples have been found in which a complete outer layer of cytoplasm exists. When this occurs, a cross section of the central sheath appears almost identical to that of a peripheral sheath (Peters, 1964a), for an outer mesaxon is present in both cases. Except for these rare examples, though, a true mesaxon is not usually present in the central sheath. The intraperiod line of the sheath terminates as the plasma membrane peels off the outermost lamella of the myelin to enclose the cytoplasm of the tongue process (Figure 6–9). At the ends of the intraperiod line, tight junctions are usually present (Schnapp and Mugnaini, 1975).

There are also differences between central and peripheral myelin sheaths in respect to the amount of cytoplasm on the inside of the sheath. Often the cytoplasm does not form a complete layer on the inside of the myelin of central sheaths. Instead it is usually confined to a small part of the circumference on each side of the internal mesaxon (Figure 6–9). In transverse sections the inner mesaxon and the outer tongue of cytoplasm are commonly located in the same quadrant of the sheath (Figure 6–9). Peters (1964a) found this condition to exist in about 75

Figure 6–9. **Myelinated Nerve Fibers, Central Nervous System.**

The figure shows complete transverse sections through two myelinated axons (Ax_1 and Ax_2), and portions of four others. The spiralled lamellae of the myelin sheaths start at the internal mesaxons (mes_1, and mes_2). Here the intraperiod line (*IL*) is produced as the outer leaflets of two portions of the plasma membrane belonging to the oligodendrocyte come into apposition. The major dense line (*DL*) alternates with the intraperiod line and is formed by apposition between the inner leaflets of the same plasma membrane. These two lines continue in a spiral and terminate on the outside of the sheaths. The major dense line terminates as the inner leaflets of the plasma membrane separate to surround the external tongue process (T_1 and T_2), and the intraperiod line terminates (*arrows*) as the external tongue process turns away from the outside of the sheath.

The mesaxon (mes_3) and external tongue process (T_3) of a third sheath are also visible.

Since the cytoplasm on the outsides of the myelin sheaths is limited, the outer surfaces of adjacent sheaths are frequently apposed. An intraperiod line is then formed between them.

In the cytoplasm of the axons microtubules (*m*) and neurofilaments (*nf*) are apparent. Note that some of the microtubules display a central dense dot.
Optic nerve of adult rat. × 200,000.

The **inset** shows the double nature of the intraperiod line (*IL*) so that a gap exists between the two apposed outer leaflets of the plasma membrane forming the sheath.
Cerebral cortex of rat. × 400,000.

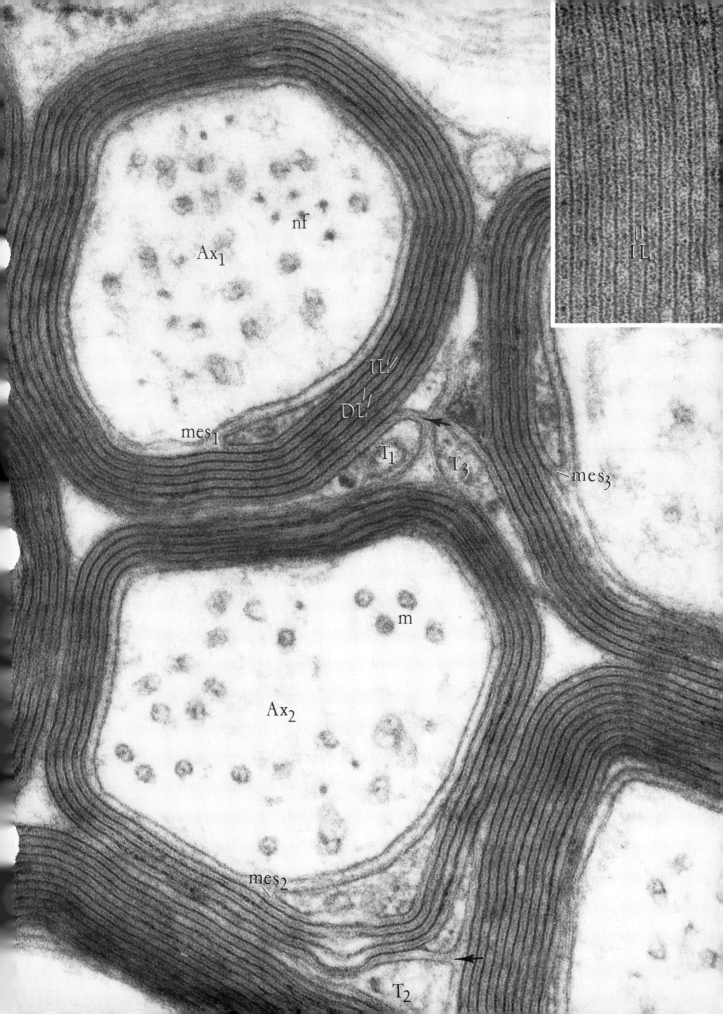

per cent of the sheaths examined from the optic nerves of mature mice and rats. A similar situation has now been shown to exist in peripheral myelin sheaths (Fraher, 1972).

The structure initially postulated by Peters (1964a) and Maturana (1960) for myelin sheaths of the optic nerves of amphibians has now been confirmed in a number of other animals and in other regions of the central nervous system. These include the diencephalon of the frog (Metuzals, 1960 and 1963), the spinal cords of cats (Bunge, Bunge, and Ris, 1961), the optic nerves of rats and mice (Peters, 1960b and 1962a; Peters and Vaughn, 1970), the inferior olive of cats (Walberg, 1964), the cerebral cortex of rats (Hirano, Zimmerman, and Levine, 1966; Hirano and Dembitzer, 1967), and in tissue cultures of the cerebellum of rats, mice, and kittens (Périer and de Harven, 1961; Ross, Bornstein, and Lehrer, 1962). Direct visualization of the spiral of central myelin has been presented in electron micrographs published by Peters (1964a), Uzman (1964), and Hirano and Dembitzer (1967).

THE FORMATION OF THE CENTRAL MYELIN SHEATH

Stages in the formation of myelin sheaths of the central nervous system have been studied in the optic nerves of rats and mice (Peters, 1960b, 1962a, and 1964b; Peters and Vaughn, 1970) and in axons remyelinating during recovery from experimental lesions (Bunge, Bunge, and Ris, 1961; Hirano, Levine, and Zimmerman, 1968; Reier and Webster, 1974).

The following description is based upon the process as seen in transverse sections of nerve fibers such as those shown in Figures 6–10 and 6–11 and represented diagrammatically in Figure 6–12. In the initial phase of myelination a thin process of the myelin-forming cell, now generally accepted to be the oligodendroglial cell (see page 208), becomes applied to the outer surface of an axon (Figure 6–12, A, and Figures 6–10 and 6–11, Ax_1), the plasma membranes of the two structures being separated by a space of about 12 nm. The process then elongates to encircle the axon completely and in some examples a mesaxon is formed at this time, as in peripheral myelination, by apposition of the free edges or lips of the growing process (Figure 6–12, B and Figures 6–10 and 6–11, Ax_2). In effect, the axon is now lying inside a tube formed by the myelin-forming cell, and it should be pointed out that neither at this nor at subsequent stages is a nucleus present in the cytoplasm of the process surrounding the axon.

It should be noted that the initial stages of this process—those establishing the satellite relationship between neuroglial cell and axon—are fundamentally different from those occurring in the peripheral nervous system. In the periphery, Schwann cells associate themselves with large numbers of axons, and by cell division which gradually increases the number of cells, they isolate a single one of the larger axons for their attention (Figure 6–8). In the central nervous system a single oligodendrocyte merely encompasses a single axon with one of its processes and straight away starts the irregular process of spiral wrapping (Figure 6–12). The intermediate stage can be eliminated because there is no compulsion to monopolize the neuroglial cell.

Next, the mesaxon, which contains the precursor of the intraperiod line, elongates so that one lip of the encircling process grows over the other, and a continuation of this growth leads to the beginning of a spiralled mesaxon (Figures 6–10 and 6–11, Ax_3, and Figure 6–12, C). In a recent study of serial sections of myelinating axons in the lumbar cord of five-day-old rats,

Figure 6–10.   **Developing Myelin Sheaths, Central Nervous System.**

Although some of these cross-sectioned axons (Ax) are still bare at this stage of development, others are becoming myelinated. In the earliest stage of development an axon (Ax_1) is enclosed by a process (P) from an oligodendrocyte. The lips of the process enveloping the axon (Ax_2) then come together to form a mesaxon (mes). As myelination continues, the enveloping process extends in a spiral around the axon. A sequence of formation of the early spiral is shown around the axons labelled Ax_3 to Ax_6 (see Figure 6–12). In this sequence the outer (Co) and inner (Ci) ends of the spiralling cytoplasmic processes are shown. Although the apposition of the plasma membranes to form the precursor of the intraperiod line occurs early in this sequence, it will be seen that the initial loss of cytoplasm in some parts of the spiral to form the major dense line is not uniform (Ax_4 and Ax_5). It usually becomes uniform, however, when three or four turns have been completed (Ax_6).

In addition to the axons, this field also shows the glycogen-containing processes of immature astrocytes (As).

Developing white matter beneath the cerebral cortex of 15-day postnatal rat. × 60,000.

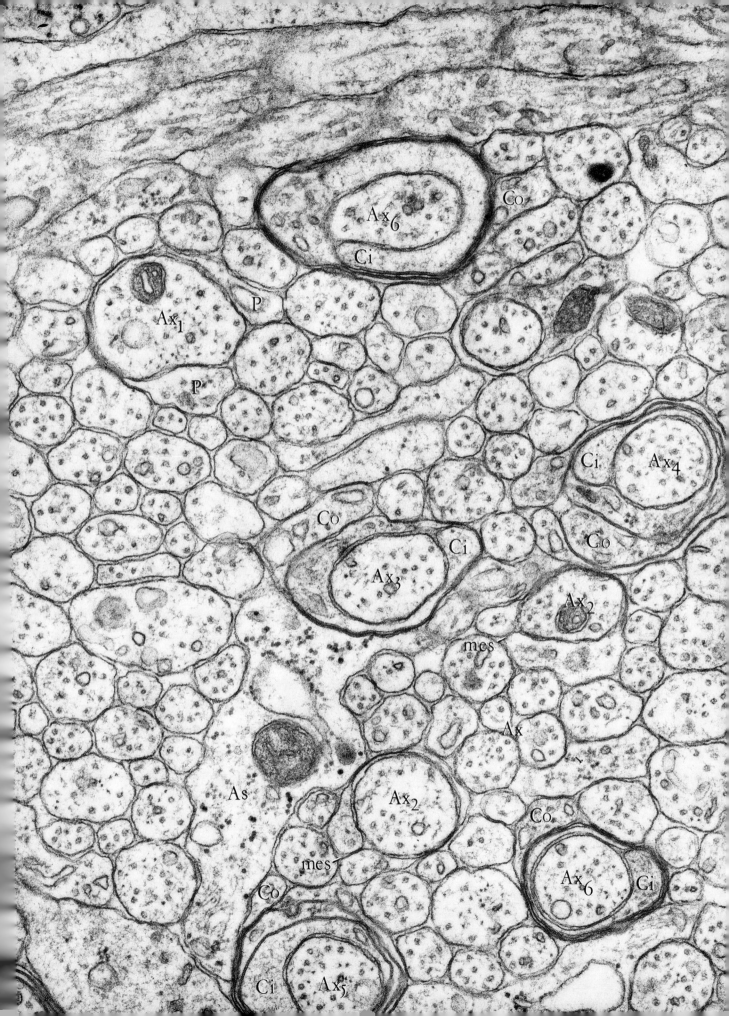

Stempak and Knobler (1972) and Knobler, Stempak, and Laurencin (1974) showed that, as in peripheral nerves (Webster, 1971), the direction in which the mesaxon elongates, clockwise or counterclockwise, can change along the length occupied by the enveloping process. Thus, on each side of a site where the lips of the myelinating process meet to form an initial and short mesaxon, one of the advancing lips occupies the outer position, while on the other side the other lip may occupy this position, so that the direction of the spiral is reversed. Quite soon, even perhaps before the mesaxon has completed a single turn, some of the cytoplasm is excluded from the myelinating process. With this event the major dense line of the sheath starts to form. The subsequent growth of the sheath is achieved by the addition of more turns to the spiral (Figure 6–10, Ax_3–Ax_5; and Figure 6–11, Ax_3–Ax_4), and although cytoplasm may persist in varying amounts within the elongating spiral, it is eventually lost completely (Figure 6–10, Ax_6, and Figure 6–11, Ax_5–Ax_7). Consequently, in the more mature sheaths, cytoplasm commonly appears only within the outer and inner ends of the spiralling process (Figures 6–9 and 6–12, D). As in developing peripheral nerves, however, a myelinating process may not completely encircle the axon at one place, while some distance away one or two complete lamellae of myelin may have formed.

As pointed out by Caley (1967) and by Caley and Butler (1974), the above sequence is not always followed. Sometimes cytoplasm is lost from the middle portion of the encircling process at a very early stage, occasionally even before the myelinating process has completely encircled the axon (Figures 6–10 and 6–11). This results in the formation of a dumbbell-shaped process in which cytoplasm is only retained at the ends (Figure 6–12, B_1). It also leads

to the early production of the major dense line, for the loss of cytoplasm brings the cytoplasmic faces of the plasma membrane on each side of the process into apposition (Figure 6–12, C_1). When the formation of myelin follows this pattern a mesaxon is usually not formed for some time, and the appearance of the intraperiod line is delayed. Consequently the elongating spiral initially has the form of loose coils in which only the major dense line exists.

As shown in a more recent study of serial sections by Knobler, Stempak, and Laurencin (1974), it is unlikely that there are some sheaths that first form intraperiod lines and others that form major dense lines. In reality one line or the other is probably formed in different parts of the same sheath, so that there are local differences in the manner in which the compact lamellae are initiated. Thus, it seems that myelinogenesis in the central nervous system is a less stereotyped process than in the peripheral nervous system, where a mesaxon is always formed first and the loss of cytoplasm is delayed until several turns of the spiral have been formed.

As in peripheral nerves, the myelin sheaths of the central nervous system are formed in segments, and the formation of these segments has been studied in tissue cultures by Hild (1957 and 1959). He described the first appearance of the sheath as a series of cuffs that form around the axon and later extend toward each other, eventually leaving only short gaps, the nodes of Ranvier, between them. In the central nervous system the sheaths never attain the same thickness as those around axons of similar diameter in the peripheral nerves, and this is well demonstrated by studying the transition in the form of the sheath as an axon enters or leaves the central nervous system. On each side of a specialized node where the transition occurs, the peripheral sheath is always thicker than the

---

Figure 6–11.   **Developing Myelin Sheaths, Central Nervous System.**

Most of the transversely sectioned axons *(Ax)* in this field are still unmyelinated but some of them are becoming myelinated. As shown in the previous figure some of the axons (Ax_1) are being enveloped by a simple process. In some cases (Ax_2) cytoplasm is lost from the middle portion of the process so that it has a dumbbelled profile. Something of the sequence in the extension of this process into a spiral is shown around the axons labelled Ax_3 to Ax_5 (see Figure 6–12). Stages in the thickening of the compact myelin sheath are also shown $(Ax_6$ and $Ax_7)$, and in these cytoplasm is retained only at the inner (*Ci*) and outer (*Co*) ends of the spiral, the latter being equivalent to the external tongue process of the mature sheath. The sheath of the axon labelled Ax_8 may be a stage in the myelination of an internode, but it could equally well be a section through a developing paranode.

At the upper right is part of the dense perikaryon of an active oligodendrocyte, from which a process (*Op*) extends across the field.

Developing white matter beneath the cerebral cortex of 15-day postnatal rat.
× 40,000.

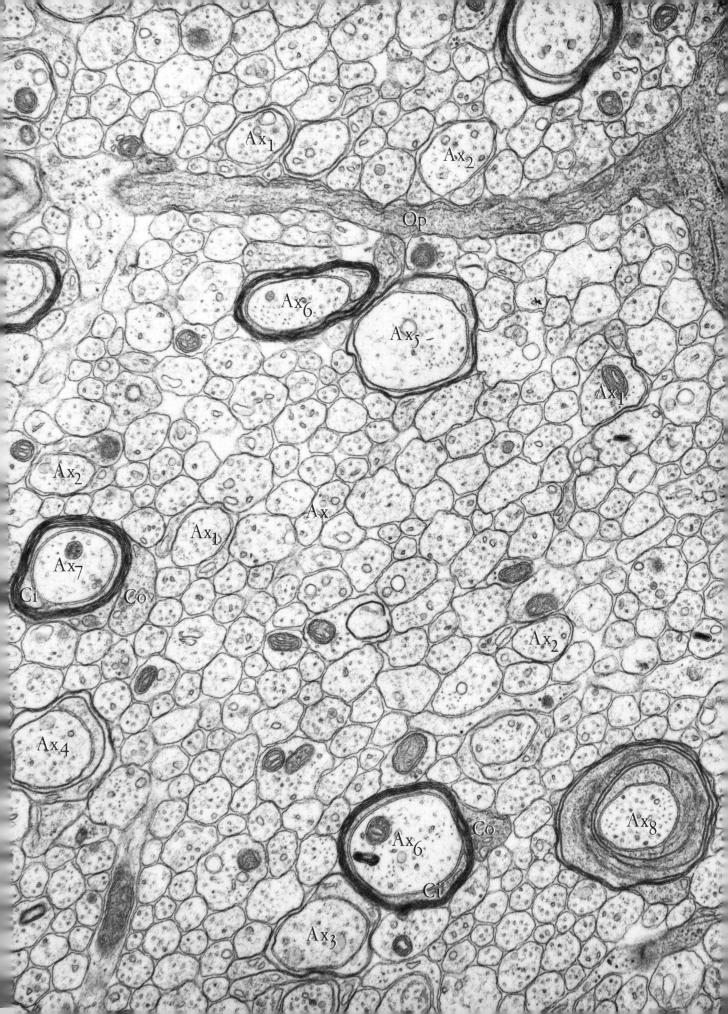

central sheath (see Maxwell, Kruger, and Pineda, 1969).

In the peripheral nervous system the myelin sheaths are formed by Schwann cells whose nuclei are intimately related to the sheath, and one Schwann cell is responsible for the formation of one internodal length of myelin. In the central nervous system, nuclei are never found in the cytoplasm of the outer tongue process (Figures 6–9 to 6–12). This suggests that the perikarya of the myelin-forming cells of the central nervous system are situated some distance away from the sheath, the two being connected by a bridging process of cytoplasm (Figure 6–13, *Op*). Such connections have been demonstrated in developing spinal cords of kittens (Bunge, Bunge, and Pappas, 1962; Bunge and Glass, 1965; Bunge, 1968) and in the optic nerves of rats (Peters, 1964b). The longest connecting processes observed were 12.3 microns in the kitten and 10.2 microns in the rat. Shorter connecting processes also exist, and in some instances continuity has been demonstrated with myelin sheaths that actually indent the perikarya of the myelin-forming cells. Except in edematous tissue (Hirano, 1968), such connections have not, however, been demonstrated in mature animals.

Bunge, Bunge, and Pappas (1962), Peters (1964b), and Bunge and Glass (1965) have given examples of single myelin-forming cells connected to two myelin sheaths, each surrounding a different axon. This observation indicates that a myelin-forming cell in the central nervous system is capable of forming more than one segment of myelin (Bunge, 1968). This concept is in agreement with the fact that although axons of the same diameter have similar internodal lengths in the peripheral and central nervous systems (Vizoso and Young, 1948; Hess and Young, 1949), the ratio of Schwann cells to myelinated fibers in peripheral nerves, where each Schwann cell forms only a single internodal length of myelin, is greater than the ratio of neuroglial cells to myelinated axons in the central nervous system tracts. In an analysis of the optic nerve of the adult rat, calculations have shown that there are 20 to 40 times as many internodes as oligodendrocytes (Peters and Proskauer, see Peters and Vaughn, 1970). In the spinal cord of the rat, the ratio is between 18 and 60 (Matthews and Duncan, 1971), while in the cranial nerves of the cat the ratio is only 2 to 3 (McFarland and Friede, 1971). These ratios pose many intriguing questions concerning the formation and maintenance of myelin in the central nervous system, for each myelin-forming cell must produce vast quantities of plasma membrane.

Hirose and Bass (1973) have studied myelin formation in the rat optic nerve and found that the number of oligodendrocytes in this nerve increase tenfold between 5 and 20 days postnatally. As indicated by changes in the amounts of cerebrosides and cholesterol present and in the appearance of myelinated fibers, it is during this period that the maximal rate of myelin deposition occurs. By 20 days the cell population of the optic nerve is similar to that of the adult and the oligodendroglia have essentially completed their differentiation.

In relation to the production of myelin sheaths of the central nervous system at the ends of neuroglial cell processes, it may be significant that in transverse sections of tracts of myelinated nerve fibers, it is common to find that profiles of nodes of Ranvier tend to occur in groups. Such groupings would be expected only if a major neuroglial cell process branched and formed sheaths around a few neighboring axons.

Figure 6–12. **Diagrammatic Representation of the Formation of Myelin in the Central Nervous System.**

In the first stage (**A**) an axon is enclosed by the process of the myelin-forming oligodendroglial cell. The process then completely envelops the axon and its lips come together to form a mesaxon. At this time the enveloping process may contain cytoplasm throughout the entire extent (**B**), or some of the cytoplasm may be lost (**B₁**) so that the cytoplasmic faces of the portions of the plasma membrane on each side of the process come together and form the beginning of the major dense line. The process then elongates (**C** and **C₁**) so that a spiral is initiated. With time the spiral becomes more extensive, and irrespective of the amount of cytoplasm retained in the early stages the end product is the same. As shown in **D**, the mature sheath has cytoplasm only in the inner and outer ends of the spiralled process. Because of the apposition of the outer and cytoplasmic faces of the plasma membrane bounding the myelinating process the intraperiod and major dense lines are formed.

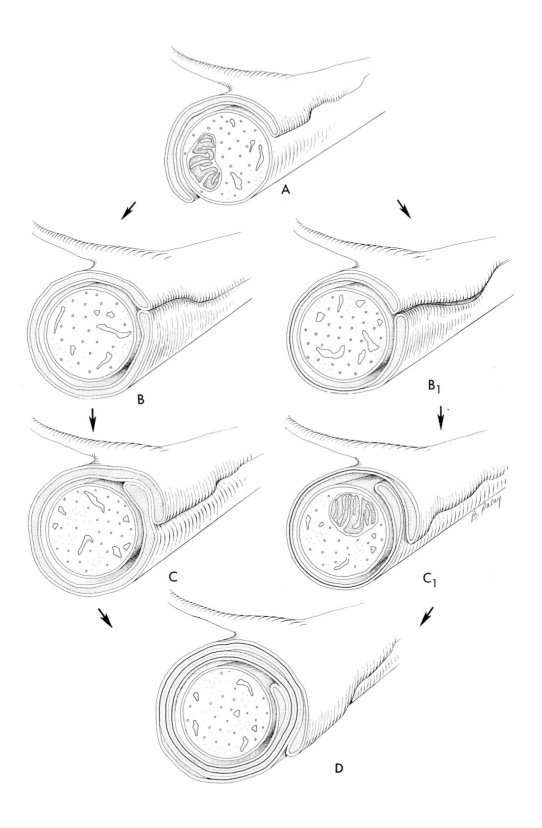

IDENTIFICATION OF THE MYELIN-FORMING CELL OF THE CENTRAL NERVOUS SYSTEM

The myelin-forming cell in the central nervous system is now generally agreed to be the oligodendrocyte. The disposition of these neuroglial cells in interfascicular rows in tracts of white matter supports this view, as does the morphology of the cells having connections with developing sheaths (Bunge, Bunge and Pappas, 1962; Peters, 1964b; Bunge and Glass, 1965) and with sheaths re-forming after a lesion (Hirano, 1968). It also agrees with the conclusions of earlier authors (e.g., del Rio Hortega, 1928; Morrison, 1931) and with the observation that in optic nerves of young rats the appearance of identifiable oligodendrocytes precedes the first myelin sheaths (Vaughn and Peters, 1971).

It is nevertheless true that the identity of the myelin-forming cell in the central nervous system can only be categorically established by demonstration of continuity between a neuroglial cell and a myelin sheath in normal, mature tissue. Attempts to find such continuity have been made in several laboratories, but so far they have been unsuccessful. For example, Metuzals (1963) showed that small myelinated nerve fibers may indent oligodendrocytes in the diencephalon of the adult frog, but he was unable to demonstrate continuity between the plasma membrane of the neuroglial cell and the lamellae of the outer tongue of the sheath. Another example portrayed by Kruger and Maxwell (1966) is also subject to alternate interpretations.

Why have attempts to find continuity between the plasma membrane of oligodendrocytes and myelin sheaths in adult tissues failed? The most probable explanation is that as the central nervous system matures and the cellular elements expand in volume, the connecting processes become longer and more tortuous. Thus, in tracts of white matter, the processes of oligodendrocytes are often quite thick and stubby during development, but in the adult they are thin and long, so that it is unusual to be able to trace an oligodendrocyte process for any distance in a single section. If mature connections are to be found, and there is no reason to doubt their existence, it will be almost certainly necessary to resort to serial sections as a means of tracing them.

Bunge, Bunge, and Pappas (1962) point out that if one could stain the ridge of cytoplasm running along the outside of an internode (the outer tongue process) as well as the cytoplasm of the connecting process, then one would see a form like that originally illustrated by del Rio Hortega (1928) and more recently by Ramón-Moliner (1958) (see also Penfield, 1932, or Bunge, 1968). These illustrations show classically stained oligodendrocytes with processes that emerge from the cell body and then divide to run in opposite directions along the lengths of nerve fibers (see Frontispiece, D). As Bunge, Bunge, and Pappas (1962) suggest, the slender processes that del Rio Hortega shows encircling the axon could correspond to areas in which cytoplasm remains between the lamellae of the sheath (also see Hirano and Dembitzer, 1967).

Although it is likely that myelin sheaths of the central nervous system are usually formed by oligodendrocytes, there are suggestions that this may not always be so. Thus, Bunge, Bunge, and Ris (1961), who examined remyelination in the spinal cords of rats, and Ross, Bornstein, and Lehrer (1962), who examined explants of newborn rat cerebellum, noted fibrils in the cytoplasm associated with the newly formed myelin. In normal nervous tissue, the presence of fibrils in the cytoplasm is usually a criterion used for the identification of astrocytes. It must be taken into account, however, that in each of these studies the myelination was taking place under experimental conditions.

Wendell-Smith, Blunt, and Baldwin (1966) and Blunt, Baldwin, and Wendell-Smith (1972) believe that astroglioblasts may partake in the formation of myelin in the optic nerves of cats. They find that in the lamina cribrosa, where myelin is present, astrocytes are the only neuroglial cells in the region. The nearest oligodendroglial cells are several millimeters away. Until observations such as these are explained

---

Figure 6–13.   **The Myelin-Forming Cell, Central Nervous System.**

In the lower half of the field are parts of two oligodendrocytes, one of which sends out a process (*Op*). This process loses its cytoplasm as the bounding plasma membranes become apposed (*arrow*) to form the lamellae of the myelin sheath surrounding an axon (*Ax*). In addition to other myelinated axons, the remainder of the field contains some axons (*Ax₁*) that have not yet started to myelinate and one axon (*Ax₂*) that has just been enclosed by an oligodendrocyte process.
Optic nerve of 15-day postnatal rat. × 61,000.

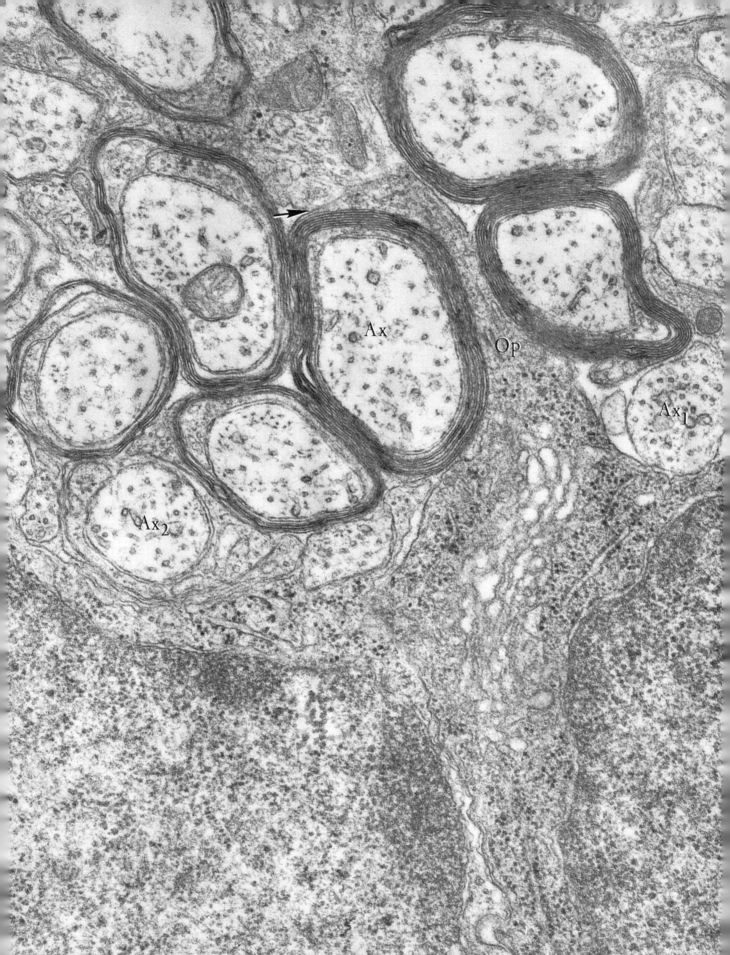

and until definite connections are established between myelin sheaths in normal and mature animals, there remains an element of doubt about whether all myelin sheaths in the central nervous system are formed by oligodendrocytes.

THE MECHANISM OF MYELIN FORMATION

How the spiralled lamellae of the myelin sheath are formed is still uncertain. In the peripheral nervous system, where one Schwann cell is related to each internode of myelin, it is attractive to think that the spiralling of the mesaxon is produced by a rotation of the Schwann cell around the enclosed axon. This idea receives some support from observations made in tissue culture (Crain and Peterson, see Murray, 1959; Pomerat, Hendelman, Raiborn, and Massey, 1967) in which movements of Schwann cell nuclei consistent with their rotation have been seen. However, Speidel (1964) stated that he failed to observe such a rotation in tadpole tails in which he studied growing nerve fibers.

Even if rotation of the Schwann cell accompanies formation of the spiral, it is clear that other mechanisms control the pattern and rate of spiral growth. The initial stages of peripheral myelination are well characterized by the measurements and three-dimensional observations of Webster (1971). He shows that the mesaxon enlarges first by adding loose spiral turns in the Schwann cell's perinuclear region. Spiral growth then extends longitudinally in an irregular fashion so that the number of turns is not uniform along the internode. According to Webster's measurements, initial growth of the myelin membrane is proportional to the area already present and is exponential. As long as the entire surface of the myelin spiral is covered by cytoplasm, exponential growth continues at an ever-increasing rate. Myelin membrane area increases initially by the addition of spiral turns rather than by growth along the axon. When three to four turns are formed, the spiral starts to become compact. During this transitional stage, when three to six turns are present, only longitudinal strips of cytoplasm continue to separate the spiral layers, and the growth rate begins to decrease. The position of these strips may change in order to increase the surface area available for membrane growth. This distribution of cytoplasm continues to favor the addition of spiral turns, and numerous irregularities reflect the rapid rate of membrane synthesis. As sheaths acquire more than six to eight spiral turns, the longitudinal strips disappear, the longitudinal extent of the sheath increases, and the enlarging spiral becomes much more uniform.

The greatest increase in myelin membrane area occurs at a relatively constant rate while the sheath is a compact lamellar spiral. Mesaxons, the Schmidt-Lanterman clefts, and the sheath's outer and inner layers probably are large enough interfaces for the addition of new membrane material from the cytoplasm at the rate required for the final stage of the sheath's growth. Webster (1971) concludes that growth of the myelin spiral does not take place at a restricted site such as one end of the spiral (Sjöstrand, 1963b); instead, it occurs by interposition of molecules into all membrane surfaces exposed to Schwann cell cytoplasm.

This concept is supported by studies in which radioactive molecules have been incorporated into the sheath. Thus, Hendelman and Bunge (1969) showed that in cultures of peripheral nerves, tritiated choline is incorporated along the entire internodal length and not preferentially at any one site. A similar observation was made by Hedley-Whyte, Rawlins, Salpeter, and Uzman (1969) who labelled myelin in young rats by injecting them with radioactive cholesterol.

Another factor which appears to affect compact sheath growth in peripheral nerves is the size of the axon. A linear increase in myelin sheath thickness that correlates with axon caliber is well documented (Friede and Samorjaski, 1968; Williams and Wendell-Smith, 1971; Fraher, 1972). However, growth patterns differ when several fiber populations from the same species are compared (Williams and Wendell-Smith, 1971). The thickness of compact myelin sheaths can also be changed by altering axon caliber experimentally. Thinner sheaths surround axons swollen by edema (Hirano and Dembitzer, 1967) or by distal compression (Friede and Miyagishi, 1972). If axon and myelin sheath growth is retarded distal to a ligature around a developing nerve, release of the ligature then accelerates the rate of both axon and myelin sheath enlargement (Friede, 1972).

The formation of central sheaths clearly does not occur by rotation of the myelin-forming cell, since the observation that myelin-forming cells of the central nervous system are connected to more than one internodal length of myelin means that rotation of the cell body to produce a continuous spiral is impossible. Furthermore, if we assume that the growth of the central myelin sheath occurs at the ends of the spiral, then the addition of new lamellae must be intermittent, rather than continuous, for examination of transverse sections of developing myelin sheaths (Peters, 1964a) reveals that the inner mesaxon and the outer tongue process are not positioned randomly with respect to each other. Instead, they tend to occur in the same quadrant of the sheath. If the growth were a continuous process, then one would expect the ends of the spiral to have no preferred disposition. Fraher (1972) noticed a similar relation between the external and internal mesaxons of developing peripheral sheaths, and remarked that the tendency for these to be present within the same quadrant increases with sheath thickness.

Whatever the mechanism for its formation, the appearance of compact myelin does not signal the end of sheath formation. The enclosed axon undergoes further increase in diameter after this compact myelin has been laid down, and this means the myelin sheath must expand to accommodate it. An increase in the internal diameter of the sheath could be effected by the myelin lamellae slipping over each other, as has been demonstrated to take place in experimental edema of central axons (Hirano and Dembitzer, 1967) and in proximal portions of axons that have swollen after a ligature has been placed around a peripheral nerve (Friede and Miyagishi, 1972).

It should also be pointed out that myelination can be inhibited by a variety of factors. Thus, cholesterol inhibitors retard myelination (Rawlins and Uzman, 1970a and b), as do undernutrition (Clos and Legrand, 1970; Hedley-Whyte and Meuser, 1971) and experimental thyroidectomy (Balazs, Brooksbank, Davison, Eayrs, and Wilson, 1969).

In a strain of dwarf mice which has multiple pituitary hormone deficiencies and secondary hypothyroidism, the separation of peripheral axons into small fascicles during development is delayed. Thus, even at 50 days of age some of the unmyelinated axons in these dwarf mice are still retained in large groups in which they are not individually segregated by Schwann cell processes (Reier, Froelich, Sawchak, and Hughes, 1974).

Another interesting fact to emerge recently is that the process of myelination in the central and peripheral nervous systems is under separate genetic control. This could have perhaps been predicted from the knowledge that different cell types are responsible for myelin formation in the two systems. However, the fact is nicely shown by a study of some mutant mice. In "jimpy" mutants, electron microscope studies (Herschkowitz, Vessella, and Bischoff, 1971) show that although sciatic nerves are myelinated normally, the cerebral cortex has almost no myelinated nerve fibers. Compared to nerve fibers of the same caliber from normal animals, in the "quaking" mutant (Samorajski, Friede, and Reimer, 1970), peripheral nerve fibers have only about half as many lamellae as nerve fibers of similar caliber in normal animals, and in the brain a smaller proportion of the axons have any myelin. Similar results have been obtained by Wiśniewski, and Morell (1971).

It should be appreciated that while myelination in the peripheral nervous system is a relatively stereotyped process, this is not true of the central nervous system. In the peripheral nervous system few developmental faults have been described; they include paranodal variations in sheath contour (Webster and Spiro, 1960) and extensive elongation of the mesaxon (Gamble, 1966). It is common in both the peripheral and central nervous systems, however, to encounter examples in which the myelin sheaths are too large for the enclosed axons. The axon is then confined to one end of the sheath which extends away into a long and flattened sheet. This type of sheath has been described a number of times in the central nervous system (e.g., Rosenbluth, 1966; Fleischhauer and Wartenburg, 1967), and occasionally the long sheets of myelin are flattened around cell bodies of either neurons or neuroglial cells (Rosenbluth, 1966; Herndon, 1964; Peters and Vaughn, 1970).

One reason for the low incidence of developmental faults in the peripheral nervous system may be that Schwann cells ensheathing axons are separated from each other by basal laminae and endoneurium. This means that when a Schwann cell is forming myelin it is subjected to no interference from uncommitted Schwann cells in the neighborhood. Within the central nervous system, however, unusual sheaths are common. Hirano, Zimmerman, and Levine (1966) and Hirano and Dembitzer (1967) have described double concentric myelin sheaths around a single axon, and Walberg (1964) has described mature sheaths in which two or three myelinated axons are themselves enclosed within a commonly shared outer sheath. The probable precursor of such situations is commonly encountered during early development, when axons are often encircled by two different neuroglial cell processes.

Finally, it is now apparent that myelination is not an entirely constructive event, for as shown by Hildebrand (1972), at least in the developing spinal cord of the cat myelination is accompanied by a disintegration of some sheaths and demyelination of short internodes, as well as degeneration of some oligodendroglial cells.

Perhaps the most remarkable fact about myelination is that the end product is such a well-ordered structure, for in well-fixed adult tissue abnormal sheaths are uncommon.

THE NODE OF RANVIER

Nodes of Ranvier occur regularly along the lengths of myelinated fibers in both the peripheral and central nervous systems. They represent the intervals between adjacent segments of myelin. The structure of the nodes is essentially similar in both the peripheral (Uzman and Nogueira-Graf, 1957; Robertson, 1959b; Elfvin, 1961; Harkin, 1964; Bargmann and Lindner, 1964; Bunge, Bunge, Peterson, and Murray, 1967; Berthold, 1968; Williams and Kashef, 1968; Phillips, Hibbs, Ellison, and Shapiro, 1972) and central (Pease, 1955; Metuzals, 1960 and 1965; Uzman and Villegas, 1960; Bunge, Bunge, and Ris, 1961; Andres, 1965b; Laatsch and Cowan, 1966b; Peters and Vaughn, 1970; Hildebrand 1971a and b; Phillips, Hibbs, Ellison, and Shapiro, 1972) nervous systems, and consequently the two forms of node will be considered together.

As the myelin sheath approaches a node, the lamellae begin to terminate. The region in which they terminate is called the paranode (Figures 6–14 and 6–15). The innermost lamellae terminate first and succeeding turns of the spiral then overlap and project beyond the one lying beneath. As the lamellae terminate, the major dense line of the sheath opens to accommodate cytoplasm (Figures 6–14 and 6–15, *P*). In longitudinal sections this paranodal cytoplasm is represented by a series of pockets arranged along each side of the axon, but in reality of course, these pockets are sections through a helix of cytoplasm, and by means of this helix continuity is established between the cytoplasm on the inside and the outside of the myelin. Within the paranodal cytoplasm are microtubules and vesicles along with some dense particles which are often aligned in the cytoplasm adjacent to the plasma membrane that abuts against the axolemma (Elfvin, 1961; Bunge, Bunge, Peterson, and Murray, 1967). Also, particularly in the peripheral nerve fibers, it is not uncommon for stacks of desmosome-like structures to be formed between the membranes bounding adjacent pockets of paranodal cytoplasm (Harkin, 1964). Since the microtubules in the paranodal cytoplasm follow the course of the helix, in longitudinal sections through the paranodal region the microtubules appear as circular profiles (see Figures 6–14 and 6–15).

The above description of a regular sequence of paranodal pockets of cytoplasm aligned in an orderly manner on each side of the axon applies only to the smaller caliber nerve fibers. In both peripheral and central nerve fibers of large size the alignment of the paranodal pockets is much more disorderly (see Berthold, 1968; Phillips, Hibbs, Ellison, and Shapiro, 1972). Here the paranodal pockets are small and only a few of them reach the axon surface (Figure 6–15). The majority are piled up or telescoped either in a

---

Figure 6–14.   **The Node of Ranvier, Peripheral Nervous System.**

The **upper picture** shows a longitudinal section of the nodal region of a myelinated axon *(Ax)*. As the adjacent lengths of myelin approach the nodal region *(Nd)* the successive lamellae terminate to enclose pockets of paranodal cytoplasm *(P)*, and processes *(arrows)* from the Schwann cells *(SC)* cover the nodal region of the axon. In this example the axon bulges out at the node. In addition to the longitudinally oriented microtubules *(m)* and neurofilaments *(nf)* in the axon, this picture also shows the arrangement of the collagen fibers *(Col)* of the endoneurium.
Sciatic nerve of adult rat. × 36,000.

The **lower left picture** is an enlargement of part of the paranodal region in the above picture. The axon *(Ax)* is on the right and the axolemma *(Al)* is indented by the pockets of paranodal cytoplasm *(P)*. These pockets arise as the major dense line *(DL)* of the sheath opens up.
Sciatic nerve of adult rat. × 110,000.

The **lower right picture** is a transverse section through a nodal axon *(Ax)*. The nodal axon is bounded by an axolemma *(Al)* which has a dense undercoating *(D)*, and its cytoplasm contains microtubules *(m)*, neurofilaments *(nf)*, and round profiles of tubular cisternae of smooth endoplasmic reticulum *(SR)*. Surrounding the axon are finger-like processes *(arrows)* from the Schwann cells that meet at the node.
Sciatic nerve of adult rat. × 60,000.

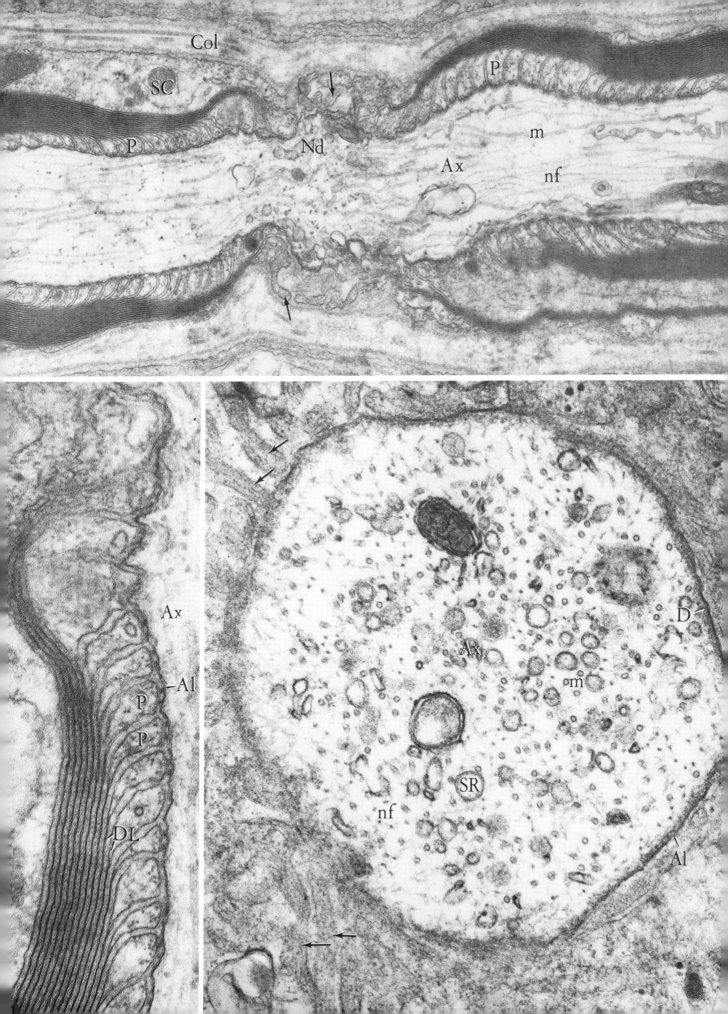

random fashion or in rather regularly arranged groups between the necks of the pockets that reach the axon surface.

Asymmetry of the paranodal regions of both sides of a node has been recorded by a number of authors (see Williams and Kashef, 1968). It is quite often found in limb nerves to muscle, for example, that the paranodal region, or bulb, nearest to the cell body giving rise to the ensheathed axon is larger than the one on the distal side of the node.

In the internodal region, the axolemma and the plasma membrane limiting the inside of the sheath are separated by a distance of not less than 12 nm, but at the paranode these two membranes are separated by a gap of only 2.5 to 3.0 nm (Figures 6–14 and 6–15). Furthermore, over the extent of the paranode the two plasma membranes run strictly parallel with each other; thus, in longitudinal sections the axolemma usually has a scalloped appearance because it follows the contours of the pockets of paranodal cytoplasm bulging into it (Figures 6–14, 6–15, and 6–18). Since the paranodal pockets are parts of a continuous helix, in smaller caliber fibers the relation between the axon and its sheath at the paranode must be akin to that between a nut and a bolt. In larger caliber fibers, although the scalloping is still evident, the piling up of the paranodal loops can often constrict the axon, so that it becomes thinner over the extent occupied by the two adjacent paranodes and the node itself.

In low power micrographs of longitudinal sections through the paranodal regions of both peripheral (see Bargmann and Lindner, 1964; Bunge, Bunge, Peterson, and Murray, 1967) and central (see Andres, 1965b; Peters, 1966; Laatsch and Cowan, 1966b; Hirano and Dembitzer, 1967) nerve fibers, a row of diffuse dots appears in the narrow interval between the axolemma and the plasma membrane bounding the inner surface of the sheath. At higher resolution, however, it is evident that these dots are regularly spaced densities related to the outer leaflet of the axolemma and bulge into the extracellular space (Figure 6–15, *inset*). Each density is about 15 nm long and the center-to-center spacing between adjacent densities is 25 to 30 nm. In obliquely oriented longitudinal sections passing through the paranodal region, these densities become displayed as a series of dense bands, or rings, that pass circumferentially around the axon (Peters, 1966).

While this image is evident in aldehyde-osmium–fixed material, Schnapp and Mugnaini (1975) have shown that in tissue fixed directly in potassium permanganate, or treated en bloc with uranyl acetate after osmication, both the axon plasma membrane and that bounding the inner surface of the paranodal pockets have the appearance of complete membranes that lie parallel to each other. The intermittent nature of the outer leaflet of the axolemma is not evident. When the Karnovsky ferrocyanide-osmium mixture (Karnovsky, 1971) is used for fixation, however, a different image is obtained; both the axonal and the paranodal myelin membranes undulate so that the crests of apposed undulations meet and appear to almost obliterate the extracellular space between them. The outer leaflets of the two membranes become closely apposed. In retrospect, it seems that these points of apposition in longitudinal sections of the paranode correspond to the dense loci where the outer leaflet paranodal axolemma is

---

Figure 6–15.   **The Node of Ranvier, Central Nervous System.**

At the node, the axon is bare and in the cytoplasm beneath the axolemma (Al) is a dense undercoating (D). On each side of the node are the terminal, or paranodal, portions of the two adjacent segments of myelin. The sheath becomes thinner as successive lamellae terminate to enclose pockets (P) of paranodal cytoplasm, which contain microtubules (m_1). The pockets indent the surface of the axon and their enclosing plasma membranes become closely apposed to the axolemma. In this uranyl block-stained preparation the intermittent densities of the outer leaflet of the axolemma are not very apparent. While the pockets of cytoplasm are regularly arranged in the paranodal region of the upper length of myelin, in the lower paranode they are piled up so that not all of them reach the axolemma.

The axoplasm of this longitudinally sectioned axon contains microtubules (m), neurofilaments (nf), and some profiles of the smooth endoplasmic reticulum (SR). *Basal ganglia of adult rat.* × 60,000.

The **inset** shows part of the paranode from a myelinated axon. This material was not stained in the block with uranyl acetate. Hence the intermittent densities (*arrows*) associated with the outer leaflet of the axolemma are apparent. *Optic nerve of adult rat.* × 100,000.

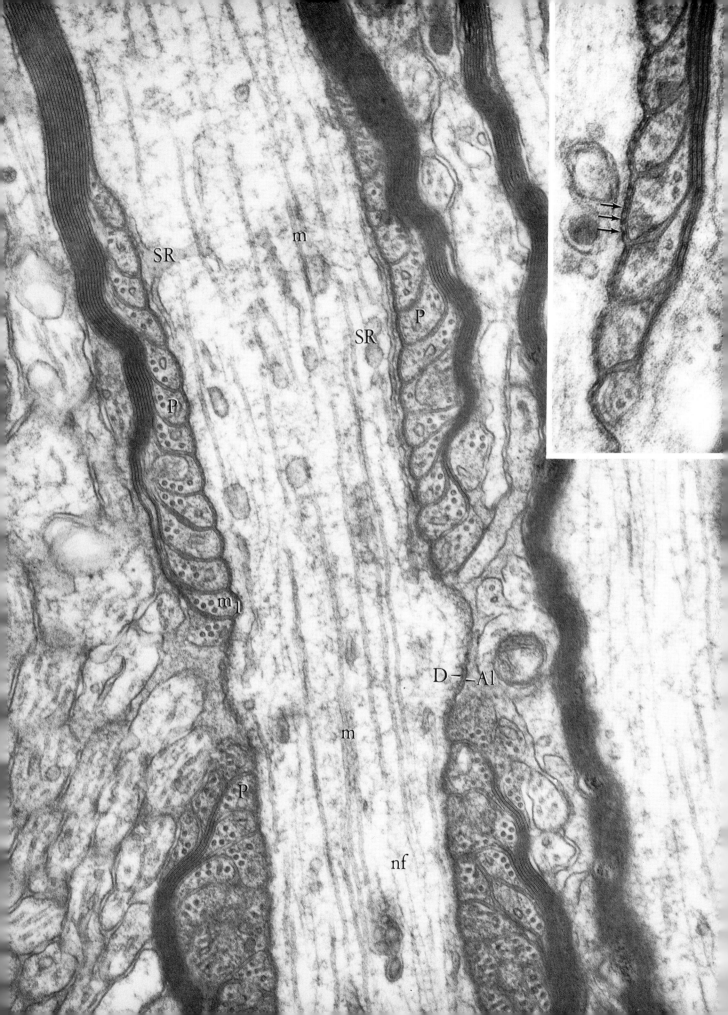

apparent in glutaraldehyde-osmium–fixed material.

Much of this appearance can be explained on the basis of freeze-cleaved preparations (Livingston, Pfenninger, Moor, and Akert, 1973; Dermietzel, 1974b; Schnapp and Mugnaini, 1975). There are some differences in these accounts and in the following discussion the presentation of Schnapp and Mugnaini (1975) will be followed (see Figures 6–18 and 6–19).

In tangential or longitudinal freeze-fractured preparations of myelinated fibers the paranode is readily identified by a set of transversely arranged scallops or broad concavities indenting the axon. These are impressions produced by the pockets of helically arranged paranodal cytoplasm bulging into the axon (Figures 6–18 and 6–19). The successive scallops are bounded by sharp crests that run transversely around the axon surface and correspond to sites where successive turns of the paranodal helix meet each other.

At the paranode the A face of the axolemma (Figure 16–19, *AlA*) shows a series of fine ridges that pass obliquely across the exposed surface at an angle to the scallops produced by the paranodal pockets. These ridges, which are 25 to 30 nm apart, correspond to the crests of the undulations seen in sections of ferrocyanide-osmium–fixed material, and to the intervals where the outer leaflet of the axolemma is deficient in sections of aldehyde-osmium–fixed material (Figure 6–15, *inset*. Alternating with the ridges on the A face of freeze-fractured material of the axolemma is a series of grooves. This A face also shows membrane particles, 8 to 15 nm, which appear to be randomly distributed in some preparations, but mainly aligned along the ridges in others. The B face of the axolemma (Figures 6–18 and 6–19, *AlB*) is complementary to the A face and is virtually devoid of particles, suggesting that the particulate components of the paranodal axolemma cleave entirely with the A face.

In this same paranodal region the A face of the plasma membrane of the myelin-forming cell also shows a system of fine parallel ridges and grooves (Figure 6–19, *B*), so that the appearance of this membrane surface is essentially like that of the apposed axolemma. However, unlike the axolemma, the membrane of the myelin-forming cell shows that the particles cleave either with the A (Figure 6–19, *A*) or the B (Figure 6–19, *B*) face, and not preferentially with one of them. Those associated with the A face, however, are absolutely confined to the ridges and on the B face to the mirroring grooves. Another difference is that in some of their replicas Schnapp and Mugnaini (1975) found that the B face of the axolemma had an unusual crystalline configuration in which the surface overlying the grooves of the A face was occupied by a chain of regularly arranged protrusions. The repeating unit of the chain is a pair of closely apposed subunits, each 6 nm in diameter, with a center-to-center spacing of 8 to 9.6 nm, and a repeat every 10 to 12 nm along the chain. The complementary view of this structure was not apparent on the axolemmal A face, and they had no counterpart in the membrane of the myelin-forming cell at the paranode. Although a comparison is difficult, it should be noted that Livingston, Pfenninger, Moor, and Akert (1973) also show a similar appearance on the B face of the axolemma.

The article by Livingston, Pfenninger, Moor, and Akert (1973) shows many of the features encountered by Schnapp and Mugnaini (1975). However, Livingston and his colleagues did not find the A and B faces of the membranes to be complementary to each other, so that they describe a system of ridges on the B face of the axolemma, but not on the A face, for example. It is apparent from both studies, however, that at the paranode the axolemma and the membrane of the myelin-forming cell are joined by a helical and ridge-like junction which is unusual in being asymmetrical in form. Schnapp and Mug-

---

Figure 6–16. **The Node and the Paranode, Central Nervous System.**

In the center of the field are two axons (*Ax₁* and *Ax₂*) sectioned in the paranodal region. Ax_1 is nearer to the node than Ax_2. The cytoplasm of these axons contains microtubules (*m*) and neurofilaments (*nf*). The axolemma (*Al*) in the paranodal region is separated from the plasma membrane of the inner surface of the sheath by only 3 nm. Thus, the two membranes come together to form a seven-layered complex (*arrow*). Two astrocyte processes (*As*) containing fibrils (*f*) insinuate themselves among the nerve fibers in the field.
Optic nerve from adult rat. × *160,000.*

Inset: At the node of Ranvier, the axon is bare and beneath the axolemma (*Al*) is a dense layer (*D*). Note the neurofilaments (*nf*) and microtubules (*m*) in the axoplasm.
Optic nerve from adult rat. × *106,000.*

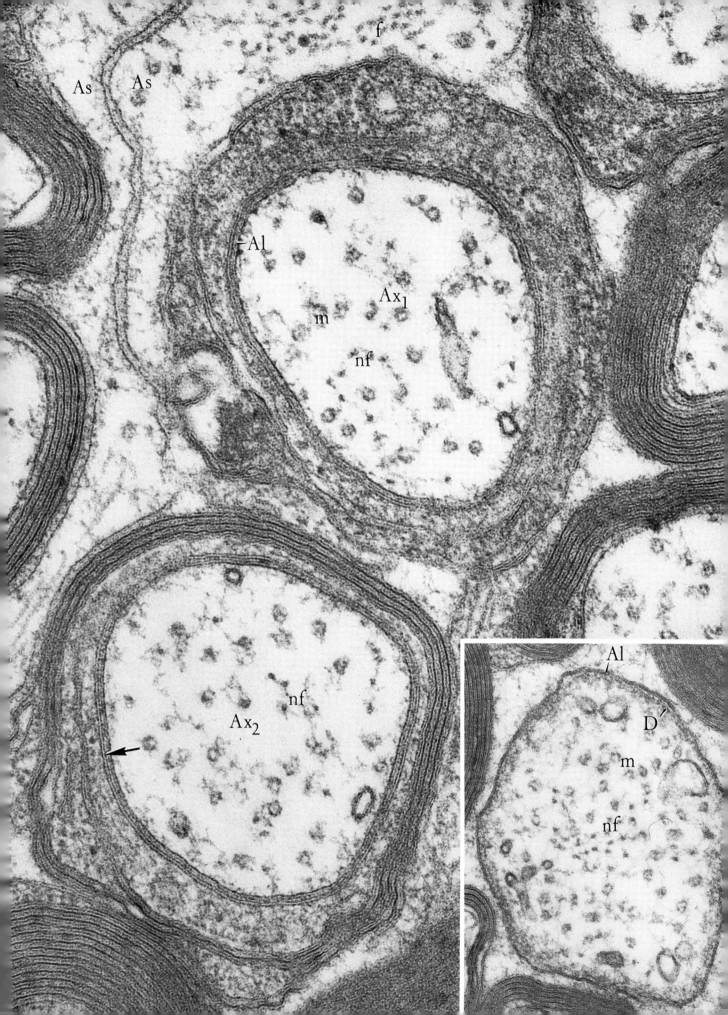

naini identify this junction as a type of septate intercellular junction.

A study by Blank, Bunge, and Bunge (1974) has shown that the integrity of the paranodal junction is dependent upon the presence of calcium ions. Thus they found that if myelinated cultures of sensory ganglia are maintained for long periods of time in media with low calcium levels, very soon there is an accumulation of fluid in the space between the axon and the myelin sheath and a lengthening of the nodes of Ranvier. The changes began with accumulation of fluid between the paranodal pockets and a stretching and shrinkage of the pockets which eventually led to breaking the paranodal junction between the Schwann cell membrane and the axolemma. These changes were reversible if the cultures were returned to media with normal calcium levels. Somewhat similar changes are also induced by treatment of cultures with trypsin (Yu and Bunge, 1975).

The existence of these junctions at the paranode initially led to the conclusion that they might obstruct the interchange of ions between the extracellular space surrounding the node and the space beneath the internodal myelin sheath, since such an obstruction would be desirable in explaining saltatory conduction. However, in both the central (Hirano and Dembitzer, 1969) and peripheral (Hall and Williams, 1971) nervous systems, lanthanum salts applied to fixed nerve fibers penetrate into the intervals between densities at the paranode, so that in longitudinal sections of the paranode the tracer appears in regularly spaced deposits. This appearance, incidentally, suggests that the densities bridging between the axolemma and the

plasma membrane of the myelin-forming cell are arranged in a helical fashion and not in closed rings, and that the lanthanum penetrates by moving along the helix. Hirano and Dembitzer (1967) suggest there are 6 to 8 separate helical bands and not a single one following a tight pitch.

Feder, Reese, and Brightman (1969) also found microperoxidase (mol wt, about 2000) to enter the periaxonal space of central myelinated fibers, although the space is inaccessible to horseradish peroxidase (mol wt, about 40,000). In peripheral fibers, Hall and Williams (1971) showed that ferritin with a molecular diameter of about 9.5 nm could not enter the gap between the axolemma and the sheath at the paranode. Thus, while this gap is accessible to small molecules it is not patent for larger ones. This indicates that the gap is not readily distensible, and if the access for molecules and ions is through a narrow helical channel, this clearly does not prevent an interchange between the two spaces, but might produce sufficient retardation of the ions to explain saltatory conduction.

In transverse sections of nerve fibers the close proximity between these two plasma membranes, that of the axolemma and that bounding the paranodal pockets, readily allows paranodal regions to be identified (Figures 6–4 and 6–16). The spiral densities around the axolemma are not readily apparent, however, although they may sometimes appear as discontinuities of its outer layer. Other features that characterize the region are the presence of paranodal cytoplasm within the sheath and the increased frequency with which microtubules tend to occur within the axon (Peters, 1967).

Figure 6–17.   **Freeze-Fractured Myelin Sheaths.**

The **left picture** shows a peripheral myelinated fiber. The cleavage plane passes across the axon (*Ax*) and its myelin sheath (*my*) at the bottom of the picture, and the fracture has peeled off the outer half of the Schwann cell membrane so that the A face of the membrane (*SCA*) is exposed on each side of the external mesaxon. The position of the mesaxon (*mes*) is evident from the location of the Schwann cell cytoplasm (*SC*) in the outer turn of the sheath. Extending downward from the site of the external mesaxon are the junctional strands of the zonula occludens (*zo*) which occurs at the end of the external mesaxon.
Chicken ophthalmic nerve. × 55,000.

The **right picture** shows a peripheral sheath in which the continuity of the tight-junctional system is demonstrated. At the bottom of the field is the nodal axon displaying the A face of the axolemma (*NdA*). Just above, and on each side, are the cross-fractured images of the outermost, and therefore last, loop of paranodal cytoplasm (*P*). The B face (*SCB*) of the outermost loop is exposed, and passing along it are the tight-junctional furrows of the zonula occludens (*zo*) that occupies the end of the external mesaxon. At their lower end these furrows (*arrow*) pass into the tight junctions that occur between the adjacent loops at the paranode, and at their upper end (*arrowhead*) enter into a Schmidt-Lanterman cleft.
Chicken ophthalmic nerve. × 50,000.

Micrographs by B. Schnapp and E. Mugnaini.

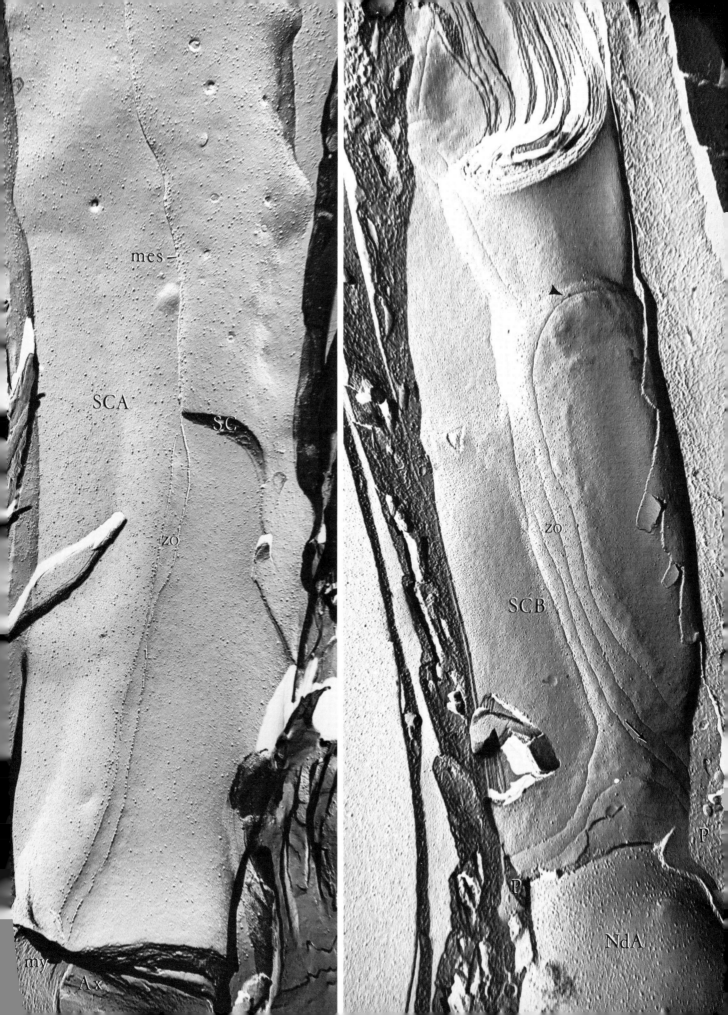

The length of the nodes of myelinated axons appears variable. Axons of the rat's optic nerve have nodes with an average length of 0.8 micron, and in fibers from the cat spinal cord the length is between 0.4 and 4.4 microns (McDonald and Ohlrich, 1971). Gray (1970) has observed nodes as long as 14 microns in frog spinal cord, and similarly, long nodes appear in the gray matter of the cerebral cortex. In the peripheral nervous system the nodes appear to be generally shorter (Hess and Young, 1952; Fraher, 1973), and in small fibers, from frog's peripheral nerve, for example, the length is only about 0.5 micron (Robertson, 1959b). In the central nervous system the nodal axon is completely bare and in many instances it is surrounded by an extracellular space that seems only slightly larger than elsewhere (Figure 6–16, *inset*). Sometimes the axon becomes thinner at the node, but in other examples it bulges outward. Unlike central nodes, the nodes of the peripheral nerves (Figure 6–14) are covered by interdigitating processes that extend from the outer cytoplasmic layers of the Schwann cells forming the myelin internodes on either side (e.g., see Robertson, 1959b; Elfvin, 1961; Webster, Spiro, Waksman, and Adams, 1961; Bunge, Bunge, Peterson, and Murray, 1967). The arrangement of the interdigitating processes is very irregular, and their outer surfaces may be covered by the basal lamina that coats the outer surface of the Schwann cell. It is worthy of note that, at least in peripheral nerves, the region immediately surrounding the nodal axolemma contains mucopolysaccharide (Langley and Landon, 1968) which binds cations (Landon and Langley, 1971).

At the node, the contours of the axolemma are usually irregular and beneath it is a layer of dense, granular material (Peters, 1966). This layer is apparent at nodes in both the central (Figure 6–16, *D*) and peripheral (Figure 6–14, *D*) nervous systems. It is not applied directly to the inner surface of the axolemma, but is separated by a distance of about 10 nm. The layer is about 20 nm thick and appears similar to the one beneath the axolemma at the initial axon segment (see page 92). In the central nervous system at least, the axoplasm at the node is also characterized by an increase in the number of microtubules.

A striking variation of the usual form of nodal axon has been shown by Waxman (1972) and Waxman, Pappas, and Bennett (1972) in the nerve fibers supplying the electric organ of the gymnotid knife fish. Where the nerve fibers enter the electric organ the nodes are similar to those present elsewhere in the peripheral nervous system, but in the electric organ they are three to five times longer, and there are extensive nodes at which the axolemma is elaborated into irregular polypoid-shaped processes. These processes markedly increase the axonal surface area, and an electron-dense undercoating of the axolemma is not present. The function of these specialized nodes, which do not generate spikes, as do those with a typical morphology, is apparently to act as a series capacitor (see Bennett, 1970 and 1971). The undercoating may also be absent or limited at nodes which form synapses or collaterals in mammals and reptiles (Waxman, 1974).

Some other features of nodes must be considered to complete the picture. At the junction between the peripheral and central nervous systems the sheath of an axon changes so that on one side of the node the sheath is formed by a Schwann cell and on the other by an oligodendrocyte. This transitional region has been examined by Maxwell, Kruger, and Pineda (1969) in the trigeminal nerve of the macaque. They find that compared to the peripheral sheath, the cen-

---

Figure 6–18.   **Freeze-Fractured Myelin Sheaths.**

The **left figure** shows a freeze-fracture plane through a node of Ranvier and the two adjacent central myelin segments. In the middle of the field is the A face of the nodal axon (*NdA*), which is studded with randomly distributed membrane particles. On each side of this are the A faces of the paranodal axolemma (*AlA*). The one at the bottom shows the scalloping (*arrows*) produced by the pockets of paranodal cytoplasm that are visible at the sides (*P*). The fracture plane then passes across the axon (*Ax*) so that the B face (*AlB*) of the axolemma on the other side comes into view. *Turtle cerebellum.* × 41,000.

The **right figure** shows freeze-fractured peripheral myelin at the level of a Schmidt-Lanterman cleft. The successive turns of the spiralled cytoplasmic tube of the funnel-like cleft are indicated by *arrows*. The *arrowheads* indicate the paired tight-junctional furrows on the B face (*B*) of a myelin lamella. This B face has many small particles. At *SCA* is the A face of the external Schwann cell membrane which has many large particles.
Chicken ophthalmic nerve. × 60,000.

Micrographs by B. Schnapp and E. Mugnaini.

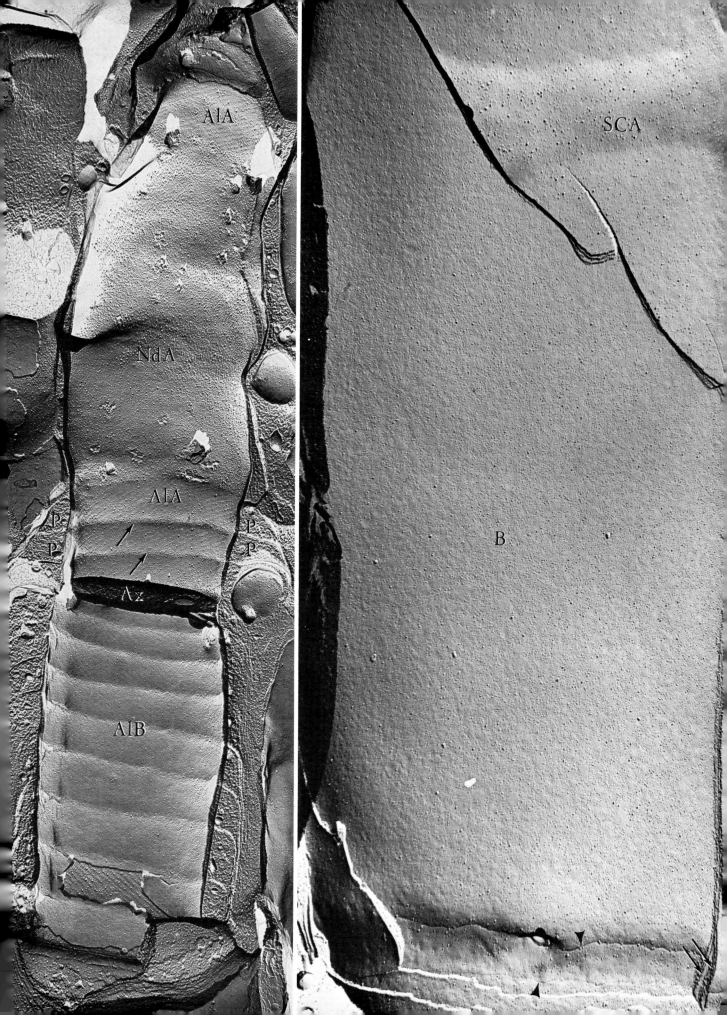

tral sheath on the other side of the node has thinner myelin, and if the peripheral part is lightly myelinated, as the axon enters the brain, it may lose its sheath altogether. The Schwann cell forming the peripheral internode abuts a dome formed by the perikarya and processes of astrocytes. This astrocytic dome is the "fibrous cone" described by light microscopists (Tarlov, 1937) and is essentially a thickened portion of the glia limitans that covers the central nervous system elsewhere. As the myelinated axons pass into the brain the basal lamina of the Schwann cells becomes continuous with that of the astrocytic dome. This transition zone requires further study.

Interesting variations on the normal morphology of peripheral nodes of Ranvier have recently been described by Hall (1973) who examined the morphology of myelin sheaths found after demyelination induced by intraneural injection of lysophosphatidyl choline. While the remyelination of most fibers resembled primary myelination, a number of atypical forms of nodes were seen. Thus, at some remyelinating paranodes, five or six lamellae extended beyond the rest so that there was an interval between sets of paranodal pockets, making the paranodes unusually long. Another variation Hall refers to as a "pseudonode," because this structure occurred within the territory of an individual Schwann cell. Such an entity consists of two sets of opposing cytoplasmic filled loops, separated from each other, but overlain by Schwann cell cytoplasm. This cytoplasm is apparently continuous with that in the loops, and as such a sheath increases in thickness, the interval between the

two sets of loops becomes covered by lamellae that are continuous across the interval. Despite the absence of discontinuity between the two apposed sets of loops, the axolemma between them seems to acquire an undercoating like a typical node.

Just before a myelinated intramuscular fiber terminates to form a motor end-plate, it loses its myelin sheath at a final node of Ranvier, or to be more precise at a heminode. From the outer layer of cytoplasm surrounding the sheath many small finger-like processes extend, rather like the ones that interdigitate over the surface of the nodal axon. These small processes have a basal lamina only on their exterior surfaces; this basal lamina becomes confluent with that of the muscle cell. Hence, it seems that it is the Schwann cell and not the cells of the perineural sheath that cover the outer surface of the terminal axon as it lies in the gutter indenting the surface of the muscle cell (see Figures 7–1 and 7–2).

In the central nervous system a nodal axon may sometimes participate in the formation of a synapse (for example, see Bodian and Taylor, 1963; Andres, 1965b; Khattab, 1966; Sotelo and Palay, 1970; Waxman, 1972; Kohno, Nakai, and Yamada, 1972). When this occurs the axon gives rise to a protuberance, like other presynaptic axon terminals, containing an accumulation of synaptic vesicles and mitochondria. So far as we are aware, no nodal axons have been shown to act as postsynaptic elements.

The branching of a myelinated nerve fiber always takes place at a node. At the site of branching three or more segments of myelin converge. The basic features of these branching

---

Figure 6–19.   **Freeze-Fractured Myelin Sheaths.**

The upper picture shows the paranodal region of a myelinated nerve fiber. The axoplasm is apparent at *Ax*. The fracture has exposed a portion of the B face of the axolemma (*AlB*) and the A face (*A*) of the myelin-forming cell. Note the undulations of the axolemmal B face and the parallel rows of particles that adorn the A face of the myelin-forming cell.
Turtle cerebellum. × *100,000.*

The lower left picture displays the B face (*B*) of the myelin-forming cell and the A face of the axolemma (*AlA*). The B face of the myelin-forming cell has parallel rows of particles, which occupy the grooves that mark its surface. The counterparts of these grooves are less obvious on the A face of the axolemma (*AlA*), but they appear to be oriented in the same direction.
Turtle cerebellum. × *100,000.*

The lower right picture shows details of the axolemmal A face (*AlA*) at the paranode. The almost horizontally disposed ridges are the markings of the boundaries between adjacent pockets of paranodal cytoplasm and crossing them are the fine scorings of parallel ridges which have particles on their crests.
Turtle cerebellum. × *72,000.*

Micrographs by B. Schnapp and E. Mugnaini.

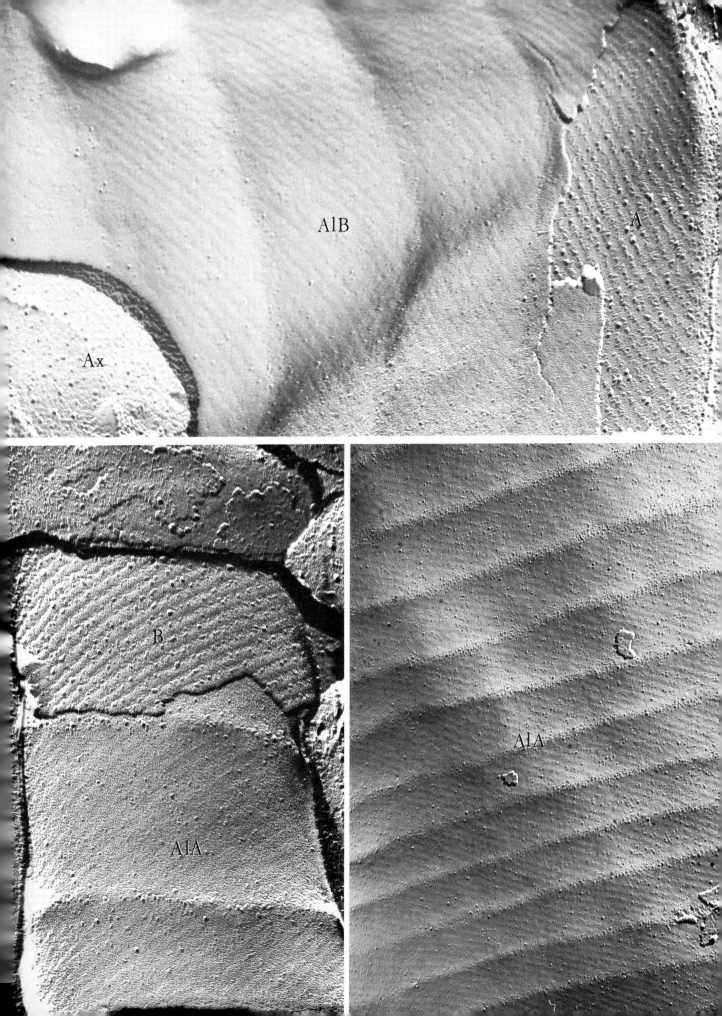

sites appear to be identical to those of the more simple nodes described above (see Ha, 1970; Lieberman, Webster, and Špaček, 1972).

SCHMIDT-LANTERMAN INCISURES

As shown in the Frontispiece (*J*), in light microscope preparations of osmic acid–fixed nerve fibers from the peripheral nervous system, the sheaths of the internodal region are interrupted by a series of oblique, funnel-like clefts, or incisures (Schmidt, 1874; Lanterman, 1877) which traverse the sheath at an average angle of 9 degrees (Friede and Samorajski, 1969). Counts along myelin segments of longitudinally sectioned nerves reveal that they are most numerous midway between the node of Ranvier and the Schwann cell nucleus (Webster, 1964). Similar incisures may also be observed in living nerve fibers examined with oblique incident light (see Hall and Williams, 1970), and so it is likely that they represent a real entity rather than an artifact produced by fixation. In an early electron microscope study of these Schmidt-Lanterman incisures, Robertson (1958a), who considered them to be shearing defects in the sheath, showed that the clefts are areas where the lamellae are separated along the major dense line so that cytoplasm intervenes between them. This same structure was also shown by Elfvin (1968). Hall and Williams (1970) demonstrated that the intraperiod line may also be split where the clefts occur and that stacks of attachments resembling puncta adhaerentia may occur between the myelin-forming membranes separated by such a split. These faces of the membranes forming the intraperiod line at a Schmidt-Lanterman cleft may also have tight junctions between them (Schnapp and Mugnaini, 1975). Thus, in many respects the structure of the incisures resembles that of the paranodal portion of the sheath.

When the incisures extend across the entire thickness of the sheath, it is apparent that they provide a pathway through which cytoplasm on the outside of the sheath is confluent with that on the inside, for, in effect, the cytoplasm of the incisure occupies a helical funnel (see Figure 6–18). Hall and Williams (1970) have shown that the incisures are subject to dilation or contraction if the nerve fibers are put into hypotonic or hypertonic solutions, respectively, but whether metabolites use this pathway is not clear. In an attempt to answer this question Friede and Samorajski (1969) injected radioactive leucine but found no preferential uptake of this label into the incisures. They do, however, show alkaline phosphatase activity (Pinner and Campbell, 1965). Krishnan and Singer (1973) demonstrated that in nerves soaked in horseradish peroxidase for periods of up to six hours, the Schmidt-Lanterman clefts and the paranodal loops may provide a pathway of access to the periaxonal space. The peroxidase is sequestered in vesicles in the Schwann cell cytoplasm before entering the cytoplasm of the clefts and of the paranode, and after prolonged incubation it appears in the periaxonal space. Ultimately, it may appear in vesicles and agranular endoplasmic reticulum of the axoplasm. In view of this discrepancy in the results of experiments using radioactive leucine and horseradish peroxidase, no clear statement can be made about the function of Schmidt-Lanterman clefts. A clue may be provided, though, by the observation that in sections of osmium-fixed nerves, the incisures increase in number where myelin segmentation begins during the onset of Wallerian degeneration (Webster, 1964). Williams and Hall (1971a) concluded that after injury, incisures dilate and do not increase in number, but they provided no counts for the *in vivo* distribution of incisures along normal and degenerating myelin segments. They saw that damage opens up the incisures so that the nerve develops undulating contours. Subsequent constriction of the sheath at the incisures leads to the formation of ellipsoidal segments of myelin like those frequently reported to occur in the first stages of Wallerian degeneration.

Until recently the existence of Schmidt-Lanterman incisures in the central nervous system has been in doubt. However, McDonald and Ohrlich (1971) and Hildebrand (1971a) demonstrated their existence in myelinated nerve fibers from the cat spinal cord, and Blakemore (1969b) studied the fine structure of incisures in fibers from the dorsal columns of the rat spinal cord and rabbit medulla. Blakemore (1969b) points out that incisures are only to be found in the sheaths of the larger fibers, with a minimum myelin thickness of 0.5 micron and an axon diameter of 2 microns. The incisures are clearly like those of peripheral nerve fibers. The fact that they are present only in the sheaths of thick fibers may explain why they were overlooked in previous studies, for such fibers are amongst the most difficult structures to fix adequately in the central nervous system.

THE DIFFERENCES BETWEEN PERIPHERAL AND CENTRAL MYELIN SHEATHS

Although central and peripheral myelin sheaths are basically similar in that they both consist of a spiral of plasma membrane derived from a myelin-forming cell, a number of important differences exist. Some of these differences, such as the amount of cytoplasm on the outside of the sheath and the form of the node of Ranvier, have already been mentioned. Others will be considered under the following headings:

The Proximity of Adjacent Sheaths

In peripheral nerves the external surfaces of adjacent Schwann cells are separated from each other by two elements. These are (1) the basal lamina that completely surrounds the external surface of each Schwann cell and (2) the collagen and reticulin fibrils of the endoneurium (Figures 6–4 and 6–5). In the central nervous system neither of these two elements exists. Consequently, the external surfaces of neighboring central myelin sheaths can lie immediately adjacent (Figure 6–9). Since the cytoplasm on the outside of a central myelin sheath is sparse, the outer surfaces of adjacent sheaths frequently come so closely in contact with each other that an intermediate or intraperiod line is formed between them. When this occurs, the periodicity of the myelin appears uninterrupted across the entire thickness of two sheaths (Peters, 1960a; Maturana, 1960; Metuzals, 1960; Rosenbluth, 1966).

This intimate contact between adjacent myelin sheaths in the central nervous system is one of the factors that led to difficulty in early attempts to interpret their structure. Similar contacts between the outer surfaces of myelin-forming cells also appear to play an important role during the formation of central myelin sheaths, for there is no structural barrier to prevent mechanical interference between the processes of different cells. Because of this, myelination in the central nervous system is a less well ordered procedure than it is in the peripheral nervous system, where adjacent Schwann cells are kept apart by their basal laminae. This difference in the separation of myelin-forming cells probably accounts for the formation of irregular or concentric sheaths of a type that is sometimes encountered in the central nervous system but never, apparently, in peripheral nerves (see page 211).

The Thickness of Myelin Lamellae

X-ray diffraction studies have shown the fundamental repeating unit of central myelin to be about 10 per cent lower than that of peripheral myelin (see Finean, 1961). This difference is also apparent when myelin is examined by other techniques. Thus, in electron micrographs of sections Karlsson (1966a) demonstrated that the repeating distance between the centers of dense lines is 12 nm in peripheral myelin and 10.6 nm in central myelin, even though the tissues from both parts of the nervous system were prepared in the same way. Some of this difference in the periodicity may be due to the known differences in the chemical composition of central and peripheral myelin (Finean, Hawthorne, and Patterson, 1957; Evans and Finean, 1965), and some to differences in the intraperiod line. Thus, in peripheral myelin it is now clear that the intraperiod line can be resolved into a pair of lines 2 nm apart. The splitting of the intraperiod line of central myelin is rather less distinct and the gap seems to be somewhat narrower (Figure 6–9, *inset*).

The difference in periodicity between central and peripheral myelin observed in sectioned material is also apparent in freeze-etched material. Bischoff and Moor (1967b) found that the periodicity of myelin from sciatic nerve was 18.5 nm, while from spinal cord it was 16 nm. In freeze-etched material the central myelin showed dark lines 16 nm apart that alternated with somewhat fainter lines. Peripheral myelin, on the other hand, showed broad, dark lines separated by intervals of 18.5 nm that contained a pair of fine lines which were themselves 4 nm apart.

Bischoff and Moor (1967a) interpreted the fracture planes in their material as passing between membranes of the myelin sheath. However, in keeping with the membrane splitting hypothesis proposed by Branton (1966), Tani, Ikeda, and Nishiura (1973) and Schnapp and Mugnaini (1975) showed that the fracture plane passes within the membranes of the myelin, revealing the internal structure (Figures 6–17 and 6–18). In cross fractures of freeze-etched central myelin in which the membranes of the sheaths are seen end-on, Tani, Ikeda, and Nishiura (1973) found a series of alternating ridges and furrows. They suggest that the ridges correspond to the intraperiod and major dense lines, and the furrows to the middle of the lipid layer of the membranes. In agreement with other studies (Branton, 1967; Bischoff and Moor,

1967a and b) these authors found the exposed surfaces of membranes in more tangentially fractured sheaths to be relatively free of globules or particles. This is contrary to the results obtained by Schnapp and Mugnaini (1975) who found particles 8 to 16 nm in diameter on fractured surfaces of compact myelin from both the central and peripheral nervous systems (Figures 6–17 and 6–18). In peripheral myelin they found that most of the particles are small and are retained with either the A or the B face, although a smaller population of larger particles remain preferentially with the A face. The A face is the inner face of a membrane, and in this case it is the one immediately adjacent to the major dense line. In central myelin most of the particles remain attached to the A face. Thus, peripheral and central myelin differ in the disposition of particles according to Schnapp and Mugnaini (1975). It should be noted, however, that although the intraperiod line has an appearance that is similar to a gap junction in sectioned material, in freeze-fractured material it does not show the close packing of particles or globules which characterize gap junctions. Consequently it is unlikely that the intraperiod line provides a low resistance pathway between adjacent myelin lamellae, and of course it should not provide such a pathway if one of the functions of myelin is to provide insulation.

On the question of the periodicity of myelin, it should be noted that Hildebrand (1972) has recently found that the myelin period measured in electron micrographs of feline spinal cord is inversely proportional to the number of lamellae present in the sheath. In glutaraldehyde-fixed material he found the sheaths with less than 10 lamellae to have a periodicity of about 11.1 nm and those with more than 60 lamellae to have a periodicity of about 9.6 nm. The significance of these measurements is not clear in terms of the molecular configuration of myelin.

The Radial Component of the Central Sheath

In transverse sections of central myelin sheaths fixed with osmic acid and stained on the section with potassium permanganate, a radial component is prominent (Honjin, 1959; Peters, 1961b and 1962b; Honjin, Kosaka, Takano, and Hiramatsu, 1963; Honjin and Changus, 1964). At low magnifications this component appears as a series of fairly regularly spaced radial lines, usually 30 to 40 nm apart, that extend either partially or entirely across the thickness of the sheath. At higher resolution it is evident that these radial lines are produced by regular thickenings in the intraperiod line of a sheath. At a thickening the width of the intraperiod line increases from 2 to 3 nm to 4 to 5 nm. The thickenings of the intraperiod line are most common in that part of the sheath underlying the external tongue of cytoplasm, but they also occur in other regions, in particular, where two adjacent sheaths come into contact with each other.

When the radial component was first observed, it was thought to have a punctate form. Later, however, examination of oblique (Peters, 1964a) and longitudinally oriented sections (Peters, 1968) of permanganate-stained sheaths revealed that the component is composed of a series of lines, or rodlike thickenings, oriented along the length of the sheath.

In the light of recent studies of freeze-cleaved preparations of central myelin sheaths by Dermietzel (1974a) and by Reale, Luciano, and Spitznas (1975) it now seems that these radial components represent the locations of junctions between the outer faces of plasma membrane in adjacent turns of myelin lamellae. Thus there are longitudinal rows of parallel particles on the A face of freeze-cleaved lamellae that are matched by furrows on the B faces. These junctions are present throughout the width of the sheaths and are most common in the part of the sheath underlying the external tongue of cytoplasm. Dermietzel failed to find similar junctions in freeze-cleaved preparations of peripheral myelin sheaths, and this is compatible with the fact that despite numerous accounts in the literature of peripheral myelin, only once has a radial component been described in them (Robertson, 1960b).

SHEATHS OF MYELINATED GANGLION CELLS

Although the majority of nerve cells of the peripheral sensory ganglia are surrounded by simple capsules composed of a single layer of Schwann cells, in certain ganglia, notably the vestibular and acoustic (spiral) ganglia, it is not uncommon for the cell bodies to be enclosed by myelin sheaths. The form of this myelin sheath has been examined electron microscopically by Rosenbluth and Palay (1961) in the goldfish, by Rosenbluth (1962a) in the rat, and by Adamo and Daigneault (1973a) in the cat.

In the goldfish the form of the sheaths surrounding the neurons in the eighth-nerve ganglion varies considerably. A few of the smaller cell bodies have simple sheaths consisting of a single layer of Schwann cell processes. Around the majority of neurons, however, the sheath consists of between 2 and 90 lamellae that represent either layers of Schwann cell cytoplasm or a mixture of loose and compact myelin. The compact myelin has a form similar to that around nerve fibers. Major dense and intermediate (intraperiod) lines are present. These alternate with each other and have a periodicity of about 15 nm. In the loose myelin, however, the lamellae consist of layers of Schwann cell cytoplasm, so that only the intermediate line exists. Such layers are generally between 10 and 100 nm thick, although any one layer can vary considerably in thickness over its full extent. When the layers of the loose myelin are thick, then cytoplasm lies between the plasma membranes bounding the lamellae, but in some places the cytoplasm may disappear so that a major dense line is formed by the coaptation of the inner surfaces of the bounding membranes.

Areas of contact also occur between the outer surfaces of the lamellae of loose myelin. These may lead either to the formation of an intermediate line or in some situations to such a close contact that even the intermediate line is obliterated. In the latter instance a compound membrane unit is formed that is only about 10 nm thick and consists of two parallel dense layers separated by a lighter zone. Rosenbluth and Palay postulate that this image represents such a complete condensation between the two apposed plasma membranes that only the cytoplasmic dark layers of each of the membranes is present; the outer dark layers have completely disappeared. Consequently, the structure has a form that is essentially similar to a single plasma membrane, although slightly thicker, i.e., 10 nm. Two other important features of the myelin sheaths of the eighth-nerve ganglion of the goldfish are that desmosomes are sometimes present between the lamellae and that each bipolar ganglion cell is contained within a single internode, which may have more than one Schwann cell related to it.

The myelin sheaths of the vestibular or spiral ganglia of the rat and cat are very similar to that of the goldfish. Again the sheaths consist of both loose and compact myelin, the amount of each type varying over the surfaces of different neurons. In the rat and cat, however, the myelin sheaths never attain the thickness of up to 90 lamellae as reported for the goldfish. Instead the maximum number seems to be between 20 and 25. Also, the number of lamellae changes over the surface of even the same ganglion cell, for each sheath may receive lamellae from more than one Schwann cell, and conversely one Schwann cell can contribute to the sheath of more than one neuron (Adamo and Daigneault, 1973a). These lamellae interweave and overlap, and each lamella may terminate anywhere within the sheath, may bifurcate, or reverse its direction.

An interesting feature of the myelinated cells of the cat spiral ganglia is that inner lamellae of the sheath may penetrate into the neuronal perikaryon (Adamo and Daigneault, 1973b). There they may envelop a portion of the neuronal cytoplasm, but whether such cytoplasm is thereby isolated or only partially enveloped is not clear from the existing description.

The myelinogenesis of such complex sheaths as those of the spiral ganglion neurons is discussed at some length by Rosenbluth (1962a). However, as he points out, the manner in which this myelin is formed will be understood only after a developmental study has been performed.

A somewhat similar sheath also occurs around perikarya in the ciliary ganglion of the chick (Hess, 1965; Takahashi and Hama, 1965).

MYELIN SHEATHS OF DENDRITES IN THE CENTRAL NERVOUS SYSTEM

It has been known for some time that dendrites in the central nervous system may be at least partially ensheathed by astroglial processes. However, contrary to what would be expected on the basis of the classical doctrines pertaining to the nervous system, Pinching

(1971) and Willey (1973) have shown that some dendrites may have myelin sheaths. These dendrites occur in the olfactory bulb, the only location in which they have so far been described. The myelin sheaths are thin and cover the primary dendrites of large mitral and tufted cells in the most superficial portion of the external plexiform layer and in the periglomerular region. From Pinching's (1971) description, the myelin sheaths appear to have a form similar to those around axons. The myelin internodes are relatively short—20 to 60 microns—and occasionally two successive internodal lengths of myelin may be present along a dendrite.

On the basis of the morphological features displayed by the myelinated processes there is little doubt about their identity, but it is not apparent which cells are forming the myelin, and this must be investigated further.

FUNCTIONS OF SATELLITE AND SCHWANN CELLS

Although the structural relationships between neurons, their processes, and the related Schwann cells have been well defined by many electron microscope studies carried out during the past 20 years, the roles of these sheath cells in the overall function of the peripheral nervous system has been less easy to clarify. Progress to date can be considered under the following headings.

BIOCHEMICAL RELATIONSHIPS

In the peripheral nervous system, the neural elements are separated from one another by a large extracellular compartment that contains collagen, fibroblasts, and a few mast cells. The chemical environment within this endoneurial compartment is determined partially by perineurial and vascular barriers (see page 330), which allow much greater tracer penetration into the parenchyma of ganglia than they permit in peripheral nerves (Kristensson and Olsson, 1973; Arvidsson, Kristensson, and Olsson, 1973). These relatively "leaky" barriers in ganglia are probably needed to fill the metabolic needs of neurons and satellite cells. They also may explain the high incidence of ganglionic lesions and the relative sparing of nerves in a number of diseases (Waksman, 1961; Kristensson and Olsson, 1973). Once in the endoneurial space, substances can diffuse much more rapidly than in the smaller extracellular compartment of the central nervous system. In spinal ganglia, it has been found that tracers pass through the satellite cell basal lamina and between the satellite cell processes and are subsequently taken up by pinocytosis into neuronal multivesicular bodies (see Rosenbluth and Wissig, 1964; Holtzman

and Peterson, 1969; review by Holtzman, 1971). Presumably, a comparable route and similar uptake mechanism are also available throughout the peripheral nervous system along the entire lengths of unmyelinated nerve fibers and at the nodes of Ranvier of myelinated nerve fibers. However, at nodes, macromolecular tracers like ferritin (mol wt, 900,000) diffuse slowly along the paranodal axolemma and do not penetrate into periaxonal spaces of the internode injected (Hall and Williams, 1971). In the central nervous system, injected microperoxidase (mol wt, 2000) enters this periaxonal space *in vivo* but horseradish peroxidase (mol wt, 40,000) rarely does (Feder, 1971). Molecular size may also determine how quickly other substances enter the periaxonal space in the peripheral nervous system, although data are lacking. The demonstration that the Schmidt-Lanterman clefts are not openings in the myelin sheath (Schmitt and Geschwind, 1957; Robertson, 1958a; Hall and Williams, 1970) undermined the earlier notion that substances could reach the internodal axon directly. However, they attain this space by traveling through the helical funnel of cytoplasm that composes the Schmidt-Lanterman cleft (Krishnan and Singer, 1973).

Movements of Schwann cells and their myelin sheaths could also facilitate exchange between axonal and extracellular compartments and also could affect axoplasmic flow. Rippling, undulating movements of myelin sheaths of developing tadpole nerve fibers *in situ* were observed years ago by Speidel (1964). Murray and her collaborators noted similar movements in mature fibers after myelination *in vitro*. Often located near myelin overgrowths, Schmidt-Lanterman clefts were thought to fluctuate and play a role in remodeling the mature sheath (Murray,

1965; Murray and Herrmann, 1968). Every 10 to 15 minutes, rippling pulsations traveled along the Schwann cells and frequently reversed direction. As each ripple passed over a partially open cleft, the cleft was squeezed shut temporarily. Singer and his collaborators (Singer and Bryant, 1969; Gitlin and Singer, 1974) suggest that these movements help substances like amino acids (Singer and Salpeter, 1966; Singer and Green, 1968) and tracers (Krishnan and Singer, 1973) to enter the Schwann cell, cross the myelin sheath, and penetrate the axon. However, when mammalian myelinated nerve fibers are examined *in vivo* for two to six hours, the number and location of incisures along internodes do not change; also, most of these incisures are "closed." A few are moderately open, but there is little change in their state of dilatation (Williams and Hall, 1971a and b; Hall and Williams, 1970). Thus, the available evidence suggests that there is relatively little movement *in vivo* of mature Schwann cells and myelin sheaths when they are located in nerve fascicles, and it seems unlikely that the described motion significantly affects axoplasmic flow or penetration of substances into the internodal axon. Still, the importance of these exchange routes is suggested by recent evidence that some of the cholesterol (Rawlins, 1973) and proteins (Giorgi, Karlsson, Sjöstrand, and Field, 1973) of the myelin sheath may originate from the axon.

Another topic of interest is the biochemistry of neurons and their satellites during neuronal activity. To date, the biochemical data, almost all of which have been obtained from central nervous tissue, are difficult to interpret. However, in one of the few studies utilizing peripheral nervous tissue, Pevzner (1965) measured the protein and nucleic acid contents of cells in the superior cervical ganglion. He found that, after exhaustive stimulation of the ganglion for three hours, there was an increase in the nucleic acid and protein content of the cytoplasm of the neurons. At the same time, the total nucleic acid content of the satellite cells decreased, although the amount of protein remained relatively constant. Thus, as far as nucleic acids (probably RNA) are concerned, it seems that with prolonged stimulation, the changes in the satellite cells are the reverse of those in the neurons. Daily injection of epinephrine extending over a period of two weeks brought about a pronounced increase in the protein and nucleic acid content of neurons and little change in their locations. This result suggests that the satellite cells support their neurons metabolically during prolonged activity.

Schwyn (1967) provided evidence suggesting that satellite cells respond to increased metabolic or synaptic activity by proliferating. He showed that if the afferent fibers to the superior cervical ganglion of a cat are electrically stimulated and if tritiated thymidine is concurrently injected into the animal, then the label is incorporated into the nuclei of the satellite cells. The incorporation is accelerated by neostigmine, an inhibitor of cholinesterase, and retarded by atropine sulfate. This latter compound is thought to compete with acetylcholine for postganglionic receptor sites of synaptic junctions.

When presynaptic endings in sympathetic ganglia (Pysh and Wiley, 1974; Birks, 1974) or neuromuscular junctions (Heuser and Reese, 1973) are stimulated and then examined electron microscopically, changes in the axolemma accompany the depletion of synaptic vesicles. Both types of ending return to normal during recovery, yet throughout this process, there appears to be little morphological change in the satellite cells of the ganglia or in the Schwann cells covering the neuromuscular junction. However, at denervated neuromuscular junctions Bevan, Miledi, and Grampp (1973) find that miniature end-plate potentials can still be recorded. Since actinomycin D can abolish this activity in the presence of otherwise normal protein synthesis, they suggest that the degenerating axon terminals stimulate the adjacent Schwann cells to produce and release acetylcholine, a function that is normally repressed.

Finally, metabolic requirements probably help determine the relationships between the volumes and surface areas of ganglionic neurons and those of their satellite cells. Yet if growth of sympathetic neurons is stimulated experimentally by the administration of nerve growth factor, a comparable hypertrophy and hyperplasia of satellite cells does not occur (Angeletti, Levi-Montalcini, and Caramia, 1971).

BREAKDOWN OF MYELIN

One of the most important functions of Schwann cells is the formation and maintenance of myelin sheaths (for example, see Causey, 1960; Peters and Vaughn, 1970; Webster, 1975). During early growth of the compact sheath, remodeling eliminates many of the initial irregularities (Webster, 1971). Also, counts and measurements of developing internodes in nerve roots of the cat show that as fiber diameter and internodal length increase, the number of short internodes (10 to 150 microns in length) decreases. Degenerative changes occurring in these short internodes include the presence of Marchi-positive ovoids and high acid phosphatase activity paranodally (Berthold, 1973a and b). In the internodes that remain and continue to lengthen, these changes are seen much less frequently.

As Waller (1850) showed more than a century ago, transection of a nerve produces changes in the myelin sheaths that are associated with degeneration of the axons distal to the lesion. Recently, these changes have been observed *in vivo* (Williams and Hall, 1971a and b). Widening of the nodal gap and dilation of incisures were apparent along some sheaths within one hour after transection. In sections of fixed nerves, fragmentation of paranodal myelin accompanies the earliest axonal changes at nodes of Ranvier (Webster, 1962), and an increase in the number of Schmidt-Lanterman clefts precedes the breakdown of the myelin sheath into ovoids (Webster, 1965), many of which show an acid phosphatase activity (Holtzman and Novikoff, 1965). It is of interest that when Wallerian degeneration is produced and observed *in vitro*, the onset of some alterations in axons and myelin sheaths can be delayed by reducing the calcium ion concentration in the medium (Schlaepfer and Bunge, 1973). Later, fragmentation of the myelin sheath is associated with hypertrophy and hyperplasia of Schwann cells (Bradley and Asbury, 1970). Myelin and axons are engulfed and sequestered by macrophages thought to originate mainly from Schwann cells (Berner, Torvik and Stenwig, 1973). The basal laminae of the Schwann cells persist as a longitudinal framework that assists in the orientation of proliferating Schwann cells and the subsequent growth of regenerating axons down the Schwann tubes (see Cajal, 1928; Thomas, 1964b). The new myelin segments formed by the remyelination process are shorter and thinner than their predecessors. Proximal to the transection site, a simultaneous series of changes occurs in the affected nerve fibers (Morris, Hudson, and Weddell, 1972a to d) and their cell bodies (axonal reaction). One of these changes is a proliferation of their satellite cells (Friede, 1967).

Alterations in number, size, and shape of Schwann cells are less striking if the myelin breakdown occurs in the presence of an intact axon (segmental demyelination). Fragmentation of paranodal myelin lamellae is followed by breakdown of the sheath within the parent Schwann cell cytoplasm. Myelin remnants are phagocytosed and sequestered by macrophages; the axon, which remains apparently normal, is displaced toward the Schwann cell surface. The initial stages of remyelination often resemble those of normal development. But, after 4 to 10 spiral layers are formed, there frequently is little additional growth of the compact sheath. The longitudinal strips of Schwann cell cytoplasm often persist between the spiral layers, and the regenerated segments remain thin and short (Webster, Spiro, Waksman, and Adams, 1961; Webster, 1964; Webster and O'Connell, 1970). If the segmental demyelination results from experimental allergic neuritis, the distribution of regenerating myelin is usually much more irregular (Allt, 1972).

OTHER FUNCTIONS

Other functions that have been ascribed to Schwann cells deserve brief mention. One of these is that Schwann cells, along with the endoneurial collagen, help provide structural support and elasticity for axons which are repeatedly stretched during limb movements. In addition, several lines of evidence suggest that Schwann cells are capable of forming collagen (Nathaniel and Pease, 1963; Harkin, 1964; Church, Tanzer, and Pfeiffer, 1973) even though recent observations continue to reaffirm their neural crest origin (Johnston and Hazelton, 1972).

Chapter VII

THE NEUROGLIAL CELLS

The neuroglia was discovered by Virchow in 1846, when he recognized a pervasive nonnervous interstitial substance in the walls of the ventricles and in the spinal cord. As this substance was "of a soft, medullary, fragile nature," contrasting with the fibrous connective tissue of nerves and other organs, he gave it the name neuroglia—"nerve glue" (see Virchow, 1860, pp. 272–280). Virchow also recognized that this interstitial material contained special stellate or spindle-shaped cells that were difficult to preserve and to distinguish from the smaller nerve cells. He observed that the neuroglia everywhere separates the nervous tissue from the blood vessels, and he was quick to perceive the great importance for physiology and pathology of the distinction between the nervous tissue proper and this interstitial substance. Virchow and his contemporaries conceived of the neuroglia as an interneuronal matrix in which characteristic cells were suspended, just as in the areolar connective tissue of other organs. In one form or another, this view prevailed until very recent times, in fact, until the advent of electron microscopic studies on tissue from the central nervous system fixed by perfusion. Only then could it be seen that the interneuronal matrix consists of the perikarya and processes of the neuroglial cells. Thus, the neuron doctrine was given a corollary proposition, that the nervous system is composed almost entirely of cells—neurons and neuroglial cells—with only a thin film of extracellular material between them.

Although the nuclei of neuroglial cells may be readily recognized in preparations of nervous tissue stained with basic dyes, knowledge of their shapes and dispositions came about only with the development of the metallic impregnation techniques. In the main, these techniques were developed by Cajal (1913 and 1916) and del Rio Hortega (1919 and 1921), and it is to them that we owe the basis for the vast light microscopic literature on neuroglia that was written in the first half of this century. In the present account it is not appropriate to give a detailed discussion of the light microscopic literature on neuroglial cells, and for further information, reference should be made to reviews such as those of Glees (1955), Windle (1958), and Penfield (1932).

In addition to the ependyma which lines the ventricular cavities and spinal canal (see Chapter VIII), light microscopists recognize two categories of supporting cells in the central nervous system, the macroglia and the microglia. The macroglia comprise the astrocytes and the oligodendrocytes. These cells, like neurons, have an ectodermal origin, but they differ from neurons in having only one type of process. They do not form synapses, and they retain the ability to divide throughout life, particularly under the influence of damage to the nervous system. In contrast, the microglia are considered by del Rio Hortega (1932) and others to have a mesodermal origin and to enter the brain in the neonatal period. Because of this different and later origin, which is itself questionable, some authors do not regard the microglia as true neuroglial cells. The microglia are the most controversial of the non-neural elements, and some of the reasons for the controversy will be discussed more fully in a later section. As their name suggests, the microglia are smaller than either the astrocytes or the oligodendrocytes. They are also capable of multiplying by mitosis under proper stimulation such as injury to the nervous system, and they are avid phagocytes. In such conditions they are recognized as "rod cells" and "gitter cells."

On the basis of light microscopic investigations, the supporting cells of the central nervous system may be classified as follows:

Macroglia
1. Astrocytes
   a. Protoplasmic
   b. Fibrous
2. Oligodendrocytes
   a. Interfascicular
   b. Perineuronal satellites
Microglia

As pointed out above, descriptions of the characteristics and dispositions of neuroglial cells at the light microscope level are based largely upon the examination of tissue stained by metallic impregnations. The techniques are very capricious, as anyone with experience of them is aware, yet it is from direct extrapolation of the results with these techniques that the identification of the different neuroglial cells in electron microscope preparations is based. In the initial phases of electron microscopy of the brain, the identification of the different neuroglial cell types was complicated by the very unsatisfactory preservation of the tissue. This situation led to a controversy about the identification of the different neuroglial cells in which extreme points of view were taken. However, as the techniques of preservation have improved over the past few years, general agreement about the identification of neuroglial cells has been reached. To pursue the early electron microscopic literature and to analyze the reasons for the controversy seem fruitless now. In the present account emphasis will be placed upon the recent literature.

THE DEVELOPMENT OF NEUROGLIA

Not a great deal is known about the formation of neuroglial cells in development and it is not even certain whether they are derived from the same neuroepithelial precursors as neurons, or whether neurons and the neuroglia have different stem cells. A review of the older literature concerning the theories of the early development of neurons and neuroglia has been provided by Langman (1968). Recent studies using tritiated thymidine as a label for dividing cells suggest that at least some of the astrocytes and oligodendrocytes are derived from the subventricular zone of the developing neural tube. To put this statement into perspective, the following abbreviated account of the development of the neural tube is presented. The account is largely based upon the reviews by Angevine (1970), Sidman (1970a), and Sidman and Rakic (1973), and for more complete details, their articles should be consulted.

In the following account the nomenclature proposed by the Boulder Committee (1970) will be used. The early neural tube is composed of a sheet of columnar epithelial cells which bridge the thickness of the tube from its eventual ventricular to pial surfaces. At this stage two zones are recognized in the thickness of the neural tube: a *ventricular zone* in which the nuclei and inner processes of the columnar cells are located, and a *marginal zone* across which the outer processes of the cells extend. The ventricular zone persists throughout development, and by progressive division of its cells, it becomes thicker and pseudostratified. The nuclei deep in the ventricular zone synthesize DNA for cell division and progressively move toward the ventricular surface, or neurocoele, where they divide. After cell division, the daughter cells then return to the deeper portion of the ventricular zone, and the generation cycle continues. In the earliest phases of development, the ventricular cells produce only more ventricular cells; consequently the sheet of cells expands, thickens and increases in cell density. As development continues, both ventricular cells and postmitotic neuroblasts are produced, but eventually the ventricular cells cease dividing and differentiate into ependymal cells and neuroglial cells (Fujita, 1963). The postmitotic neuroblasts migrate out as the neural tube thickens, and with their migration, another zone, the *intermediate zone*, appears between the ventricular and marginal zones. At least in the developing cerebral cortex, some cells, the spongioblasts or radial glia, which can be regarded as early neuroglial cells, continue to span the thickness of the cerebral vesicle (hemisphere) at this and later periods of development, and it seems that these cells act as guides along which the postmitotic neuroblasts migrate toward the outside of the hemisphere to form the cortical plate (Rakic, 1972; Peters and Feldman, 1973; Sidman and Rakic, 1973).

Eventually, another population of cells appears between the intermediate and ventricular zones, and these make up the *subventricular zone*. The cells in this zone differ from those in the intermediate zone in that they continue to divide, and unlike the cells whose nuclei are contained in the ventricular zone, their nuclei do not move back and forth as they pass through a generation cycle.

Neurons and most of the population of astrocytes and oligodendrocytes appear to be derived from cells in the subventricular zone (Smart and Leblond, 1961; Altman, 1966). But it is not clear whether the neurons and the neurog-

lial cells arise from a common precursor. As neuroglial cells are formed, and it is thought that they form somewhat later than the majority of neurons, they migrate outward and continue to divide. Thus it appears that though some neuroglia are present early in development, their generation cycles are longer than those of neurons and at least in the rat, the greatest proliferation of neuroglial cells occurs after birth. In the spinal cord of the rat, for example, the number of neuroglial cells increases sixfold during the first two postnatal weeks (Gilmore, 1971). It is of interest that in the deeper portions of the cerebral cortex, the subependymal cells may give rise to neuroglial cells even in young, mature rats (e.g., see Lewis, 1968a and b).

It is commonly considered that although the macroglia are formed from cells in the neural tube, the microglia have a mesodermal origin. This question will be discussed later.

ASTROCYTES

As a result of studies carried out with the gold-sublimate method of Cajal (1913), it may be stated that in light microscope preparations, astrocytes are recognized as star-shaped cells (see Frontispiece), whose processes extend into the surrounding neuropil. At least some of the processes from each cell form expansions that are applied to the surfaces of blood vessels, where they form the so-called "end-feet" or "sucker processes" (Figures 10–1 to 10–3). Other processes extend to the surface of the central nervous system to form similar expansions that constitute the glial limiting membrane (glia limitans) (Figure 13–4). As demonstrated by Weigert (1895), the astrocytes in white matter have numerous fibrils within their cytoplasm and so are referred to as fibrous astrocytes. The astrocytes in the gray matter, on the other hand, generally contain few fibrils and consequently have been called protoplasmic astrocytes. It should be mentioned that, although few fibrils occur in normal protoplasmic astrocytes, masses of them may be formed in pathological conditions.

These two criteria—the presence of fibrils within the cytoplasm and the formation of end-feet, both at the surfaces of blood vessels and at the periphery of the brain—are the main features that have been used to identify astrocytes

in electron microscope preparations. Cells possessing these features are very susceptible to edema and are among the first elements of the central nervous system to swell in poorly fixed preparations. Because such swelling was prevalent in the earlier electron microscope preparations of central nervous tissue, it led to the impression that astrocytes were cells with a "watery" cytoplasm, in which the organelles are clumped. This view is no longer tenable. In well-fixed tissue from normal material, the cytoplasm of these cells is not "watery," and as in other cell types, the organelles are evenly distributed throughout the cytoplasm, although they may sometimes be relatively sparse (see Mugnaini and Walberg, 1964; Wendell-Smith, Blunt, and Baldwin, 1966; Palay, 1966; Kruger and Maxwell, 1967; Vaughn and Peters, 1967, 1971; Mori and Leblond, 1969b; King and Schwyn, 1970; Palay and Chan-Palay, 1974).

FIBROUS ASTROCYTES

In electron microscope preparations fibrous astrocytes are characterized as cells whose appearance is light in comparison with the other cells present in white matter (Figures 7–1 and

7–7). The nuclei (Figure 7–1, *Nuc*) are often bean-shaped or irregular and the nuclear envelope may be thrown into deep folds. The karyoplasm generally has a fairly even density, although there may be some clumping immediately adjacent to the nuclear envelope, and occasionally a nucleolus is present.

The most prominent cytoplasmic component of the fibrous astrocyte is the numerous fibrils or filaments that occur throughout the perikaryon and extend as parallel arrays into the processes. The filaments are 8 to 9 nm in diameter and in transverse sections they appear to be hollow, for they have a dense wall 2 to 2.5 nm thick that surrounds a light center (Figures 4–7 and 7–3). Transverse sections of the filaments show that their wall contains a number of dense subunits, four in number according to Wuerker (1970), embedded in a somewhat lighter matrix. The filaments do not have absolutely smooth outlines, for thin wisps arise from their outer surfaces. These short appendages sometimes give the appearance of forming cross-bridges between adjacent filaments, but this point is difficult to establish. Hence as individual units the astrocytic filaments bear a close resemblance to neurofilaments. Their dimensions are somewhat smaller though, and unlike neurofilaments the astrocytic filaments commonly occur in closely packed bundles. The composition of the filaments is not known, but it is apparent that they are much thinner than the neuroglial fibrils observed in light microscope preparations. According to Vaughn and Pease (1967) and to Mori and Leblond (1969b), it is upon bundles of the 8- to 9-nm filaments that gold is deposited by the Cajal (1913) gold sublimate stain for the light microscope visualization of the astrocytes.

The usual organelles occur in the cytoplasm of fibrous astrocytes, but they are sparse in comparison with those of other types of cell. With the exception of the mitochondria, the organelles are mainly confined to the perikaryal region, where they are interspersed with the filaments (Figure 7–1).

The rough-surfaced endoplasmic reticulum is represented by a relatively small number of short cisternae unevenly, but prominently studded with ribosomes (Figure 7–1, *ER*). The cytoplasmic surface of the outer nuclear membrane also has an uneven studding of ribosomes, and only a few free ribosomes occur in the perikaryon, either as individual granules or rosettes and spirals. The Golgi apparatus (Figure 7–1, *G*) is located in the region of the cell where the cytoplasm is most abundant, but it is confined to a few stacks of cisternae. The cisternae of the Golgi apparatus usually appear to be empty, and like the rough-surfaced cisternae, they do not extend far beyond the bases of the processes that issue from the perikaryon.

The mitochondria of the fibrous astrocytes are generally elongated (Figure 7–1, *mit*), and their fine structure conforms to the common pattern for most cell types, including the presence of dense matrix granules. A great variety of shapes exists, however; some branch so that they have the form of a letter "Y." Within the perikaryon the mitochondria are randomly dispersed; in the processes they are usually oriented parallel to the long axes of the processes and, consequently, parallel to the filaments.

According to Mugnaini and Walberg (1964) the mitochondria have the same distribution as the gliosomes that have been described in light microscopic literature on astrocytes, a conclusion that was expressed earlier by Fieandt (1910) and Nageotte (1910). The gliosomes more likely correspond to the unusual forms that have been described for mitochondria in the electron microscope literature. Mugnaini (1964), for example, has reported that in the rat some mitochondria in astrocytes of the corpus striatum have widely dilated intercristal spaces filled with long, parallel fibrils. Each fibril consists of a 3-nm filament coiled into a regular helix, 14

Figure 7–1. **Fibrous Astrocytes.**

This transverse section contains two fibrous astrocytes and part of a much darker cell, an oligodendrocyte (*O*). The nuclei (*Nuc*) of astrocytes are homogeneous in density and irregular in shape. Their cytoplasmic organelles are relatively sparse, and only a few profiles of mitochondria (*mit*) and cisternae of the granular endoplasmic reticulum (*ER*) and of the Golgi apparatus (*G*) are present. Most prominent are the fibrils (*f*). These occupy a large proportion of the cytoplasm and extend into the processes (*AsP*) extending from the cell body. In the optic nerve the main astrocytic processes divide into smaller ones, which come together to form sheets (*AsP₁*) that group the nerve fibers into bundles.
Optic nerve of adult rat. × *17,000.*

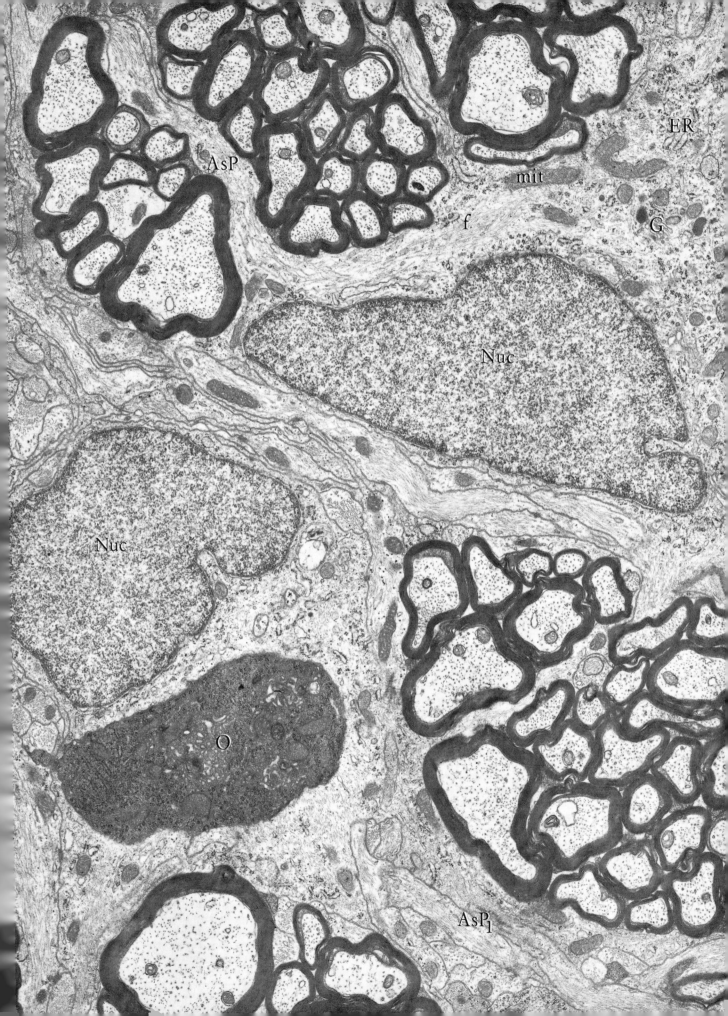

nm wide. In astrocytes from the brains of amphibia Szebro (1965) has described large mitochondria which have an electron-opaque or granular matrix surrounded by a periphery of canaliculi, which may be small cristae. These structures he terms type 1 gliosomes. A second type, type 2, contains parallel and regularly arranged, longitudinally oriented lamellae. Since no transverse sections of this type of mitochondria are illustrated by Szebro, it is not clear that the longitudinally oriented structures are lamellae. Gliosomes with either a granular or a lamellar matrix have also been described by Donelli, D'Uva, and Paoletti (1975) in the hypothalamic region of the lizard. These authors analyzed the diffraction patterns obtained from these different types of gliosomes and conclude that their matrix is in a more or less advanced state of crystallization. Morales and Duncan (1971) illustrated mitochondria from astrocytes of cats and hamsters that had a similar appearance in longitudinal section, but in transverse section the parallel structures appeared to be long, prism-shaped cristae, embedded in a matrix of filaments oriented parallel to the cristae. These appear similar to the mitochondria that Gray (1960) described earlier in the astrocytes of lizards. Hashimoto (1969) encountered mitochondria in the spinal cord of the cat which were similar to the two types described by Szebro (1965). Hashimoto followed their development and found that at birth such mitochondria have a finely granular matrix and dispersed cristae. Subsequently these mitochondria enlarge, and simultaneously the filamentous content increases and becomes organized. While these changes are occurring, cisternae of granular endoplasmic reticulum appear to be closely associated with the mitochondria.

Homogeneous dense bodies are present in the cytoplasm of fibrous astrocytes, and as Mugnaini and Walberg (1964) have noted, heterogeneous dense bodies also occur. Both of these inclusions probably correspond to the various types of lysosomes. Small dense granules limited by a membrane have been described by Holtzman and his colleagues (1973).

Smaller dense granules with diameters of 20 to 40 nm lie free in the cytoplasm and appear to represent glycogen (Figure 7–6, *gly*). In material fixed by perfusion, these granules are most common in the end-feet of both protoplasmic and fibrous astrocytes at the surfaces of capillaries. It is known that glycogen is difficult to fix for electron microscopy, and since perfusion allows the fixative to reach the end-feet first, it may be suspected that under optimal conditions glycogen would be observed throughout the cytoplasm of fibrous astrocytes. Some indication of the validity of this expectation comes from the study of Phelps (1972) who found prolonged anesthesia with barbiturates to produce large increases in the amount of glycogen in astrocytes. He concluded that the greatest accumulation of astrocytic glycogen occurs in areas of high synaptic density and near neuronal perikarya. Phelps (1972) also reviewed the literature showing that such diverse conditions as trauma, x-irradiation, hibernation and hypothermia, synaptic degeneration, and administration of a number of depressant drugs can lead to glycogen accumulation in astrocytes.

Only a few microtubules are interspersed with the fibrils in the cytoplasm of mature astrocytes. But in the immature fibrous astrocytes of the optic nerve in the early postnatal rat, microtubules are very numerous (Peters and Vaughn, 1967; Vaughn and Peters, 1967). As maturation proceeds, the microtubules decrease in number, and their place is taken by the typical astrocytic fibrils, which are almost entirely absent at birth.

Centrioles occur in the perikarya of fibrous astrocytes, and it is quite common to find the profile of a cilium embedded in the cytoplasm. These cilia, apparently only one to a cell, seem to be similar to those emerging both from neurons and from cells in the choroid plexus:

Figure 7–2. **Protoplasmic Astrocyte.**

At the bottom of the field is the nucleus (*Nuc*) of a protoplasmic astrocyte. This shows condensations of karyoplasm beneath the nuclear envelope. Arising from the top of the cell body is a thick process that contains a bundle of filaments (*f*). Other organelles present in the cytoplasm include mitochondria (*mit*), microtubules (*m*), free ribosomes (*r*), rather short cisternae of the granular endoplasmic reticulum (*ER*), and two lysosomes (*Ly*).

The outline of this astrocyte is very irregular and is partially picked out with *triangles*, which show that its contours follow those of the dendrites and axons in the surrounding neuropil. Sheet-like processes (*asterisks*) from neuroglial cells such as this one pervade the neuropil and are recognized by their irregular contours. *Cerebral cortex of adult rat. × 20,000.*

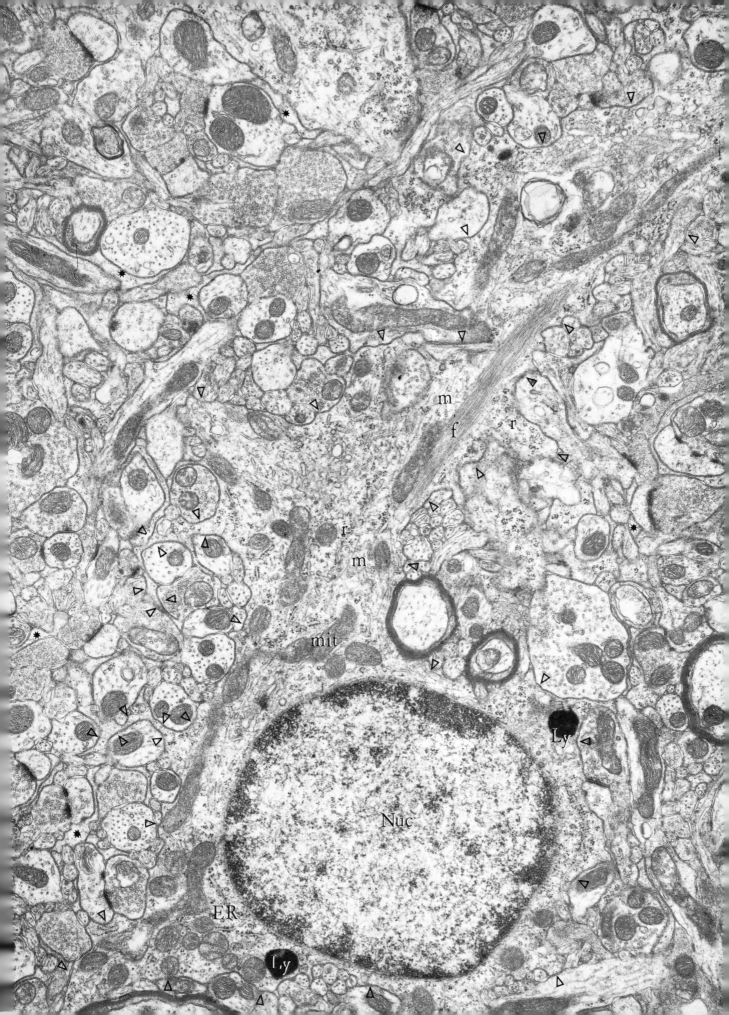

that is, the central pair of microtubules is lacking, so that only the nine peripheral pairs exist.

Each broad process arising from the perikaryon of a fibrous astrocyte branches to form a number of smaller processes (Figures 7–1 and 7–6, *AsP),* whose cytoplasm contains little beyond numerous fibrils, mitochondria, and glycogen granules and a few vesicles. In the optic nerve, in which the fibrous astrocytes have been most thoroughly studied, the main processes emerge from the cell body in a predominantly radial pattern. These, and the smaller processes into which they divide, assemble with similar processes of other cells to form laminae that group the nerve fibers into bundles (Figure 7–1). A few processes also invade the bundles of nerve fibers.

In contrast to the protoplasmic astrocytes, which will be described subsequently, the individual processes of fibrous astrocytes in white matter do not themselves have the form of sheets. Instead, they are elongated, cylindrical processes and in the transverse plane have rounded, square, or oval profiles (Figure 7–1). Furthermore, they do not have the highly irregular contours of protoplasmic astrocyte processes and show little tendency to conform to the shapes of the surrounding neuronal elements with which they intertwine

As pointed out earlier, the processes of fibrous astrocytes form expansions, or end-feet, at the surfaces of the capillaries passing through white matter (Figure 7–6). As far as can be determined, these end-feet form a complete layer that is interposed between the nerve fibers and the endothelial cells. The width of this astrocytic layer varies. Sometimes it is several processes thick, but frequently it is formed either by a single thin process or by the cell body of an astrocyte. Separating the plasma membrane of the neuroglial element from that of the endothelial cell nearby is a gap of 40 to 100 nm (Figure 7–6) which is occupied by a basal lamina. In regions of greatest separation the basal lamina splits into two layers, one applied to the outside of the endothelial cell and the other to the neuroglial element. In the space between the two layers, collagen fibers and pericytes can occur. A parallel situation exists at the surface of the central nervous system, where the limiting membrane may be up to 15 microns thick in the cat (Haug, 1971). Here again, either the end-feet or cell bodies of astrocytes form a complete layer, the glia limitans, in this instance separating the nervous components from the pial elements. As at blood vessels, the outer surfaces of the astrocytic components are covered by a basal lamina. In the rat, at least, it is common to find patches of cytoplasmic density associated with the plasma membrane adjacent to the basal lamina. These patches, which resemble hemidesmosomes (Figure 7–6, *arrows,* and Figure 13–4), are also present in Rhesus monkeys, in which Bondareff and McLone (1973) observed a filamentous layer, 50 to 70 nm thick and composed of microfilaments, beneath the plasma membranes of the most superficial astrocytic processes in the glia limitans. The presence of these microfilaments, which have been implicated in contractile processes in other cellular systems (see page 114), suggests to Bondareff and McLone (1973) that the glia limitans may have the capacity of motility, since they must continually adjust themselves to changes in the pressures exerted by the fluid-filled spaces surrounding them.

In the rat the outer surfaces of the astrocyte processes comprising the glia limitans seem to

---

Figure 7–3. **Protoplasmic Astrocytes.**

The **upper picture** shows a protoplasmic astrocyte lying next to a neuron (*N*). Except for condensations beneath the nuclear envelope, the nucleus (*Nuc*) of the astrocyte exhibits a homogeneous karyoplasm. The cytoplasm is confined to a relatively thin rim and contains bundles of filaments (*f*). Other organelles in the rather lucent cytoplasm are microtubules (*m*), mitochondria (*mit*), cisternae of the granular endoplasmic reticulum (*ER*), free ribosomes (*r*), and a portion of the Golgi apparatus (*G*).
Lateral geniculate nucleus of cat. × 25,000.

The **lower picture** shows parts of two adjacent processes (*AsP* and *AsP₁*), one of which contains two bundles of filaments (*f*). For most of their extent the plasma membranes (*arrows*) of these two processes are separated by a wide interval, but to the right they come closer together to form a gap junction (*g*). At the gap junction the outer leaflets of the apposed membranes are about 3 nm apart. In this instance the gap seems to be bridged by striations.
Rat cerebral cortex. × 150,000.

Micrograph by D. W. Vaughan.

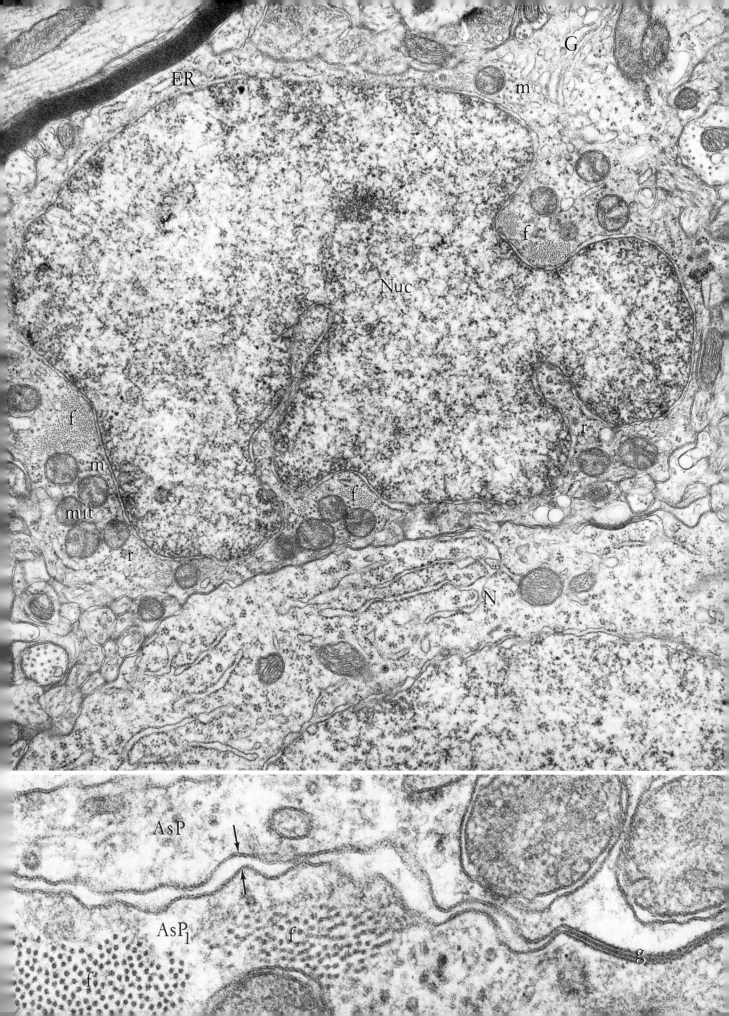

follow the contours of the pial cells (Figure 13–4). According to Ramsey (1965), this situation does not exist at the surface of the human cerebral cortex. Instead, the glia limitans and the pial cells do not appear congruent but are frequently separated by spaces containing both collagen fibers and cell processes.

In most instances the plasma membranes of adjacent astrocytic cell bodies and processes are separated by a distance of 15 to 20 nm. The space can be larger, but sometimes it seems to be completely obliterated in specimens prepared by conventional means, so that the outer leaflets of adjacent membranes appear apposed. The studies of Brightman and Reese (1969) have shown, however, that these are not zonulae occludentes as thought previously (Peters, 1962b) but *gap junctions* in which there is an interval of 2 to 3 nm between the outer leaflets of the apposed plasma membranes (Figures 7–3 and 7–6, *g*). This gap in the junction is open to penetration by horseradish peroxidase and lanthanum (Brightman and Reese, 1969; Brightman, 1967). When lanthanum-penetrated gap junctions are viewed *en face* the gap is seen to be occupied by an array of polygonal subunits, with a center-to-center spacing of about 10 nm, each faintly outlined by a thin rim of lanthanum, the rim being about 2 nm wide.

In a study of freeze-fractured astrocytic membranes Landis and Reese (1974a) showed that 7- to 12-nm globular particles are present on both the A and B faces, although they are most frequent on the A face. In addition, there are distinctive arrays, or assemblies, of smaller particles on the A face. These assemblies are rectangular in outline, and each contains 4 to 60 particles packed in an orthogonal array with a periodicity of about 6 to 7 nm. This is also the approximate diameter of each particle. Not all the astrocytic membranes possess such assemblies. For example, the astrocytic processes investing the axon layer immediately adjacent to the glomerular layer of the olfactory bulb are devoid of them, as are the Bergmann astrocyte cell bodies in the cerebellum. The highest concentration of particle assemblies were found in the plasma membranes of perivascular and subpial astrocytic processes facing away from the neurous tissue. The significance of these assemblies is not understood.

The pictures of Landis and Reese (1974a) suggest that the gap junctions between astrocytic plasma membranes are similar to those present elsewhere, in that at such sites the A faces of the involved plasma membranes show aggregates of 7- to 12-nm particles. This was reported in the study by Tani, Nishiura, and Higashi (1973), who also showed that while gap junctions are present between astrocytes involved in the formation of astrocytomas of the human brain, they are markedly decreased in number in glioblastoma multiforme. In these latter the particles associated with the gap junctions are also packed more loosely. On the basis of their observations Tani, Nishiura, and Higashi (1973) conclude that the decrease in gap junctions in human glioblastoma multiforme results in a decrease in coupling between the cells and that this is correlated with the malignancy of the tumor. Similar reductions in the number of gap junctions have been recorded in tumors in other locations, although there appears to be no simple correlation between the number of gap junctions and the proliferative activity of the cells involved.

Also occurring between the plasma membranes of adjacent astrocytes are punctate adhesions that have some features in common with *zonulae adhaerentes* (Farquhar and Palade, 1963), and are therefore called *puncta adhaerentia* (see page 6). At such *puncta* the distance

---

Figure 7–4. **Golgi Epithelial Cells and the Purkinje Cell.**

Four Golgi epithelial cells (protoplasmic astrocytes) lie in an arc around the perikaryon of a Purkinje cell (*N*) at the left. The nucleus (*Nuc*) of this astrocyte appears homogeneous, and the thin rim of cytoplasm surrounding it contains only a few organelles. Fibrils are rarely present. Like astrocytes in other regions of gray matter, these cells have very irregular contours, which fit into those of the surrounding cellular processes. The outline of one cell is indicated by *triangles*. Thin, sheet-like processes extend into the surrounding neuropil, and some of them form a sheath (*arrows*) around the Purkinje cell. This sheath is penetrated only by axon terminals (*At*) that synapse upon the neuron.
Cerebellar cortex from adult rat. × 15,000.

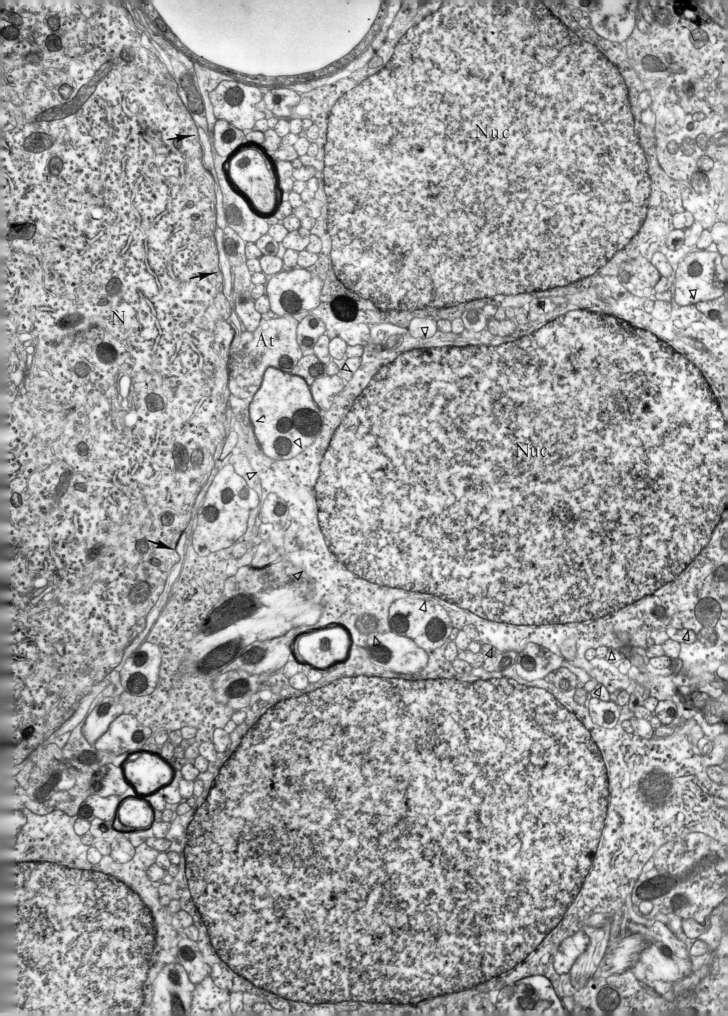

between adjacent membranes increases to about 25 to 30 nm, and the two plasma membranes come to lie exactly parallel to each other. No central line is apparent in the interval between the adjacent membranes, but these adhesions are characterized by some increase in electron density both within the gap and in the cytoplasm immediately on each side of the adhesions.

PROTOPLASMIC ASTROCYTES

The protoplasmic astrocytes occur in gray matter, and as with fibrous astrocytes, their most characteristic feature is the presence of cytoplasmic fibrils (Figures 7–2 and 7–3). There are fewer fibrils, however, than in fibrous astrocytes. They do not fill the cytoplasm but tend to occur in bundles (Figures 4–7, 7–2, and 7–3). Further, the number of fibrils in protoplasmic astrocytes varies widely in different parts of the brain, even in the same animal. In the Golgi epithelial (Fañanas) cells of the cerebellum, for example (Herndon, 1964; Palay, 1966; Palay and Chan-Palay, 1974), it is not uncommon to obtain sections of cells in which fibrils are entirely absent (Figures 7–4 and 7–5). At the other extreme are astrocytes like those in the inferior olive of the cat, which have so many fibrils in their cytoplasm that Scheibel and Scheibel (1955) and Walberg (1963) consider them to be fibrous astrocytes even though they occur in gray matter.

The main features of protoplasmic astrocytes are shown in Figures 7–2 to 7–5. As in the fibrous astrocytes of white matter, the endoplasmic reticulum of protoplasmic astrocytes is not very extensive. It consists of relatively few small cisternae, and since there are not many free ribosomes, the cytoplasm is light in appearance. Again, granules of glycogen are common, and

the cytoplasm also contains a number of large and elongated mitochondria in addition to microtubules, the occasional centriole, and sometimes a cilium.

All these cytoplasmic components occur in the larger processes of protoplasmic astrocytes, but in the smaller processes mitochondria, endoplasmic reticulum, and microtubules are usually absent. Consequently, the only structures commonly found in the small processes are ribosomes, glycogen granules, and bundles of fibrils.

Unlike fibrous astrocytes, the cell bodies and processes of protoplasmic astrocytes are usually irregular in outline. Their shape appears to be imposed upon them by the surrounding elements of the neuropil, whose outlines they conform to and between which they send processes. Indeed, one of the means of distinguishing profiles of protoplasmic astrocytes from those of axons and dendrites is that the former rarely have rounded profiles. Very often the smaller processes have the form of sheets and they can be so thin that the plasma membranes bounding each side of the sheet are separated by only a few tens of nanometers. Frequently these sheets surround synapses, and sometimes they overlap each other to form laminae, such as those around the synaptic glomeruli of the thalamus (Figure 5–18). The form of some astrocytic processes is well shown in the articles by Stensaas and Stensaas (1968) and by Špaček (1971), who have reconstructed their form from serial thin sections.

Like fibrous astrocytes, the protoplasmic astrocytes form end-feet at the surfaces of capillaries (Figures 7–5 and 10–1 to 10–3) and partake in the formation of the glia limitans at the surface of the brain (Figures 10–4 and 13–4). Their processes may also have "gap" junctions between (Fig 7–3, g) them as well as the

---

Figure 7–5.   **Golgi Epithelial Cell and a Capillary.**

On the right of the field is part of the perikaryon of a Purkinje cell (*N*). This cell is surrounded by a sheath composed of laminar processes (*AsP*) of protoplasmic astrocytes. The sheath is penetrated only by axons whose terminals (*At*) synapse with the neuron.

A portion of a protoplasmic astrocyte extends diagonally across the picture toward the wall of a capillary on the left. Except for an almost complete absence of fibrils, these neuroglial cells are similar to the protoplasmic astrocytes elsewhere within the central nervous system. They have a relatively homogeneous nucleus (*Nuc*), only a sparse population of cytoplasmic organelles, and an irregular shape (*arrowheads*). Like the processes of other astrocytes, some of the processes (*AsP₁*) of these cells surround blood vessels. Such processes remain separated from the endothelial cells (*End*) by a basal lamina (*B*).
Cerebellar cortex from adult rat. × 23,000.

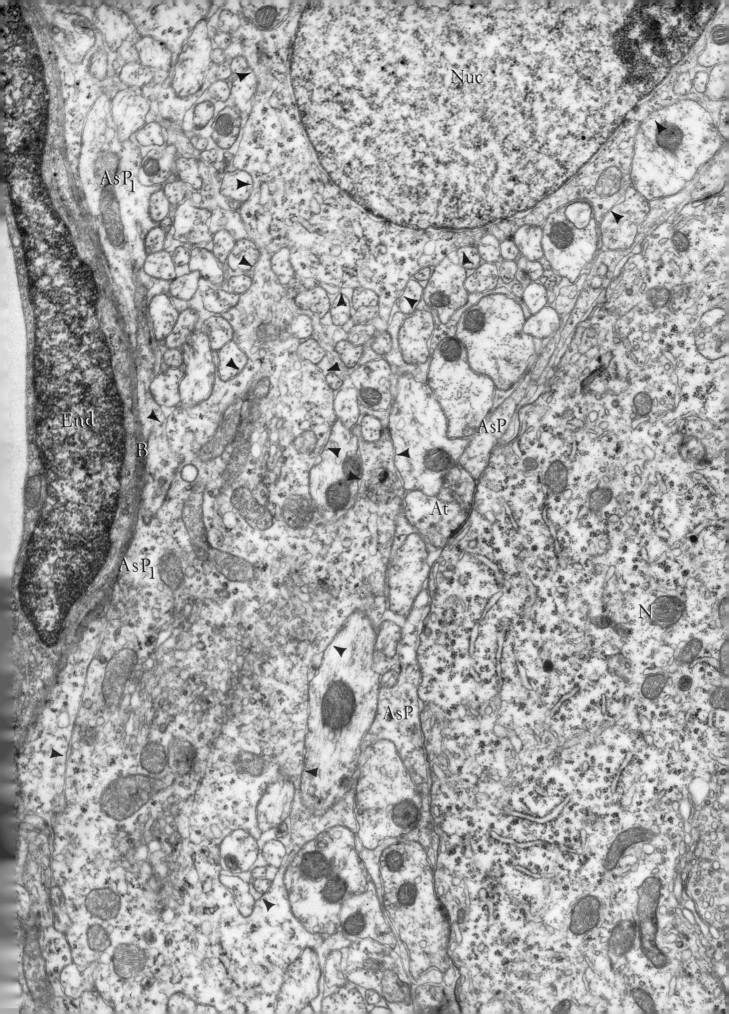

punctate adhesions described previously. The nuclei of protoplasmic astrocytes are also homogeneous in appearance (Figures 7–2 to 7–5). They tend to be round or oval but are less frequently indented than those of fibrous astrocytes.

In their detailed study of the cerebellum Palay and Chan-Palay (1974) showed that some of the astrocytes have extremely thin, veil-like extensions from the larger processes. Because of this very distinctive feature, Palay and Chan-Palay (1974) called such cells *velate astrocytes* to distinguish them from protoplasmic astrocytes which lacked such appendages. In the cerebellar cortex a velate form is assumed by two types of supporting cells, the Golgi epithelial cells (Figures 7–4 and 7–5) and the astrocytes commonly present in the granular layer. The veil-like form of the processes of these two cell types is well displayed in Golgi-impregnated preparations of these cells examined in the high voltage electron microscope (Chan-Palay and Palay, 1972b; Palay and Chan-Palay, 1974). The thin processes are also encountered in electron micrographs of thin sections (Figures 7–4 and 7–5) when they are seen to pass through the neuropil as sheets and to encapsulate both individual neurons and synaptic nests. Although similar detailed studies of other parts of the central nervous system have not been carried out, it can be assumed that astrocytes with a similar velate form are common in the neuropil, for sheet-like extensions of protoplasmic astrocytes are frequently encountered (see Figure 7–2). As will be discussed later these extensions seem to serve to compartmentalize groups of elements in the neuropil.

FUNCTIONS OF ASTROCYTES

Since the discovery of neuroglial cells in the middle of the last century many functions have been attributed to astrocytes. Despite the many recent studies, however, there is still a great deal of uncertainty about their function. Most of the recent theories are elaborations of older hypotheses and can be brought together under a number of headings, as listed below. Before these various functions are considered though, it should be mentioned that even in apparently normal tissues, astrocytes are not completely static cells. Despite their apparently well-differentiated appearance they are able to divide. This property has been shown by Mori and Leblond (1969b), who, using tritiated thymidine, were able to show dividing astrocytes with fully developed cytoplasmic characteristics in the corpus callosum of young rats.

Structural Support

The concept that astrocytes, and indeed neuroglial cells in general, play a role as structural supporting elements within the central nervous system was put forward by Weigert in 1895. He emphasized that in the central nervous system neuroglial cells fill the space that is not occupied by neurons and their processes.

Although direct evidence for this concept is still lacking, some features of fibrous astrocytes may be mentioned in its favor. First, astrocytes and their processes provide sheaths on all outer surfaces of the central nervous system. Second, at many sites adjacent processes of astrocytes are

---

Figure 7–6. **The Perivascular Glia Limitans.**

The lower portion of this transverse section is occupied by part of a large capillary that is situated at the periphery of the nerve. The endothelial cells (*End*) are bounded by a basal lamina (*B*). Streaming toward the capillary are processes (*AsP*) of fibrous astrocytes whose cytoplasm contains fibrils and dense glycogen granules (*gly*). These processes terminate in end-feet (*AsP₁*), which form a complete layer around the capillary. They are bounded by their own basal lamina (*B₁*), which is separated from that of the endothelial cells by a space containing collagen fibers (*Col*). Note that where the plasma membrane of an end-foot is covered by the basal lamina, localized cytoplasmic densities occur (*arrows*). These densities resemble hemidesmosomes and probably serve as attachment sites between the end-feet and the basal lamina (*B₁*). In some places where adjacent astrocytic processes come together, gap junctions (*J*) may be found between their plasma membranes but in other places (*g*) the interspace is widened and is filled with a dark material. The dark cell lying in the middle of the field is an interfascicular oligodendrocyte (*O*).
Optic nerve from adult rat. × 40,000.

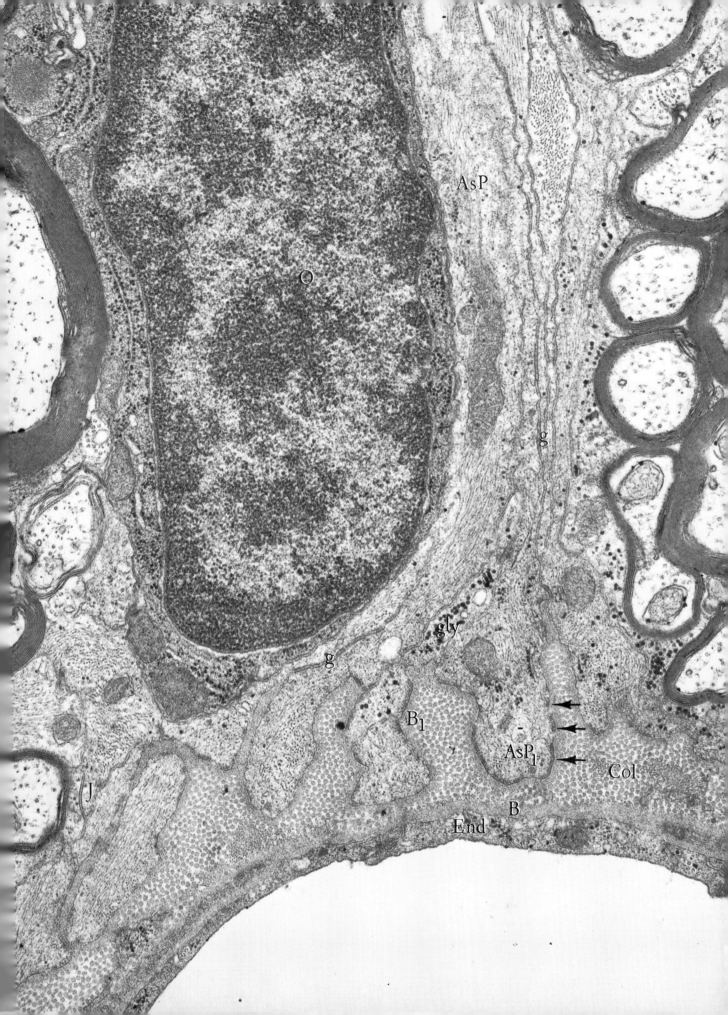

held together by junctions between their plasma membranes. Although typical desmosomes seem to be absent between the astrocytes in mammalian central nervous tissue, they do occur between astrocytes in amphibians and between the neuroglial cells that resemble astrocytes in invertebrates. Finally, in white matter—for example, in the optic nerve of the adult rat (Figure 7–1)—the astrocytes contain fibrils arranged in bundles. These fibrillar bundles are arrayed parallel to the lengths of the many processes that arise from the astrocytic perikarya and come together to form groups, which interweave with the nerve fibers. Since the groups of astrocytic processes generally pass at right angles to the direction of the nerve fibers, an analogy might be drawn with the warp and weft of a fabric.

Repair

When lesions are made in the central nervous system, neuroglial cells, especially the astrocytes, repair the defect by proliferating and filling the spaces that were occupied by neurons and their processes. The sequence of events in the repair of brain damage has been studied by many light microscopists, and the literature on this subject is voluminous. For the present purposes, however, we shall confine ourselves to a few examples from the electron microscope literature. Schultz and Pease (1959) showed that when stab wounds are inflicted on the cerebral cortex, astrocytes proliferate and form a core in the center of the lesion. They also wall off the damaged area of the brain from the overlying leptomeningeal cells. Maxwell and Kruger (1965a) demonstrated that after the cerebral cortex is damaged by alpha particle radiation, the astrocytes undergo a sequence of reactive changes. Initially there is a marked increase in the amount of glycogen in the cells. Later the astrocytes hypertrophy and come to contain large numbers of filaments. Maxwell and Kruger also show that there is an increase in the number of fatty inclusions in the cytoplasm of the reactive cells. As they point out, although such inclusions are sometimes thought to be indicative of phagocytosis, there is no direct evidence in their material that astrocytes ingest extracellular debris. In a study of the responses of astrocytes to Wallerian degeneration of the optic nerves of rats, Vaughn, Hinds, and Skoff (1970) showed that the scar formation by astrocytes is not achieved by a significant increase in the number of astrocytes but rather through an increase in

their size. These reactive astrocytes have larger nuclei than normal and have many dense bodies in their cytoplasm. At the same time the Golgi apparatus becomes more elaborate. These same features are also displayed by developing astrocytes and so may be a response to the production of the large numbers of filaments that are produced by the cells during scar formation. Vaughn and Pease (1970) also found the astrocytes to contain myelin fragments and lipid droplets, and they suggest that although the astrocytes are not the primary phagocytes in degenerating optic nerves, they may remove debris from sites of scar formation where some nerve fibers have become entrapped and are inaccessible to other phagocytes. In a discussion of the role of astrocytes as phagocytic cells, it must not be forgotten that in most cases in which axon terminals have been made to degenerate by experimental lesions, the degenerating terminals are usually sequestered by astrocytic processes (see Chapter XI).

In a study of Tay-Sachs disease Terry and Weiss (1963) also identified reactive macroglial cells, whose content of fibrils suggests that they are astrocytes. These cells contain numerous dense bodies composed of granules, vesicles, membranes, and homogeneous material, which the authors consider to be derived from the enzymatically degraded neuronal lipid. There is also a fibrous astrocytosis in Tay-Sachs disease.

Crushing the facial nerves of rats at birth leads to changes in the facial nerve nucleus. Torvik and Söreide (1972) found that the proliferating astrocytes of the neuropil have what they term a "sheet-reaction." This is characterized by the penetration of sheet-like processes of astrocytes between other processes of the neuropil (see also Barron, Chiang, Daniels, and Doolin, 1971; Torvik, 1972). This reaction appears to be an exaggeration of the normal tendency on the part of astrocytes to isolate neuronal surfaces.

Blood-Brain Barrier

The concept that a physiological barrier exists between the blood and the brain is useful, for there is ample evidence to suggest that certain substances circulating in the blood reach equilibrium with the brain tissues at a very slow rate. The literature on this subject is very extensive, and for detailed information reference should be made to the reviews of Friedemann (1942), Bakay (1956), Brierley (1957), Dobbing

(1961), Kuffler and Nicholls (1966), Reese and Karnovsky (1967), Brightman and Reese (1969), Brightman, Klatzo, Olsson, and Reese (1970), and Westergaard and Brightman (1973).

If substances are retarded in their passage from the blood to the neural elements, then the site of the so-called barrier could be (1) the endothelial cells in the wall of the blood vessel, (2) the basal lamina between the endothelial cells and the astrocytic end-feet, or (3) the astrocytic end-feet themselves (Figures 7–4 to 7–6 and 10–1 to 10–4). Any or all of these structures could be involved.

Early electron microscope studies to ascertain the site of the blood-brain barrier were carried out by Dempsey and Wislocki (1955) and by van Breemen and Clemente (1955). They put silver nitrate in the drinking water of rats and mice and found that very little silver appeared around the capillaries in the cerebral cortex, medulla, and cerebellum. There was, however, an accumulation of silver around the capillaries in the area postrema, the neurohypophysis, pineal body, and intercolumnar tubercle, parts of the brain where the barrier is apparently absent. Unlike the capillaries in regions where the barrier is present, those in the area postrema are fenestrated and are surrounded by an extensive extracellular space (e.g., Leonhardt, 1967a). These results suggest that the endothelial cells of the vessels present a barrier in most parts of the brain, but in regions like the area postrema silver passes through the endothelium and is deposited in the enlarged perivascular spaces.

Concerning the barrier provided by the astrocytic end-feet, there are two questions to be asked. How complete is the layer formed by adjacent end-feet, and how consistently do occluding junctions occur between adjacent end-feet? Most studies indicate that while the end-feet form a relatively complete layer, the junctions between these end-feet are not continuous or of the occluding type.

The most recent evidence on the site of the blood-brain barrier comes from the studies using electron-dense markers such as lanthanum and horseradish peroxidase (see Brightman, 1965a and b, 1967a and b, 1968; Reese and Karnovsky, 1967; Brightman and Reese, 1969). These studies have shown that when such tracers are injected intravenously they do not penetrate between the vascular endothelial cells. This passage is prevented by the presence of tight junctions, or zonulae occludentes, that are formed between the plasma membranes of adjacent endothelial cells near to the luminal surface (Figure 10–2).

These junctions appear rather punctate in sections, but because of their occluding properties they must be extensive in their longitudinal dimension and form belts around the cells. At such junctions, the outer leaflets of the contributing pair of plasma membranes are apparently fused together. After an intravenous perfusion some endothelial cells do have a few micropinocytotic vesicles containing marker (Reese and Karnovsky, 1967), but these vesicles do not appear to discharge their contents into the basal lamina or into the space outside the capillaries. When the tracers are introduced into the ventricles of the brain, on the other hand, they pass between the ependymal cells and move readily into the extracellular spaces of the neuropil, including junctions between the perivascular end-feet of astrocytes, as far as the perivascular basal lamina.

Consequently, in answer to the two foregoing questions, it is apparent that the junctions between astrocytes are not zonulae occludentes but gap junctions (Figure 7–3), and even if the end-feet of astrocytes do form a complete layer, substances can pass between them. Hence the perivascular end-feet of astrocytes do not appear to provide an effective barrier even if substances should pass through the endothelial cells into the brain neuropil. Indeed, based upon the evidence of experiments using electron-dense markers, the blood-brain barrier function rests at the level of the endothelial cells and is the result of the existence of an extracellular obstruction, the zonulae occludentes, and the absence of active vesicular transfer of substances from the luminal to the abluminal face of the endothelium.

Related to the earlier hypothesis that astrocytic end-feet play a role in the blood-brain barrier is the concept that astrocytes function somehow in the transfer of substances from the blood to the neurons (see De Robertis and Gerschenfeld, 1961). This concept was put forward on the basis of early electron microscopic observations, when astrocytes appeared to be cells with a watery cytoplasm that extended from the surface of blood vessels into the neuropil. In view of the recent evidence presented above and that cited by Kuffler and Nicholls(1966) to show that large molecules can pass readily through the intercellular spaces of the central nervous system, it is improbable that astrocytes play an important role in the transport of substances in the central nervous system. Calculations indicate that within an intercellular space 15 to 20 nm deep, the rate of diffusion for large molecules, such as sucrose, is only slightly less than in free solution.

Isolation of Receptive Surfaces

Some 60 years ago Cajal favored the concept that neuroglial cells play an isolating role within the central nervous system. He proposed that neuroglial cells are always distributed in such a way as to prevent the flow of impulses from neurons in a hapazard manner.

In a study with the electron microscope Palay and Peters (see Peters and Palay, 1965; Palay, 1966) studied the disposition of the processes of protoplasmic astrocytes in different parts of the central nervous system and concluded that they are arranged in discernible patterns. Although the patterns vary, the observations indicate that in each part of the central nervous system the processes are disposed in such a way as to segregate, or isolate, the receptive surfaces of neurons (i.e., the perikaryon and dendrites) from nonspecific afferent influences. Thus, it seems that when the afferent terminals on the surfaces of a group of neurons are not all derived from the same source, then the different terminals are ensheathed by astrocyte processes to prevent them from affecting neighboring neurons. For example, in the spinal cord the axon terminals synapsing on the surfaces of anterior horn cells are segregated, either individually or in small groups, so that in effect they lie in compartments (Figures 5–4, 5–9, and 11–3). In other parts of the central nervous system, neurons such as Purkinje cells (Figures 3–2, 7–4, and 7–5) and those in the substantia gelatinosa are individually and completely covered by astrocytic sheaths that are penetrated only by the axon terminals specifically synapsing with

them. Other examples may be seen in the thalamus, where the synaptic glomeruli are surrounded by astrocytic sheets that form capsules several layers thick (Figure 5–18), and in the cerebellum, in which the glomeruli are also enclosed by astrocytic processes (Figure 5–17). Conversely, only a few astrocytic processes may be present in those parts of the brain where individual synapses are widely separated by other neuronal but not synaptic elements. This situation obtains in the intervals between rows of Purkinje cells in the molecular layer of the cerebellum.

On the basis of observations such as these, Palay and Peters suggest that by preventing axon terminals from influencing neighboring and unrelated receptive neuronal surfaces, the astrocytes ensure that the terminals act in a discrete and localized manner.

As pointed out earlier, it now seems likely that this segregation of components of the neuropil is achieved by the processes of velate astrocytes (Chan-Palay and Palay, 1972; Palay and Chan-Palay, 1974) which have very extensive, sheet-like processes.

Pollen and his coworkers (see Pollen, 1973) have concluded that alterations in the normal neuroglial-neuron relationship may result in focal epilepsy. Thus, they found that focal spiking appeared in the border zones of most neuroglial scars made in cat brains by the freezing technique of lesioning, and at the borders of chronic epileptic foci, Wilder, Schimpff, and Collins (1972) observed that the relations between apparently normal neurons and their neighboring neuroglial cells were markedly altered. Pollen considers that the epileptic foci may result from the astroglia of a scar failing to play a normal role in the sequestering and distribution of potassium ions.

OLIGODENDROCYTES

GENERAL MORPHOLOGY

The term oligodendroglia was introduced by del Rio Hortega in 1921 to describe those neuroglial cells that show few processes in material stained by the metallic impregnation techniques (see Frontispiece). The processes radiate from a spherical or polygonal cell body and are rather more delicate than those of astrocytes. In

preparations stained with basic dyes the nuclei of oligodendrocytes are smaller, more regular, and more chromophilic than the astrocytic nuclei.

Oligodendrocytes most commonly occur in the following sites:

1. In white matter, where they may be aligned in rows between the nerve fibers. These are the interfascicular oligodendrocytes.

2. In gray matter, where they are also associated with groups of myelinated nerve fibers.

3. In gray matter, where they are frequently satellite cells in close association with neurons. It should be mentioned that astrocytes and microglial cells can also assume a similar position, but their occurrence has been less commonly recognized.

In recent electron microscope studies (Bunge, Bunge, and Ris, 1960; Mugnaini and Walberg, 1964; Schultz, 1964; Wendell-Smith, Blunt, and Baldwin, 1966; Kruger and Maxwell, 1966) oligodendrocytes are pictured as moderately dense cells that contrast with the rather lucent astrocytes (Figures 7–1 and 7–6 to 7–8). The nucleus can be round, oval, or irregular, and the nuclear chromatin tends to clump. Clumping seems to be more frequent in interfascicular oligodendrocytes (Figures 7–6 and 7–7) than in those of gray matter, where the karyoplasm has a generally homogeneous appearance (Figure 7–8). In interfascicular oligodendrocytes a rim of clumped material usually lies immediately beneath the nuclear envelope. The perinuclear cisterna tends to swell in most preparations, so that it appears larger than it does in astrocytes.

Since the nucleus usually lies in an eccentric position, a large mass of cytoplasm can occur at one pole of the cell, but in most planes of section the nucleus appears to be surrounded by only a thin rim of cytoplasm (compare Figures 7–6 to 7–8). In the perikaryon the rough-surfaced endoplasmic reticulum of the oligodendrocyte (Figures 7–7 and 7–8, *ER)* is well developed, and the cisternae, which are flattened, tend to be arranged in a circumferential manner around the nucleus. Single cisternae are common, but stacks of them are seen frequently, especially in the abundant cytoplasm at one pole of the cell. Ribosomes also stud the outer surface of the nuclear membrane (Figure 7–7, *r),* and relatively large numbers of free ribosomes occur in the cytoplasm, sometimes grouped to form rosettes (Figure 7–8, *r).* Although there are many ribosomes, both free and associated with membranes, these particles do not entirely account for the density of the cytoplasm in electron microscope preparations. The cytoplasmic matrix has an intrinsic density, which is produced by large numbers of small, pallid granules that occupy all the open space between the other organelles.

The Golgi apparatus of oligodendrocytes is generally well developed, and its cisternae and vesicles occur throughout the perikaryal cytoplasm, although, like the granular endoplasmic reticulum, it tends to aggregate at one pole (Figures 7–7 and 7–8, *G).* Because of the density of the cytoplasm, the mitochondria are rather inconspicuous. They show no unusual features. Most of them are short, and the cristae are arranged transversely.

Unlike astrocytes, oligodendrocytes have few cytoplasmic fibrils and glycogen granules. Microtubules, however, are conspicuous components of oligodendrocytes. Like those in neurons, these microtubules are about 25 nm in diameter, and they show no preferential orientation within the perikaryal cytoplasm. Microtubules are also very abundant in the oligodendrocyte processes, where they are arranged parallel to one another (Figure 7–7, *inset).* Because of the abundant microtubules, it is sometimes difficult to distinguish profiles of oligodendrocyte processes from those of dendrites. Differentiation is usually made possible by the fact that oligodendrocyte processes have no synapses upon their surfaces. Furthermore, unlike dendrites, their cytoplasm has an inherent density. As would be expected from light microscopy, the processes of oligodendrocytes are not numerous, and in electron microscope sections it is unusual to see them emerging from the cell body.

Dense bodies are sometimes encountered in the cytoplasm of oligodendrocytes. Most of these have a homogeneous appearance, but others contain granules, filaments, membranous components, and droplets. Other dense bodies, first described by Bunge, Bunge, and Ris (1960), have a heterogeneous appearance and contain one or two clear rectangular areas. Similar heterogeneous inclusion bodies seem not to occur in astrocytes.

Oligodendrocytes can exhibit a spectrum of morphological variation involving their cytoplasmic density and the clumping of the nuclear chromatin. This has been emphasized by Kruger and Maxwell (1966) and by Mori and Leblond (1970). Mori and Leblond (1970) recognize three types of oligodendrocytes: light, medium, and dark. In the order listed, there seems to be a tendency for the dark type to be smallest and to have the most dense chromatin and dense cytoplasm. Cells in this category are most likely to be confused with microglia. On the basis of labelling the proliferating neuroglia of the corpus callosum of young rats with tritiated thymidine, Mori and Leblond (1970) suggest that the cells make up a gradient in which the light oligodendrocytes are the most actively dividing cells and that oligodendrocytes become progressively darker as they mature. This is in agreement with the studies of Vaughn (1969) and Vaughn and Peters (1971) who found the immature, or active oligodendrocytes of the developing optic nerve to be large cells, with prominent cytoplasmic processes that appear just prior to myelination.

Despite these variations in the appearance of the oligodendrocytes there are certain features that consistently distinguish oligodendrocytes from astrocytes. These are (1) the greater density of both the cytoplasm and the nucleus, (2) the absence of fibrils and glycogen in the cytoplasm, and (3) the presence of large numbers of microtubules in the processes. The distinction between oligodendrocytes and microglial cells is less apparent and will be considered when the microglial cells are described.

The satellite oligodendrocytes have essentially the same morphological characteristics as interfascicular ones. Satellite oligodendrocytes are most commonly associated with the larger neurons of the central nervous system, and they usually appear to be closely applied to the surface of a neuron. Sometimes the plasma membranes of the neuron and its satellite oligodendrocyte lie in direct apposition, separated from each other by a distance of about 20 nm (Figure 7–8). The appositional surfaces are smooth and display no morphological specializations. Thus far, no morphological evidence has been discovered to indicate that exchange of substances takes place between the neuron and its satellite. Sotelo and Angaut (1973) have shown in the deep cerebellar nuclei of the cat that the plasma membranes of adjacent oligodendrocytes may form gap junctions.

As pointed out above, oligodendroglial cells are not the only cells to assume a satellite position. Both microglia and astrocytes can also be satellites (see Figures 7–3 and 7–9). Sotelo and Palay (1968) have shown that in the lateral vestibular nucleus of the rat, oligodendrocytes only rarely approach the surface of Deiters neurons. The oligodendrocytes often seem to be separated from the neurons by thin sheets of astrocyte processes.

THE FUNCTIONS OF OLIGODENDROCYTES

The two functions usually ascribed to oligodendrocytes are the formation of myelin and the nutrition of neurons.

The role of oligodendrocytes in myelin formation has already been considered in an earlier section (see page 208) and evidence in favor of this concept is based upon the following observations: (1) oligodendrocytes first appear immediately prior to the time when myelination begins (see Davison, 1968; Vaughn, 1969) and the most rapid rate of myelin formation, at least in the rat optic nerve, is synchronous with the mitotic proliferation and cellular differentiation of the oligodendrocytes (Hirose and Bass, 1973); and (2) in developing tissue, connections have been demonstrated between immature sheaths and young oligodendrocytes (Figure 6–13). Such connections, however, have not yet been found in adult tissue. Certainly, the external tongue process of the mature sheath resembles the cy-

---

Figure 7–7.   **Interfascicular Oligodendrocyte.**

The chromatin of this oligodendrocyte (*Nuc*) is clumped beneath the nuclear envelope, on the outer surface of which are attached ribosomes (*r*). Because of the inherent density of the oligodendrocytic cytoplasm, the organelles are not prominent. However, profiles of cisternae of the granular endoplasmic reticulum (*ER*) are discernible in addition to the well-defined Golgi apparatus (*G*) and the mitochondria (*mit*). Surrounding most of the oligodendrocyte are the lighter processes of fibrous astrocytes (*As*).
Optic nerve of adult rat. × 50,000.

Inset: Transverse section of the process of an oligodendrocyte. The cytoplasm of the process contains two mitochondria and many microtubules (*m*), some of which show a central "dot." The cytoplasmic matrix of the process shows the fine, dense particles that are responsible for the overall density of oligodendrocytes.
Optic nerve of adult rat. × 80,000.

Micrograph by J. E. Vaughn.

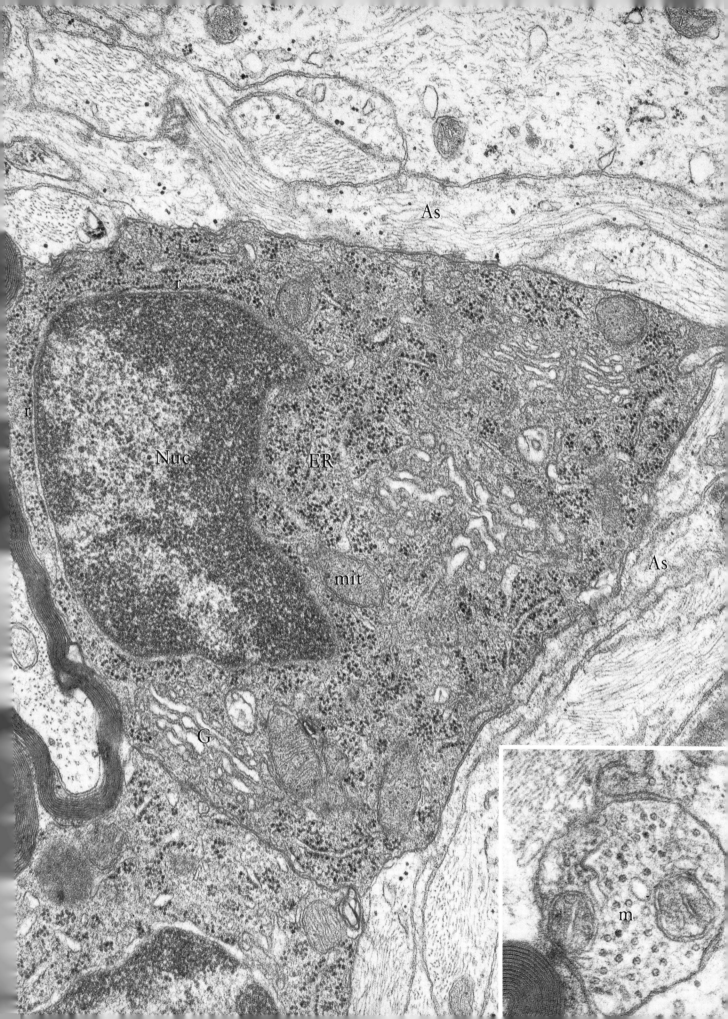

toplasm of the oligodendrocyte, but until continuity between the two has been directly visualized, the role of these cells in the sustenance of adult sheaths may still be questioned.

The idea that oligodendrocytes play a role in the nutrition and maintenance of neurons is largely based upon the observation that frequently these neuroglial cells are satellites to neuronal cell bodies. Although this concept has most recently been elaborated upon by Hydén and his coworkers, the theory of a symbiotic relationship between neurons and neuroglia is an old idea that was first expounded by Holmgren (1900) and by Cajal in 1913 (see Cajal, 1928).

In their studies of the symbiotic relationships between neurons and their associated neuroglial cells, Hydén and his coworkers (see Hydén, 1959; Hydén and Pigon, 1960; Hydén, 1967) have made extensive use of the giant neurons from the Deiters nucleus. By a delicate method of microdissection giant neurons are separated from their associated neuroglial cells, and each of these two elements is analyzed separately (see Hydén, 1967). In the earlier studies Hydén (see Hydén, 1959; Hydén and Pigon, 1960) considered that a giant cell from the Deiters nucleus is enclosed by a neuroglial envelope formed of about 35 to 40 oligodendrocytes and a proportion of astrocytes not exceeding 10 per cent of the total. More recently Hamberger (1963), using the same method, has found that the specimens he considers to represent the neuroglial envelope contain seven to eight neuroglial cells. However, he agrees that the proportion of astrocytes in such a specimen is only about 10 per cent of the total.

Using these specimens, Hydén and his collaborators have analyzed such factors as the content of oxidative enzymes and the base composition of nucleic acids in the neuroglial cells as

compared with the giant cells of Deiters. He has examined these factors under normal and experimental conditions such as learning and forced activity. For example, in the control animal Hydén finds twice as much cytochrome oxidase and succinoxidase activity in the neuroglia as in an equal mass of Deiters neurons (Hydén and Pigon, 1960). Similar results have been obtained in respect of the ATPase activity (Cummins and Hydén, 1962). Conversely, the neuroglia contain only about 10 per cent of the RNA found in the neuron, but under certain conditions of chemical stimulation and forced activity the base compositions of the nuclear RNA in the neurons and neuroglial cells are reported to change in opposite directions (Hydén and Egyházi, 1963).

Although studies of this type may indicate a symbiotic relation between neurons and neuroglial cells, it is unfortunate that few modern investigators have dealt with the identification of the neuroglial cells associated with the neurons and with the morphological relations that exist between them. Astrocytes, microglia, or oligodendrocytes can assume a satellite position to neurons, and in the spinal cord and the cerebral cortex, for example, all may be in immediate contact with the same neuronal perikaryon. In a detailed electron microscopic analysis of the lateral vestibular nucleus of the rat, Sotelo and Palay (1968) found that oligodendrocytes rarely approach the surface of Deiters perikarya. This is contrary to the findings of Hydén and his collaborators. The two types of cellular components that immediately surround Deiters cell bodies are (1) axon terminals synapsing upon their surfaces and (2) delicate sheets of astrocytic cytoplasm. These latter sheets always separate oligodendrocytes from the surface of the giant neuron. Although this does not invalidate the symbiotic theory, it does affect the pertinence of cytochemical data supporting the theory and

---

Figure 7–8.　**A Satellite Oligodendrocyte.**

This picture shows an oligodendrocyte occupying a satellite position with respect to an anterior horn cell. As is apparent in both this figure and Figure 7–7, oligodendrocytes are much darker than neurons. The darkness of the nucleus (*Nuc*) is due to a high concentration of chromatin, and that of the cytoplasm to small, dense granules in the cytoplasmic matrix. These granules are much smaller than the ribosomes (*r*) that lie free within the cytoplasm or stud the outer surfaces of the granular endoplasmic reticulum (*ER*) and the nuclear envelope (*Nev*). The presence of the small granules renders organelles such as the Golgi apparatus (*G*), microtubules (*m*), and mitochondria (*mit*) rather inconspicuous.

No special features mark the areas where the plasma membranes of the neuron and its satellite come into opposition (arrows).
Spinal cord of adult rat. × 35,000.

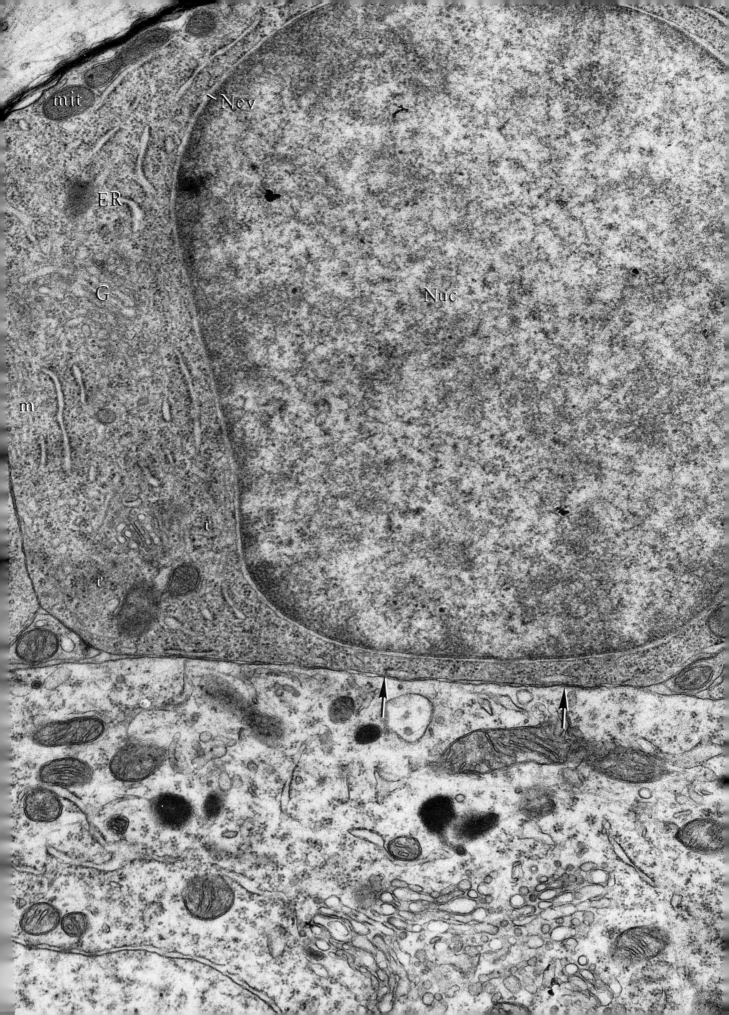

makes the results difficult to interpret. It further emphasizes the necessity for strict morphological evaluation of samples used for biochemical studies of neuronal and neuroglial interactions. Other criticisms concerning the experimental procedures and conclusions of Hydén and his collaborators are presented by Kuffler and Nicholls (1966).

A full consideration of the role of neuroglial cells in the metabolism of neurons is beyond the scope of this volume, and for more information on this subject reference should be made to reviews such as those of Hydén (1962, 1967), Giacobini (1964), Koenig (1964), Friede (1965),

Kuffler and Nicholls (1966), and Hydén and Lange (1970).

It should be added that quite early Ferraro and Davidoff (1928) studied Wallerian degeneration by using silver stains and came to the conclusion that oligodendroglia are the phagocytic cells. In a more recent study of Wallerian degeneration in the monkey and cat optic nerves Cook and Wiśniewski (1973) also implicated the oligodendroglia in the phagocytosis of degenerating material. However, their evidence is rather tenuous, and the basis for referring to the phagocytosing cells as oligodendroglia is not clear.

NEUROGLIAL CELLS INTERMEDIATE BETWEEN ASTROCYTES AND OLIGODENDROCYTES

No definite conclusions seem to have been reached on the question of whether there are forms of neuroglia that are intermediate between astrocytes and oligodendrocytes. Cells considered to be intermediate in character have been described by light microscopists (e.g., Penfield, 1924; Ramón-Moliner, 1958) using metallic impregnation methods, and in an early study of the neuroglia in the cerebral cortex Farquhar and Hartmann (1957) came to the same conclusion. This view has also been reiterated by Hartmann (1962). More recent electron microscopic work does not substantiate the existence of intermediate types. Thus, Wendell-Smith, Blunt, and Baldwin (1966) observe that in the optic nerve of the cat, neuroglial cells with fibrils or

glycogen never have a dense cytoplasmic matrix. Consequently, Wendell-Smith and his colleagues contend that these features are mutually exclusive and consider that most forms previously described as intermediate should now be classified as organelle-rich astrocytes. Mugnaini and Walberg (1964) arrived at essentially the same conclusion, as did Maxwell and Kruger (1965b).

Transitional forms of neuroglia do appear to exist in pathological conditions such as those examined by Bunge, Bunge, and Ris (1960 and 1961). They designate these cells, which have a dense cytoplasm and contain fibrils, as "reactive macroglia."

MICROGLIA

Cajal (1909–1911) classified the neuroglial cells into three categories. The first two corresponded to varieties of astrocytes, and the last to a "third element," a group of cells comprising what are nowadays referred to as oligodendrocytes and microglial cells. Although microglial cells (rod cells, mesoglia, Robertson-Hortega cells, Hortega cells) had previously been described by a number of authors, including Nissl (1899), Robertson (1900), and Alzheimer (1904), it was not until del Rio Hortega (1919 and 1932) introduced his silver carbonate method that microglial cells and oligodendroglial cells could be

more completely visualized and separated from each other on the basis of their structure. According to the accounts of del Rio Hortega and others (see del Rio Hortega, 1932), microglial cells are small in comparison with astrocytes. They have elongated or triangular nuclei which stain deeply with basic dyes, and from the scanty perikaryon arise wavy processes which branch and give off spine-like projections. Such cells occur in both white and gray matter, but on the whole they are more abundant in gray matter. According to del Rio Hortega (1932), many microglial cells are scattered at random in the central nervous system, but others are preferentially situated near neurons and blood vessels. From the consensus of available data, it seems that in light microscope preparations of the cerebral cortex, for example, about 5 to 10 per cent of the neuroglial cells are microglia. The most favored animal for the study of microglia is the rabbit.

The microglial cells are commonly said to have a mesodermal origin and to invade the developing central nervous system at the time when the vascular supply of the brain is being elaborated. The major sources of these cells are usually considered to be the pia mater, the walls of the vascular elements, and the tela choroidea. In the normal adult brain the microglial cells seem to be inactive. That they are a normal component of the brain and not induced by brain injury is borne out by Cammermeyer's (1970) demonstration that these cells are present in germ-free rats. The microglia are, however, activated by any inflammatory or degenerative lesions of the nervous system. Under such conditions the microglial cells undergo rapid proliferation, as may histiocytes from the meninges and blood vessels. Both types of cells retract their processes and migrate toward the site of the injury, where they turn into macrophages and remove the debris. At this time, the cells may assume either a rod-like form or rounded and globular shapes as they become laden with lipids and cell remnants. Once they have phagocytosed the debris, the further fate of the macrophages is uncertain. They transport the debris to the vicinity of blood vessels, but whether they discharge their contents into the blood vessels, or themselves pass through, is uncertain. Microglial cells are also capable of ingesting vital dyes such as trypan blue, so that in effect they react in the same way as macrophages in the reticuloendothelial system. A review of the literature pertaining to microglia has recently been presented by Cammermeyer (1970).

Before continuing with this account it would be helpful to insert a few remarks based on the preceding description of microglia. In considering the "resting" microglia, that is, the inactive cells existing in the normal brain, it seems clear that one is dealing with a specific type of cell, whose shape and distribution can be defined. In the case of the "reactive" microglia, on the other hand, it is likely that one is dealing with a variety of cells, some derived from the resting microglia and others that invade the brain from the vascular system. The sources of the macrophages probably depend upon the

extent of the lesion and whether the vascular supply to the area has been affected (see Stenwig, 1972).

It has been suggested (Peters, Palay, and Webster, 1970) that there may be two reasons for the failure of electron microscopists to identify microglial cells in the normal nervous system, one reason being that in the normal brain the cells do not exist as a separate entity. This question was raised by Maxwell and Kruger (1965b) who inferred from their studies dealing with the effects of ionizing radiations on the cerebral cortex that the appearance of large macrophages in the brain depended upon the resulting perivascular reaction. They concluded that the macrophages were derived from the pericytes of the small vessels and not from any pre-existing neuroglial element in the neuropil. Other studies have also indicated that not all macrophages activated as a result of brain injury are derived from pre-existing neuroglial cells but may have origin from the vascular walls or the blood itself (see Cammermeyer, 1965a and b; Konigsmark and Sidman, 1963; Kitamura, Hattori, and Fujita, 1972; Stenwig, 1972). In this context, it is important to note, however, that Cammermeyer (1970) using silver-stained light microscope preparations showed microglia to be present even in the brains of germ-free rats. In this type of animal the microglia could not have been induced as a result of a pathological process, so that the cells do indeed seem to be a normal constituent of the central nervous system.

The second reason given for the failure to find microglial cells in earlier electron microscope studies was that these cells may not have been distinguished from oligodendrocytes. In light microscope preparations the same silver techniques are used to stain both oligodendrocytes and microglial cells, and generally the two types of cells appear simultaneously in the same preparations (see Cammermeyer, 1966). Consequently, differentiation between these cells may be difficult, even with the light microscope. The similarity in staining affinities indicates that oligodendroglia and microglia may have similar chemical properties, and perhaps a similar appearance in the electron microscope (see Matthews and Kruger, 1973b).

In retrospect, this second reason seems to explain the delay in the identification of microglia in electron microscope studies of normal tissue. A neuroglial cell that seems to have most of the attributes of the microglial cells described in normal tissue studied in light microscope preparations is that which Vaughn and Peters (1968) referred to in their initial description as a "third neuroglial cell." This initial noncommittal terminology was used because at the time there were insufficient data available about the cell to warrant a more specific name. Since then, however, a number of investigators have recognized this cell in both normal tissue (e.g., Mori and Leblond, 1969a; Barón and Gallego, 1972) and injured tissue (e.g., Vaughn, Hinds, and Skoff, 1970; Blinzinger and Kreutzberg, 1968; Torvik, 1972; Price, 1972; Kerns and Hinsman, 1973b). Mori and Leblond (1969a), who described this type of cell in the corpus callosum of the rat, showed it to stain by a modification of the del Rio Hortega method for microglia and so were able to conclude that this cell is the equivalent of the classical microglial cell in normal tissue.

Before this cell is described it is pertinent to consider previous descriptions of microglial cells. In the earliest electron microscope studies the criteria for the identification of microglial cells appear to have been arrived at by a process of elimination (Schultz, Maynard, and Pease, 1957; Farquhar and Hartmann, 1957). Thus, it was found that after cells had been classified as either astrocytes or oligodendrocytes there remained a third form of cell. This was a small cell with a very dark cytoplasm and a correspondingly dark nucleus. It was also characterized by highly irregular contours, giving it a somewhat crenated appearance. A similar description for microglial cells was later given in a review by Mugnaini and Walberg (1964) and in a report by Herndon (1964). However, the crenated appearance of these cells and the compacting of the cytoplasmic organelles suggest that in reality these descriptions refer to cells that

have been damaged either osmotically or in the handling of the tissue (see Mugnaini, 1965). In respect of this point it is probably significant that, as methods for the fixing and handling of central nervous tissue have improved, few accounts of dark cells have appeared in the recent literature. This conclusion is supported by a recent study of Stensaas, Edwards, and Stensaas (1972). These authors found that dark neurons can result from a premature handling of the tissue after fixation by perfusion. They also concluded that dark cells can be produced by subjecting neurons to mechanical trauma while the animal is alive.

GENERAL MORPHOLOGY

In normal tissue, the cells identified in recent studies as microglia make up 4 to 5 per cent of the total population of neuroglial cells in white matter, about 18 per cent in the gray matter of the rat cerebral cortex (Vaughan and Peters, 1974), and about 6 per cent in the anterior horn of the rat spinal cord (Kerns and Hinsman, 1973a). Such cells are frequently located immediately beneath the glia limitans and in the vicinity of blood vessels where they can lie adjacent to the astrocytic end-feet surrounding a capillary. On the other hand, microglia often lie in a perineuronal position, and in the cerebral cortex, for example, they are often separated from the neuron by a thin astroglial process (Figure 7–9). However, the presence of such processes is not a diagnostic feature, for satellite oligodendrocytes may also have astrocytic processes interposed between themselves and an adjacent neuron. These three locations are those in which microglial cells are found in

---

Figure 7–9.   **A Perineuronal Microglial Cell.**

The rather dark microglial cell in this picture lies close to a pyramidal neuron. For the most part the two cells are separated by a thin astrocytic process (*AsP*). The nucleus (*Nuc*) of the microglial cell is oval and has large clumps of chromatin beneath the nuclear envelope. The dark cytoplasm forms only a thin rim around most of the nucleus, so that the organelles are contained in the cytoplasm at the two ends of the cell. There the cytoplasm shows mitochondria (*mit*), as well as the characteristic long cisternae of endoplasmic reticulum (*ER*) and dark inclusions that appear to be lipofuscin (*Lf*).

This microglial cell resembles an astrocyte in that the outline of the cell is irregular and follows the contours of the elements in the surrounding neuropil. However, unlike astrocytes these cells do not have thin and sheet-like processes.

Cerebral cortex of adult rat. × 17,500.

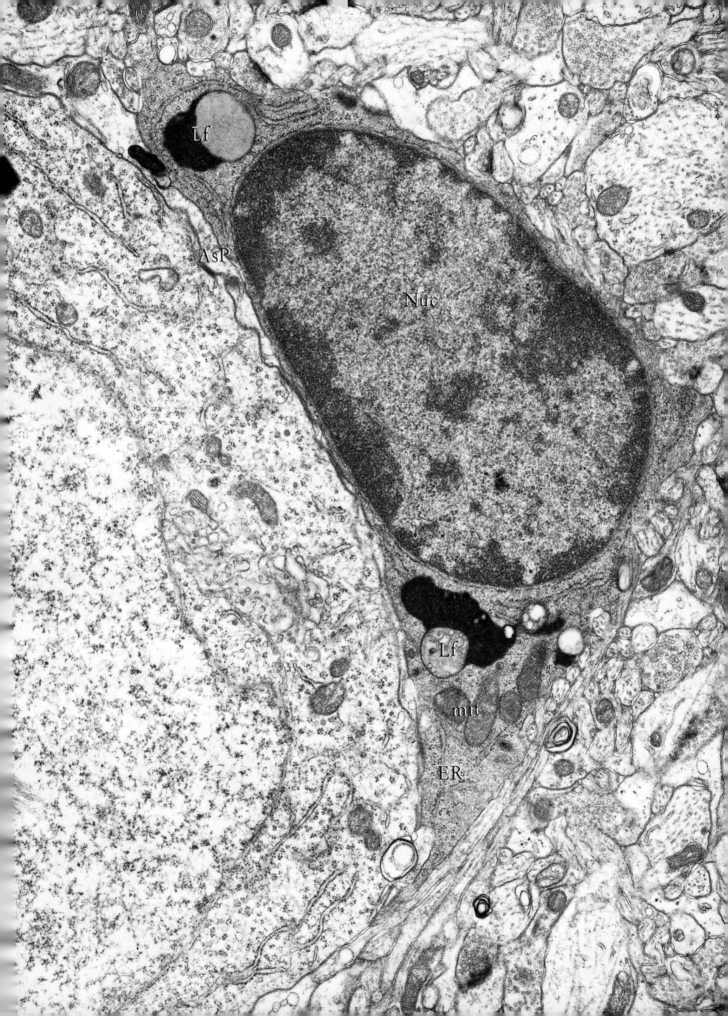

classically stained preparations (del Rio Hortega, 1932).

A microglial cell (Figures 7–9 and 7–10) is generally smaller than either an astrocyte or an oligodendrocyte, and its nucleus is usually oval or elongate with clumps of chromatin beneath the nuclear envelope and throughout the nucleoplasm (Figures 7–9 and 7–10). In some respects the nucleus resembles that of the oligodendrocyte, but the chromatin clumps of the microglial cells are generally more prominent and occupy a larger proportion of the nuclear volume. Hence, the cell often has a darker nucleus than the oligodendrocyte when examined in light microscope preparations stained with basic dyes. The cytoplasm of the microglial cell forms a thin rim around the nucleus (Figure 7–9), but often extends out in quite broad processes (Figure 7–10). When cells are in perineuronal positions these processes seem to partially encompass the neuron (Figure 7–9), but when microglial cells are lying free (Figure 7–10), the processes invade the surrounding neuropil so that the cell has a basically irregular shape that conforms to the contours of the surrounding neuropil, as does an astrocyte. The density of the cytoplasm, however, parallels that of the oligodendrocyte, but it contains fewer microtubules and has none of the glycogen granules and bundles of filaments that characterize an astrocyte. Perhaps the most distinctive feature of the microglial cell is the form of its granular endoplasmic reticulum, for the cisternae are long and narrow, almost stringy, and are often seen to wind tortuously through the cytoplasm (Figure 7–9, *ER*). This is quite unlike the granular endoplasmic reticulum of an oligodendrocyte, which generally has the form of short cisternae (Figure 7–8).

The Golgi apparatus is usually prominent at one pole of the perikaryon (Figure 7–10, *G)*, where it often surrounds the end of the nucleus.

Dense laminar bodies, homogeneous droplets, lysosomes, and lipofuscin are quite commonly encountered in the cytoplasm (Figures 7–9 and 7–10), much more commonly than in either oligodendrocytes or astrocytes. It should be pointed out that Cammermeyer (1970) suggests that in light microscope preparations, clustering of PAS-stained granules in the vicinity of the nucleus, or at sites of branching of processes, is typical of normal, "resting" microglial cells, and that in the absence of any other criteria, the presence of such bodies, which are prominent in older animals, is indispensable for the identification of microglia. In this context, recent electron microscope studies of the cerebral cortex of aging rats (Vaughan and Peters, 1974) have shown a significant increase in the dense inclusions present in the cytoplasm of cells identified as microglia on the basis of the morphology given in the preceding account. Another incidental observation is that these cells abound in the cerebral cortices of rats which are suffering from pneumonia, and it may be significant that the animal most commonly chosen for the study of microglia is the rabbit, which commonly suffers from respiratory infection. Perhaps the number of these cells contained in the brains of apparently normal animals is partially dependent upon the animal's previous history of infections, for it is becoming apparent that while the brains of some animals have quite large numbers of these cells, in the brains of other animals of the same species and comparable age, there are relatively few.

The cells that Stensaas and Stensaas (1968) refer to as microglia in the spinal cord of the toad bear some resemblance to the cells that have been described in the mammalian nervous system. The general shapes of the cells and their nuclei are similar, but the microglia from the toad have a rather lighter cytoplasm. The account by Stensaas and Stensaas (1968) should be

---

Figure 7–10. Microglial Cell.

This microglial cell has its nucleus (*Nuc*) at one end of the perikaryon, where it is surrounded by a thin rim of cytoplasm. Most of the cytoplasm is at the other pole of the cell, and it contains large inclusion bodies that have the characteristics of lipofuscin (*Lf*). Other organelles in the cytoplasm are the Golgi apparatus (*G*), mitochondria (*mit*), a few cisternae of the endoplasmic reticulum (*ER*), and free ribosomes (*r*).

The contours of this dark cell are much more irregular than those of an oligodendrocyte.

Cerebral cortex of adult rat. × 20,000.

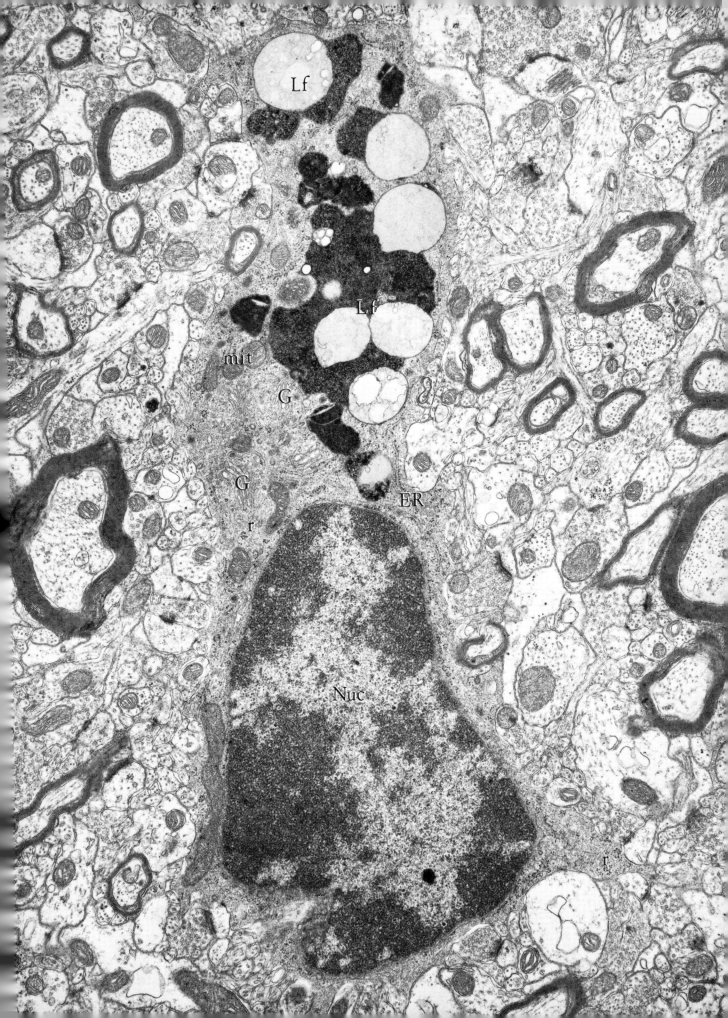

consulted, if only for the interesting drawings of the shapes of microglia, astrocytes, and oligodendrocytes.

FUNCTIONS

In considering the functions of microglia, we will restrict our discussion to what is known of the cells just described. Because of the striking resemblance of their "third neuroglial type" now more appropriately termed microglia, to presumed neuroglial precursors in the optic nerve of fetal neonatal rats, Vaughn (1969) and Vaughn and Peters (1968 and 1971) consider that in the adult, the microglial cells may be multipotential elements that are retained, just as are multipotential cells in other tissues. The existence of such cells could account for some of the low level of glial cell formation that takes place throughout life (Hommes and Leblond, 1967; Dalton, Hommes, and Leblond, 1968). Evidence for this concept is indicated by the fact that in adult optic nerves undergoing Wallerian degeneration, these cells increase in number, surround degenerating myelin fragments, and come to contain many lipid inclusions. Indeed in later postoperative stages, such cells appear to be very like the "gitter" cells of classical studies, for they enlarge and their cytoplasm becomes filled with debris (Vaughn, Hinds, and Skoff, 1970).

Similar cells, identified as microglial cells in light microscope studies (see Cammermeyer, 1970; Torvik, 1972), proliferate rapidly in the initial phase of the response of motor neurons to section of their axons. In the facial nucleus of the rat (Blinzinger and Kreutzberg, 1968) and in the anterior horn of the spinal cord of frogs (Price, 1972) and rats (Kerns and Hinsman, 1973a and b), the microglial cells proliferate by mitosis and extend over the surface of chromatolytic motor neurons, apparently displacing synaptic boutons. This observation may be correlated with the results of Hamberger, Hansson, and Sjöstrand (1970), who using a scanning electron microscope found the surfaces of isolated, chromatolytic neurons to have a reduced number of particles (synaptic boutons) upon them. In some instances (Price, 1972; Torvik, 1972) processes of the microglial cells may penetrate deeply into the neuronal cytoplasm and apparently begin to phagocytose pieces of it. This process becomes more apparent if the motor neuron is degenerating. On the other hand, when a neuron recovers after chromatolysis, the synaptic boutons are replaced on its surface and there are fewer microglia (also see Torvik and Söreide, 1972).

DISCUSSION

The literature concerning microglia is rather confused and, on the basis of present knowledge, is difficult to interpret, especially since most of it is concerned not with microglia in normal tissue but with the reactions of cells to injury. There is little point in attempting to review the microglial literature in any detail in the present context, for that has recently been effected very adequately by Cammermeyer (1970). The problem of the origins of these cells during development and during their proliferation following injury or insult is not made easier by recent electron microscope studies. However, in an attempt to bring out some of the difficulties and to consider how they may be reconciled, two of the main problems will be discussed.

The Origin of Microglia

One problem concerns the normal origins of the microglia during development of the central nervous system. According to the classical views propounded by del Rio Hortega (1932), the microglia have a mesodermal origin, and hence differ from the other neuroglial types, whose origin is generally considered to be ectodermal. del Rio Hortega (1932) considered that the microglia enter the brain at the end of embryonic development, at a time when the vascularization commences. He believed that these cells first appear in some areas of the brain immediately below the pia and later appear in paraventricular and subependymal sites. The pial adventitia of the large and medium-sized blood vessels were also regarded as sites of origin.

So far as we can discern, the reason for del Rio Hortega's (1932) view of the mesodermal origin of microglia from the meninges and ependyma, as well as from the tela choroidea and choroid plexus, was the finding of irregular, small cells resembling lymphocytes at the interface between the meninges and the central nervous system proper and at the ependymal surfaces. In later stages cells deeper in the nervous system also became impregnated by silver carbonate and developed the characteristic morphology of resting microglia. The whole process of migration of these cells into the central nervous system was supposed to be accomplished within a few days.

While these views have been subsequently shared by a number of investigators and are widely quoted in almost every text dealing with the nervous system, others have taken a different view and consider microglia, like other neuroglial cells, to be derived from the subependymal zone (periventricular matrix layer). Thus, Pruijs (1927) described the microglia as originating from the ependymal regions of fetal and newborn rabbits, and Rydberg (1932) found a similar origin in a wide variety of animals.

Fujita (1965) has pointed out that Hortega's silver carbonate methods not only stain macrophages but immature forms of neuroglial cells if staining is carried out in the developmental period. In a recent study of the developing human spinal cord Fujita (1973) applied these methods and concluded that the cells frequently described by others as microglioblasts are really glioblasts which have differentiated from the ventricular or matrix zone. Some of these cells may transform into microglia, but others would be expected to produce astrocytes and oligodendrocytes. At the end of his discussion Fujita (1973) concluded that there is no evidence for the migration of cells of mesenchymal origin into the brain, at least during the development of the human spinal cord.

Cells like the cuboidal cells described by del Rio Hortega (1932) have been found by Vaughn (1969) and by Vaughn and Peters (1971) to be present at the surface of the developing rat optic nerve. Such cells were always on the neural side of the glia limitans surrounding the nerve and never outside it. A careful search revealed no cells entering the optic nerve from the outside. In this study, there was no indication of cells entering the nerve from the adventitia of the blood vessels.

Consequently, Vaughn and Peters (1968) suggested that microglial cells differentiate from glioblasts present early in development. Indeed they concluded that the multipotential glial cells, or early microglia, are the precursors of other glial cell types. This conclusion is contrary to that of Mori and Leblond (1969a), Barón and Gallego (1972), and Sturrock (1974). Essentially these latter authors conclude that microglia make their first appearance as well-differentiated cells and are derived from pericytes.

We will now consider the inner surface of the brain. As described earlier, during development a subventricular zone of dividing cells appears between the ventricular zone and the intermediate zone in most regions of the central nervous system (see Angevine, 1970). When these cells are labelled with tritiated thymidine it is apparent (Sidman, 1970b) that they incorporate the label and do not have intermitotic migrations as do cells that originate earlier in development. Such cells differentiate into both neurons and neuroglia (Smart and Leblond, 1961; Altman, 1967), but whether they are an early source of microglia has not been investigated.

Later in development, as the cells of the ventricular zone differentiate into ependymal cells, the subventricular zone, now in the mature brain referred to as the subependymal layer, may continue to show a high mitotic activity, especially in the angle between the pallium and the caudate nucleus in the wall of the third ventricle. Lewis (1968a and b) has shown that if the brains of young rats are labelled by an intraventricular administration of tritiated thymidine, labelled neuroglial cells, some of which are identifiable as microglia and astrocytes, are derived from the subependymal layer. Two weeks after injection of the label, such neuroglial cells can be found throughout the deeper portions of the cerebral hemispheres, although not in the cortex itself. Blakemore (1969), following Lewis's study, examined the fine structure of the subependymal layer and in his electron microscope study was able to identify microglia in this region. Cammermeyer (1965a) also showed classically stained microglia to be present in the subependymal region and believes that they take origin from cells located outside the basement membranes of blood vessels. However, Stensaas and Gilson (1972) were not able to find direct evidence for the origin of microglial cells through mitosis of either subependymal or ependymal cells in the caudato-pallial junction of neonatal rabbits, although they were able to confirm the presence of microglia in this region.

In view of these observations there is at least reason to question the classical concepts of the origin of microglia in development, and the time is now ripe for a re-evaluation of the origins of these cells using labelling techniques in conjunction with electron microscopy.

The Origins of Phagocytes

The second problem concerns the origins of cells that proliferate and undertake phagocytosis when an insult is inflicted upon the brain. Under such circumstances studies using classical stains indicate that microglia in the brain proliferate and that there may also be an invasion of the area by phagocytes from other sources.

In studies of an injury not involving the blood vessels in the vicinity of the site where degeneration is taking place—for example, in the case of Wallerian degeneration of nerve fibers some distance from the site of the lesion—phagocytes seem to be mainly provided by a proliferation of microglia already existing in the area (e.g., Vaughn, Hinds, and Skoff, 1970; Stenwig, 1972). However, if the vascular supply to the area is directly affected, as for example by a stab wound or by freezing, then the phagocytes may be derived mainly from the blood, this source being mobilized under certain conditions (see Stenwig, 1972). Thus, Konigsmark and Sidman (1963) arrived at the conclusion that a stab wound of the cerebral cortex led to a situation in which at least two-thirds of the macrophages appearing in the lesion site were derived from mononuclear leukocytes (monocytes). As to the origin of the remaining third, they were uncertain but considered it most likely that they were derived from neuroglial cells present in the brain before wounding. On the basis of some interesting experiments in which blood cells were labelled, Oemichen, Grüninger, Saebich, and Narita (1973) concluded that a great number of the microglia and pericytes in experimental brain damage in rabbits and rats derive from blood monocytes. In addition, they were able to demonstrate a proliferation of the microglia and pericytes which had been in the locale before the damage was inflicted. Kitamura, Hattori, and Fujita (1972) arrived at a somewhat different conclusion, namely that the macrophages which invade a stab wound are all monocytes, and that pericytes, neuroglial cells, and other types of cell do not contribute. They do state, however, that the monocytes undergo a marked transformation as they leave the blood vessels and migrate into the damaged area, and it is interesting that one of their illustrations of a transformed monocyte looks remarkably like a microglial cell.

Matthews and Kruger (1973a and b) studied cellular changes in the thalamus of the rabbit after making lesions in the cerebral cortex. They found a distinct increase in the number of perivascular cells within the basal laminae surrounding capillaries and venules in the thalamus. The cells within the perivascular space were of various kinds. In addition to the indigenous pericyte population there were many agranular leukocytes and a few plasma cells and eosinophils. Some of these cells seemed to be penetrating the walls of the vessels. In the neuropil of the thalamus Matthews and Kruger (1973b) encountered cells with a morphology distinct from astrocytes and oligodendrocytes, but with sufficiently diverse forms so that Matthews and Kruger were unable to identify them specifically. With time those cells accumulated vacuoles and dense bodies in their cytoplasm. In the article, which reviews the sources of phagocytes in the neuropil, the authors come to the conclusion that the phagocytic cells are derived from a number of sources.

In rather sharp contrast to the conclusions of Matthews and Kruger are the results of Adrian and Williams (1973). They carried out electron microscopic autoradiography on specimens from the spinal cords of mice that had been injured with stab wounds and injected with tritiated thymidine on the second day after injury. When the tissue was examined two hours following the thymidine injection, the type of cell most frequently labelled, both at the site of injury and away from it, was the microglial cell. Such cells were also frequent two days after injection of the label, but their number was almost equalled by a second type of labelled cell resembling an astrocyte.

In another study Blakemore (1972) examined the response of cells in the cerebral cortex to cold lesions. On examining the lesion during the first two days after operation, before there was any large influx of hematogenous cells, he found that it was possible to follow the sequence of changes undergone by the microglia in the area. The resting microglia had a typical morphology, but within 24 hours of the injury they had become activated and had acquired membrane-bound inclusions in their cytoplasm. By three days the microglia could no longer be identified with any certainty in and around the lesion because a large influx of hematogenous cells had occurred. Between three and seven days the activated microglia and the invading hematogenous cells had a similar appearance.

The point to be made here is that when

blood vessels have been damaged, both the microglial cells intrinsic to the area and cells derived from the vascular system are involved in the repair process. Furthermore, cells from these two sources seem to adopt a similar morphology as they turn into phagocytes. Hence, in discussing the "reactive microglia" one is dealing with a population of cells derived from more than one source. Around this fact revolves much of the problem of equating the recent fine structural studies with those carried out earlier using the classical techniques of staining. Hence it is apparent that the term "microglia" has to be redefined, for at present the term has different meanings to different authors. In our opinion it would be best if the term microglia were used to refer to the resting or minimally active forms of these neuroglial cells normally present in the central nervous system, and to refer to cells responding to an insult as *phagocytes*. The use of this latter term is preferred since it has no implication of origin of the cells. This is important since it is now apparent that the phagocytes may be derived from the microglia, from monocytes, and perhaps from pericytes and other sources, depending upon the extent and form of the lesion, and particularly upon whether blood vessels are disrupted.

Chapter VIII

THE EPENDYMA

The ependyma is a layer of epithelial cells lining the walls of the ventricles of the brain and the central canal of the spinal cord. Beneath the ependyma may be a second layer, the subependyma, which separates the ependyma from the underlying periventricular neuropil.

In mammals the ependyma is derived from the ventricular zone (Boulder Committee, 1970), which appears early and persists throughout development (see page 232). Initially, the cells of the ventricular zone produce only more ventricular cells, but during the active growth of the brain they also produce neuroblasts and neuroglia. Ultimately, the ventricular zone cells finish dividing and differentiate into ependymal cells. During the perinatal period in the rabbit (Tennyson and Pappas, 1962), the ependyma of the cerebral aqueduct is a thick stratified layer of rather undifferentiated cells. Microvilli are present at their luminal surfaces, and cilia form just before birth. Soon after birth, the ependyma changes to a pseudostratified columnar layer with the nuclei disposed at different levels. At that time it begins to resemble the ependyma of the mature animal. Eventually it becomes a regular, simple epithelium.

During development, some of the ventricular cells have processes that extend to the outer, or pial surface of the central nervous system. Cells of this type are referred to as spongioblasts. In some regions of the central nervous system such cells may persist throughout life, especially where the distance between the ventricles and the outside surface of the brain is short, as for example in the lateral lobe of the hypothalamus of the dogfish. Cells retaining this form in the mature brain are referred to as tanycytes (Horstmann, 1954). Tanycytes also persist in the walls of the third ventricle of mammals. They occur throughout the dorsoventral extent of the third ventricle but are most numerous ventrally (Millhouse, 1971). Because of their similarity to the spongioblasts of the developing brain, tanycytes might be interpreted as undifferentiated cells remaining in the ependyma and capable of forming ependymal cells and neuroglia. But as will be shown later, the tanycytes have also been implicated in a number of other functions.

As pointed out in the brief account of the formation of neuroglial cells (see page 232), during development a population of cells appears just deep to the ventricular zone, separating it from the intermediate zone of migrating neuroblasts. This population of cells constitutes the subventricular zone, and while this zone has only a transitory existence in some of the phylogenetically older parts of the brain, it may persist as a pronounced subependymal layer in regions such as the lateral angle of the lateral ventricle where there may be coarctation of the apposed ependymal layers (Westergaard, 1970). In brains of neonatal and young mature mammals, this layer continues to be a region of active cell proliferation.

The ependymal cells constitute the greatest population of cells in the lining of the ventricles and central canal of the spinal cord of mammals. They are cells with essentially epithelial characteristics, and their bases do not project into the periventricular neuropil. Tanycytes seem to be mainly confined to the third ventricle in mammals and have long basal processes extending into the neuropil and sometimes reaching the outer surface of the brain. Unfortunately, a distinction between these two cell types is not always made in accounts of the ependyma, and consequently some confusion can arise in the interpretation of published data.

It should be mentioned that other cells may also be present in the ventricular wall. In addition to typical ependymal cells and tanycytes, Knowles (1972) lists the three following components: (1) liquor-contacting neurons, which are neurons with processes, and sometimes perikarya, in contact with the cerebrospinal fluid, (2) neurosecretory neurons, which are best observed in fishes and secrete substances into the ventricles, and (3) glandular epithelial cells, which contain considerable amounts of PAS-positive material that in some cases seems to be discharged into the ventricles. These three components are largely confined to the walls of the third ventricle in the region of the hypothalamus, and for further details of their occurrence the review by Knowles (1972) should be consulted. Some mention of these three types of cells will be made in the following account, but it will become apparent that this classification is not rigid. For example, some of the liquor-contacting neurons seem to discharge substances into the ventricles and so could equally well be considered as neurosecretory.

THE MORPHOLOGY OF EPENDYMAL CELLS

In mature animals the ependyma consists of a single layer of squamous, cuboidal, or columnar cells, depending upon their location, and when viewed *en face* in whole mount light microscope preparations stained with silver nitrate, the cells are shown to have polygonal shapes (Bruni, Montemurro, Clattenburg, and Singh, (1973). In the adult mouse the ependymal cells are tallest at the front of the anterior horn of the lateral ventricle and are flattest where they overlie white matter (Westergaard, 1970). In light microscope preparations, typical ependymal cells show numerous cilia at their luminal surfaces. The cilia and their basal bodies were first described by Purkinje (1836), whose account subsequently was elaborated upon by other observers (see Agduhr, 1932). The cilia, which spring from basal bodies located in the apical cytoplasm, tend to be clustered toward the center of the free surface of the cell. In the rat (Brightman and Palay, 1963), the cilia are 15 to 20 microns long and about 0.4 micron in diameter (Figures 8–1 and 8–3). Each contains nine peripheral pairs of microtubules surrounding a central pair, a pattern which is common to most cilia (Klinkerfuss, 1964), but the basal bodies of the cilia are rather unusual in that each one is surrounded by an array of fine filaments encompassed by a cloud of finely granular material (Figure 8–3).

Attached to each basal body are a ciliary rootlet and a basal foot, similar to appendages found in many types of ciliated epithelium. A detailed account of these is given by Anderson (1972). The ciliary rootlet (Figure 8–3, x) is a short, conical collection of straight filaments, cross striated with a periodicity of about 90 nm. The basal foot which projects from the side of each basal body is a stumpy, cone-like structure which often bears a spherical mass of amorphous material at its tip (Figure 8–3, *arrow*). The profiles of these structures may sometimes be confused with the fibrillogranular aggregates which are also present in the apical cytoplasm (Figures 8–1 and 8–3, *fg*). The fibrillogranular aggregates have a variety of shapes, but their profiles are either more or less straight or folded. They consist of a core of fibrillar material bounded on each side by relatively evenly spaced dense granules. A thread-like condensation of the fibrillar material forms a central axis to each aggregate. According to Sorokin (1968), who studied ciliogenesis in mammalian lungs, the fibrillogranular aggregates give rise to deuterosomes which organize the growth of procentrioles around them and so give rise to the basal bodies of additional cilia.

The movements of the cilia, which were first described by Purkinje (1836) and subsequently recorded by a number of other observers (see Worthington and Cathcart, 1963, Cathcart and Worthington, 1964), are rapid and produce movements of the cerebrospinal fluid. Within the fourth ventricle the effective stroke seems to be toward the lateral apertures and roof (Cathcart and Worthington, 1964).

Located between the cilia are many shorter and thinner finger-like projections. Some of them resemble microvilli, but others are more irregular, being little more than simple extensions of the surface plasma membrane. Some of these projections contain small vesicles and fine filaments (Figures 8–3 and 8–5).

Regional differences in the surfaces of ependymal cells can be readily studied with the scanning electron microscope (Figure 8–2), since the ependyma is one of the few parts of the brain accessible to this form of microscopy (see Scott, Kozlowski, and Sheridan, 1974). In a study of the third ventricle of the mink, for example, Scott, Kozlowski, and Dudley (1973) found that the dorsal third of the ventricle was covered by a dense feltwork of cilia arranged in a repetitive wave-like pattern, which suggested that the cilia were beating in metachronal waves at the time of fixation. These cilia were so densely packed that they obscured the apical surfaces of the ependymal cells. Toward the middle third of the wall, there was a substantial reduction in the number of cilia and the convex apices of the ependymal cells could be discerned. In the lowest third of the wall and in the floor of the ventricle, cilia were almost absent, and the surfaces of the cells displayed numerous small, blunt processes that were interpreted as the thinner, microvillous processes shown in transmission electron microscope studies. Similar observations have also been made on the third ventricles of rabbit, cat, mouse, and human brains (Clementi and Morino, 1972; Scott, Paull, and Dudley, 1972; Bruni, Montemurro, Clattenburg, and Singh, 1972).

Supraependymal cells are sometimes found lying on top of the ependymal cells. Clementi and Morini (1972) have shown that in the lateral recess of the floor of the third ventricle supraependymal cells have a triangular shape, while those lying over the nonciliated areas of the preoptic and infundibular recesses appear more rounded (Coates, 1973a and b). In these latter areas the supraependymal cells have many branching processes that extend over the ependymal surface and enter into crevasses and holes in the ependyma. Such cell processes are proba-

bly different in form from the long, thin and beaded processes described by Scott, Paull, and Dudley (1972), for the latter can probably be equated with the neuronal processes, axons, and boutons that have been described in a number of transmission electron microscope studies (e.g., Westergaard, 1970; Leonhardt and Lindemann, 1973b; Coates, 1973b).

In the caudal portion of the third ventricle, near the region where it enters the aqueduct, in the cat there is a distinct difference in the patterns formed by cilia above and below the sulcus limitans. Dorsal to the sulcus limitans the cilia have a relatively uniform and dense distribution, while ventral to the sulcus the cilia are more sparse and form tufts. Similar tufts are also present in the lateral ventricles of all animals so far examined (e.g., Noack, Dumitrescu, and Schweichel, 1972; Kozlowski, Scott, and Krobisch-Dudley, 1973; Allen and Low, 1973) and in the floor of the fourth ventricle. Between the tufts of cilia the apical surfaces of the ependymal cells with their felt-like microvillous protrusions are evident (Figure 8–2).

It should be mentioned that many of the published studies on the appearance of the surfaces of cells in the ependyma have employed air-dried material, which leads to an agglutination of the cilia. Critical point drying (Anderson, 1951) produces more discrete images, and this technique should be used in preference to air-drying of tissue to be examined in a scanning electron microscope. Studies using the critical point drying technique include those of Coates (1973a), Allen and Low (1973), Hoyosa and Fujita (1973), and Peters (1974).

The significance of these differences in the distribution of cilia in the ventricles is not understood, and it would be worthwhile to make a complete survey of the ventricular surface in a brain to determine if regional differences in ciliary pattern can be correlated with the movements of cerebrospinal fluid.

In transmission electron microscope prep-

Figure 8–1. **The Ependyma.**

Ependymal cells have rather light nuclei (*Nuc*) in which the chromatin is evenly dispersed. Sometimes a filamentous inclusion (*f*) is present. The cytoplasm is also light and contains mitochondria (*mit*) and a Golgi apparatus (*G*). At their apical ends the cells show rather short and uneven microvilli (*mv*), as well as tufts of cilia (*cil*). The cilia arise from basal bodies (*bb*) and these sometimes have fibrillogranular aggregates (*fg*) associated with them.

In the subependymal layer are both astrocytic (*As*) and microglial (*M*) processes. This layer sometimes contains labyrinthine spaces which are occupied by a basal lamina (*B*) that is apparently derived from adjacent capillaries. Some of the profiles at the apical surfaces of these cells appear to be axons (*Ax*).

Rat lateral ventricle. × *12,000.*

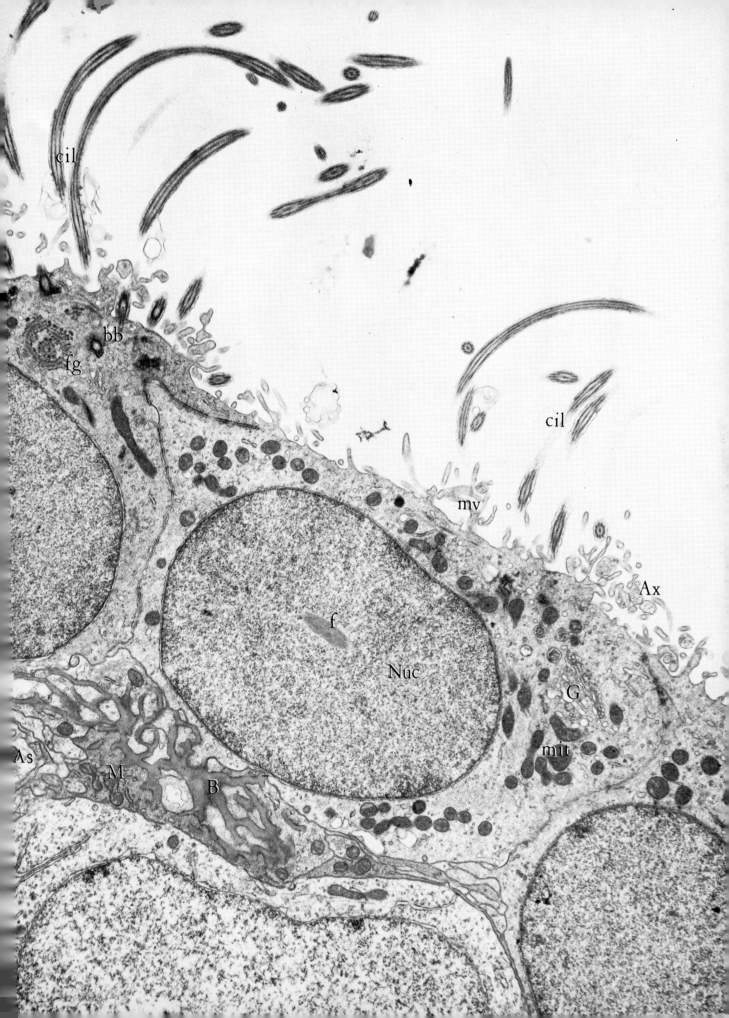

arations the lateral surfaces of the ependymal cells are relatively simple in form, but the plasma membranes of neighboring cells may interdigitate and exhibit pits and vesicles, some of which are coated (Figures 8–4 and 8–5). Near the apices of the cells, light microscope examination shows the presence of terminal bars, and with the electron microscope it is apparent that these consist of two types of junction, *gap junctions* and *fasciae* or *zonulae adhaerentes* (Brightman and Palay, 1963; Klinkerfuss, 1964; Brightman, 1965a; Brightman and Reese, 1969; Blakemore and Jolly, 1972). The fasciae adhaerentes, which are more extensive junctions than zonulae adhaerentes (Brightman, 1965a), occur in groups of two and three in the rat (Brightman and Palay, 1963), but in the cat they appear to involve a more extensive area of the apposed faces of ependymal cells (Klinkerfuss, 1964). These junctions (Figures 8–4 and 8–5), at which adjacent plasma membranes are separated by a distance of about 23 nm, seem to completely encircle the cells. Each junction is made prominent by the 30-nm thick plaque of dense material applied to the cytoplasmic surfaces of each of the participating plasma membranes (Figures 8–4 and 8–5, *za*). The gap junctions, which were originally thought to be zonulae occludentes (Brightman and Palay, 1963; Westergaard, 1970), occasionally occur at the ventricular end of the interface between adjacent ependymal cells, but more frequently they are situated between two fasciae adhaerentes, at some distance from the free surfaces of the cells and independent of the fasciae. These junctions do not form a complete girdle around the ependymal cells and so do not occur in every section of the ependymal cell interface. Often they occur where one cell bulges into its neighbor to form a stud-like adhesion (Figure 8–5, *g*). The outer surfaces of the apposed plasma membranes are separated by a gap of 2 to 3 nm that is open to penetration by horseradish peroxidase and by lanthanum (Brightman and Reese, 1969).

At their basal ends the lateral surfaces of adjacent ependymal cells may be separated by a band of dense material which is contained in a space with many finger-like processes indenting into the ependymal cells (Figure 8–1, *B*). Booz and Desaga (1973) refer to these spaces as basal membrane labyrinths and state that the material contained in them originates from the basement membranes of capillaries situated nearby (see also Westergaard, 1970). It should also be mentioned that sheet-like cytoplasmic processes sometimes extend from the basal ends of ependymal cells. Such cytoplasmic processes extend laterally and so pass beneath adjacent ependymal cells, separating them from the underlying subependymal layer, which in the lateral ventricle of the rat appears to consist mainly of the processes of astrocytes and microglial cells (Figure 8–1).

It should be noted that while the majority of ependymal cells have gap junctions between their lateral faces, as described above, in certain areas tight junctions, or *zonulae occludentes,* do exist. Examples of such areas are those overlying the area postrema and the median eminence (Brightman and Reese, 1969).

The nuclei of ependymal cells usually have a simple, regular, oval shape. They occupy a relatively large portion of the cell volume and usually lie in a central position. The nucleolus is commonly eccentric and embedded in a rather light and finely granular chromatin, which may contain a filamentous inclusion (Hirano and Zimmerman, 1967; and Figure 8–1, *f*). In the cytoplasm the usual galaxy of organelles is to be found, although these may have an uneven distribution (Figures 8–1 and 8–3 to 8–5). For example, the mitochondria, which generally have an elongate form and resemble those of astrocytes, are most numerous at the apical poles of the cells. This arrangement is reflected by the distribution of succinic dehydrogenase in ependymal cells (Friede and Pax, 1961; Chason and Pearse, 1961; Thomas and Pearse, 1961). The Golgi complex is also largely confined to the apical portion of each cell and overlies the nucleus. It consists of the usual system of flattened cisternae surrounded by numerous small vesicles. These small vesicles resemble many others that occupy the cytoplasm and form part of the extensive smooth endoplasmic reticulum. In contrast, the granular endoplasmic reticulum is rather sparse and consists of

Figure 8-2. **Ependymal Surface.**

In scanning electron microscope preparations the ventricular surface of each ependymal cell shows a tuft of cilia (*cil*) rising out of a field of short microvilli (*mv*). This material was dried by the critical point method.
Rat lateral ventricle. × *13,500.*

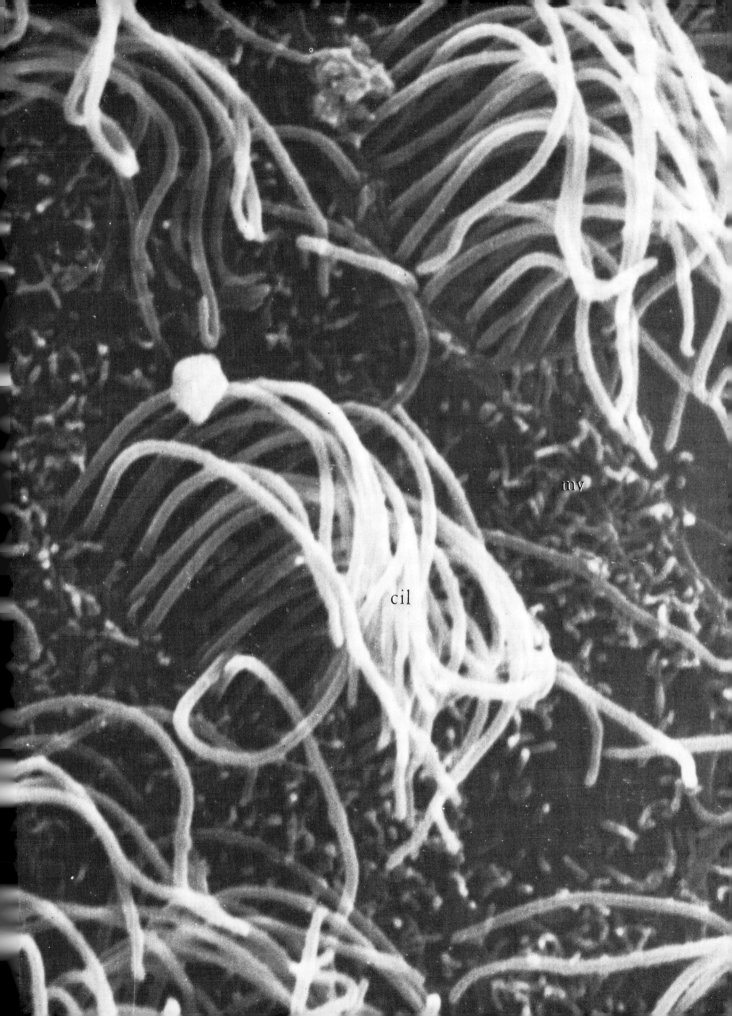

only a few small cisternae, although clusters of free ribosomes are widely distributed in the cytoplasm.

The most conspicuous organelles of the ependymal cells are the 8- to 10-nm filaments (Figures 8–3 and 8–4), which are sometimes arranged in large fascicles that swirl through the cytoplasm. In their dimensions and in the manner in which they form bundles, these filaments resemble those in the cytoplasm of astrocytes (see page 234) and serve to accentuate the similarity in appearance of astrocytes and ependymal cells. In addition to these bundles, however, similar filaments run as individuals or in smaller fascicles of 4 to 10 members throughout the cytoplasm, interlacing with all the other organelles (Figure 8–4). They even extend into the superficial cytoplasm at the bases of the microvillous folds. Besides these 8- to 10-nm filaments the cytoplasm is pervaded by a cottony network of microfilaments which provide the cytoplasm with a matrix of homogeneous density (Figure 8–4). These microfilaments tend to be concentrated beneath the plasma membrane of the microvilli, where they may be considered to form a kind of terminal web (Figure 8–3). Microtubules are relatively sparse in these cells and show no preferred orientation.

Osmiophilic, dense bodies are also a feature of the cytoplasm of ependymal cells. In the main, these dense bodies are of two varieties and occur in the apical cytoplasm. One variety contains both fine granules and somewhat larger granules that Brightman and Palay (1963) suggest might be ferritin. The second variety of dense body has a heterogeneous content of granules, vesicles, and lamellae; these are probably lysosomes.

THE MORPHOLOGY OF TANYCYTES

The basal ends of cells in the ependyma are variable, and depending upon their form, Tennyson and Pappas (1964) distinguish three types of cell: (1) simple ependymal cells of the type just described, which have flattened or ovoid bases, (2) ependymal tanycytes, which are ependymal cells with long, radially oriented and unbranched basal processes, and (3) ependymal astrocytes which have a basal process that branches several times. The basal process of the latter two types of cell reach at least as far as the subependymal capillaries, where they form endfeet separated from the endothelial walls by a basal membrane (Leonhardt, 1966; Hirano and Zimmerman, 1967). The ependymal tanycytes, which may even extend to the outer surface of the brain, are the concern of this section. As noted above, tanycytes were first recognized in the brains of elasmobranchs (Horstmann, 1954), in which the walls of the brain are relatively thin. They also constitute the principle supporting, or neuroglial, element in the hagfish and lamprey, which have an avascular central nervous system. In mammals tanycytes have been encountered principally in the walls of the third ventricle; especially in the thin floor.

In Golgi preparations of the walls of the third ventricle of rodents, Millhouse (1971) showed that tanycytes occur in clusters. For the purposes of description, each tanycyte can be regarded as consisting of a somatic, a neck, and a tail portion. The somatic portion lies in the ependyma and contains the nucleus. This part of the cell frequently has many lateral cytoplasmic extensions, as does the neck portion that sticks into the periventricular layer of neuropil, where it appears to contact a blood vessel. According to Millhouse (1972) the tail portion is devoid of cy-

Figure 8–3. **The Cilia of Ependymal Cells.**

Each ependymal cell has a tuft of cilia. Each cilium contains long microtubules (*m*) which take origin from a basal body (*bb*) that has a laterally protruding basal foot (*arrow*) and a ciliary rootlet (*x*). The striated rootlet may be confused with the fibrillogranular aggregates (*fg*) which also lie in the apical cytoplasm. These aggregates show a core of fibrillar material bounded on each side by evenly spaced granules.

The apical end of the ependymal cell shows mitochondria (*mit*), short cisternae of the granular endoplasmic reticulum (*ER*), free ribosomes (*r*), vesicles (*v*), microtubules (m_1), and multivesicular bodies (*mvb*), which are embedded in a cytoplasm containing thin filaments often aggregated into bundles (*f*).
Rat lateral ventricle. × 38,000.

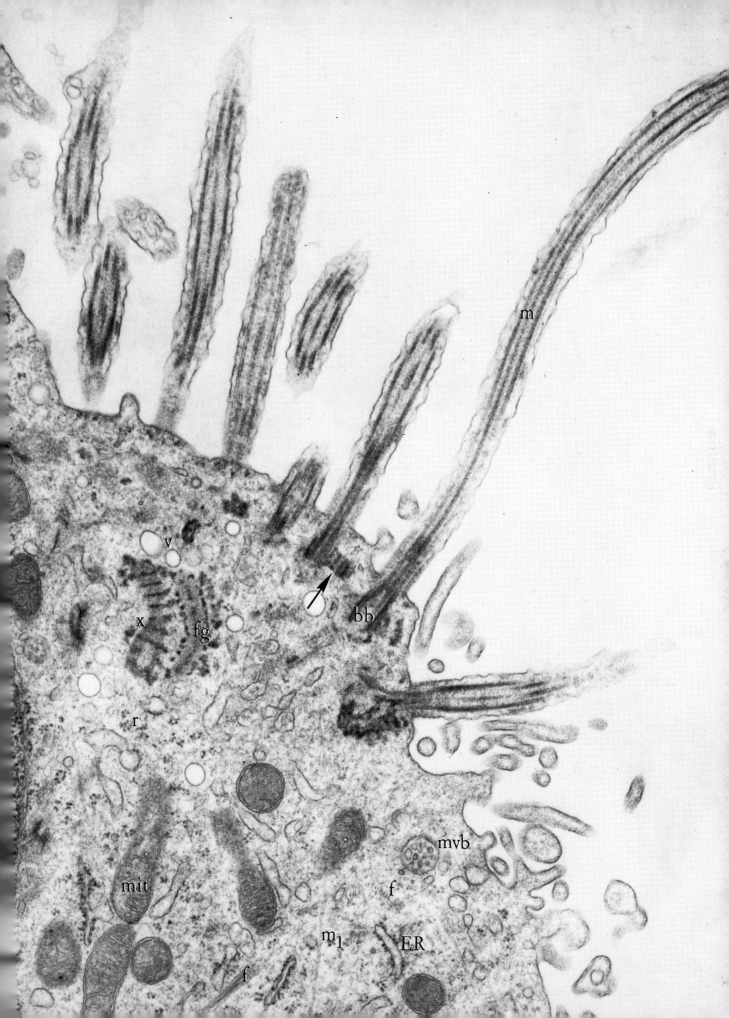

toplasmic extensions and courses through the hypothalamic nuclei to form small bulbous swellings, or end-feet, that terminate either on blood vessels or at the pial surface of the brain. Thus, these cells have some resemblance to astrocytes.

In another study of the morphology of tanycytes, Bleier (1971) used the Golgi-Cox method of impregnation to show that in a number of animals the tails, or basal processes, of tanycytes in the third ventricle extended into every cell group of the hypothalamus. Unlike Millhouse (1971), she found a great variation in the form of the tail processes, for although some were smooth, others bore spines and knobs. Also, while some cells had unbranched processes, others had processes that divided to form two or three thinner ones. A large number of the processes appeared to end on capillaries and neurons.

The clustering of tanycytes is confirmed in electron microscope studies (Leonhardt, 1966; Millhouse, 1972; Brawer, 1972). These studies show the tanycytes to have irregular or oval-shaped nuclei that contrast with the well-rounded nuclei of ependymal cells. Also the cytoplasm of the tanycytes may be somewhat darker than that of ependymal cells because of a rather flocculent, dark matrix (Millhouse, 1972), although such a difference in density is less obvious in the study by Brawer (1972). Other differences from ependymal cells are that swirling bundles of filaments are not present in the cytoplasm of tanycytes, while microtubules are more common. The cytoplasm of tanycytes contains free ribosomes arranged in groups, and the granular endoplasmic reticulum is represented by only a few, isolated cisternae. Profiles of the Golgi apparatus are numerous, and lysosomes are a common feature.

The ventricular surfaces of tanycytes have many thin, and occasionally branching, cytoplasmic extensions of relatively uniform dimensions projecting into the ventricle. These are rather like those of ependymal cells, but more nu-

merous. Sometimes the cytoplasmic processes appear to fuse at their tips to enclose drops of cerebrospinal fluid. Cilia are less common than at the apices of ependymal cells.

The wispy processes that are seen to arise from the apical soma and neck regions of tanycytes in Golgi preparations are recognized in the electron microscope as thin processes that interweave with those of adjacent tanycytes. These processes form plications which are frequently oriented parallel with the surface of the ventricle, and zonulae adhaerentes occur between them. Similar interdigitating processes exist between the lateral surfaces of embryonic ependymal cells (Tennyson and Pappas, 1962), but in the adult, the lateral surfaces are smoother.

Profiles of unmyelinated axons and dendrites are frequently wedged between the tanycytes' somata (Millhouse, 1972; Brawer, 1972). Sometimes a small fascicle of neuronal processes may be entirely surrounded by tanycytes, but more frequently, astrocytic processes partially separate the fascicles from the tanycytes. Millhouse (1972) failed to find any synapses involving a cell in the ependyma and the neuronal processes passing between them. Astrocytes also stretch between the basal portions of tanycytes and seem to form sheaths around their necks.

In his study, Brawer (1972) found the peripheral processes of tanycytes to be long and tapering and to project through the neuropil of the arcuate nucleus to form end-feet on either arcuate capillaries or at the surface of the brain lateral to the median eminence. These processes are distinguished from other elements of the arcuate nucleus by many longitudinally oriented microtubules running parallel to their lengths. The processes are rather irregular in shape and, in addition to microtubules, contain oriented mitochondria, lipid droplets, and accumulations of smooth endoplasmic reticulum in the form of concentric lamellae arranged in rings.

The peripheral processes of tanycytes

Figure 8–4. **Ependymal Cell Cytoplasm.**

The ependymal cells in this picture display the filamentous components of the cytoplasm. At the apical surface the cells show a microfilamentous (*mf*) network. This network pervades the entire cytoplasm, producing a cottony background. Other filaments are rather thicker (*f*) and aggregate into fascicles that swirl through the cytoplasm. The apical end of the intercellular junction (*J*) is marked by zonulae adhaerentes (*za*). Lower down the apposed plasma membranes show no junctional specializations. It is common, however, to observe coated vesicles (*cv*) in this region. *Rat lateral ventricle.* × 26,000.

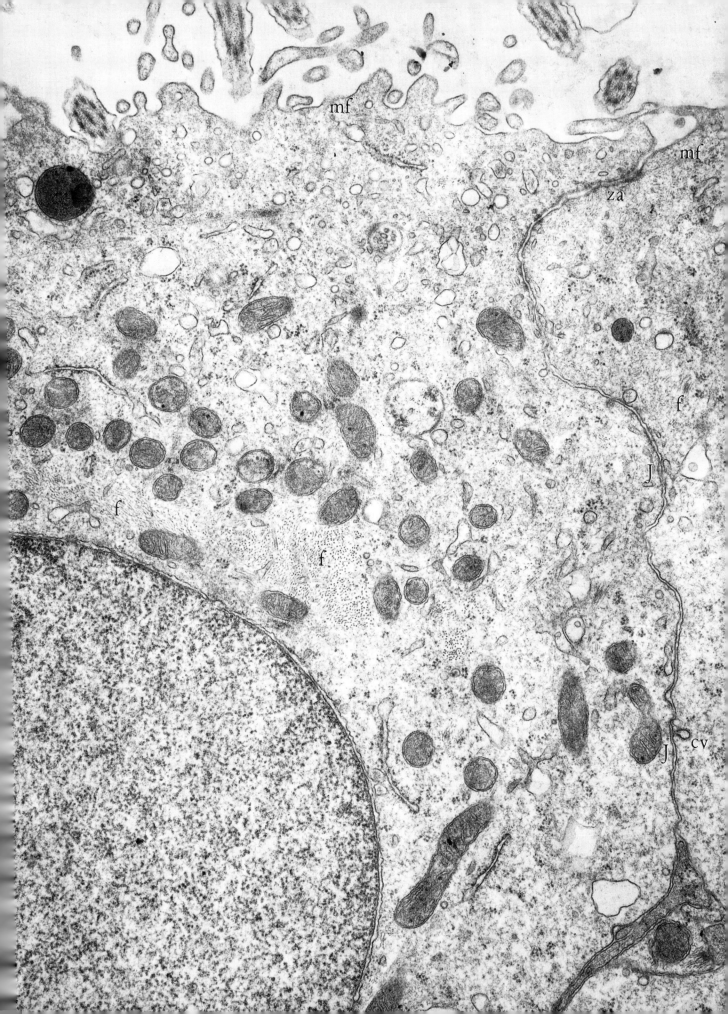

which form end-feet at the surfaces of blood vessels are separated from the endothelial cells by a basal lamina, in much the same fashion as astrocytic end-feet. Knigge and Scott (1970) state that processes of tanycytes from the infundibular recess of the third ventricle abut the capillary perivascular space and contain a spectrum of irregularly shaped vesicles and inclusions. These authors also conclude that terminals of the arcuate-tuberoinfundibular fibers come into contact with tanycytes and neuroglial cells and fre-

quently form junctions that resemble chemical synapses. Brawer (1972) also found some of the pericapillary tanycyte processes to contain vesicles and granules. These were sparse in some end-feet but abundant in others. The inclusions in the end-feet do not constitute a uniform population, for many of them appear to be short tubules of smooth endoplasmic reticulum, while others are circular, elliptical, club-shaped, or pleomorphic.

INTRAVENTRICULAR NERVE ENDINGS

In their description of the ependyma of the rat, Brightman and Palay (1963) called attention to groups of neuronal processes between the lateral aspects of adjacent ependymal cells and to some neuronal processes lying at the free surface of the ependyma. Similar fine intraventricular processes have also been observed by Rinne (1966) and by Leonhardt and his coworkers.

In the third and fourth ventricles of the brain of the rabbit, Leonhardt and Lindner (1967) encountered a great number of unmyelinated nerve fibers (Figure 8–1, Ax), some in bundles that run parallel to the ventricular surface where they form bulb-like endings containing both clear (40 to 80 nm) and dense-cored (65 to 100 nm) vesicles. Similar results have been obtained by Westergaard (1972), who examined the lateral ventricles of rats. Other endings of nerve fibers (Leonhardt and Prien, 1968) contain large numbers of long and thin mitochondria which are unusual in each having a single crista oriented parallel to the length of the mitochondrion. These nerve endings appear to form synapse-like contacts with ependymal cells (Leonhardt and Backhus-Roth, 1969), although the vesicles in the nerve endings are not conspicuously accumulated close to the site of contact. Other contacts between nerve endings and ependymal cells resemble maculae adhaerentes (desmosomes) and the impression is gained that the relation between the nerve endings and the ependymal cells is like that between nerve fibers and smooth muscle cells or glands, rather than the type of chemical synapse that is typically present between two neuronal components. Sometimes the nerve fibers are myelinated (Leonhardt, 1968), and as the myelin sheath is lost, a fiber appears to branch and to approximate the surfaces of ependymal cells.

In addition to the small, bulb-like endings on the anterior wall of the fourth ventricle—opposite the area postrema—Leonhardt (1967b) found nerve cells with large swellings, or bulbs, protruding into the ventricle. Each swelling contains large numbers of mitochondria, as well as clear and dense-cored vesicles, and in the lateral ventricles of the rat brain Richards, Lorez, and Tranzer (1973) showed that the nerve terminals selectively accumulate 5-hydroxydopamine, which indicates that they are monoaminergic. In another study using formaldehyde-induced fluorescence Lorez and Richards (1973) studied the distribution of these supraependymal nerve terminals, and on the basis of assessing the factors which affect the fluorescence, they concluded that the transmitter in the terminals is probably 5-hydroxytryptamine. The perikarya of the neurons forming the swellings are synapsed upon by small axon terminals. Somewhat similar neuronal bulbs are also present at the surface of the paraventricular organ of the soft-shelled turtle (Takeichi, 1967). The paraventricular organ is situated two-thirds of the way up the wall of the third ventricle and the tips of the bulbs in this region also contain both clear and dense-cored vesicles. In both cases, the authors consider that the vesicles contained in these bulbs might be discharged into the cerebrospinal fluid, although what is being secreted is unknown.

More complex endings protruding into the ventricles are encountered in lower vertebrates and for a further discussion of these structures reference should be made to the reviews by Agduhr (1932) and Fleischhauer (1972) and to the article by Vigh-Teichmann, Vigh, and Koritsanszky (1970).

THE SUBEPENDYMA

In mature carnivores and primates, the ependyma of most regions of the cerebral ventricles is separated from a layer of large astrocytic perikarya by a feltwork of astrocytic processes. The astrocytes and their processes make up the framework of the subependymal layer (Figure 8–1, *As*). Fleischhauer (1972) described the numerous astrocytic processes beneath the ependyma as being well oriented. In some parts of the third ventricle, for example, the processes are mainly oriented parallel to the surface of the ventricle, while in other regions, two or more systems of astrocytic processes cross over each other. Some regional differences in the structure and orientation of subependymal astrocytes are also discussed by Merker (1970).

As pointed out earlier (see page 264), in some parts of the ventricular wall and particularly in the anterior horn of the lateral ventricles of mammals, the subependymal layer contains small cells. In the mature rat at the angle between the caudate nucleus and the corpus callosum (Privat and Leblond, 1972) this subependyma is three to five cells deep and separated from the lumen of the ventricle by a single layer of ependymal cells. On its other side the subependymal layer is covered by a narrow border layer that separates it from the underlying neuropil. Privat and Leblond (1972) describe the subependymal cells as being smaller than ependymal cells and having darker nuclei. The observation that the subependymal cells are often in mitosis fits in with the tritiated thymidine studies showing the subependyma to be an actively proliferating zone postnatally, and indeed this layer seems to be a remnant of the embryonic subventricular zone that produces many cells in the later phases of embryonic brain development. According to Globus and Kuhlenbeck (1944), these active cells may be a source of certain forms of brain tumor.

Blakemore and Jolly (1972) studied the ependyma and subependyma in the anterior part of the caudate nucleus of the dog. They found that in addition to the small and dark cells which are sometimes referred to as "subependymal plate cells," the subependyma also contains cells with pale nuclei. This latter group of cells seems to be composed of a mix of astrocyte-like cells, tanycytes, and ectopic ependymal cells. The latter possess both cilia and microvilli, but these do not extend to the ventricular surface; they either fit between adjacent cells, or extend into small cystic cavities unconnected with the ventricles (see also Westergaard, 1970). Both dark and pale cells are sometimes concentrated into nests containing up to 30 or more cells. Some nests contain only pale cells or dark cells, while others contain mixtures of the two. Blakemore and Jolly (1972) also record the presence of cells in mitosis in the subependymal layer.

Blakemore (1969a), Stensaas and Gilson (1972), and Privat and Leblond (1972) have all identified microglia in the subependymal layer (Figure 8–1, *M*). In the border between the subependymal layer and the underlying neuropil Privat and Leblond (1972) find many scattered elements among neuronal and neuroglial processes which appear to be neuroblasts, or astrocytes, or cells with features intermediate between subependymal cells and oligodendrocytes. Privat and Leblond (1972) conclude that the subependymal layer is composed of actively dividing immature cells, whose progeny migrate through the border layer. They begin to differentiate in this layer before ultimately entering the neural tissue to complete their differentiation (see also Paterson, Privat, Ling, and Leblond, 1973). Perhaps not all cells produced by the subependymal layer migrate into the neural tissue, however, for Blakemore and Jolly (1972) consider that some of the pale cells undergoing division might be used to replace cells of the ependyma.

From the discussion given by Fleischhauer (1972) it is clear that there are many regional differences in the morphology of the ventricular wall with respect to both the shapes of ependymal cells and the length of their cilia, as well as in the composition of the underlying subependymal layer. These differences are strongly accentuated in certain areas of the ventricles, where the so-called ventricular organs occur. These organs are the hypophysis, pineal gland, subcommissural organ, subfornical organ, area postrema, and the vascular organs of the hypothalamus and the lamina terminalis (supraoptic crest). In contrast to other parts of the brain, all of these regions stain with vital dyes such as trypan blue, and their blood supply is described as thin-walled sinusoids which often loop in arcades (Duvernoy and Koritké, 1965). The reader is referred to the article by Fleischhauer (1972) for a further discussion of this topic, for almost nothing is known of these regional differences at the electron microscope level.

Note should be made of the observation by Leonhardt (1970) that in the wall of the posterior horn of the lateral ventricle of the rabbit brain the subependymal layer beneath the simple cuboidal ependymal cells contains many large capillaries and veins. These are surrounded by a basement membrane and lie in labyrinthine spaces that are also lined by a basement membrane.

FUNCTIONS OF CELLS IN THE EPENDYMA

In considering the functions of cells in the ependyma, it is difficult to determine in some instances whether the author is referring to ependymal cells proper, or to tanycytes in the sense defined in this account. Hence, there is frequently some confusion about the type of cell being considered. However, a brief summary of the functions that have been proposed for cells in the ependyma may be discussed in terms of the following headings.

MOVEMENTS OF CEREBROSPINAL FLUID

The cilia of the ependymal cells are known to beat rapidly during life, and it is believed that their activity may bring about movements of the cerebrospinal fluid in the ventricles (Cathcart and Worthington, 1964).

PROLIFERATION

As pointed out earlier, the ependyma is derived from the ventricular zone of the embryonic nervous system, and this is the zone from which an active proliferation of cells takes place early in development. Later some of this proliferative activity is assumed by the subventricular zone that forms the subependymal layer of the mature brain. In some areas, notably the angle between the pallium and the caudate nucleus of the lateral ventricles, the subependymal layer remains mitotically active in the brains of young mature mammals (Lewis, 1968a and b) and seems to be a source of neuroglial cells. In experiments in which tritiated thymidine was injected over a period of 30 days, Kraus-Ruppert, Laissue, Bürki, and Odartchenko (1973) showed that up to 60 per cent of the cells in the subependyma of the lateral ventricles of young adult mice became labelled. In addition, Privat (1970) injected tritiated thymidine into the ventricles and found the subependymal cells to be labelled with increasing time after injection. Cells in the caudate nucleus and corpus callosum were found to be labelled. These studies indicate that some glial cells originate in the subependyma postnatally and then migrate into surrounding structures (see also Privat and Leblond, 1972). In lower animals, more of the subependyma seems to retain a generative capacity and appears to be even capable of regenerating parts of the brain that have been experimentally ablated.

SUPPORT

Whether the ependyma of mammals has a supporting function, much like that attributed to astrocytes, is uncertain. It has been held that the long processes of the tanycytes give some support to the brain, especially in the lower vertebrates (Agduhr, 1932), and in the opinion of Merker (1970) the well-oriented processes in the subependyma of primates prevents collapse of the ventricular lumen.

Figure 8–5. **Ependymal Cell Junctions.**

The junctions between ependymal cells are rather complex. At the ventricular and basal ends are zonulae adhaerentes (*za*) which may occur in a series. These appear to encircle the cells. Between them, a cell can indent its neighbor to produce a stud-like arrangement, where the adjacent plasma membranes form a gap junction (*g*). These cells also display the cottony cytoplasmic matrix in which mitochondria (*mit*), the Golgi apparatus (*G*), the granular endoplasmic reticulum (*ER*), and clusters of free ribosomes (*r*) are embedded. Part of the nucleus (*Nuc*) of one cell is shown at the bottom right.
Rat lateral ventricle. × 75,000.

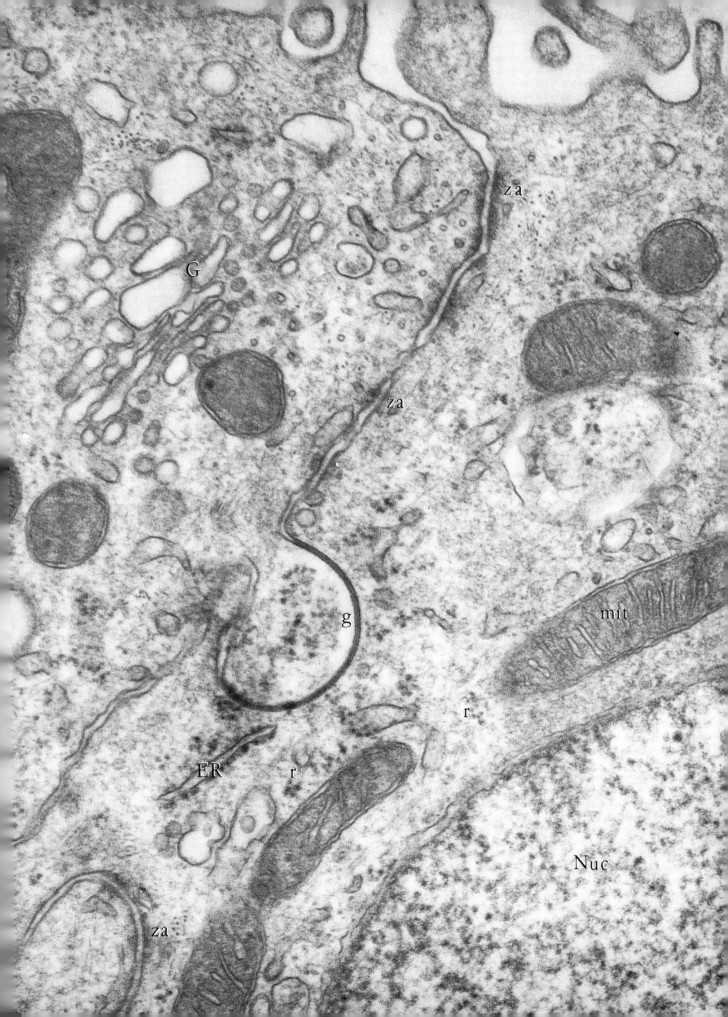

SENSORY FUNCTION

The suggestion that some elements of the ependyma may have a sensory function springs from the early light microscope observations of nerve endings in the ependyma and in the ventricles overlying the ependyma (see Agduhr, 1932). There is no indication of the type of information that might be gleaned by these nerve endings, but in lower vertebrates there are complex nerve endings such as those in the salamander (Arnold, 1970). These nerve endings have bulbs which project into the ventricles and bear stereocilia-like processes, so that the endings have some resemblance to the hair cells on the vestibular epithelium. It is reasonable to suppose that the free nerve endings projecting into a fluid-filled space might be concerned with sensing some specific or general property of the fluid.

SECRETION

Several authors have attributed a secretory function to some ependymal cells, and for a review of the rather extensive literature pertaining to this subject reference should be made to the accounts by Agduhr (1932), Knowles (1972), Fleischhauer (1972), and Leonhardt and Lindemann (1973b). In the present discussion we shall confine ourselves to some of the electron microscope evidence. As pointed out in the description of the nerve endings in the ventricles, some of the neuronal processes extending into the ventricles contain vesicles and granules, which might be discharged into the cerebrospinal fluid. There is little direct evidence for such a secretion, however, and its nature is unknown.

There is more evidence for secretion from ependymal cells overlying specialized areas of the ventricles. Thus, in their consideration of the subfornical organ of the rabbit brain, Leonhardt and Lindemann (1973a) showed that in scanning electron microscope preparations the ventricular surfaces of some cells are covered by a secretory material having an appearance like worm casts. Examination of sectioned tissue indicates that this secretion is derived from the emptying of large vacuoles which occur at the apices of some of the ependymal cells. Other evidence for secretion comes from the experiments presented by Schechter and Weiner (1972), who examined the ependymal cells overlying the median eminence. These authors found that if

epinephrine or dopamine were injected directly into the third ventricle of the rat brain, the ependymal cells in the floor and lateral recess of the third ventricle displayed an increase in the number of bleb-like protrusions at their apical surfaces. The blebs are present in increased numbers up to 5 minutes after the injection, but within 15 minutes they are no longer apparent. Schechter and Weiner (1972) conclude that the blebs represent a secretory process, whereby fragments of the ependymal cell cytoplasm are released into the cerebrospinal fluid.

In this same context, it should be noted that Knowles and Anand-Kumar (1967) have shown bulbous ventricular protrusions of tanycytes to become especially large in female Rhesus monkeys at mid-estrus and to disappear almost completely at, or about, menstruation (see also Knowles, 1972). In addition, Kobayashi, Matsui, and Ishii (1972) state that the ependymal cells of the rat median eminence have cellular protrusions which may absorb substances from the cerebrospinal fluid. They also noted that ovariectomy of rats followed by estrogen treatment leads to an increase in the number of apical protrusions.

In an effort to obtain more information about the function of tanycytes Brawer, Lin, and Sonnenschein (1974) studied the ventricular surfaces of the cells lining the ventral basal region of the third ventricle of the female rat with the scanning electron microscope at different stages in the estrous cycle. At mid-diestrus the surfaces of the tanycytes were devoid of microvilli and other surface extensions. At late diestrus the cells sprouted microvilli that were prominent at the borders of the cells, and these microvilli increased in number during proestrus. They persisted through estrus and then disappeared in early or mid-diestrus, when presumably the cycle continued again. These authors also found the numbers of supraependymal cells to alter. They were most common in early diestrus.

This study seems to indicate that the tanycytes of the third ventricle are sensitive to changing levels of gonadal steroids, although the significance of the cycle of structural events is not known.

TRANSPORT OF SUBSTANCES

As shown by Brightman (1965a and b) and Brightman and Reese (1969), ferritin and horseradish peroxidase injected into the ventricles of the brain pass between ependymal cells to gain access to the intercellular spaces of the underlying neuropil. When labelled substances are injected into the ventricles it is apparent from a number of studies (see Fleischhauer, 1972) that their rates of penetration into the brain are not uniform over the whole ventricular surface. Generally, penetration is deepest into regions composed of gray matter and shallowest into places composed of white matter.

In addition to the passage of materials between ependymal cells, some electron-dense label passes into the ependymal cells to be sequestered into vesicles and multivesicular bodies. It has been suggested that some substances normally present in the cerebrospinal fluid may be handled in this same fashion. The cells especially implicated are the tanycytes of the third ventricle, which it is thought might transport the substances to their end-feet at the surfaces of blood vessels. Thus, the cells in the ependyma overlying the median eminence, where incidentally there are zonulae occludentes between ependymal cells (Brightman and Reese, 1969), have been implicated in relating hypothalamic to adenohypophysial activity on the assumption that cells lining this part of the third ventricle might release substances from their end-feet into the portal vessels that lead primarily to the adenohypophysis (see Löfgren, 1959; Knowles and Anand-Kumar, 1967; Wittkowski, 1969; Scott and Knigge, 1970; Knigge, Scott, and Weindl, 1972). It has been suggested that the tanycytes themselves might produce such substances, or that the tanycytes transport material between the cerebrospinal fluid and the blood (Leonhardt, 1966; Scott and Knigge, 1970; Ondo, Mical, and Porter, 1972). But in either case it must be borne in mind that the end-feet of the tanycytes are separated from the circulating blood by both a basal lamina and the endothelial cells of the vessel walls.

Support for the idea that the tanycytes might be involved in the transport of substances from the ventricles to the blood is largely derived from their morphology. Thus, the apical ends of these cells have many microvillus-like processes, and Kobayashi, Wada, Uemura, and Ueck (1972) have shown that ependymal cells over the median eminence of mice take up peroxidase injected into the ventricle. In addition, the basal ends of tanycytes impinging upon blood vessels contain large numbers of vesicles and granules, rather like those contained in the cytoplasm of neurosecretory cells.

Knigge and Scott (1970) consider it possible that terminals of the arcuate-tuberoinfundibular fibers might form synapses upon the end-feet and processes of both tanycytes and neuroglia in the external zone of the median eminence of the monkey. Wittkowski (1969) also observed the presence of synapse-like contacts between axons of the tuberohypophysial tract and tanycytes in the mouse. Wittkowski considers that at such contacts substances are passed from the nerve endings to the tanycytes. He believes these substances form accumulations of pale vesicles in the tanycytes and eventually become part of the vesicle-containing protrusions at the free surface of ependymal cells before being discharged into the cerebrospinal fluid.

At present it is clear that the role of tanycytes in transporting substances between the cerebrospinal fluid and either the blood or the neuropil is largely based upon conjecture. A great deal of circumstantial evidence seems to be in favor of tanycytes playing such a role, however, and this area deserves continued attention.

Chapter IX

CHOROID PLEXUS

In the following description, the term choroid plexus will be used to refer to a vascular fold of the pia mater covered on its outer surface by an epithelium derived from the ependymal lining (lamina epithelialis) of the ventricles. The vascular fold of the pia mater contains blood vessels embedded in a connective tissue stroma, and in some texts this vascular fold alone is referred to as the choroid plexus, while this together with the epithelium is named the tela choroidea. This latter terminology is more accurate, but the term choroid plexus, as used here to include both the pial and the epithelial components, is the most widely used term in current texts.

There are four choroid plexuses, one each in the roofs of the third and fourth ventricles and in the medial wall of each lateral ventricle. At its free edge a choroid plexus is invaginated into the ventricle, and its surface is greatly increased by many fine frond-like projections (Figure 9–1). Such a frond consists of tiny villous processes composed of an enclosing single layer of epithelial cells surrounding a central core containing a capillary and a small amount of loose connective tissue. Supplying each choroid plexus are arteries. These break up into the capillaries, one to each villus, which then join together to form an efferent vein. All of these blood vessels are supported by a connective tissue stroma. An historical review of the choroid plexus has recently been presented by Dohrmann (1970).

During development the pia mater, along with blood vessels present in the subarachnoid space, invades the roof of the third and fourth ventricles and the medial walls of the cerebral hemispheres. In these sites it pushes the epithelial lining of the ventricles in front of it so that the whole structure bulges into the ventricle. At this early phase (see Shuangshoti and Netsky, 1966; Netsky and Shuangshoti, 1970; Kappers, 1958; Tennyson and Pappas, 1968) the choroid plexus is a simple fold covered by a pseudostratified, columnar epithelium, while the mesenchymatous stroma is filled with blood cells and strands of angioblasts forming capillaries. Next the choroid plexus becomes lobulated, and in the case of the cerebral hemispheres, it almost fills each lateral ventricle. At this time, the epithelium comes to consist of only a single

---

Figure 9–1. **Scanning Electron Micrographs of the Choroid Plexus.**

In the **upper micrograph,** the choroid plexus dissected from the lateral ventricle is seen to consist of a series of more or less longitudinal folds of variable length. Their surfaces display rounded protrusions, each one of which is a choroidal cell. *Lateral ventricle of adult rat.* × *350.*

The **lower micrograph** shows the surfaces of the choroidal cells at a higher magnification. Each cell is domed and has thin, irregular, and tightly packed microvilli. *Lateral ventricle of adult rat.* × *8000.*

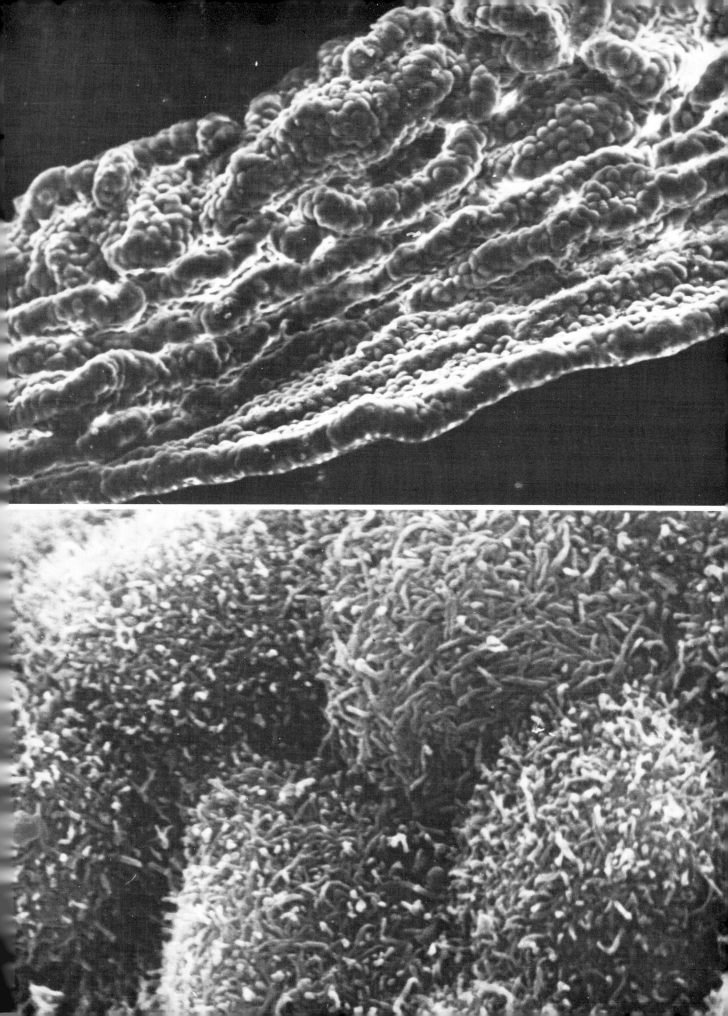

layer of cells that are rich in glycogen (Tennyson and Pappas, 1964). During the later phases of growth the epithelial cells, although still containing glycogen, come to resemble those of the mature animal, for they assume a cuboidal or squamous shape. By now the choroid plexus is lobulated and starts to develop the numerous fronds and villi which characterize the mature structure. Concomitant with these alterations in the epithelium, the fibrillar connective tissue appears and the amorphous ground substance of the stroma decreases. Because of the origin of the vascular core of the choroid plexus, it is assumed that the central core of connective tissue

is arachnoidal in origin, while the stroma of the villi arises from the pia mater.

For the purposes of description, the choroid plexus, whose fine structure has been presented by a number of authors (e.g., Dempsey and Wislocki, 1955; Van Breemen and Clemente, 1955; Millen and Rogers, 1956; Maxwell and Pease, 1956; Wislocki and Ladman, 1958; Case, 1959; Millen and Woollam, 1962; Tennyson and Pappas, 1961, 1964, and 1968; Davis, Lloyd, and Milhorat, 1973), may be regarded as consisting of two parts. These are the choroidal epithelium and the vascularized core of connective tissue.

THE CHOROIDAL EPITHELIUM

The choroidal epithelium of the brain has basically a simple cuboidal structure, although foci of pseudostratification and stratification seem to be still present (Netsky and Shuangshoti, 1970). The rather pale and rounded nuclei are located in the centers of the cells and have relatively homogeneous chromatin. At their free luminal surfaces the cells have uneven borders consisting of thin cytoplasmic processes which are very like irregular and tightly packed microvilli (Figures 9–1 to 9–3, *mv*). However, the surface projections are too pleomorphic to be considered as constituting a brush or stratified border. Cilia are consistently present, and while they may occur singly, they are more often found in groups of three or more (Figure 9–5). The cilia originate from basal bodies embedded in the apical cytoplasm of the cells. In most studies, the cilia are described as having a 9 plus 2 configuration, but in the cat, Santolaya and Rodríguez-Echandía (1968) report that while the peripheral 9 pairs of microtubules are present, the central pair is replaced by filaments, so that the cilia have a 9 plus 0 form known to occur in some neurons and sensory cells (see pages

43 to 44). The same is also true of the cilia of the rat choroid plexus.

In scanning electron microscope studies (Clementi and Morini, 1972; Scott, Paull, and Dudley, 1972; Chamberlain, 1973; Scott, Kozlowski, Paull, Ramalingen, and Dudley, 1973; Peters, 1974) the individual choroidal epithelial cells appear as well-defined bulges, each about 10 microns in diameter, forming a rather regular pattern of domes on the surface of the choroid plexus (Figure 9–1). These ventricular surfaces of the epithelial cells show many fine and irregular projections that are the cytoplasmic processes seen in transmission electron microscope studies. In the adult animal, the cilia cannot be differentiated from the other projections of the cell surface for they are of similar width and length.

In both the transmission and scanning electron microscope preparations some of the cells have rather more bulbous surface projections. In the transmission electron microscope preparations such projections are associated with cells having a somewhat more lucent cytoplasm than others. These are probably the more actively

---

Figure 9–2. **The Choroid Plexus.**

Microvilli (*mv*) project from the ventricular surfaces of the choroid cells. The basal ends of the cells rest on the basal lamina (*B*), beneath which is a thin layer of attenuated cell processes (*x*). Deeper still are endothelial cells (*End*) making up the walls of a fenestrated capillary (*Cap*). The choroidal cells have pale nuclei (*Nuc*), and mitochondria (*mit*) are concentrated at their apical ends. The Golgi apparatus (G) is represented by small stacks of cisternae. Also conspicuous in the cytoplasm are short cisternae of the granular endoplasmic reticulum (*ER*) and many clear vesicles (*v*). The cell on the left contains two lysosomes (*Ly*). The intercellular junction (*J*) displays many complex infoldings (arrow) at its basal end.
The lateral ventricle of adult rat. × 12,000.

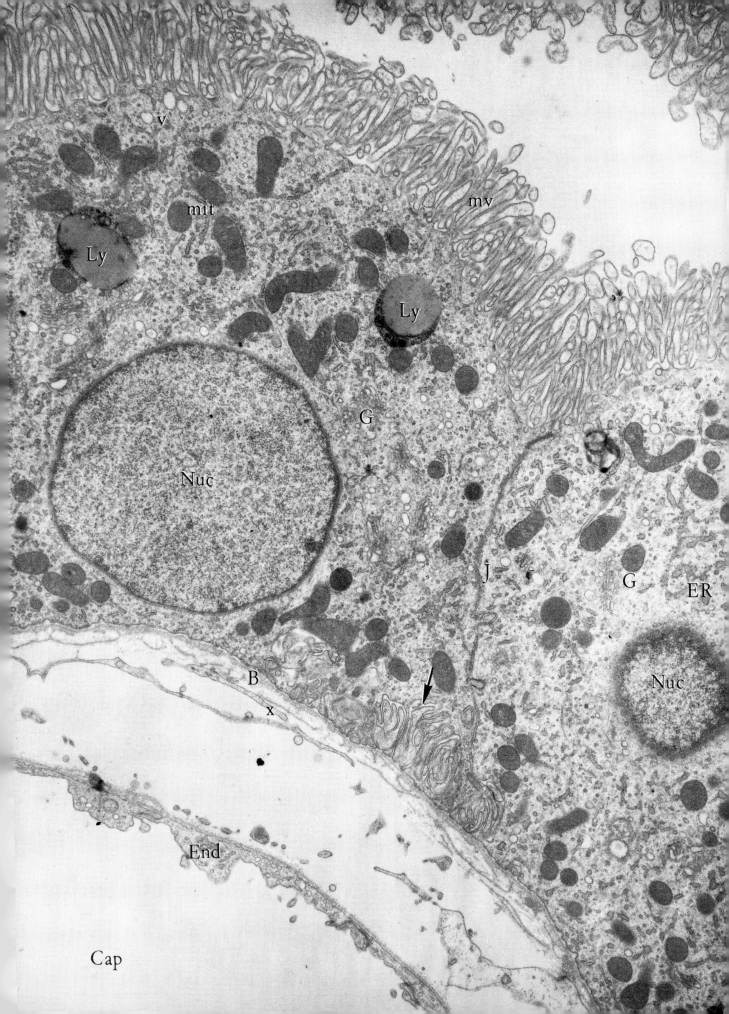

secreting cells, for Santolaya and Rodríguez-Echandía (1968) have shown that if cerebrospinal fluid production is stimulated by pilocarpine injection, the microvilli at the apical ends of the choroidal epithelial cells become more regular in shape and size. Stimulation by extraction of cerebrospinal fluid from the ventricles leads to an increase in the luminal surface, which becomes organized into a complex labyrinth of ridges and microvilli with expanded tips. Injection of adenosine triphosphatase (ATPase) into the ventricles produces a similar effect to cerebrospinal fluid extraction, and in each experimental condition there is an increase in the intercellular gaps between the lateral surfaces of the cells. Because of these changes that can be brought about in the appearance of the luminal surfaces of choroidal epithelial cells, Santolaya and Rodríguez-Echandía (1968) suggest that the elaborations are transient and indicative of a highly dynamic surface.

The cytoplasm of the choroidal epithelial cells is light, although some cells are more watery in appearance than others (Figure 9–2). Large numbers of mitochondria are present, and these seem to be most concentrated at the apical ends of the cells (Figures 9–2 and 9–4). It is assumed that the mitochondria are responsible for the high respiratory metabolism of the epithelial cells and that they provide the energy necessary for the active transport which the cells undertake during their secretion of cerebrospinal fluid. The granular endoplasmic reticulum consists of short, irregular and dilated cisternae which are studded with ribosomes and occur throughout the cytoplasm where they have clustered ribosomes scattered between them (Figure 9–3, ER). The Golgi apparatus is rather ill-defined and is represented by numerous small stacks of cisternae which are prominent at the apical ends and sides of the nucleus. The smooth endoplasmic reticulum is represented by a large number of tubules and vesicles which are most prominent in the more lucent cells

(Figure 9–2). Throughout the cytoplasm many clear vesicles, 30 to 40 nm in diameter, are encountered. Such vesicles are especially numerous at the apical ends of the cells where many of them are coated and occur in the cytoplasm in the angles between the bases of the cytoplasmic processes (Figures 9–3 and 9–4, cv). Here they are embedded in a cytoplasm through which pass thin microfilaments preferentially oriented parallel to the cell surface rather like those at the apices of absorptive cells in the small intestine (Figures 9–3 to 9–6, mf). In some choroidal epithelial cells these microfilaments seem to form part of a system of filaments that are also aggregated into bundles which pass in the perinuclear cytoplasm more or less parallel to the surface of the nuclear envelope.

Most of the clear vesicles in the cytoplasm of the choroidal epithelial cells seem to take origin, by pinocytosis, from the basal ends of the cells (Figure 9–6) and then move to the luminal surface to be discharged into the cerebrospinal fluid. Thus, Brightman (1968) has shown that if peroxidase is injected into the blood supply, the marker crosses the endothelium of the choroid plexus to enter the perivascular connective tissue space. Appreciable amounts of the marker penetrate the basal lamina upon which the choroidal epithelial cells rest and become incorporated into numerous pits and vesicles at the bases and basolateral walls of the cells. The marker is also present in numerous vesicles, some of which are clearly coated, and in multivesicular bodies. The marker, thus sequestered, moves into the interior of the cells and tends to migrate toward the free, luminal surface. Electron-dense markers introduced into the cerebrospinal fluid (Tennyson and Pappas, 1961; Brightman, 1965a and b and 1968) are also taken up into vesicles at the free luminal surfaces of the choroidal epithelial cells, but in less amounts than are taken up at the basal ends. This suggests that the net transport of materials in vesicles is from the basal to the apical poles

Figure 9–3. **Choroid Plexus.**

The apical ends of choroidal cells have many microvilli (*mv*), beneath which is a network of microfilaments (*mf*). Mitochondria (*mit*) are concentrated in the apical cytoplasm, which also contains cisternae of the granular endoplasmic reticulum (*ER*), many clusters of free ribosomes (*r*), and vesicles (*v*), some of which are coated (*cv*) and appear (*cv₁*) at the bases of the microvilli. The intercellular junction shows a zonula occludens (*zo*) at its apical end, and beneath this is a zonula adhaerens (*za*). Deeper, the intercellular junction exhibits dilatations (*x*) and the two plasma membranes diverge (*arrow*) where the basal infoldings commence.
Lateral ventricle of adult rat. × 54,000.

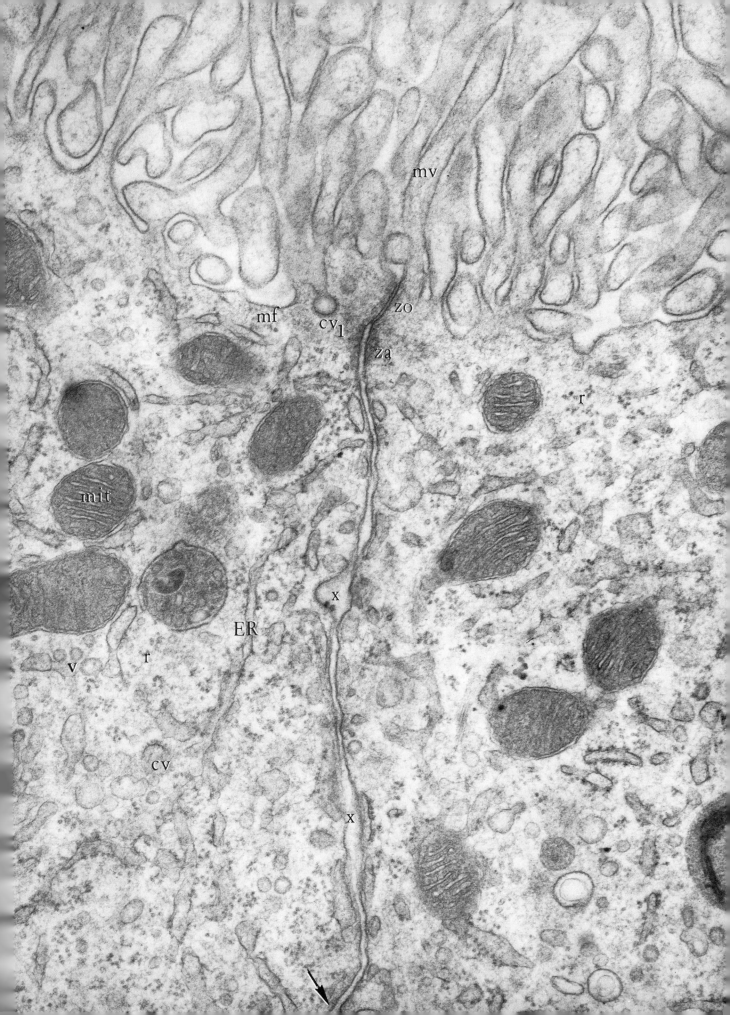

of the cells. Such a transport is nicely shown when ferritin is administered ventricularly and peroxidase is simultaneously administered intravenously. Then the number of ferritin-containing vesicles in the apical cytoplasm is small in contrast to the number of peroxidase-containing vesicles arising from the basal ends of the cells (Brightman, 1968).

It should be noted that in this type of experiment no colloidal label passes between the adjacent epithelial cells in discernible amounts in either direction. The reason for this is found in the relation between the lateral surfaces of adjacent cells (Figures 9–3 and 9–4). At their apical ends the lateral faces of contiguous epithelial cells form zonulae occludentes, or tight junctions (Brightman, 1968; Brightman and Reese, 1969), at which the intercellular space is obliterated by an apparent fusion of the outer leaflets of the apposed plasma membranes (Figures 9–3 and 9–4). These occluding junctions apparently form girdles around the apical ends of the cells (see also Bohr and Møllgård, 1974).

In a more recent study of the cat choroid plexus Castel, Sahar, and Erlij (1974) raise the question of whether the tight junctions may be leaky. They found that when buffered lanthanum chloride solutions are perfused into the carotid arteries lanthanum deposits occur in the lumina of the choroidal blood vessels, the perivascular space, and along the lengths of the junctions between adjacent choroidal cells. Occasional lanthanum deposits were also present in the ventricular lumen. When injected into the ventricle the tracer also penetrates past the tight junctions. Since Castel, Sahar, and Erlij did not find that the lanthanum bypassed the tight junctions by transport in pinocytotic vesicles, they concluded that the tight junctions of the choroidal epithelium may be leaky and that the passage may occur through narrow and tortuous channels that penetrate the tight junctions. Simi-

lar leaky tight junctions also seem to occur in the gallbladder and intestine (Machen, Erlij, and Wooding, 1972).

Just beneath the zonulae occludentes are zonulae adhaerentes (Figures 9–3 and 9–4, za), and beneath these junctions the plasma membranes of adjacent cells run more or less parallel to each other in most cases. The intercellular space may be dilated, however, and it is not unusual to find mitochondria and cisternae of granular endoplasmic reticulum aligned parallel to the plasma membranes of these lateral cell surfaces. Near the basal regions of the cells there are more complex infoldings formed by extensions from adjacent cells, so that the area of their surfaces available for the exchange of materials is greatly increased (Figures 9–2 and 9–6). Electron microscope histochemical techniques have shown adenosine triphosphatase to be localized in these infoldings (Torack and Barrnett, 1964; Yasuzumi and Tsubo, 1966).

In contrast to their lateral edges, the basal ends of epithelial cells are relatively smooth and rest upon a basal lamina that does not enter into the basolateral infoldings (Figures 9–2 and 9–6). This basal lamina is not a barrier to the penetration of lanthanum and horseradish peroxidase, but it seems to act as a diffusion barrier to silver particles (Dempsey and Wislocki, 1955) and to thorium dioxide particles (Tennyson and Pappas, 1968).

A variable number of membrane-bound dense bodies, probably lysosomes, also occur in the cytoplasm of the epithelial cells (Figure 9–2) and Case (1959) described the presence of hemosiderin-containing inclusions which might be the products of the breakdown of red blood cells. The number of dense bodies is greatly increased if an electron-dense marker is administered into the ventricles, for then these bodies may come to contain such substances as silver particles (Wislocki and Ladman, 1958), thorium

---

Figure 9–4. **Choroid Plexus.**

The plane of this section passes through the apices of two choroidal cells and so displays the apical portion of the intercellular junction that girdles them. At each end of the junctional profile are portions of the zonula occludens (zo), and toward the middle is the zonula adhaerens (za) with its associated accumulation of dense filamentous material. This filamentous material appears to be continuous with the microfilamentous network (mf) that passes beneath and into the microvilli (mv). In the meshes of this network coated vesicles (cv) are apparent. The cell on the right shows the apical mitochondria (mit), short cisternae of the granular endoplasmic reticulum (ER), and free ribosomes (r).

Lateral ventricle of adult rat. × 55,000.

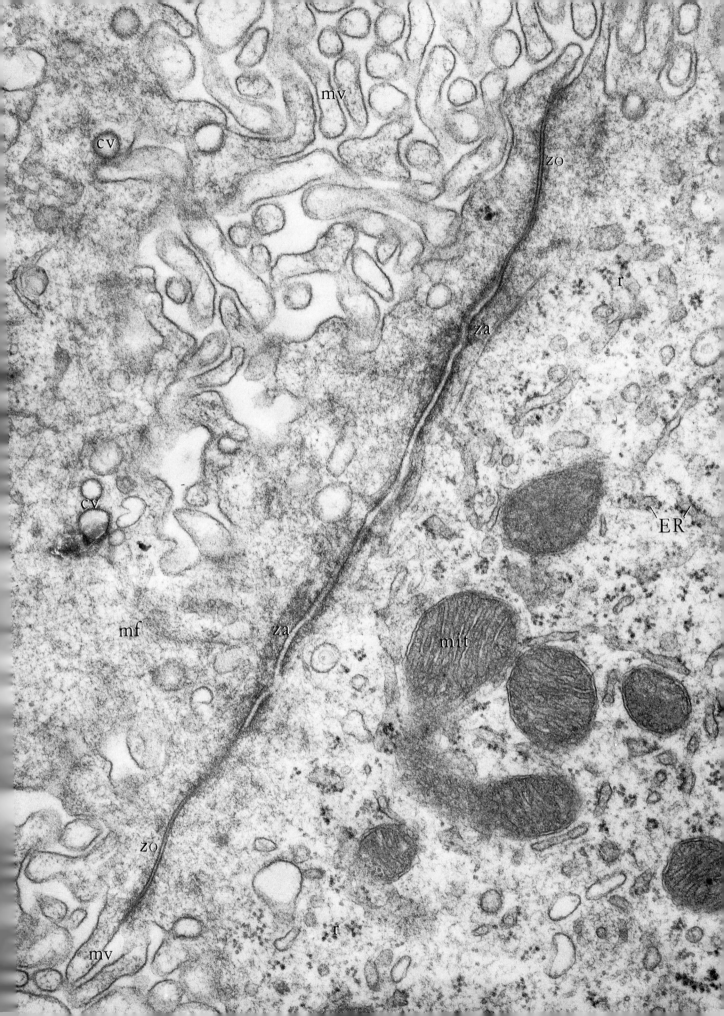

dioxide particles (Tennyson and Pappas, 1968), or lanthanum and horseradish peroxidase (Brightman, 1968; Brightman and Reese, 1969).

In the rat some free cells lie on the surface of the choroidal epithelium. In scanning electron microscope preparations these cells are very obvious (Hoyosa and Fujita, 1973; Peters, 1974; Chamberlain, 1974) and have rather amoeboid shapes with a number of processes, some of which are very long and thin (Figure 9–7). These free cells clearly represent the macrophages first described in lower vertebrates by Kolmer (1921). In a later study of these same cells in higher vertebrates Kappers (1953) designated them as "epiplexus cells." In an electron microscope study of the Kolmer or epiplexus cells in the cat Carpenter, McCarthy, and Borison (1970) found them to rest on the microvilli of the choroidal cells and to sometimes have their plasma membranes indented by the tips of the microvilli and cilia of the choroidal cells. In the rat, the Kolmer cells also rest on the tips of the microvilli, but these processes do not appear to indent these macrophages. The general morphology of the Kolmer cells in the lateral ventricle of the rat is shown in Figure 9–7. In their cytoplasm the Kolmer cells may contain membrane-limited vacuoles and lysosomes. In the rat these become more numerous with age, and in older rats the cytoplasm of some cells may be so full of inclusions that the cells are bloated. Such cells seem to have fewer processes than the cells with fewer vacuoles that predominate in young rats. The identity of these Kolmer cells as macrophages is well demonstrated in the study by Carpenter, McCarthy, and Borison (1970) in which it was shown that under experimental conditions they rapidly ingest tracer particles introduced into the cerebrospinal fluid. Thus, their function may be to keep the surfaces of the choroidal cells free of debris.

THE VASCULARIZED CONNECTIVE TISSUE CORE

The choroidal epithelial cells rest on a basal lamina beneath which are a few pale cells whose flattened processes produce a thin and attenuated layer (Figures 9–2 and 9–6). Beneath this cell layer is the connective tissue core of the choroid plexus which is composed of a loose network of collagen fibers that are condensed beneath the epithelium and at the bases of the villi. These collagen fibers are produced by fibroblasts present in the connective tissue stroma. The bulk of the central core of the choroid plexus is occupied by blood vessels, however, and in addition to small arteries and arterioles there are large venous sinuses and capillaries. The walls of the small arteries and arterioles have a muscular media of smooth muscle cells surrounding them. The walls of the venous sinuses are much thinner than those of veins, and although they do not possess smooth muscle cells, they are covered by elastic fibers that make wide, intertwining spirals around them (Agdhur, 1932). These sinuses do not appear to have been studied with the electron microscope.

In the villi themselves are capillaries of unusually large diameter for the brain. They are also unusual in that they are fenestrated and have very thin endothelial walls (Figures 9–2, 9–6, and 10–2). At the fenestrations the walls of the endothelial cells are essentially collapsed but not perforated, for each fenestration is bridged by a thin diaphragm (Brightman, 1968; Tennyson and Pappas, 1968). If horseradish peroxidase is injected intravenously the dense

Figure 9–5. Choroid Plexus.

The apical end of this choroidal cell shows the tubules and vesicular profiles of the smooth endoplasmic reticulum (*SR*) enmeshed in the microfilamentous network (*mf*). A tuft of cilia (*cil*), which arise from basal bodies (*bb*), is intertwined with the microvilli (*mv*).

The **inset** shows transverse sections of the choroidal cilia. At their proximal ends (*cil₁*) these cilia possess a peripheral ring of 9 pairs of microtubules and a core of fibrous material. More distally (*cil₂*) one of the peripheral pairs of microtubules moves into the vacant position giving an 8 + 1 configuration, and in a profile nearer the tip (*cil₃*) one of the peripheral pairs of microtubules is lost so that a 7 + 1 pattern results.

Lateral ventricle of adult rat. × *40,000.*

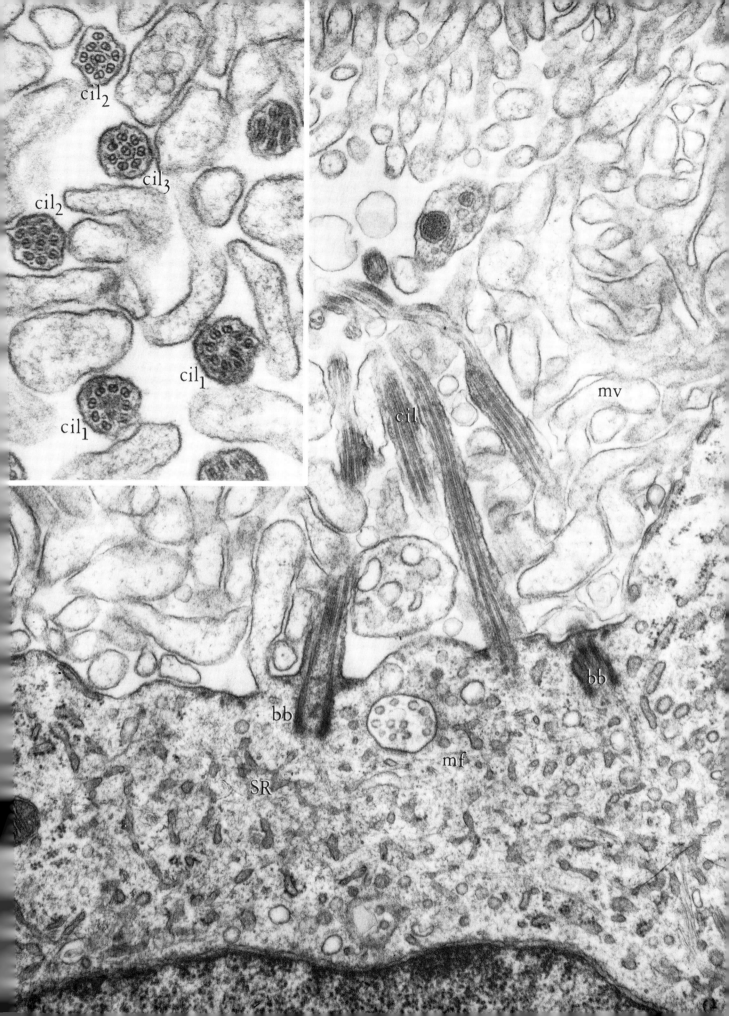

reaction product usually appears as a coating on the entire luminal surface of the endothelial cells (Brightman, 1968). Some of the peroxidase is taken up into the endothelial cells by pinocytosis, so that their cytoplasm may be filled by dense vesicles. In most instances the peroxidase does not appear to pass between the endothelial cells, although Brightman (1968) observed some examples in which it occupied most of the interendothelial junction. Neither did the peroxidase seem to penetrate intact fenestrae, but often the fenestrae burst and then the peroxidase leaked out to the basal lamina surrounding the capillary. At present there is uncertainty about just how peroxidase passes across the fenestrated endothelial cells, although Brightman (1968) considers it possible that the passage takes place by pinocytosis and by intercellular migration along endothelial cell junctions. It should be noted that thorium dioxide also enters the endothelial cell junctions (Pappas and Tennyson, 1962). If the passage is by vesicular transport, then it probably takes place across those parts of the capillary wall where the endothelium is at least 30 nm thick, since the more attenuated parts of the endothelium do not contain pinocytotic vesicles.

Although the presence of nerve fibers in the choroid plexus has been reported by a number of investigators (see Millen and Woollam, 1962), these do not appear to have been considered in any electron microscope studies. One group of nerve fibers seems to be related to the adventitia and media of the blood vessels and another to the choroidal epithelium. It is generally believed that the nerve fibers are postganglionic (see Edvinnson, Nielsen, Owman, and West, 1974), since they degenerate after cervical sympathectomy.

Neither does attention appear to have been paid to the fine structure of the psammoma of the choroid plexus. These concentric laminated bodies have been recorded in the choroid plexuses of a number of animals. They increase with age (Millen and Woollam, 1962) and probably arise from a laying down of successive layers of material around a central core. The bodies have been recorded to contain cholesterol, calcium carbonate, and calcium and magnesium phosphate, but their origins and functions are unknown.

FUNCTIONS OF THE CHOROID PLEXUS

It is generally accepted that the choroid plexus is primarily concerned with the formation of cerebrospinal fluid (CSF) (see Dohrmann, 1970). The newly formed CSF mixes with that already present in the ventricles and passes into the subarachnoid space to be absorbed into the blood, either through the walls of the subarachnoid vessels or via the cranial and spinal arachnoid villi. Reviews of the manner in which CSF is produced have been recently presented by Davson (1967 and 1972), Netsky and Shuangshoti (1970), and Cserr (1971), who investigated the question of whether the production of CSF is by active secretion or by a passive dialysis.

According to Netsky and Shuangshoti (1970) both processes appear to occur, but at present the conditions under which these two processes operate are not clear.

Morphologically, in terms of their content of numerous mitochondria, pinocytotic vesicles, convoluted basolateral surfaces and the existence of zonulae occludentes between their lateral faces, the structure of the choroidal epithelial cells favors a secretory mode (Figures 9–2, 9–3, 9–5, and 9–6). In possessing these features, cells of the choroidal epithelium resemble those present in the ciliary body of the eye, the salivary glands, and the renal tubules, each of

---

Figure 9–6. **The Basal Ends of Choroidal Cells.**

The choroidal cells rest on a basal lamina (*B*) and the plasma membranes of the basal ends are coated by microfilaments (*mf*), which extend into the cytoplasm. Some coated vesicles (*cv₁*) open at this surface and others (*cv*) occur in the deeper cytoplasm, which displays some large multivesicular bodies (*mvb*), mitochondria (*mit*), free ribosomes (*r*), and cisternae of the granular endoplasmic reticulum (*ER*). At its basal end the intercellular junction (*J*) has complex infoldings (*X*). A thin layer of tenuous cellular processes separates the choroidal cells from the fenestrated endothelium (*End*) of the blood vessels in the core of the choroid plexus.
Lateral ventricle of adult rat. × 30,000.

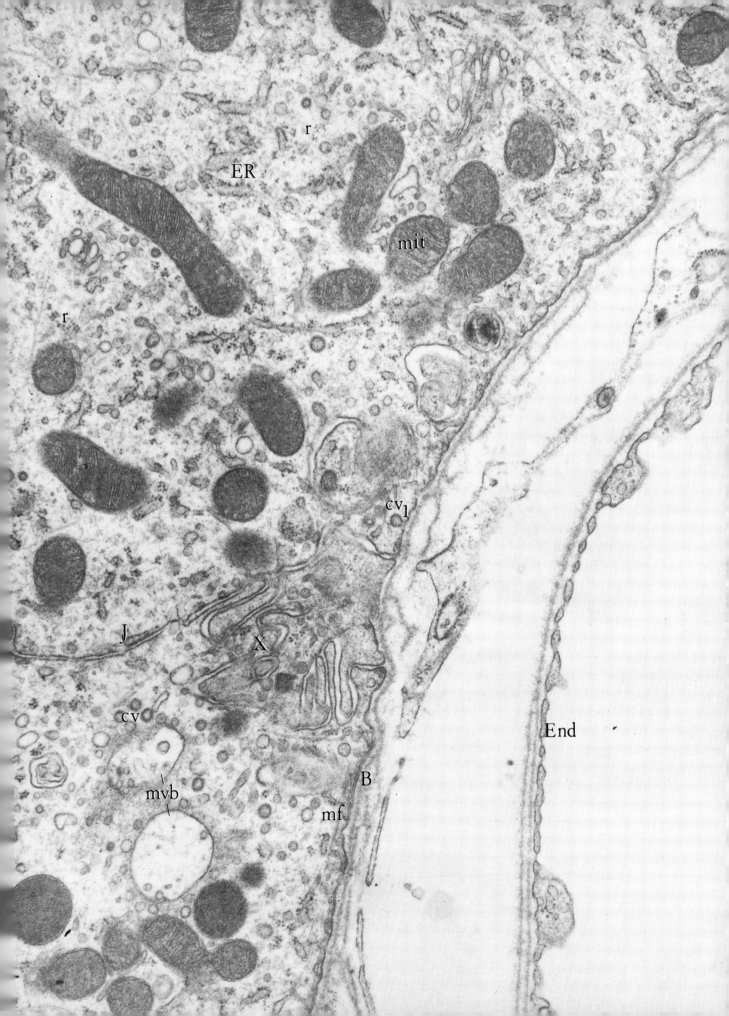

which is known to undertake secretion. Also the physiological characteristics of the cells clearly show a permeability barrier in respect to substances such as sodium and urea.

The site of the sodium pumps involved in sodium secretion by the choroid plexus has recently been investigated by Quinton, Wright, and Tormey (1973). They used the frog choroid plexus and took advantage of the fact that ouabain is a potent and specific inhibitor of the enzymes involved in sodium transport, arguing that determination of the site of ouabain action should reveal the location of the sodium pump. They found ouabain to be bound at the apical surfaces of the choroidal cells where the microvilli occur, but not on their lateral or basal surfaces. Consequently, the results of Quinton, Wright, and Tormey (1973) support the idea that sodium from the blood enters the choroidal cells passively, down an electrochemical gradient, after which it is subsequently pumped actively across the apical surface membrane into the cerebrospinal fluid.

In terms of the rate of production of CSF, it is interesting that in all animals so far studied about 0.5 per cent of the total CSF volume is replaced every minute (Davson, 1967). This means that an amount of CSF equal to that of the total volume present is produced every 200 minutes.

Perhaps the first demonstration that the choroid plexuses secrete CSF was that of Cushing (1914) and other neurosurgeons, who saw fluid being extruded from the choroid plexuses at craniotomy. Such observations have since been criticized because under these conditions the choroid plexuses are exposed to air and the intraventricular pressure is lowered by incision of the ventricles. Additional evidence for active secretion appeared to come from the experiments of Dandy (1919) who blocked the aqueduct and then plugged the foramen of Monro on one side after removing the choroid plexus from the lateral ventricle of that same side. The ventricle containing the choroid plexus enlarged, while the one from which the choroid plexus had been removed and the foramen blocked, collapsed. Hence it seemed that the pressure of the secreted CSF was the force leading to hydrocephalus. Later, however, Bering (1962) performed a similar experiment but did not block the foramen of Monro. Despite the free communication between the ventricles he found hydrocephalus to still occur in the ventricle containing the intact choroid plexus, while the other ventricle still did not enlarge. The reason for this is not yet known.

On the basis of recent studies, there is little doubt that CSF is produced by secretion. The composition of newly formed CSF has been examined and shown to be different from that of an ultrafiltrate of plasma. It also seems that changing the hydrostatic pressure in the ventricles has no significant effect on CSF production. The question about whether CSF is produced only by the choroid plexus is still open, for there is some suggestion that the ependyma may also be a source of the fluid.

In addition to its secretory activity, the choroid plexus has also been implicated in absorption from the ventricles, for a number of substances have been shown to be taken up by it under experimental conditions (see Cserr, 1971). For example, Diodrast and phenolsulfonphthalate can be actively transported out of the CSF into blood against a concentration gradient (Pappenheimer, Heisey, and Jordan, 1961). Consequently the eventual composition of the CSF may result from a combination of secretory and reabsorptive processes, rather like the manner in which the ultimate composition of urine is determined. Indeed, the choroid plexus may be essentially involved in the production of CSF which serves as a medium for the exchange of substances between the blood

---

Figure 9–7. **Kolmer Cells.**

The **upper picture** is a transmission electron micrograph of a Kolmer cell resting on the tips of the microvilli (*mv*) of a choroidal cell. The nucleus (*Nuc*) of the Kolmer cell is oval and has condensations of chromatin located mainly beneath the nuclear envelope. In the rather dark cytoplasm the granular endoplasmic reticulum (*ER*) consists of a few long cisternae. Some vesicles (*v*) and vacuoles (*vac*) are also present. *Choroid plexus from rat lateral ventricle.* × 15,000.

The **lower picture** is a scanning electron micrograph showing a Kolmer cell resting on the domed surfaces of the choroidal cells. The Kolmer cell has many fine processes extending from its perikaryon. *Choroid plexus from rat lateral ventricle.* × 3000.

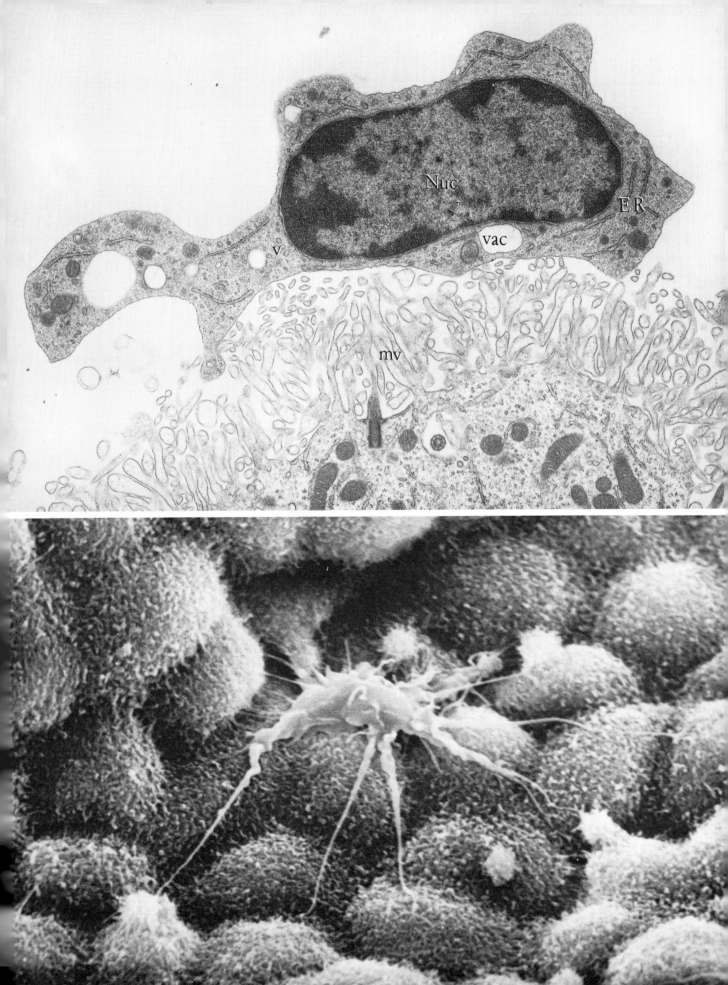

and the neurons, and it may provide a constant environment for the neurons. It may also be the medium through which some excretory products from the brain are transported away (see Millen and Woollam, 1962), for substances can pass rather freely between the CSF and the extracellular space of the central nervous system; there are no occluding junctions between most ependymal cells.

A function of the CSF which must not be ignored is its role in providing buoyancy for the brain to prevent the full weight of the brain from pulling on the emerging nerve roots, blood vessels, and meninges. Thus, it is of interest that while the weight of the human brain is about 1500 gm in air, it is only 50 gm when immersed in cerebrospinal fluid (Livingston, 1949).

Chapter X

BLOOD VESSELS

The blood vessels most commonly encountered in electron microscope preparations of the central nervous system are capillaries, which form a rich vascular bed that is richer in gray than in white matter. The blood supply to the central nervous system is provided by a relatively small number of main arterial trunks. These enter the subarachnoid space and then divide before perforating the substance of the nervous tissue to form smaller arterioles and ultimately the capillary bed. In most mammals this capillary bed has no end arteries, so that there is a free communication throughout most of the vascular tree of the brain and the spinal cord, with the capillaries forming numerous anastomoses before coming together into venules and veins. The veins from the brain then empty into a number of venous sinuses.

It should be emphasized that the central nervous system has no lymphatics. Perhaps the system of cerebrospinal fluid that is derived from the blood and secreted by the choroid plexus can be regarded as being the equivalent of the lymphatic system present elsewhere.

Although the topic will not be considered here, it is important to realize that the blood vessels supplying the central nervous system form rather definite patterns in its various subdivisions. Thus, studies of the distribution and con-

centration of blood vessels show some laminae—of the cerebral cortex and the cerebellum, for example—to be more richly vascularized than others. In addition, certain groups of neurons throughout the brain stem and spinal cord receive what is essentially their own discrete vascularization. In general the density of the capillary network is greater in regions containing groups of neuronal perikarya than in white matter, and is greater still in regions containing large numbers of synapses. In effect, the richness of the vascularization is directly related to the concentration of synapses present in a region. Further information on this point can be gained by reference to the review by Cobb (1932).

Apart from the presence of zonulae occludentes between the adjacent endothelial cells, the majority of blood vessels in the central nervous system do not differ fundamentally from those in other tissues. Reviews of the structure of blood vessels may be found in current histology texts and in the articles by Fawcett (1963), Florey (1969), and Rhodin (1962 and 1968).

The blood vessels of peripheral nerves will not be considered in this chapter, but reference to the properties of those contained within the endoneurium will be considered later (see page 330).

CAPILLARIES

The capillaries in the central nervous system have been specifically studied by a number of authors (e.g., Maynard, Schultz, and Pease, 1957; Donahue and Pappas, 1961; Wolff, 1963; Lange and Halata, 1972). The cerebral capillaries have walls which are thickened in the region of the rather flattened and elongate nuclei but attenuated elsewhere (Figure 10–1). The nuclei of the cells have a relatively homogeneous chromatin which condenses beneath the nuclear envelope. In the vicinity of the nucleus is the Golgi apparatus, which is composed of flattened sacs or cisternae, usually lying parallel to the plasma membrane and often indenting one side of the nucleus. Most of the mitochondria are also located in the vicinity of the nucleus, but occasional mitochondria occur throughout the cytoplasm, and again, because of the attenuation of the cells, these tend to lie parallel to the cell surface. The matrix of the endothelial cell cytoplasm is rather dense and appears granular (Figures 10–1 and 10–2). Some of this cytoplasmic granularity is due to the presence of fine filaments, 4 to 6 nm thick, that might represent microfilaments. Ribosomes are not prominent in the cytoplasm, but a few free clusters are present and others sparsely stud the small and infrequent cisternae of the rough endoplasmic reticulum as well as the outer nuclear membrane. Pinocytotic vesicles are less numerous than in capillaries in most other tissues and it is rare to find dense and multivesicular bodies in the cytoplasm.

The junctions between adjacent endothelial cells vary greatly in extent. Sometimes the contiguous endothelial cells, or the two ends of the same endothelial cell completely surrounding the capillary lumen, simply abut (Figure 10–2, upper figure). In other situations there is an overlap (Figure 10–2, middle figure), and it is frequently found that at the luminal end of the junction a thin fold or flap formed by one or both cells projects into the lumen. At a junction the two apposed plasma membranes lie parallel to each other, being separated by an interval of about 15 nm. However, near the luminal end of each junction the two plasma membranes always come together to form zonulae occludentes (Figure 10–2, zo), in which the outer leaflets of the membranes appear to fuse and the intervening intercellular space is obliterated (see Muir and Peters, 1962; Reese and Karnovsky, 1967; Brightman and Reese, 1969). Although these zonulae appear rather punctate in most sections of capillaries, they must completely girdle the cells, for studies with lanthanum and horseradish peroxidase show that when these substances are injected into the blood, they do not penetrate between endothelial cells of the blood vessels in the central nervous system except in a few specialized regions (Reese and Karnovsky, 1967; Brightman and Reese, 1969; Brightman, Klatzo, Olsson, and Reese, 1970). In fact, so far as electron-dense markers can tell us, the presence of the occluding junctions seems to be the morphological basis for the blood-brain barrier (see page 246). In freeze-fractured preparations Connell and Mercer (1974) showed that the zonulae occludentes between endothelial cells of capillaries in mouse cerebral cortex are like tight junctions present elsewhere (see Friend and Gilula, 1972; Wade and Karnovsky, 1974). Thus, at a junction the A face of a plasma membrane shows a network of 10-nm wide ridges which are matched by grooves on the corresponding B face.

Figure 10–1. **Capillary and Pericyte.**

The **upper figure** shows a transverse section through a capillary. The capillary wall is formed by thin endothelial cells (*End*). The only site of thickening is where the nucleus (*Nuc*) is located. The cytoplasm of the endothelial cells is quite dark and shows few organelles except mitochondria (*mit*) and short cisternae of the granular endoplasmic reticulum. In contrast to capillaries in other tissues, those in the central nervous system show few pinocytotic vesicles. Surrounding the capillary is a basal lamina (*B*), beyond which is a complete covering of astrocytic processes (*AsP*). *Cerebral cortex of rat.* × 15,000.

The **lower figure** shows a pericyte partly surrounding a capillary (*Cap*). The pericyte is completely enclosed within a basal lamina (*B*). The nucleus (*Nuc*) of the pericyte has some clumping of the chromatin beneath the nuclear envelope, and the cytoplasm is marked by lysosomes (*Ly*) and several empty vacuoles (*vac*). Other organelles in the cytoplasm are portions of the Golgi apparatus (*G*), mitochondria (*mit*), the granular endoplasmic reticulum (*ER*), and coated vesicles (*cv*). *Lateral geniculate nucleus of cat.* × 14,000.

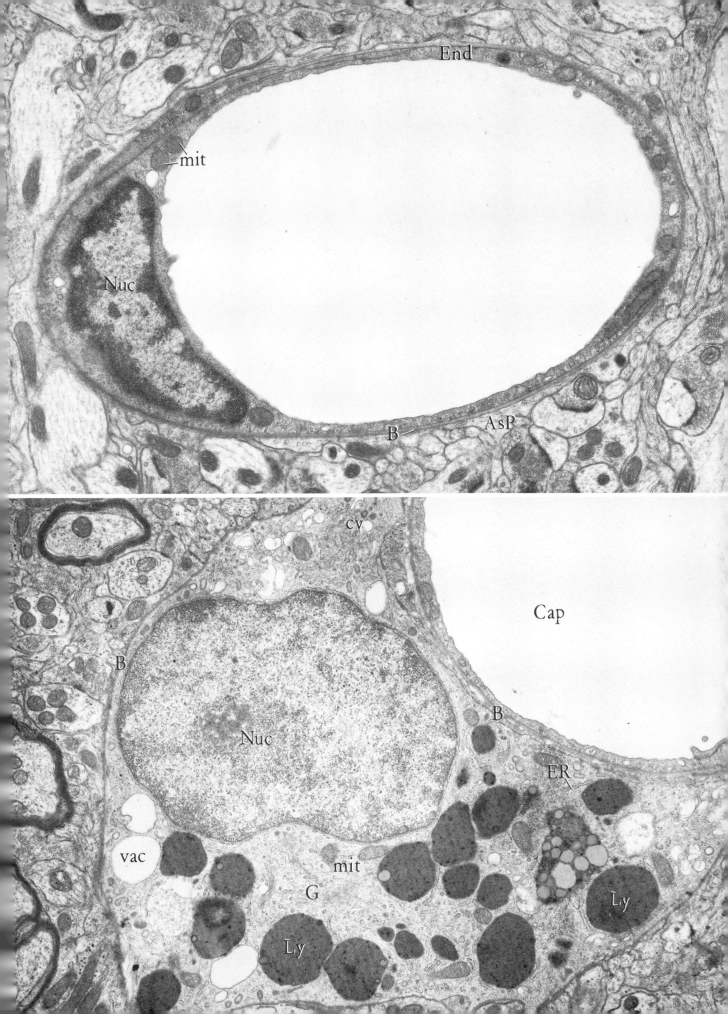

The existence of the blood-brain barrier also depends on a failure of substances to pass across the endothelium of cerebral capillaries due to both an absence of fenestrations in the endothelial cells and an absence or lack of a marked transport by pinocytotic vesicles. Compared to the capillaries in muscle, for example, cerebral capillaries have very few and rather irregular vesicles when sections of them are examined (Figure 10–1). In addition, when peroxidase is injected into the blood system only a few of the vesicles in cerebral endothelial cells take up the marker. Unlike the cerebral capillaries, some of the cerebral arterioles do transfer protein from the blood into the perivascular basal lamina, so that if sufficient time (24 to 48 hours) is allowed after injection of a marker, the intravenously injected protein appears in the extracellular and cerebrospinal fluids (see Westergaard and Brightman, 1973).

Under certain conditions the tight junctions of the cerebral endothelium can be opened. Thus, either infusion of hyperosmotic 3 molar solutions of urea into an internal carotid artery or the topical application of urea on the pia mater leads to the opening of tight junctions. Horseradish peroxidase will pass through junctions opened by such treatment and enter the extracellular fluid spaces of the brain (Brightman, Hori, Rapoport, Reese, and Westergaard, 1974). Most of the vessels affected by the hyperosmotic urea are capillaries. Other factors affecting the permeability of cerebral vessels are discussed by Brightman, Klatzo, Olsson, and Reese (1970).

It is worth mentioning that when transverse sections of cerebral capillaries are examined it is not uncommon to fail to find a junction throughout the entire circumference of a capillary wall (Figure 10–1). Sometimes this must be simply due to a junction being so oblique in orientation that it does not form a clear image. Wolff and Bär (1972) have used the term "seamless" to refer to capillaries that do not show interendothelial junctions in their walls. In the rat cerebral cortex Wolff and Bär (1972) find a significant increase in the number of seamless capillaries present between the ninth and twentieth postnatal days, by which time they account for about 20 per cent of the total number of capillary profiles encountered. Wolff and Bär (1972) estimate that about half of this number can be attributed to sections passing through capillary loops and suggest that the probable location of the seamless endothelial cells is near the venous ends of capillaries.

Lying outside the endothelial cells of cerebral capillaries is a thin and continuous basal lamina, similar to that around capillaries in other tissues (Figures 10–1 and 10–2, B). This basal lamina is 30 to 40 nm thick. In some instances the basal lamina of the capillary is separated by a narrow perivascular space from the true basal lamina of the parenchyma upon which the endfeet of astrocytes rest (see page 238). In this space collagen fibers are not uncommon, although these are more frequent in the cat than in the rat. Sometimes the endothelial and parenchymal basal laminae fuse to form one continuous lamina, so that the perivascular space is obliterated (Figures 10–1 and 10–2). However, two basal laminae are always present in places where pericytes occur, for these cells reside in the perivascular space and are always com-

---

Figure 10–2.   **Capillaries.**

In the **upper figure** is a junction (*J*) between two endothelial cells (*End*) in the wall of a capillary. At the junction the outer leaflets of the two apposed plasma membranes come together to form zonulae occludentes (*zo*). A basal lamina (*B*) separates the endothelial cells from the underlying astrocytic processes (*As*).
Basal ganglia of rat. × 200,000.

The **middle figure** shows a more extensive junction (*J*) between two endothelial cells (*End*). Along most of the junction the endothelial cell plasma membranes are separated by an interval of about 15 nm, but zonulae occludentes (*zo*) are apparent in some places where the outer leaflets of the apposed plasma membranes become apposed. A basal lamina (*B*) separates the endothelial cells from the adjacent glia limitans of astrocytic processes (*As*).
Auditory cortex of rat. × 120,000.

Micrograph by D. W. Vaughan.

The **lower figure** shows the thin wall of a fenestrated capillary (*Cap*) from the choroid plexus. At the fenestrae (*arrows*), the capillary walls are essentially collapsed, but they are not perforated, for a thin diaphragm is present. Outside the capillary is a thin basal lamina (*B*) separating the endothelial cells from the surrounding collagen-containing (*Col*) connective tissue core of the choroid plexus.
Choroid plexus of rat. × 30,000.

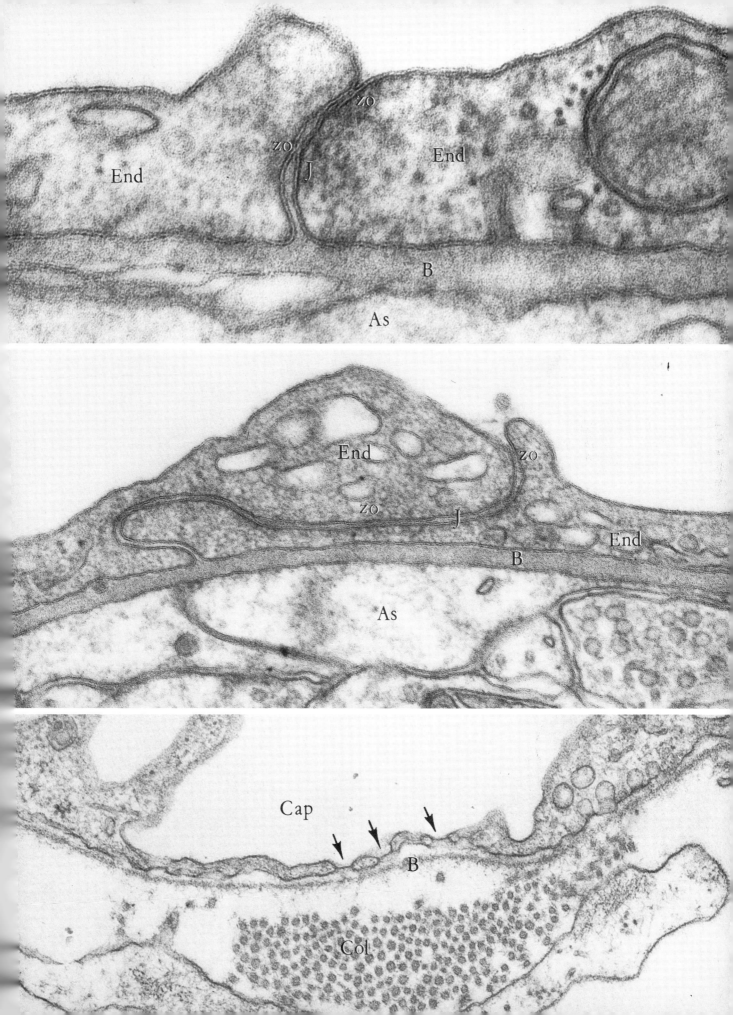

pletely bounded by a basal lamina (Figure 10–1, *lower figure*). Although the end-feet of astrocytes usually form a complete limiting membrane beneath the parenchymal basal lamina, the processes and perikarya of other cells occasionally rest directly against the basal lamina (Lange and Halata, 1972).

Pericytes have processes that extend around the capillary wall and have fusiform or elongate nuclei that conform to the shape of the underlying blood vessels (Figure 10–1). Their chromatin is rather clumped beneath the nuclear envelope (see King and Schwyn, 1970), and their cytoplasm is as dense as that of endothelial cells, which they also resemble in their content of organelles. However, unlike endothelial cells, pericytes very often contain dense bodies resembling lysosomes, and these may almost fill the cytoplasm (Figure 10–1, *Ly*). At present the functions of the pericytes are not clear, although some authors (e.g., Barón and Gallego, 1972) consider that they transform into microglia (see page 262).

Caley and Maxwell (1970), Bär and Wolff (1972), Phelps (1972a), and Hannah and Nathaniel (1974) have studied the formation of capillaries in the central nervous system. In the embryo, vascularization of the central nervous system begins as a superficial network of sinusoidal blood vessels which lie in the perineural parenchyma surrounding the brain vesicles and the neural tube (see Strong, 1961 and 1964). The superficial vessels form capillary sprouts that consist initially of virtually solid cords of cells (angioblasts). The immature intracerebral vessels develop by sprouting from pre-existing vessels, and no paired vessels are observed, as would be expected if the internal vascularization started by penetrating loops (Bär and Wolff, 1972). At the tip of each cord are pseudopod-like cytoplasmic protrusions, and it is presumed that by these cytoplasmic protrusions, the cords progress into the neuropil. Initially, the lumen of a capillary either is not apparent or has the

form of a small slit. Even at the time of the first appearance of a capillary anlage, zonulae occludentes are present between adjacent cells. Eventually, probably when a growing capillary establishes contact with another vessel which is patent, the lumen opens and becomes filled with blood. Initially no astrocytic end-feet are present around the growing capillaries, which are usually surrounded by a quite large perivascular space. Indeed, the formation of the end-feet appears to be coincidental with the opening of the capillary lumen, a narrowing of the perivascular space, and the formation of a basal lamina. Pericytes are present quite early. With the formation of the basal lamina and the decrease in the width of the perivascular space, they become included in the vascular wall (Bär and Wolff, 1972).

In the rat cerebral cortex, the capillaries are surrounded by perivascular glia at the end of the first postnatal week. Bär and Wolff (1972) consider that the final differentiation of the cerebral capillaries begins at the end of the second postnatal week, when the walls of the capillaries become thinner and the number of pinocytotic vesicles and profiles of rough endoplasmic reticulum decrease (see also Hannah and Nathaniel, 1974). Later, the basal lamina becomes thicker. In the cerebral hemispheres the internal sprouting finishes by three or four weeks postnatally. Further growth takes place by the elongation of the capillaries, which also undergo more extensive branching. A quantitative study of the growth of capillaries in the neocortex of the rat has been published by Bär and Wolff (1973).

Exceptions to the general lack of perivascular space around cerebral capillaries occur in specialized areas of the brain where there is no blood-brain barrier (see Dobbing, 1961). If the vital dye trypan blue is injected into an animal, the brain as a whole remains unstained, but the dye is taken up in the few areas that lack a blood-brain barrier. These areas, such as the area postrema, subfornical organ, epiphysis, neurohy-

Figure 10–3. **Small Blood Vessel.**

This transversely sectioned blood vessel is larger than a capillary and is either a small arteriole or a venule. The circular lumen of the vessel is surrounded by a thin endothelial cell layer *(End)* which is only thickened where the nucleus *(Nuc)* occupies the cytoplasm. On the outside of the endothelial cell layer is a smooth muscle cell *(SM)*, which gives rise to a thin process on the left. Two other small smooth muscle cell processes *(arrows)* are present on the other side of the vessel wall. The smooth muscle cells lie inside a basal lamina *(B)* that also separates the vascular elements from the glia limitans *(As)* bounding the surrounding components of the cerebral cortex.
Rat cerebral cortex. × 20,000.

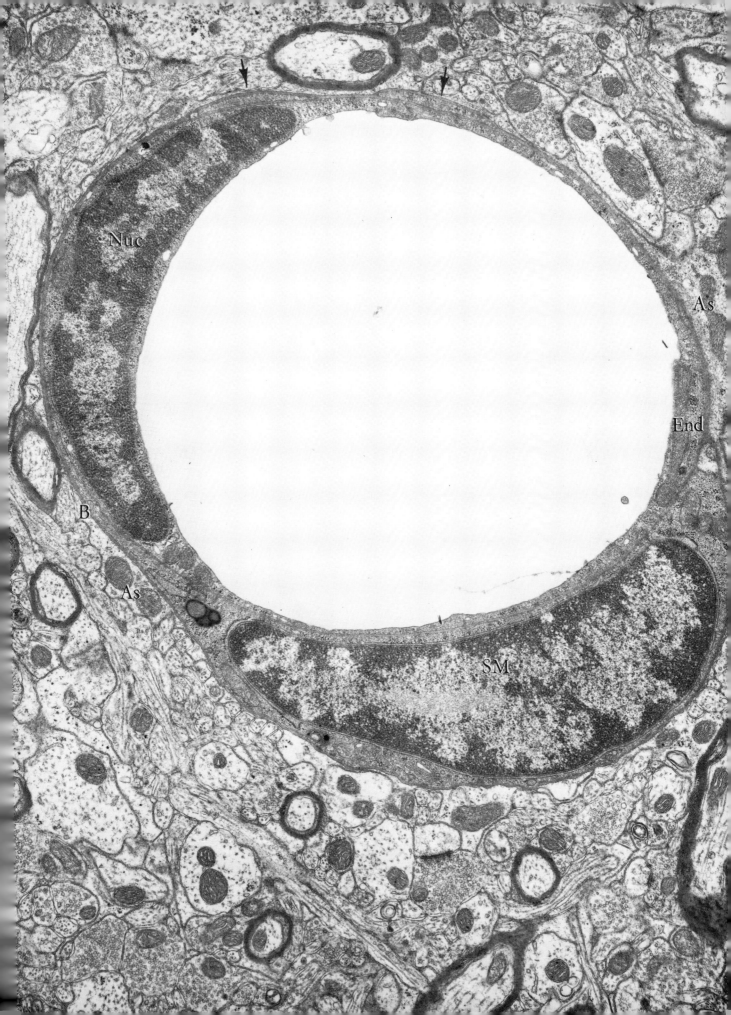

pophysis, median eminence, and pineal gland, have capillaries surrounded by quite large perivascular spaces, often containing collagen fibers and fibroblasts. It is common to find that the parenchymal lamina penetrates between the elements of the immediately surrounding neuropil, so that in low power micrographs it seems to have the form of a number of dense fingers.

In the area postrema (Leonhardt, 1967a; Rohrschneider, Schinko, and Wetzstein, 1972; Dempsey, 1973), neurohypophysis (Palay, 1955; Lederis, 1965), epiphysis (Wolfe, 1965) and subfornical organ (Rohr, 1966), and the choroid plexus (Figure 10–2, *lower figure*) the capillaries also have fenestrations, and the endothelial cells may contain quite large numbers of pinocytotic vesicles. At the fenestrae the walls of the capillaries are not perforated, for the fenestrae are bridged by thin diaphragms with a slight central thickening (Figure 10–2, *lower figure, arrows*). The diaphragms do not appear to be formed by the apposition of the plasma membranes bounding the two sides of the endothelial cells, however, for each diaphragm is even thinner than a single plasma membrane. The diaphragms may be formed by fusion of the two outer leaflets of the plasma membranes on the luminal and outer surfaces of an endothelial cell, but this has not been established.

The basis for the absence of a blood-brain barrier in these specialized areas of the central nervous system has not yet been determined. However, in the rat, Joó and Csillik (1966) find that while most cerebral endothelial cells stain intensely for butylcholinesterase, this enzyme is not present in endothelial cells in areas like the choroid plexus, the pituitary, and the area postrema which are not protected by a blood-brain barrier. Neither do the capillaries in these areas show a nucleoside phosphatase activity (Marchesi and Barrnett, 1964).

A rather unusual situation in respect of the permeability of blood vessels in the brain parenchyma exists in elasmobranchs (Brightman, Reese, Olsson, and Klatzo, 1971). In these fishes only some of the endothelial cells are connected by zonulae occludentes. Others are linked by open junctions at which the outer leaflets of adjacent endothelial cells are about 4 nm apart. Thus, when peroxidase is injected into the blood vessels of these animals it passes between endothelial cells into the perivascular space occupied by the basal lamina. It is retained in this space, and passage into the brain parenchyma is apparently prevented by the perivascular neuroglial end-feet, which are linked by both gap and tight junctions. Hence in elasmobranchs the blood-brain barrier to protein seems to lie at the level of the limiting membrane formed by the neuroglial cells rather than at the level of the capillary endothelium.

ARTERIES AND ARTERIOLES

Arteries and arterioles predominate in the superficial rather than the deeper portions of the brain and spinal cord. These vessels differ from capillaries by being larger in diameter and having one or two layers of smooth muscle in their walls (Figure 10–3 and 10–4) The smooth muscle cells are oriented more or less transversely with respect to the long axis of the vessel, and it

---

Figure 10–4. **Intracerebral Arterioles.**

In the **upper figure** is the wall of an arteriole that has just penetrated the cerebral cortex. The lumen of the arteriole is at the upper right, and it is bounded by a tunica intima composed of a single layer of endothelial cells (*End*). This layer is separated from the transversely oriented smooth muscle cells (*SM*) by a thick basal lamina (*B₁*). A basal lamina (*B₂*) also penetrates between adjacent smooth muscle cells and separates their outer faces from the extension of the subarachnoid space, which contains collagen fibers (*Col*) and leptomeningeal cell processes (*X*). On the other side of this space is the glia limitans of astrocytic processes (*As*).
Cerebral cortex of rat. × 45,000.

The **lower figure** shows a longitudinal section of the wall of an arteriole that has penetrated deeper into the cerebral cortex. The tunica intima of endothelial cells (*End*) is still complete, but the smooth muscle cells (*SM*) of the tunica media have become thinner and more sparse. The extension of the subarachnoid space between the arteriolar wall and the glia limitans (*As*) is now narrower and the leptomeningeal cell processes (*X*) are more attenuated.
Cerebral cortex of rat. × 22,000.

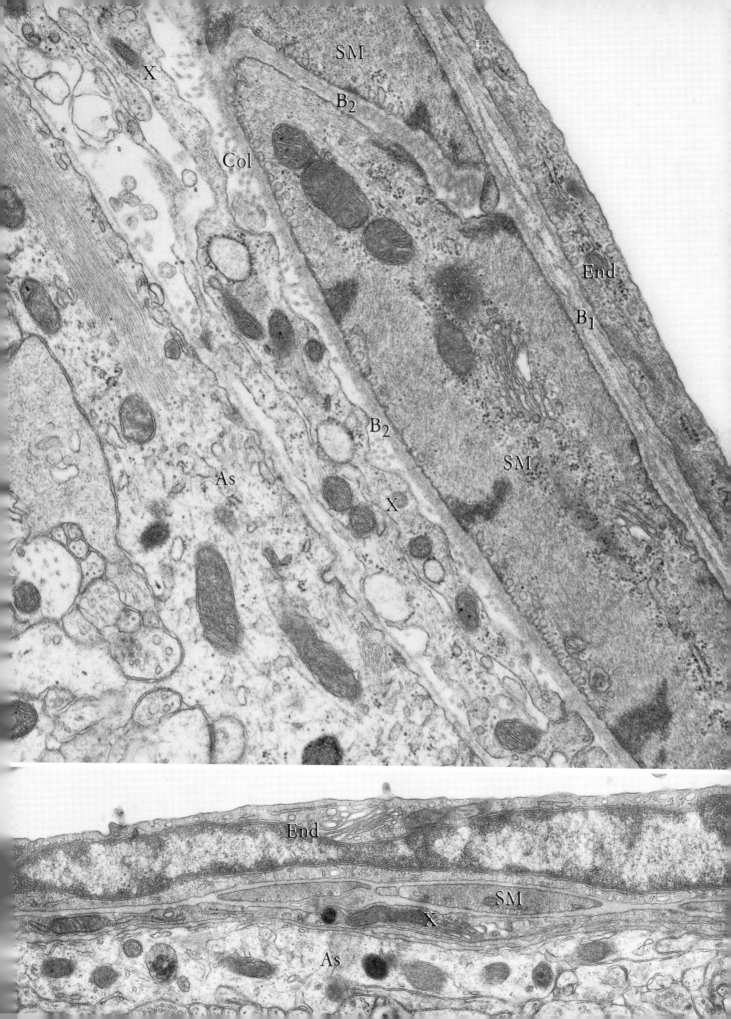

is common to find collagen fibers in the thick basal lamina.

In the cat and monkey (Pease and Molinari, 1960) and in the rat (Samarasinghe, 1965; Frederickson and Low, 1969) arteries in the subarachnoid space of the cerebral cortex have three coats. On the outside is a tunica adventitia which is extremely thin and usually consists of a single layer of cells, which may be regarded as being derived from the leptomeninges (Figure 13–4). Collagen separates the adventitia from the tunica media, which is formed by one or two layers of smooth muscle cells in the rat, but which is thicker in the cat and monkey. There are no nerves or nerve endings in the tunica media (Pease and Molinari, 1960). Between the tunica media and the tunica intima of endothelial cells is a thick basal lamina containing collagen and elastic fibers. In the walls of the larger vessels the elastic fibers form a nearly continuous internal elastic membrane, but in smaller arteries the elastic fibers form a more fragmented layer.

At the site of entry of such a blood vessel into the cerebral hemisphere (Figure 10–4, *upper figure*), it is surrounded by a continuation of the subarachnoid space (Millen and Woollam, 1961). This space is bounded on its outer side by a single layer of leptomeningeal cells, and beyond this is a basal lamina upon which the end-feet of the astrocytic processes of the glia limitans rest (see Maynard, Schultz, and Pease, 1957; Frederickson and Low, 1969; Dahl, 1973b). The inner limit of the space is lined by another layer of leptomeningeal cells that form the tunica adventitia of the artery. As the vessel penetrates deeper into the central nervous system the coating of smooth muscle cells becomes thinner and the subarachnoid space between these two leptomeningeal layers becomes narrower (Figure 10–4, *lower figure).* Finally it ends as the two leptomeningeal layers fuse (Patek, 1944; Millen and Woollam, 1962; Frederickson and Low, 1969; Rascol and Izard, 1972).

Dahl (1973b) found that in the cerebral cortex of the Rhesus monkey myoendothelial junctions occur in the intracerebral arterioles. These junctions are produced at sites where either endothelial cells or smooth muscle cells of the tunica media protrude through the intervening basal and elastic laminae. Lateral membrane-to-membrane contacts are also commonly seen between adjacent smooth muscle cells. Because of an absence of nerve fibers associated with these intracerebral vessels, Dahl (1973a) concludes that the tone of these vessels is regulated through the myoendothelial junctions.

Deeper in the cerebral cortex, the smooth muscle cells are lost and the basal laminae of the endothelial cells and of the glia limitans now oppose each other or become fused. Concomitant with the loss of the smooth muscle cells, pericytes make an appearance, so that the vessel assumes the features of a typical cerebral capillary (Jones, 1970). The depth at which these transformations occur depends upon the size of the entering vessel.

In the cat, Jones (1970) found no evidence for leptomeningeal components surrounding vessels entering the cortex. He did, however, find some cells with a foamy cytoplasm accompanying them and suggests that these may be modified pia-arachnoid cells, for their appearance indicates that they are phagocytic. It is known that when vital dyes are injected into the subarachnoid space many leptomeningeal cells become rounded, are set free into the subarachnoid space, and ingest particulate matter (Woollard, 1924).

Samarasinghe (1965) and Dahl (1973a) also examined the basilar and middle cerebral arteries from the rat and monkey, respectively. They found the lumina of the vessels to be lined by a single layer of endothelial cells. A subendothelial space separates the endothelial cells from an internal elastic lamina containing islets of elastic tissue and collagen fibers. The tunica media has four or five layers of smooth muscle cells in the basilar artery and two or three in the middle cerebral artery. The tunica adventitia is between 2 and 7 microns thick, and according to Samarasinghe (1965) and Dahl (1973a) it contains fibroblasts, collagen fibers, and nerve bundles. Dahl (1973a) considers the extracerebral arteries to be segmentally innervated and finds that all such vessels have an abundant nerve supply. In contrast, intracerebral arteries seem to lack any innervation.

VEINS

The venules formed by the coming together of capillaries attain quite a large diameter before leaving the substance of the central nervous system. According to Maynard, Schultz, and Pease (1957) and Frederickson and Low (1969), the venules resemble very large capillaries and have no more in their walls than endothelial cells resting upon a basal lamina. Consequently, it is difficult to identify the transition from a capillary to a vein, for the only essential difference between them lies in the diameter of the lumen (see Figure 10–3).

Frederickson and Low (1969) have shown that as a small vein leaves the central nervous system leptomeningeal cells surround it and soon form two layers, one applied to the vein and the other to the parenchyma, while between them is the subarachnoid space. Thus, the manner of exit of a vein from the brain is in essence the reverse of what happens when an artery enters the brain. Although there appear to be no fine structural observations on this point, it can be assumed from the review of Cobb (1932) that veins in the subarachnoid space may acquire a muscular coat, but whenever they lie in the subarachnoid space an outer leptomeningeal layer always surrounds them.

For an account of the fine structure of veins in other tissues, the review of Rhodin (1968) should be consulted.

Chapter XI

THE NEUROPIL

Neuropil is a term given to the areas of the central nervous system that contain a feltwork of intermingled and interconnected processes of neurons. It is in the neuropil that most of the synaptic junctions occur. At first sight the intermingling of the axons and dendrites appears to be random, but more careful study shows that the functional connections between these neuronal processes are very specific and precise. This organization would be anticipated from our knowledge of the exact manner in which the nervous system functions. Moreover, the precision of these connections is confirmed by the detailed electron microscope studies that have been carried out in the neuropil of different regions of the central nervous system.

The electron microscopic analysis of the neuropil is not an easy task. Not only is it necessary to identify the profiles of dendrites and axons sectioned in various planes, but it is also necessary to recognize the neuroglial processes that pass between them. As a result of investigations in which the same types of processes have been studied in different areas of the central nervous system, criteria have now been established for the identification of "typical" profiles. But in the case of dendrites, for example, subtle variations always exist. These variations depend upon such factors as the distance of the dendrite from the parent cell body, the sizes of dendrites arising from different neurons, and the functions of the part of the central nervous system under consideration. Consequently, although the typical features of a certain kind of process, either neuronal or neuroglial, can be described, it must not be expected that any particular process will

exhibit all these features. Neither must it be expected that the features will remain constant even from one portion to another of the same process. In other words, it is not possible to generalize completely. A full analysis of electron micrographs from a given area of neuropil can only be expected after some familiarity has been established with the organization of the region.

Detailed and useful analyses of the neuropil involve surveys of many hundreds of electron microscope sections. Generally though, this in itself is insufficient. The thinness of the sections and the small amount of material that can be effectively surveyed pose serious problems. Consequently, in almost every case the results of an electron microscope study must be supported by data obtained from other techniques. For the electron microscopist interested in the structure and connections of the central nervous system, perhaps the most useful of these supplementary techniques is the Golgi method. This shows a few neurons in their entirety and in sufficient detail to provide valuable clues to the morphology and characteristics of the processes of specific neurons in electron microscope preparations.

A relatively new technique which has been used to display neurons in their entirety is that of the iontophoretic injection of substances through fine-tipped hollow electrodes (see Kater and Nicholson, 1973). Either before or after a neuron has been penetrated by the electrode it is possible to determine the electrical properties of the cell. A number of substances have been introduced into individual neurons in this way.

One of the most commonly used substances is Procion yellow (see Stretton and Kravitz, 1968 and 1973; Purves and McMahan, 1972; Kellerth, 1973; Kelly and Van Essen, 1974). This dye is strongly fluorescent and does not appear to diffuse out of the injected cell, but its use in electron microscopy is limited by the fact that it is not electron-dense. Consequently, micrographs of injected neurons have to be prepared from thick light microscope sections and then compared with electron micrographs of thin sections in which profiles of similar shapes can be found. A potentially more useful dye for electron microscopy is Procion brown (MX5-BR) which has recently been introduced by Christensen (1973). Each molecule of this dye contains one atom of chromium, and although the dye does not fluoresce, it can be identified by its pink color in light microscope sections and by its electron density in thin sections. Thus, in thin sections, injected neurons can be distinguished from adjacent and uninjected neurons.

Another substance which has been used to inject individual neurons is cobaltous chloride (e.g., Pitman, Tweedle, and Cohen, 1972). After injection, the metal is precipitated as the sulfide by immersion of the tissue in ammonium sulfide. Although the resultant precipitate is black-brown in the light microscope and is also electron-dense, the disadvantage of this method appears to be that the ammonium sulfide leads to a distortion of the ultrastructure. A marked improvement in the use of cobaltous chloride seems to be gained by a modification recently introduced by Gillette and Pomeranz (1973). They use 3,3'-diaminobenzidine tetrahydrochloride (DAB) which turns the cobalt-injected neurons dark blue. After fixing the tissue in aldehydes followed by osmic acid, a dense polymer is found to accumulate beneath the plasma membranes of injected cells examined by electron microscopy.

Thus, these new methods make it possible to record from neurons which can subsequently be examined by light and electron microscopy to determine their morphology.

THE IDENTIFICATION OF PROFILES IN THE NEUROPIL

So far in this book, the parts of neurons and neuroglial cells have been described mainly as individual entities. The purpose of this section is to offer a brief guide to the identification of some of the different profiles that may be encountered in transmission electron microscope studies of the neuropil. Particular reference will be made to Figures 11–1 to 11–4, which are examples of the neuropil from the cerebellum, the cerebral cortex, and the anterior horn of the spinal cord of the rat and from the lateral geniculate nucleus of the cat.

In the neuropil, profiles of transversely sectioned dendrites (Figure 11–1, *Den;* Figure 11–3, *Den, Den₁*) can usually be recognized by their homogeneous content of microtubules. Mitochondria are also present along the length of a dendrite, but except for large dendrites there are few, if any, neurofilaments (Figure 11–1, *nf*). Other organelles that may be present are the cisternae of granular and smooth endoplasmic reticulum (Figures 11–1 and 11–3, *SR*) and ribosomes. Most of these organelles are shown in the apical dendrites (*Den*) of pyramidal neurons in Figure 11–3. At a greater distance from the perikaryon, the concentration of organelles other than microtubules and mitochondria is greatly reduced. In most situations the justification for labelling dendrites as farther away from a neuronal perikaryon is largely based upon the gradation in sizes of their profiles.

In the identification of longitudinally sectioned dendrites (Figure 11–2, *Den*; Figure 11–3, *Den₂*) their microtubular content is less useful, for small unmyelinated axons (Figures 11–2 and 11–3, *Ax*) also contain microtubules. Consequently, reliance must be placed upon other criteria. One of these is that, unlike axons beyond the initial segment, dendrites usually contain ribosomes. But the ribosomes may be sparse or even absent in small dendrites some distance from the parent cell body (Figures 11–1 and 11–3). Another useful criterion for the identification of longitudinally sectioned dendrites is that they often have irregular contours (Figure 11–2, *Den*; Figure 11–3, *Den₂*).

In addition to their cytoplasmic contents and irregular contours, an important characteristic of dendrites is that they commonly have axon terminals (Figures 11–1 to 11–3, *At*) synapsing upon their surfaces. Again, this feature is not unique to dendrites, for axo-axonal and dendro-dendritic synapses (Figure 11–4) also exist, but they are much less common than axo-dendritic synapses (Figures 11–1 to 11–3).

In some regions of the central nervous system, such as the anterior horn of the spinal cord (Figure 11–1), most of the axon terminals (*At*) form synaptic junctions (*s*) with the main stem of the dendrite. When this occurs, the neuropil has a relatively ordered appearance. In other areas, though, most of the axon terminals synapse with the spines and thorns that project from the dendrites (Figures 11–2 and 11–3). In thin sections, from the cerebral cortex, for example (Figure 11–3), the dendritic spines (*sp*) are only occasionally seen to be continuous with the parent dendrite. Most commonly they occur as isolated profiles in the area between the dendrites. Unlike the dendrites from which they arise, the spines in the cerebral cortex only rarely contain microtubules and neurofilaments. Instead, they characteristically contain a feltwork of fine interwoven fibrils, and sometimes a spine apparatus (*sa*). In size the spines (*sp*) often match the axon terminals (*At*) that synapse upon them.

Reference to Figure 11–2, which is from the molecular layer of the cerebellar cortex, shows that the thorns (*t*) in this neuropil are very similar to the spines of the cerebral cortex. The cytoplasm contains the same fine feltwork of fibrils, but unlike those of the cerebral cortex, the thorns in the cerebellum never contain a spine apparatus. Instead, they contain small tubules or other elements of the smooth endoplasmic reticulum. Again, the thorns are usually represented in the section by isolated profiles.

Axons in the neuropil are of two kinds, myelinated and unmyelinated. The myelinated processes are normally readily identified as axons (Figures 11–1 and 11–3, Ax_1), since myelinated dendrites have only so far been identified in the olfactory bulbs of the cat and monkey. Transverse sections through the paranodal regions of myelinated axons (Figure 11–1, Ax_2) may be distinguished from internodal regions by the presence of paranodal cytoplasm between

the myelin and the enclosed axon, and by the close apposition between the plasma membrane of the axon (axolemma) and the plasma membrane bounding the paranodal pockets of cytoplasm. The nodal regions of myelinated axons are marked by a dense undercoating of the axolemma (Figures 6–15 and 6–16). The initial segment of an axon (Figures 4–1 to 4–3) also exhibits this same undercoating, but in this case the microtubules are arranged in fascicles, whereas at the node they are evenly distributed.

Boutons en passant may occur at nodes of Ranvier. At these sites the cytoplasm contains synaptic vesicles and an increased number of mitochondria. Thus far there have been no descriptions of boutons synapsing upon the nodal axon.

Most of the preterminal branches of axons usually have a smaller diameter than that of any branch of a dendrite. They may measure only 0.1 to 0.2 micron. Also it is common to find small unmyelinated axons coursing through the neuropil in bundles (Figures 11–2 and 11–3, *Ax*). Dendrites usually occur as individuals, and groups of them have only been described in the cerebral cortex and in the spinal cord, but even here the bundles are much less compact. Further, the only parts of dendrites to attain the small diameter of preterminal axons are the spines or thorns, but these usually betray themselves by displaying a fine fibrillar network within their cytoplasm and by forming synapses with axon terminals.

Still, the most reliable morphological characteristic that can be used for the identification of an axon is the presence of synaptic vesicles somewhere in the axoplasm. These vesicles occur either along the length of an axon as it forms *boutons en passant* (Figure 11–2, *arrows*) or at terminations, where the axon enlarges into a *bouton terminal* (Figure 11–4, *At*). Of these two, the *bouton en passant* is the more common type of presynaptic structure, but the relative proportion of the two types of bouton in the neuropil of any particular region can be assessed

---

Figure 11–1.   **The Neuropil, Anterior Horn, Spinal Cord.**

Extending into the neuropil are dendrites (*Den*) whose cytoplasm contains microtubules, neurofilaments (*nf*), and cisternae of the smooth endoplasmic reticulum (*SR*). The preterminal unmyelinated axons (*Ax*) of this region give rise to terminals (*At*) that form synapses (*s*) with the dendrites. Other axons within the field are myelinated (Ax_1 and Ax_2). Passing between the neuronal components are processes of protoplasmic astrocytes (*As*), some of which have fibrils (*f*) within their cytoplasm.

See the text for further description.
Spinal cord from adult rat. × 23,000.

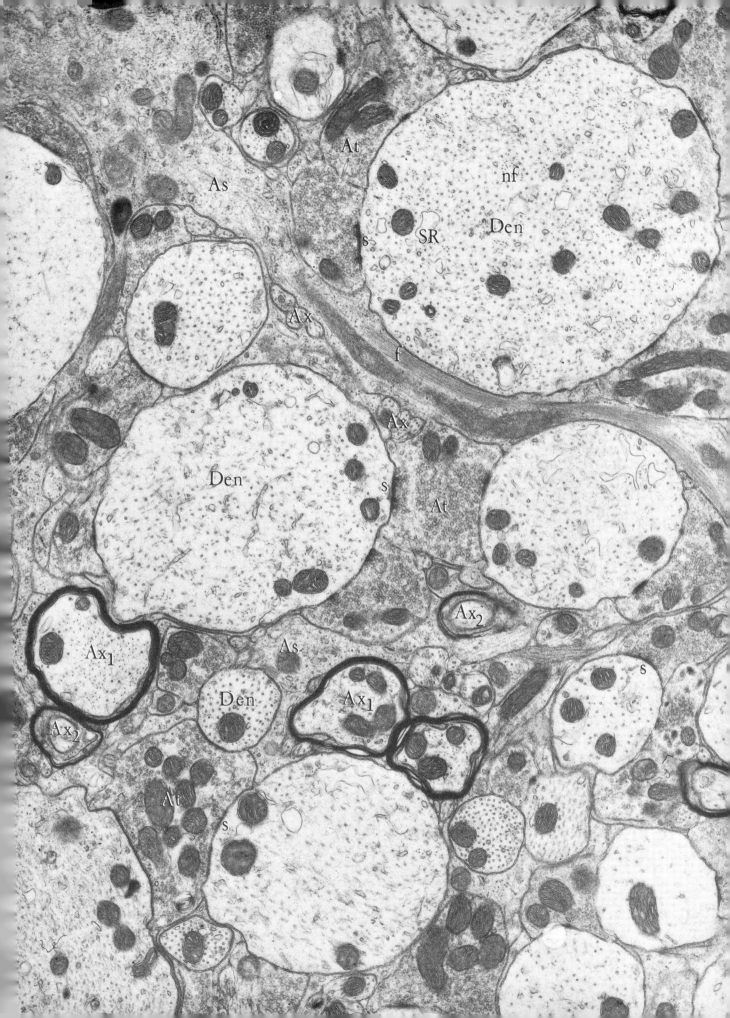

only from a critical survey of tissue sectioned in different planes. A comparison of Figure 11–2 with Figures 11–1 and 11–3 suggests that *boutons en passant* are much more common in the molecular layer of the cerebellum than in either the cerebral cortex or the spinal cord. However, this is so only because the section in Figure 11–2 passes through a favorable plane containing large numbers of straight and parallel axons that bear *boutons en passant*.

In Figure 11–2 most of the boutons en passant (*arrows*) are unilateral in which the synaptic vesicles are confined to one side of the axon, sometimes within an outpocketing. In other situations the vesicles occupy a symmetrical swelling of the axon and surround a central core of neurofilaments and microtubules (Figure 11–4, *Ax*).

It is now apparent that synaptic vesicles are not confined to axons, but may also occur in dendrites, as particularly evidenced in studies of the olfactory bulb and the thalamic nuclei. In the case of presynaptic dendrites, however, vesicles are often seen to occur in quite small groups in localized regions of processes which show other features which are characteristic of dendrites, such as a relatively large diameter, a content of microtubules, and the presence of some ribosomes in their cytoplasm. The vesicle-containing terminal portions of dendrites most frequently have the form of enlargements at the end of spinous processes and look very much like axonal boutons. This is exemplified by the gemmules or spines of the granule cells of the olfactory bulb (Figure 3–7) and, as seems likely, some of the boutons in the glomeruli of the thalamic nuclei (see Figure 11–4). Differentiation of these vesicle-containing terminals of dendrites from axonal boutons is very difficult in random electron micrographs, as can be seen in Figure 11–4. Only a careful study of correlated Golgi preparations or of serial thin sections will reveal the true identity and origin of the termi-nals. Fortunately, the occurrence of dendritic boutons is relatively rare, but their existence should always be borne in mind when carrying out studies on various parts of the nervous system.

The majority of evidence accumulated in the past few years has led to the concept that when only one of the neuronal components involved in the formation of a synapse contains synaptic vesicles, then it is the presynaptic element. Furthermore, when the synapse (Figures 11–1 to 11–3) is formed between two neuronal processes, then it is most likely that the postsynaptic component is a dendrite, since axo-dendritic synapses are the most common. But axo-axonal and dendro-dendritic synapses also exist, as described in Chapter V. In the examples of axo-axonal synapses so far described in the literature, the postsynaptic component is either an axon initial segment or the vesicle-containing preterminal portion of an axon close to the site where it itself synapses with a third component. In this latter situation, two of the three processes in the series contain vesicles. Then at each interface it is conventional to consider that the presynaptic element is the one in which at least some of the vesicles are concentrated close to the synaptic junction. Thus, the intermediate component is postsynaptic to the first component and presynaptic to the third, but as explained on page 162, there is a distinct possibility that the second vesicle-containing component of a serial synapse may sometimes be a dendrite (see Figure 11–4). So far this possibility has only been raised in the case of serial synapses in the thalamic glomeruli, but it would be worth while to re-examine other examples of supposed serial axo-axonal synapses, since the majority of them were described before the occurrence of vesicle-containing dendritic boutons was suspected.

Chemical synapses may be distinguished from similar junctions that are believed to be

---

Figure 11–2. **The Neuropil, Cerebellar Cortex.**

In the upper left of this picture from the molecular layer is part of a stellate cell from which a dendrite (*Den*) arises. Parallel fibers (*Ax*) passing through the neuropil are seen in transverse section. These fibers result from the dichotomy of the primary stems of granule cell axons (*Ax₁*), which in this plane are sectioned longitudinally. Close to the points of bifurcation the main stems (*Ax₁*) of the granule cell axons enlarge and come into synaptic relation (*arrows*) with thorns (*t*) projecting from the dendrites of Purkinje cells. At frequent intervals along their lengths the parallel fibers (*Ax*) form *boutons en passant* (*At*) that also synapse with the thorns (*t*) of Purkinje cell dendrites. Synapsing with the perikaryon of the stellate cell is an axon terminal (*At₁*) derived from a collateral of a climbing fiber.

Most of the astrocytic processes within this field (*As*) form sheaths around the synapses.

See the text for further explanation.
Cerebellar cortex from adult rat. × *16,000.*

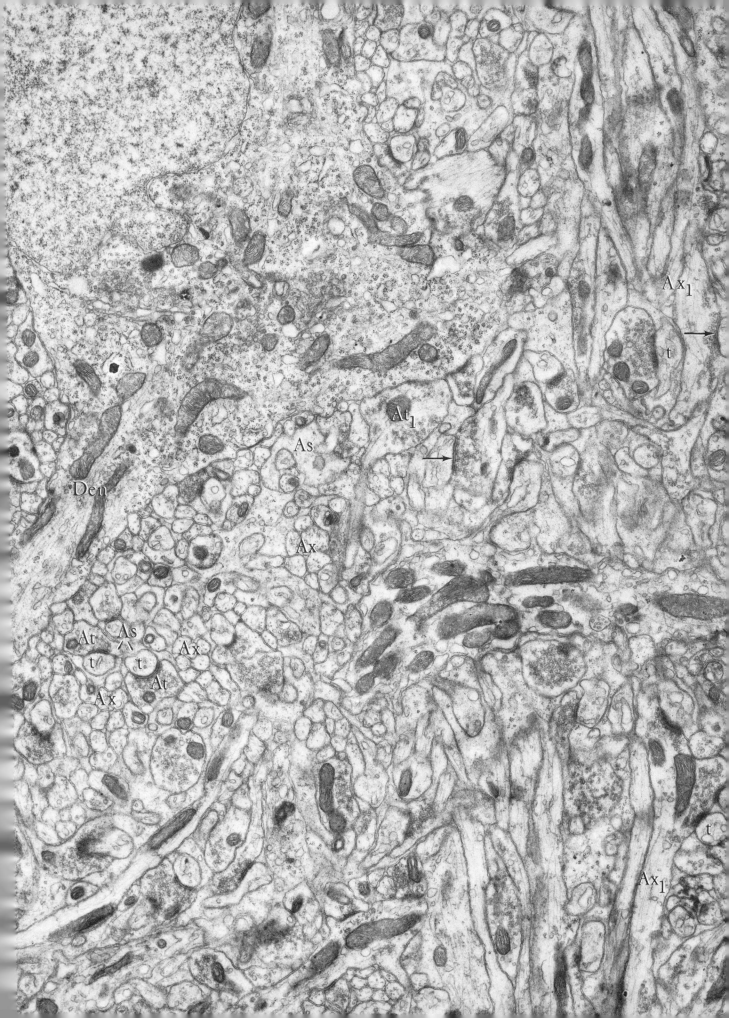

nonsynaptic by the fact that at least one of the partners contains synaptic vesicles. The nonsynaptic junctions, *puncta adhaerentia,* occur between both neuronal and non-neuronal components, and they resemble *zonulae adhaerentes* in structure. The density associated with the cytoplasmic surfaces of the two plasma membranes taking part in the *puncta adhaerentia* is usually symmetrically distributed, and the extracellular space between the membranes contains a centrally placed dense line.

Although electrical synapses, as opposed to the chemical ones described above, may occur in the mammalian nervous system, it seems that they are rare. Data derived mainly from lower vertebrates indicate that the presence of such a synapse may be suspected when the plasma membranes of two neuronal profiles are arranged exactly parallel to each other and form a gap junction. Then, the extracellular space between the neuronal profiles is reduced to 2 to 3 nm. In mixed synapses of the type occurring in the lateral vestibular nucleus and some parts of the nervous systems of lower vertebrates, the electrical junctions are interspersed with chemical junctions (see Figure 5–19).

Gap junctions also occur between astrocytic (see Figure 7–3) and oligodendroglial processes. Consequently, the identity of the components taking part in the formation of a gap junction must be ascertained as neuronal before an electrical synapse is suspected.

The processes of fibrous astrocytes in white matter can readily be identified by the bundles of fibrils within their cytoplasm (Figure 7–1). The processes of protoplasmic astrocytes may also contain fibrils (Figure 11–1, *f*), but in general, fibrils are less common than in fibrous astrocytes and it is not unusual for them to be completely absent. Fortunately, the profiles of the processes of protoplasmic astrocytes can frequently be recognized by their irregular shapes (Figures 11–1 to 11–4, *As*). They adapt themselves to the contours of the surrounding neuronal elements and only rarely have the rounded shapes that are typical of dendrites and axons.

Processes of protoplasmic astrocytes may be encountered anywhere in the neuropil. Often they form thin sheets that surround synapses (Figures 11–1 to 11–3). This is particularly evident when a number of neuronal processes are aggregated into a glomerulus. In addition, the processes of astrocytes always seem to provide a complete sheath around capillaries (Figures 10–1 and 10–2) and, indeed, around the central nervous system as a whole (Figure 13–4).

Profiles of oligodendrocyte processes can be readily confused with those of dendrites; both are rounded in outline and in both the microtubules are homogeneously dispersed (Figure 7–7). Oligodendrocyte processes are, however, usually much smaller than dendrites and have a higher concentration of microtubules. Another feature useful in distinguishing between the two is that oligodendrocyte processes have a dense cytoplasm (Figure 11–3, *Op*). The density is produced by the presence of small granules, which make an oligodendrocytic process appreciably darker than the adjacent dendrites.

The cells recently identified as microglia (Figures 7–9 and 7–10) may easily be confused with oligodendrocytes (Figures 7–7 and 7–8). Microglia occur throughout the neuropil and are common in the vicinity of blood vessels, beneath the glia limitans, and in perineuronal positions. The processes of the microglia are rather broad and generally somewhat lighter than those of oligodendrocytes. They contain fewer microtubules, frequently have elongate

Figure 11–3. **The Neuropil, Cerebral Cortex.**

In this tangentially oriented section of the cerebral cortex are the transverse profiles of five large dendrites (*Den*), probably sections of the apical dendrites of pyramidal neurons. Their cytoplasm contains regular arrays of microtubules (*m*) embedded in a fine matrix, which also contains mitochondria (*mit*) and cisternae of the smooth endoplasmic reticulum (*SR*). Smaller transversely sectioned dendrites (*Den₁*) are also present in the neuropil, as well as some dendrites (*Den₂*) that are sectioned obliquely. Many of these dendrites give rise to spines, although in this field none of these are seen to be attached to their parent dendrites. Some of the spines (*sp*) form synapses with axonal boutons (*At*), but others (*sp₁*) do not show their synapses. Other axon terminals (*At₁*) synapse on the shafts of dendrites.

The terminals arise from small unmyelinated axons (*Ax*). The field also contains two myelinated axons (*Ax₁*).

Interspersed with the neuronal components are astrocytic processes (*As*) and extending around the large dendrite in the top right corner of the field is an oligodendroglial process (*Op*).

See the text for further explanation.

Cerebral cortex of rat. × 20,000.

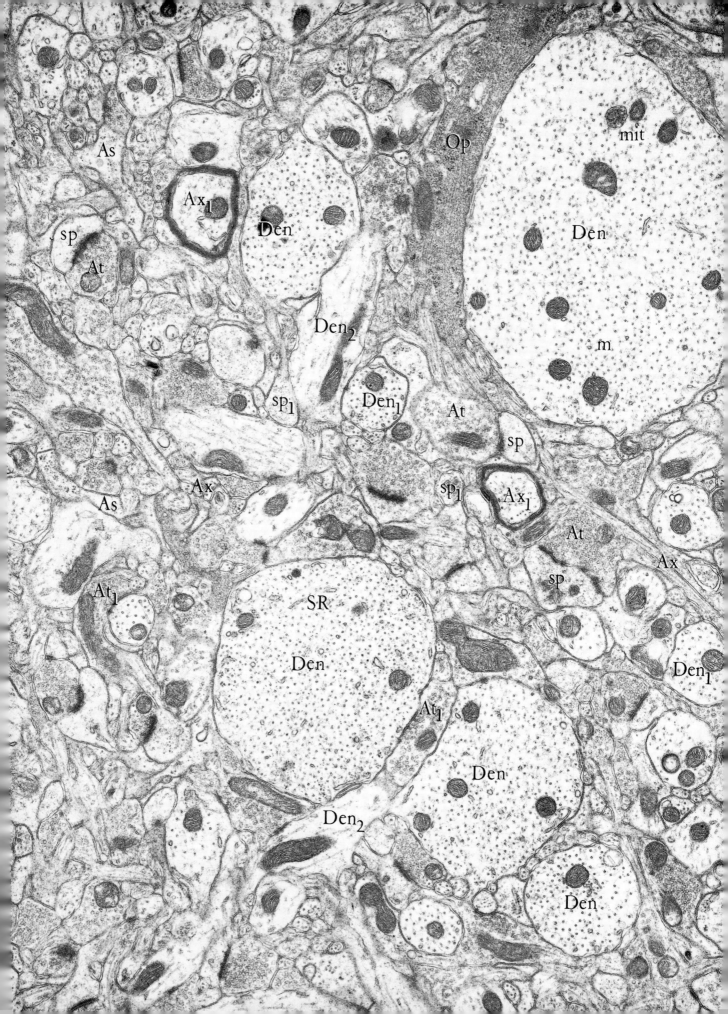

profiles of granular endoplasmic reticulum, and have shapes that resemble the processes of astrocytes in that their contours tend to conform to the outlines of the components of the neuropil through which they pass. In addition the microglia commonly show lysosomes and lipofuscin granules (Figures 7–9 and 7–10), especially in older animals. It may be stated that because of the similarities between oligodendrocytes and microglial cells many of the perineuronal satellites previously categorized as oligodendrocytes are in reality microglial cells. At least in the cerebral cortex, microglia are often partially separated from the neuronal surfaces by flattened astrocytic processes, whereas oligodendrocytes are more directly apposed to the neurons. Whether this difference between these two dark forms of neuroglial cells is true elsewhere in the central nervous system has not yet been established.

Finally, a word about pericytes. As pointed out in the chapter on blood vessels (Chapter X), pericytes are always completely enclosed within a basal lamina (Figure 10–1). In contrast, neuroglial cells reside within the neuropil, and so when they are adjacent to the blood vessels, only the perivascular face ever abuts the basal lamina. The other surfaces of the perivascular neuroglial cells lie directly adjacent to neuronal or other neuroglial profiles.

The foregoing account is presented as a guide to the identification of the profiles that may be encountered in electron microscopic preparations of areas of the neuropil. It is not a definitive key to all situations and relations within the central nervous system, for it is based upon present knowledge, which covers only a few parts of the nervous system in a limited number of animal species. As more regions of the central nervous system are examined, new and unusual relationships between the components will undoubtedly be encountered. Then, just as now, we shall need to resort to common sense, past experience, and the correlation of electron microscopy with data derived from other disciplines.

THE ORGANIZATION OF THE NEUROPIL

To study a given part of the central nervous system further and to determine the exact relationships between its components, one must examine more closely the features displayed in electron micrographs. To achieve this end, it is first necessary to determine the criteria that can be used to distinguish between the various types of neurons present. This effort must begin with a light microscope study of Nissl-stained and Golgi-impregnated preparations, as well as of thick sections taken from electron microscope blocks. On the basis of such preparations an evaluation can be made of the frequency, shapes, sizes, and Nissl patterns of neurons in the population under consideration. It is then necessary to transfer this information to the electron microscope level. Even then a correlation between the appearance of neurons in light and electron microscope preparations may not be possible, so that one must resort to additional lines of approach.

One of these approaches is the electron microscope examination of Golgi-impregnated neurons previously identified in the light microscope (e.g., see Stell, 1965). Initially the Golgi-impregnated neurons may be examined either on the cut surface of a plastic-embedded block by using incident light (see Blackstad, 1970; Ramón-Moliner and Ferrari, 1972), or in thick plastic sections by transmitted light (see West, 1972; LeVay, 1973). After study, the impregnated neurons can be thin sectioned. At present

---

Figure 11–4. **Lateral Geniculate Body Glomerulus.**

This synaptic glomerulus contains a large central axon (*Ax*) replete with synaptic vesicles (*sv*), neurofilaments (*nf*), and mitochondria (*mit*). This axon is the presynaptic element in synapses (*arrows*) with two other major components of the glomerulus. One of these components (*Den₁*) is a typical dendritic process. The other (*Den₂*) is also dendritic but contains synaptic vesicles (*sv*) and so was originally regarded as an axon. These vesicle-containing dendritic terminals also synapse (*arrowhead*) with the typical dendritic processes through dendro-dendritic synapses. The junctions that have no synaptic vesicles associated with them are puncta adhaerentia (*pa*).

A portion of the astrocytic covering of the glomerulus is visible at the top right. *Dorsal nucleus of lateral geniculate body of cat. × 40,000.*

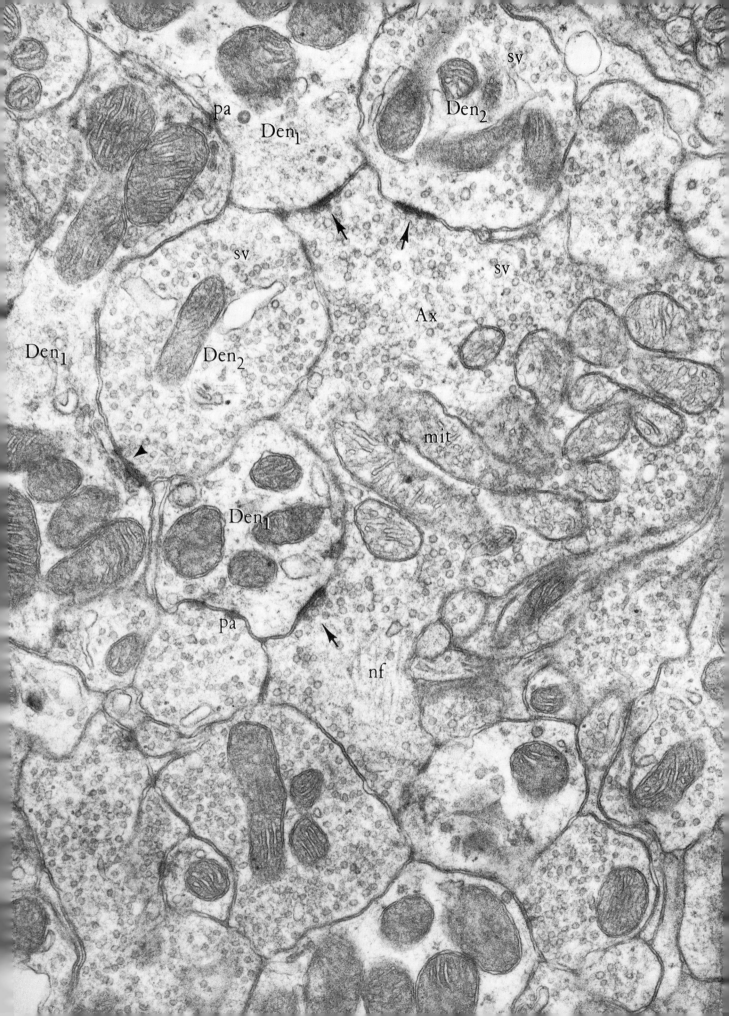

these techniques are in their infancy and have not been fully perfected or exploited. The general fixation of the Golgi-impregnated tissues is usually poor, and the granules of the heavy metal precipitate of silver chromate (Chan-Palay, 1973h) contained in the cytoplasm can make sectioning difficult. Another problem arises when the sections are examined in the electron microscope. Heating of the heavy metal granules can make the sections very unstable in the electron beam and may lead to distortion of the cytoplasmic features. Some useful progress may result from examining 1- to 5-micron thick sections of Golgi-impregnated material in the high voltage electron microscope (see Chan-Palay and Palay, 1972a and b; Palay and Chan-Palay, 1973). Finer details of the shapes of impregnated cells and their processes can be gained by using this technique, although visualization of the intervening unimpregnated components of the neuropil has not yet been achieved (see Scott and Guillery, 1974).

So that a direct comparison can be made with the components apparent in Golgi-impregnated material, another useful approach in determining the forms of neuronal processes is to make reconstructions from serial thin sections. This method also allows the relations between specific neuronal processes and other components of the neuropil to be established. Such an approach has been employed by a number of investigators (e.g., Pinching and Powell, 1971a and b; White, 1972; Famiglietti and Peters, 1972; Vaughan and Peters, 1973; Hinds and Hinds, 1974), but it is fraught with a number of technical problems. Not the least of these is the preparation of a sufficiently long and continuous series of thin sections. For it must be remembered that if sections are cut at an average thickness of 50 nm, 20 sections are required to reconstruct a slab of tissue 1 micron thick. Another problem occurs when structures are less than about 1 micron thick, as are many unmyelinated axons, for then it is often impossible to follow their profiles from section to section. This is especially true when the structures pass obliquely through the series of sections, for they are often lost because of the superimposition of their images onto those of adjacent elements. At present, reconstructions are made by tracing individual profiles visually, but ultimately it should be possible to speed up the reconstruction process by automatically scanning the micrographs with a small light beam and feeding the information into a computer. A number of laboratories are proceeding along these lines.

Once the various forms of neurons and their processes have been identified in a given region of the nervous system, attention may be turned to the synapses which they form. As a first approach, the different forms of boutons received and the patterns they form on the postsynaptic component can be studied. This type of analysis can be initiated on the basis of the sizes and shapes of the boutons present, the character of their vesicles after aldehyde fixation, the types of junctions in which they participate, and the features of the pre- and postsynaptic sides of the junctions and their sites. When studies of this kind have been attempted they have generally proved to be useful.

Examples of this kind of approach are certain studies of the cerebral cortex (e.g., Colonnier, 1968; Jones and Powell, 1970a to e), the anterior horn of the spinal cord (e.g., Conradi, 1969a and b; Conradi and Skoglund, 1969a and b; Bodian, 1972), the lateral vestibular nucleus (Sotelo and Palay, 1970), and the deep cerebellar nuclei (Chan-Palay, 1973d and f).

Taking this type of study further, as a next step, it is possible to quantitate the frequency of occurrence of different forms of boutons, both in terms of the percentage of each form present and the numbers per unit area of postsynaptic neuronal surface (e.g., see Conradi, 1969a; Lemkey-Johnston and Larramendi, 1968b; Cragg, 1967; Kaiserman-Abramof and Peters, 1972). Because of the rather irregular shapes of neurons, figures for the absolute number of boutons present on either portions of neurons or on entire neurons are difficult to obtain, and so few values are available. Yet some quantification must be achieved if we are eventually to assess the effects of various inputs on the activity of neurons.

The ultimate step is to construct the circuitry of a region. This requires the identification of the afferent terminals according to their source as well as the different parts of the intrinsic nerve cells receiving the inputs. Such studies require careful correlation of results from all available microscopic methods. Examples of this stage of analysis are, of course, relatively few and the retina (Dowling and Boycott, 1966; Dowling, 1968; Dowling, 1970;) and the cortex of the cerebellum (e.g., Mugnaini, 1972; Palay and Chan-Palay, 1974) are at the most advanced stage of study. At a somewhat less advanced stage are studies of the deep cerebellar nuclei (Chan-Palay, 1973a to g), the basal ganglia (e.g., Fox, Andrade, Qui, and Rafols, 1974), the lateral geniculate nucleus (e.g., Guillery, 1969;

Famiglietti and Peters, 1972; Wong-Riley, 1972), the olfactory bulb (e.g., Price and Powell, 1970a and b; Pinching and Powell, 1971a and b; Shep-herd, 1974), the hippocampus (Gottlieb and Cowan, 1972), and the cochlear nucleus (Brawer, Morest, and Kane, 1974).

EXPERIMENTAL APPROACHES

To determine the origins of boutons synapsing with neurons in a given part of the nervous system experimental techniques are necessary. The most common of these techniques employs degeneration. Boutons formed by afferent nerve fibers are made to degenerate as the result of a lesion which interrupts the parent nerve fibers or destroys their cells of origin. To effect lesions it is best to make use of a stereotactic head holder so that the tip of the lesioning electrode can be accurately placed. For most purposes lesions can be made by electrical or thermal co-agulation, and in general no recordings are taken from the neurons prior to their being interrupted. When such recording can be made, however, then there is no doubt that more accurate and repeatable lesions can be effected. Once a lesion has been made, it is usual to allow the animal to recover from the operation and to wait for a period of one to five days so that the boutons emanating from the affected nerve fibers have had time to reach a state in which their degeneration can be recognized in tissue fixed for morphological examination.

Before studying the degenerating boutons with the electron microscope, it is best to carry out a preliminary light microscope study of the pattern of degeneration produced. Perhaps the best method for achieving this aim is by the Fink-Heimer technique (Fink and Heimer, 1967) in which the degenerating boutons are impregnated with silver so that they show up as black dots in the light microscope (see Heimer and Peters, 1968). It should be remembered, however, that it is not sufficient to study only the region containing the degenerating boutons. A careful assessment must always be made of the locations of the lesions used to bring about the terminal degeneration and the path taken by the lesioning electrode. Consequently, in each case light microscope sections, usually frozen sections stained by the Nissl method, must be taken through the lesion site. Without such an assessment the experimenter has no assurance that the lesion was actually made in the intended site.

Once the appropriate sites for making lesions have been determined with the light microscope and the optimal times for producing adequate degeneration of boutons have been determined, attention can be turned to an electron microscope study of the distribution patterns of degenerating boutons. After a suitable post-operative period has elapsed, the nervous system should be perfused and blocks for electron microscopy taken from the region containing the degenerating terminals. Again, the positions of the lesions must be carefully assessed with the light microscope. Before taking thin sections from the areas containing degenerating boutons, it is useful to take a number of thick (1 to 2 microns) sections that can be stained for degenerating boutons by the Fink-Heimer modification for plastic sections (see Heimer, 1970; Figure 11–5).

Two primary kinds of degeneration have been encountered in electron microscope preparations containing boutons which have been experimentally isolated from their parent neurons (e.g., see Gray and Guillery, 1966; Guillery, 1970; Raismen and Matthews, 1972). One kind may be termed *electron-dense degeneration* and the other *neurofilamentous hypertrophy*.

Electron-dense degeneration is most common, and as the name suggests, it is characterized by a darkening of the isolated axon terminals (Figure 11–5). The degenerating terminals first show a slight increase in density and a tendency for the synaptic vesicles to become more closely packed together. Later the darkening is more pronounced, the terminals assume irregular outlines, and their contents of mitochondria and synaptic vesicles become less recognizable (Figure 11–5). At about this time the degenerating terminals become obviously surrounded by astrocytic processes, which may show glycogen in their cytoplasm (Figure 11–5, *As*). Whether this prominence of the astrocytic processes is due to a hypertrophy of the processes that normally surround the synapses or due to the formation of new processes has not been established. In any case, after the appropriate postoperative time has elapsed the astrocytic reaction is very apparent, and the degenerating terminals become engulfed by astrocytic processes, which isolate them from the surrounding neuropil. Even at this stage the synaptic junction remains intact so that the form of both the junction and the postsynaptic component of the synapse can still be recognized. In most systems this degree of degeneration is usually attained between two and seven days postoperatively and is the best stage for analytical purposes. Later the degenerating terminals become more fragmented and are gradually detached from their synaptic components so that the number of readily recognized boutons is reduced. The eventual fate of the terminals appears not to have been established.

In the kind of degeneration accompanied by *neurofilamentous hypertrophy* there is a progressive increase in the number of neurofilaments in the terminals (Figure 11–6, *upper picture*). First, within one to seven days following a lesion the affected terminals become almost entirely filled by a dense tangle of neurofilaments. Concomitantly, the synaptic vesicles gradually disappear, and those that do remain tend to crowd toward the synaptic junctions. Sometimes, as in the superior colliculus (Lund, 1969) and in the ventrobasal complex of the thalamus (Ralston, 1969), the filamentous change occurs initially and later proceeds to dense degeneration.

Both kinds of degeneration just described occur in the central nervous system, but in the peripheral nervous system degenerating axon terminals show a somewhat different pattern of changes. In the preganglionic terminals in the superior cervical ganglion, for example (Rais-

man and Matthews, 1972), there is first a clumping of the synaptic vesicles toward the centers of the terminals, some of which begin to display dense bodies in their cytoplasm. The presence of these dense bodies suggests that some form of autophagocytic process may be taking place. The degeneration of these peripheral axon terminals is also characterized by the formation of multiple concentric wrappings which the Schwann cells produce around them. Subsequently, the axon terminals swell, the wrappings disappear, and ultimately the terminals become phagocytosed by the surrounding Schwann cells.

Although the placing of lesions is a very widely employed and invaluable technique for neuroanatomists, it must be used with care, and it must be determined that the changes are not produced by unspecific effects such as mechanical or vascular damage. The method also has severe limitations in that it cannot be used to examine short fiber systems such as the terminations of intrinsic neurons, for small enough lesions cannot be placed. Indeed, the determination of the connections of intrinsic neurons remains one of the most outstanding problems to be solved.

Another problem in using lesions is that not only may neurons at the site of a lesion be affected, but any nerve fibers passing through that site may be also involved. One means of avoiding this problem is to label nerve terminals specifically by injecting radioactive amino acids, such as proline and leucine, at the level of their neuronal perikarya (see review by Cowan, Gottlieb, Hendrickson, Price, and Woolsey, 1972). These amino acids can be either injected or

---

Figure 11–5. **Degenerating Boutons.**

The **upper picture** is a light micrograph of a vertical section through part of layers IV and V in area 17 (visual cortex) of the rat cerebral cortex. A lesion was made in the dorsal lateral geniculate nucleus, and the animal was allowed to survive for three days before fixation. The tissue was then fixed by aldehyde perfusion, and after osmication it was embedded in an Araldite-Epon mixture. This 2-micron thick section was then stained by the Fink-Heimer method. This displays the degenerating terminals of the geniculocortical afferent axons as dense dots (*arrows*). It will be seen that the degenerating boutons are most prominent in layer IV.
Area 17 of rat cerebral cortex. × 800.

Micrograph by M. L. Feldman.

The **lower picture** is an electron micrograph showing a degenerating axon terminal (*At*) from the same tissue block as that used to prepare the light micrograph shown above. This dark degenerating axon terminal is in layer IV and is forming asymmetrical synapses (s_1 and s_2) with two dendritic spines (sp_1 and sp_2). Note the astrocytic processes (*AsP*) surrounding the degenerating terminal.
Area 17 of rat cerebral cortex. × 50,000.

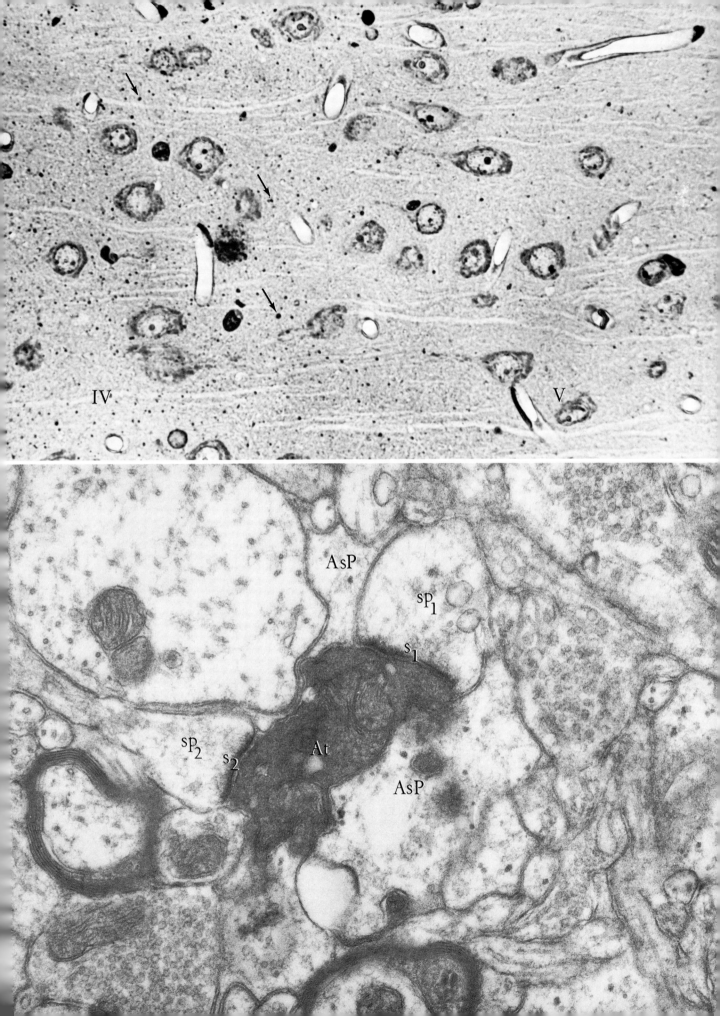

electrophoresed into the areas containing the perikarya, which take up the amino acids and transport them along the axons to the terminals. As discussed in Chapter IV, in the section on axonal flow, there are two rates of axonal flow: slow and fast. By selecting an appropriate post-injection survival time, the presence of the labelled amino acids or their derivatives can be demonstrated by autoradiography both along the paths of the axons and at their terminals. However, it should be recognized that the introduction of a quantity of a radioactive amino acid around neuronal perikarya does not constitute a pulse label, for the amino acids remain available for uptake by the neurons for an extended period of time. While the exposure times for light microscope autoradiography may be only one to three weeks, a month or more seems necessary for electron microscopic localization of photographic grains over axon terminals in thin sections. Despite this disadvantage, however, the absence of degeneration makes it possible to assess the normal morphology of the terminals derived from axons projecting to the area in question.

Use of either the degenerative or radioactive techniques allows the projection of the axons of neurons to be determined. As mentioned in Chapter IV, however, injected horseradish peroxidase is taken up by axon terminals and transported to their parent cell bodies (Figure 11–6, *lower picture.*). Hence this technique can be used to ascertain the positions of neurons giving rise to axon terminals. So far, horseradish peroxidase has been employed in only a few but steadily increasing number of studies (e.g., Jones and Leavitt, 1973; Ralston and Sharp, 1973; La Vail and La Vail, 1974; Nauta, Pritz,

and Lasek, 1974; 1974; Maciewicz, 1974), although little use has been made of this marker at the electron microscope level.

Turner and Harris (1974) injected horseradish peroxidase into the subdural space and found that the material spread through the glia limitans and into the cerebral cortex. If the neurons were damaged, they found that the horseradish peroxidase was taken up from the extracellular space into the neuronal perikarya by pinocytosis to become sequestered in coated vesicles. From there it seems to enter sacs and tubules of the endoplasmic reticulum, and multivesicular bodies as well as lysosomes. Axon terminals also pinocytose the tracer, and by 24 hours as many as 10 per cent of the myelinated axons in the area contained horseradish peroxidase. As an interesting side issue, Turner and Harris found that the cytoplasm of damaged neurons became flooded with peroxidase. This finding also emerges from the studies of Nauta, Pritz, and Lasek (1974) and could explain the observation of Adams and Warr (personal communication) that if nerve fibers are severed and horseradish peroxidase injected at the site of the lesion, the marker is transported in two directions: toward the parent perikarya and toward the axon terminals formed by the nerve fibers. In addition, in the future it can be expected that use will be made of combinations of these techniques for marking neurons and their processes. An example of this is provided by the light microscope study of Graybiel and Devor (1974) who simultaneously electrophoresed horseradish peroxidase and tritiated proline into the cerebellar vermis of the rat. They found radioactively labelled fibers that could be traced to the fastigial nucleus and located horseradish

---

Figure 11–6.   Filamentous Degeneration and Horseradish Peroxidase–Labelled Neurons.

The **upper figure** shows a synaptic glomerulus from the lateral geniculate body of a cat three days after enucleation of the eye. In the middle of the field is the terminal (*Ax*) of an optic nerve axon. This shows an early stage of filamentous degeneration characterized by an accumulation of filaments (*f*) and the appearance of glycogen particles (*gly*). If this glomerulus is compared with the one shown in Figure 11–4, it will be seen that the terminal has lost most of its synaptic vesicles (*sv*), although some of the synaptic junctions (*arrows*) still persist.

Beginning at four to five days after enucleation, the optic axon terminals progress to a "secondary" phase of dense degeneration.
Dorsal nucleus of lateral geniculate body of cat. × 25,000.

Micrograph by F. V. Famiglietti.

The **lower picture** is a light micrograph showing the dense granules produced by the horseradish peroxidase reaction in the perikarya and dendrites of neurons in the superior olivary complex. The horseradish peroxidase was injected into the cochlea. It was taken up by axon terminals and transported in a retrograde direction to these efferent neurons.
Superior olivary complex of kitten. × 1500.

Micrograph by W. B. Warr.

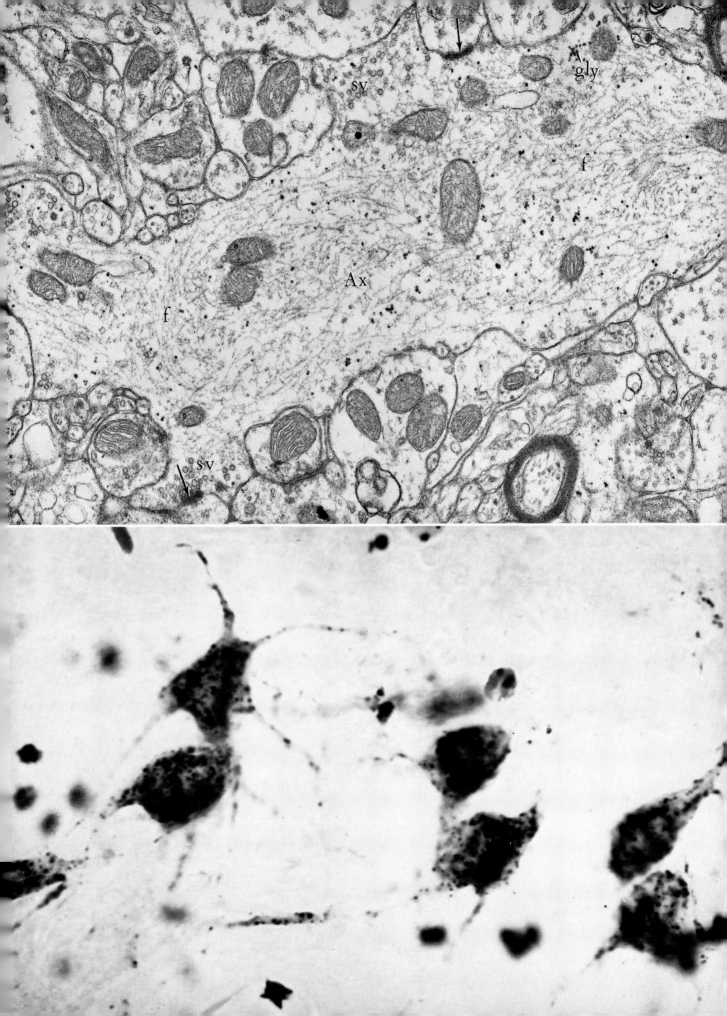

peroxidase in neurons of the inferior olivary complex and pontine gray matter contralateral to the injection site.

Finally, with respect to axon terminals, differentiation among various types may be made on the basis of the kinds of transmitter which they contain. Unfortunately, there is no means by which acetylcholine can be detected in synaptic boutons *in situ*, but in the case of γ-aminobutyric acid (GABA) and glycine it is possible to demonstrate boutons containing these transmitters by soaking pieces of tissue in solutions containing tritiated forms of either the transmitters or their precursors. These chemicals are then sequestered within specific boutons whose identity can be established by autoradiography (e.g., Iversen and Bloom, 1972; Matus, and Dennison, 1971). These labelling techniques have not been fully worked out, but the methods seem to be promising. A different technique is that of Saito, Barber, Wu, Matsuda, Roberts, and Vaughn (1974), who used a rabbit antiserum to purified mouse brain glutamate decarboxylase for demonstrating γ-aminobutyric acid contained in sections of boutons in the rat cerebellum. Glutamate decarboxylase is the enzyme that forms γ-aminobutyric acid. The sections were then incubated in peroxidase-labelled goat antibody against rabbit immunoglobulin, and the glutamate decarboxylase-containing sites were made visible in the sections by means of the peroxidase activity. The reaction product is also visible in electron microscope preparations (McLaughlin, Wood, Saito, Barber, Roberts, and Wu, 1974), and in the rat cerebellum for example, it is localized in presumed Golgi cell endings in the glomeruli and in basket cell endings on Purkinje cells.

With these new approaches for studying the connections of neurons, the types of transmitters in their terminals, and the potential correlation between the synaptic junctions and forms of neurons, electron microscopy of the nervous system can be expected to gain momentum. The future possibilities are exciting and provide a strong reason for continued morphological study of the details of the organization of the neuropil, for in the absence of these details, the new techniques cannot be employed in a manner which will allow their full potential to be explored.

Chapter XII

CONNECTIVE TISSUE SHEATHS OF PERIPHERAL NERVES

As described in Chapter VI, axons of the peripheral nervous system are embedded in Schwann cells and are either myelinated or unmyelinated. Such nerve fibers pass in or out of the central nervous system as the cranial and spinal nerves and become aggregated into fascicles that make up the peripheral nerves. The nerves have three separate connective tissue sheaths, first described by Key and Retzius (1876) and by Ranvier (1878), and the descriptive terminology advocated by Key and Retzius is in current usage. Thus, as shown in the upper picture of Figure 12–1, on the outside of each peripheral nerve is a collagenous *epineurium (Ep)* and beneath that a *perineurium (Per)* which surrounds each fascicle of nerve fibers. Individual nerve fibers are embedded in an *endoneurium (En)*, which completely fills the space bounded by the perineurium.

These three connective tissue sheaths are all present around the larger peripheral nerves, which are composed of numerous fascicles of nerve fibers. As a peripheral nerve divides and the number of fascicles in the resultant branches is reduced, the connective tissue sheaths become progressively thinner. It is usually stated that around monofascicular nerves the epineurium is lacking, intermittent, or merged with the perineurium and so can no longer be distinguished as a separate entity. More distally, before the individual nerve fibers terminate, their sheaths thin out and are no longer distinguishable from the general connective tissue.

For the light microscopic appearance and composition of the connective tissue sheaths in general, reference should be made to the accounts by Causey (1960), Sutherland (1965), and Shantha and Bourne (1968), while details about the form of the endoneurium can be obtained from the reviews by Nageotte (1932) and Young (1942).

The following description of the fine structure of the connective tissue sheaths of peripheral nerves is based upon the articles by Thomas (1963 and 1964a), Gamble (1964), Gamble and Eames (1964), Burkel (1967), and Gray (1970). The sheaths enclosing peripheral nerve ganglia have been examined by Andres (1961) and by Lieberman (1968) and appear to have an essentially similar form to those surrounding the nerves.

323

EPINEURIUM

The epineurium (Figures 12–1 and 12–2) contains connective tissue fibers and fibroblasts as well as blood vessels and some small nerve fibers which innervate the vessels. This outermost sheath encloses the fascicles of nerve fibers and is generally accepted as having a mesodermal origin. However, facial mesenchyme, including sheaths of nerves to the face, is derived from cranial neural crest cells (Johnston and Listgarten, 1972; Johnston, Bhakdinaronk, and Reid, 1973). The components of the epineurium, the most prominent of which are collagen fibers (Figures 12–1 and 12–2, *Col*), are mainly oriented longitudinally. Collagen fibers are between 70 and 85 nm thick in the rabbit gastrocnemius nerve (Thomas, 1963) and 60 to 100 nm in the human sural nerve (Gamble and Eames, 1964). The collagen fibers are identified by their regular periodic banding of about 64 nm, although in high resolution micrographs several additional bands can be resolved within each major period. Elastin fibers are also present, and these are much stouter than the collagen fibers, since they are each between 250 and 500 nm thick. In electron micrographs it is usual to find that elastin fibers are most darkly stained at their peripheries and are embedded in a ground substance containing finer filaments about 10 nm thick (Thomas, 1963). Other 10-nm filaments are intermixed with the collagen and are independent of the elastin fibers.

Scattered throughout the epineurium are the fibroblasts (Figure 12–2, *Fb*) which form the connective tissue fibers. These cells have fusiform perikarya and send out elongate processes between the connective tissue fibers. They lack a basal lamina. Their elliptical nuclei contain a generally light chromatin with some clumps beneath the nuclear envelope. The long and thin mitochondria are mainly concentrated in the perikaryon where an inconspicuous Golgi apparatus is also confined.

As pointed out, the epineurium does not form a continuous coat around the small bundles of nerves, and in such situations most light microscope accounts state that it is absent. However, Burkel (1967) considers an epineurium to be present, although discontinuous, around small nerves to the eye muscles, where it looks no different from the loose connective tissue sheaths surrounding muscle fibers and blood vessels.

PERINEURIUM

The perineurium (Figures 12–1 to 12–3, *Per*) lies beneath the epineurium and separately encloses each fascicle of nerve fibers. It is distinctive in being composed of flattened or squamous cells; the number of layers of such cells seems to depend upon the size of the nerve fascicles ensheathed and their proximity to the central nervous system (Shantha and Bourne, 1968). As many as 10 concentric layers, or sleeves of cells, may be present around large

---

Figure 12–1.   **Connective Tissue Sheaths of Nerves.**

Upper picture: This light micrograph includes part of a transversely sectioned peripheral nerve at low magnification. In the epineurium *(Ep)*, which surrounds the nerve and lies between fiber bundles, there are slender processes of fibroblasts *(Fb)*, blood vessels *(Bv)*, and fat cells *(Fa)*. Collagen fibers *(Col)* fill the spaces between cells. Smaller vascular branches *(arrow)* penetrate the perineurial sheath *(Per)* and are the only elements *(arrowheads)* of the endoneurium that are easily seen at this magnification.
Guinea pig sciatic nerve. × 410.

Lower picture: Transverse section of the sheath of the trigeminal nerve. To the right is the perineurium *(Per)* with its thin layers of closely apposed fibroblast processes. These concentric layers of cell processes alternate with layers of collagen fibers. Occupying most of the field is the epineurium, which shows a looser arrangement of connective tissue cells embedded in collagen *(Col)*. This portion of the nerve sheath is unusual in that it contains groups of small, unmyelinated axons *(Ax)* surrounded by slender processes of epineurial fibroblasts. While the function of these small axons is not known, they probably innervate blood vessels contained within the connective tissue sheath of the nerve.
Rat trigeminal nerve. × 12,000.

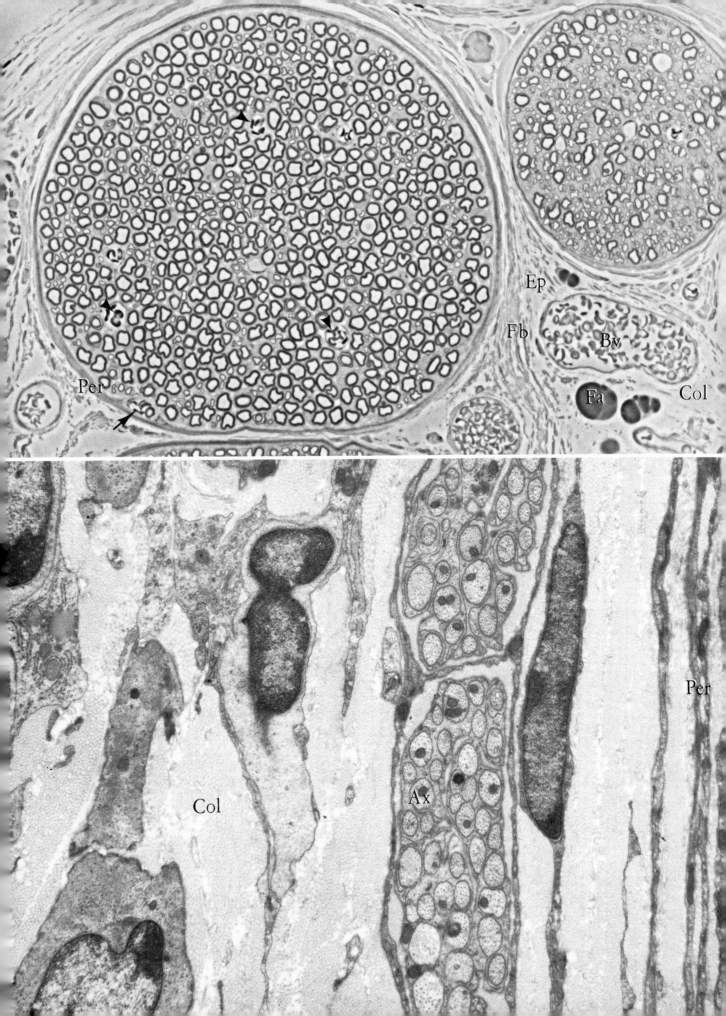

fascicles of nerve fibers (Thomas, 1963), but around smaller nerves such as those to eye muscles (Burkel, 1967), the perineurium may be formed of only three cell layers. Burkel finds that as the termination of a nerve is approached and it begins to branch, the perineurial sleeve becomes reduced to a single layer of cells which finishes in an open cuff near the ends of the individual nerve fibers. Kerjaschki and Stockinger (1970) also observed the perineurium to end openly as small tracheal and mesenteric nerves reach their terminations. On the other hand, Shantha and Bourne (1968) conclude that the perineurium extends as the capsule around nerve terminals in such organs as Pacinian and Meissner's corpuscles, Golgi tendon organs, and muscle spindles (see Schoultz and Swett, 1972).

Perineurial cells have a basal lamina on each side of them (Figure 12–3). Sometimes this may be quite thick, and at hemidesmosomes filaments pass from it toward the dense patches on the cytoplasmic faces of the plasma membranes of the cells (Thomas and Jones, 1967; Lieberman, 1968). In the larger peripheral nerves the concentric layers of cells alternate with layers of collagen fibers arranged longitudinally like those of the epineurium (Figure 12–2). The collagen fibers are rather smaller than those of the epineurium (see Figure 12–2), for they have average diameters of only about 50 nm and only a few elastic fibers are scattered between them (Thomas, 1963; Thomas and Jones, 1967). In the delicate nerves to the eye muscles, the amount of collagen is quite small, so that the concentric layers of cells, which can be as thin as 0.1 micron, become closely approximated (Burkel, 1967).

An important feature of the perineurium is that within a single layer, or sleeve, the edges of adjacent cells often dovetail together and interlock (Figure 12–3, *arrow*). At such sites, zonulae occludentes, or tight junctions, are present. As will be shown when the functions of the connective tissue sheaths are considered, these zonulae prevent tracers from penetrating between the perineurial cells to reach the enclosed nerve fibers, so that a blood-nerve barrier is produced. Similar zonulae may also occur between successive layers of the perineurium when their cells are in close approximation (Burkel, 1967).

In the nodose ganglion (Lieberman, 1968) thin perineurial laminae extend into and compartmentalize the endoneurium. Although it has not been established, it is possible that groups of nerve cells with similar peripheral functions are segregated by these partitions.

ENDONEURIUM

The endoneurium immediately surrounds the Schwann cells in a peripheral nerve and is composed of all the connective tissue elements lying inside the perineurium (Figure 12–1). The collagen fibers are mainly oriented longitudinally (Figures 12–3 and 6–14). In the nerve to the median head of the gastrocnemius muscle of the rabbit (Thomas, 1963), the collagen fibers are generally thinner than those in the epineurium, but similar to those in the perineurium, being only 30 to 60 nm thick (see Figure 12–2). Collagen fibers of similar dimensions are also present in the human sural nerve (Gamble and Eames, 1964).

For the most part, the collagen fibers are concentrated in a zone beneath the perineurium and around the nerve fibers and blood vessels contained in each fasciculus. The connective tissue fibers are separated from the surfaces of the Schwann and endothelial cells by basal laminae which are about 25 nm thick (Figure 12–3). Frequently, as in the nerve to the median head of the gastrocnemius muscle in the rabbit (Thomas, 1963), the connective tissue fibers surrounding

Figure 12–2. **Epineurial and Perineurial Sheaths.**

The longitudinally sectioned epineurium (*Ep*) is to the left, and in the picture are a few fibroblasts (*Fb*) situated between bundles of longitudinally and obliquely oriented collagen fibrils (*Col*). The collagen fibrils in the bundles in the perineurium (*Per*) and endoneurium (*En*) are smaller in diameter than those in the epineurium. At the right lower margin, part of a longitudinally sectioned myelinated axon (*Ax*) is shown next to an endoneurial fibroblast.
Rat sciatic nerve. × 11,000.

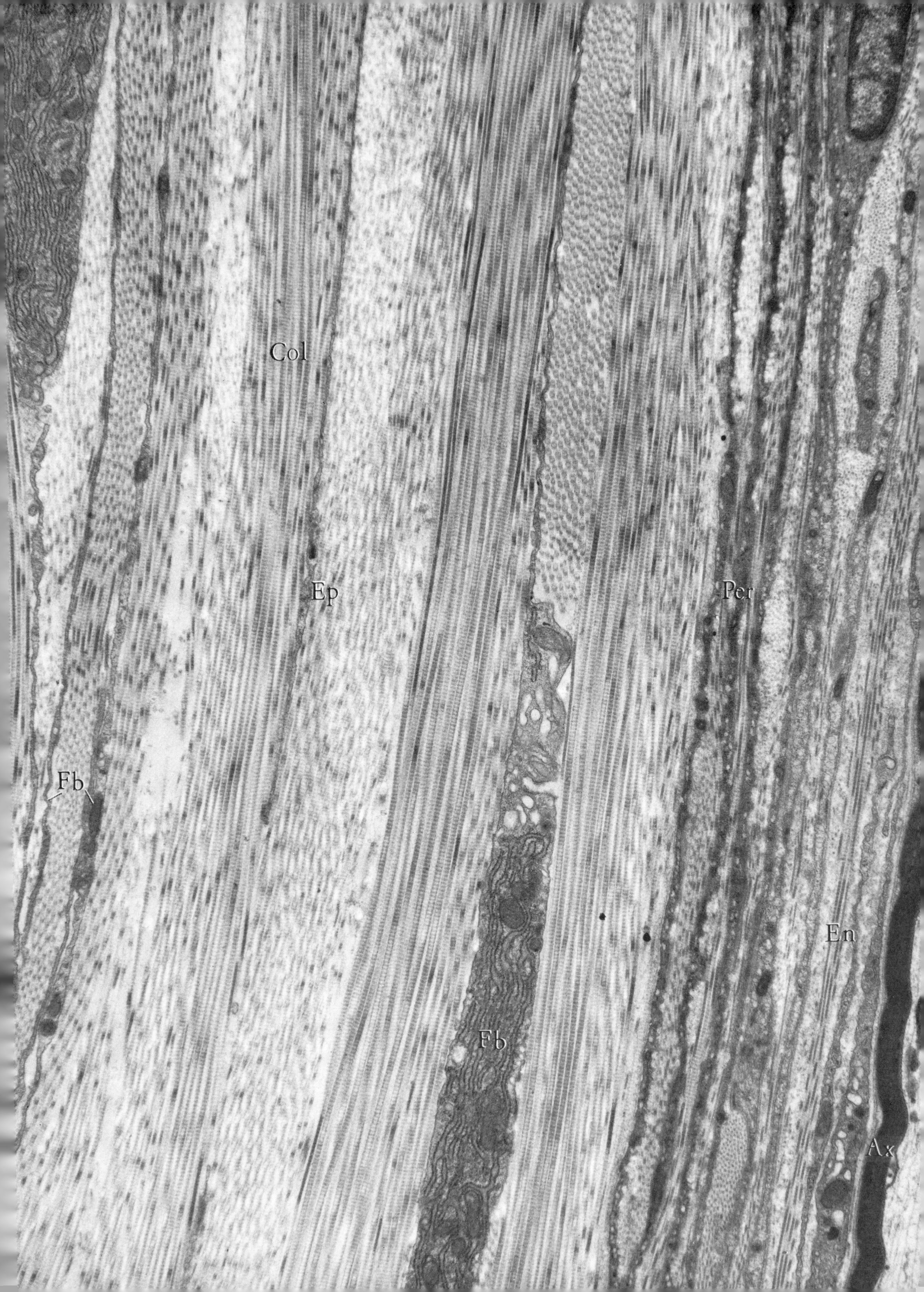
Col
Ep
Per
Fb
En
Fb
Ax

large myelinated axons form two distinct layers. The outer endoneurial layer consists of predominantly longitudinally oriented collagen fibers which are closely packed together, while the inner layer, immediately against the nerve fiber, is composed of thinner connective tissue fibers oriented randomly. Thomas (1963) noticed two similar layers to be sometimes present around smaller myelinated fibers and even around some unmyelinated axons. But on the whole, the endoneurial sheaths of these latter types of nerve fiber are less well organized. Gamble (1964 found the inner endoneurial sheaths to be less apparent in the sacral spinal roots of the rat.

So that the description given here may be equated with those appearing in some current textbooks, it should be pointed out that the outer endoneurial sheath, as defined here, corresponds to the sheath of Key and Retzius (1876), also sometimes called the sheath of Henle; the inner sheath corresponds to the sheath of Plenk and Laidlaw (Plenk, 1927; Laidlaw, 1930). Compared to the connective tissue fibers of the outer endoneurial sheath, those of the inner endoneurial sheath are thinner and argyrophilic, a property probably conferred upon them by their being embedded in a carbohydrate matrix. In our present state of knowledge, it would be appropriate to abandon the terms "sheath of Key and Retzius" and "sheath of Plenk and Laidlaw," for while these terms are still used frequently, they have no real value other than in an historical context. Yet another commonly used and confusing term is "neurilemma." Young (1942) points out that even as early as 1873 Key and Retzius suggested that this term no longer be employed. It appears to be used indiscriminately by different authors to refer to the endoneurium, to the layer of Schwann cell cytoplasm outside a myelin sheath, and to the limiting membrane of the axon, which we now call the plasma membrane or the axolemma. For the sake of clarity we would like to discard the name "neurilemma" and retain the term "sheath of Schwann" for the first, cellular layer intimately enclosing an axon or nerve cell in the peripheral nervous system. The terms "basal lamina" and "endoneurium" can then be applied to the successive condensations of connective tissue ensheathing the nerve fiber.

We shall now return to our description of the endoneurium. The fibroblasts account for about 25 per cent of the nuclear profiles encountered in the endoneurium in transverse sections of the nerve to the median head of the gastrocnemius muscle of the rabbit (Thomas, 1963). This is considerably higher than the 5 per cent figure recorded by Causey and Barton (1959) in the sural nerve. Thomas (1963) considers that the difference may be accounted for by the fact that the sural nerve contains larger numbers of unmyelinated axons and that the myelinated nerve fibers present are thinner, so that proportionally more Schwann cells are encountered. When they are sectioned transversely, endoneurial fibroblasts have triangular or rectangular perikarya, but where one partially encircles a nerve fiber it has a crescentic shape. Extending from the perikarya are processes that interweave with the collagen fibers and interdigitate with the processes of other fibroblasts. The nuclei of the fibroblasts are rather pale, and the cytoplasm is characterized by a prominent rough endoplasmic reticulum. Like fibroblasts in the epineurium, they lack a basal lamina and so their identification can be readily assured (Figure 12–3).

Mast cells also occur in the endoneurium. These are characterized by large cytoplasmic granules (Olsson, 1968). In light microscope preparations, the granules are metachromatic, and in the electron microscope it is apparent that they are bounded by a membrane and have either a granular or heterogeneous content, depending upon the species of animal being studied. According to Gamble (1964), mast cells are absent from nerve roots central to the sensory ganglia.

Nerves have a rich vascular supply (Figure 12–1) and in a recent study of the vasa nervorum Marcarian and Smith (1968) showed that in the ulnar nerve of the cat 92 per cent of the vessels had a diameter of less than 10 microns. The ratio of blood vessels to myelinated nerve fiber profiles was 1:25 and remained relatively constant at different levels of the nerve.

Figure 12–3. **Perineurium and Endoneurium of Peripheral Nerve.**

In this transverse section of the perineurium the processes of fibroblasts (*Fb*) alternate with layers of collagen fibrils (*Col*). The cytoplasm of the fibroblasts contains many organelles, including microfilaments (*mf*). Between adjacent fibroblasts of the same layer there are intercellular junctions (*arrow*). The surfaces of the fibroblasts (*Fb*) of the perineurium are covered by a basal lamina (*B*). A basal lamina also covers the Schwann cells (*SC*) surrounded by the endoneurium (*En*), but this lamina is not present around the endoneurial fibroblasts (*Fb*₁).
Rat sciatic nerve. × 50,000.

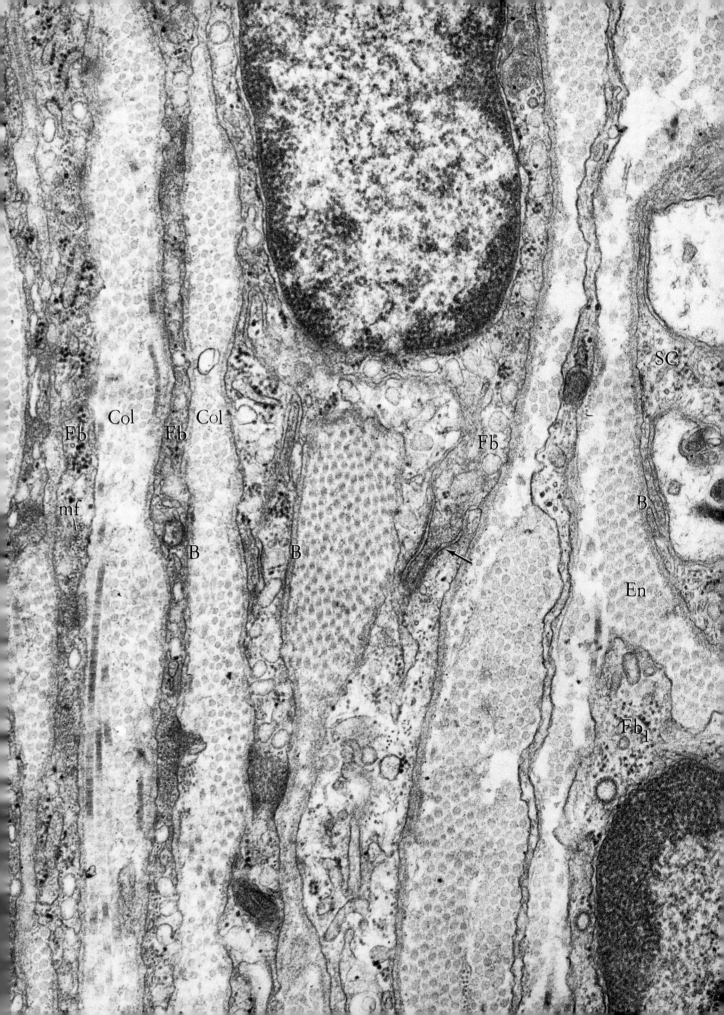

The capillaries that are frequently encountered in the endoneurium are also often covered by an outer and an inner endoneurial sheath. It seems that as a capillary enters the endoneurium, it carries a short extension of the perineurium with it. This sleeve probably helps to maintain the integrity of the perineurial barrier. Entry of substances into the endoneurium is also prevented by a vascular barrier formed by the tight junctions between adjacent endothelial cells (Olsson and Reese, 1971). In some species, however, this barrier is not complete (Olsson, 1971), and it is not present in roots or ganglion, where the endothelial cells may be either fenestrated or joined by junctions of the open type (Olsson, 1968; Olsson and Reese, 1971). Like capillaries elsewhere, those of the endoneurium have pericytes associated with them, and as usual, these cells are completely enclosed in a basal lamina.

Occasionally the endoneurium of nerves may contain hyaline bodies. These bodies are named "Renaut bodies" after Renaut (1881a and b) who first described them. In a recent article Asbury (1973) showed the bodies to be cylindrical with diameters of 20 to 150 microns and lengths of several hundred microns. The bodies are composed of randomly oriented collagen fibers, fine fibrils, and attenuated, spider-like fibroblasts whose processes bound the bodies and traverse through their substance.

FUNCTIONS OF CONNECTIVE TISSUE SHEATHS

The available evidence indicates that the functions of the connective tissue sheaths change as they form and mature. Perineurial cells are the first to appear, and initially they contain many glycogen granules, lack a basal lamina, and are not joined by the tight junctions that form a barrier in the adult (Gamble and Breathnach, 1965; Kristensson, 1970; Ochoa, 1971; Kristensson and Olsson, 1971c). These immature perineurial cells probably participate in providing and transporting nutrients to the axons and Schwann cells they surround, for at this stage there are no endoneurial blood vessels. Initially the endoneurium is limited to narrow clefts that occur between columns of Schwann cells and contain only a few collagen fibrils (see Figures 6–6 and 6–7). Since these fibrils are present before endoneurial fibroblasts appear, they are probably formed by the Schwann cells. As insulin secretion is initiated in the embryo, and as vessels invade the nerve parenchyma, the amount of glycogen in the perineurial fibroblasts decreases (Ochoa, 1971; Duckett and Scott, 1972). The amount of endoneurial collagen increases dramatically as fibroblasts appear and multiply in the endoneurium.

One obvious function of the connective tissue sheaths in the mature animal is to provide structural support to a peripheral nerve and to contribute to the elasticity which allows a nerve to be stretched during body movements (see Sutherland, 1965). In addition, the endoneurium seems to provide a constant environment for the nerve fibers embedded within it, and this constant environment is probably ensured by the rather special properties of both the surrounding perineurium and the blood vessels in the endoneurium. In effect, there is a blood-nerve barrier which protects the nerve fibers from various noxious agents and might control the passage of ions into the endoneurium.

The existence of a blood-nerve barrier was shown by Doinikow (1913) who noticed that if rabbits and rats are given repeated injections of trypan blue, the Schwann cells of a peripheral nerve do not take up the stain, and little dye enters the endoneurium. In contrast a great deal of dye appears in the perineurium and epineurium, where it is taken up by fixed connective tissue cells, by histiocytes and macrophages, and by fat cells (Figure 12–1, *Fa*). Waksman (1961) showed that in a number of species—rabbits, rats, hamsters, and monkeys—there is a barrier which effectively prevents access of a variety of large molecular weight substances to the nerves and endoneurium. Waksman (1961) also showed that rabbit peripheral nerves have a resistance to experimental diphtheritic and allergic encephalitis and concluded that this resistance could be attributed to a failure of the toxins to enter the nerve from the blood. It was later shown by Olsson (1968 and 1971) that albumin labelled with a fluorescent dye and injected intravenously does not leak out of blood vessels into the endoneurium, but does leak out of blood vessels within both the epineurium and the perineurium, so that it appears both within and around the vessels in these two sheaths.

In an effort to localize the site of the blood-nerve barrier at a fine structural level, Waggener, Bunn, and Beggs (1965) used ferritin, which has a molecular diameter of about 10 nm.

They showed that ferritin applied to the outside of a peripheral nerve passes into the epineurium but stops abruptly at the outer border of the perineurium. With extended exposures of three hours, the ferritin penetrates into the deeper layers of the perineurium but still does not enter the endoneurium. Hence, the perineurium appears to be the structure which impedes penetration of ferritin into the endoneurium from the outside. This observation was confirmed by Klemm (1970), who found that when peroxidase is injected into either the endoneurium or the epineurium it does not pass between the cells of the perineurial sheath. It will be remembered that these cells are joined together at their edges by zonulae occludentes. The only peroxidase passing across the perineurium is that which is transported in pinocytotic vesicles.

A similar conclusion has also been drawn by Olsson and Reese (1971), who employed both horseradish peroxidase and lanthanum hydroxide as electron-dense markers. Their electron microscope studies demonstrated that when these markers are injected intravenously they are confined to the lumina of the endoneurial blood vessels but leak out through the perineurial and epineurial blood vessels. Hence the endoneurial vessels act as a barrier, to at least horseradish peroxidase and lanthanum, by preventing their passage between the endothelial cells. In addition, the markers are not transported to any extent in vesicles. In contrast to those of the endoneurium, the endothelial cells forming the walls of blood vessels in the epineurium and the perineurium are joined not by zonulae occludentes but by gap junctions. As noted, there are both topographic (Olsson, 1968) and species (Olsson, 1971) differences in this barrier, which does not exist early in development (Kristensson and Olsson, 1971c).

In this connection, a number of authors (e.g., Burkel, 1967; Lieberman, 1968) have found that blood vessels penetrating into the endoneurium frequently carry a single layer of perineurium with them for some distance.

Thus, both the perineurium and the walls of the capillaries within the endoneurium are designed to prevent the passage of certain substances into the extracellular space immediately surrounding nerve fibers in the endoneurium. Burkel (1967) points out, however, that the integrity of the perineurium may be compromised in the three following sites: (1) near the termina-

tions of nerve fibers, where the perineurium has an open end, (2) at the entry of blood vessels into the endoneurium where the perineurial sleeve surrounding them comes to an end, and (3) where reticular fibers pierce the perineurium. The open ends of the perineurial sleeves may be the portals through which viruses enter the nerve.

Most of the studies on the function of the perineurium have been carried out on large peripheral nerves of mature animals. However, Kristensson and Olsson (1971c and 1973) studied the permeability of the perineurium in immature animals and found that it in rats younger than two to three weeks of age this sheath does not act as an efficient diffusion barrier (see also Malmgren and Brink, 1975). At this age, tracers such as Evans blue and horseradish peroxidase can easily pass through into the endoneurium from the outside. This appears to be due to presence of gaps between the cells of immature perineurium.

The importance of the perineurium is further emphasized by studies of Morris, Hudson, and Weddell (1972d). Between seven days and six weeks after damage to the rat sciatic nerve, they found the regenerating nerve to contain a series of small fascicles of nerve fibers, each one surrounded by a perineurium (see also Thomas and Jones, 1967). They refer to this process of enclosing regenerating nerve fibers as "compartmentation." It appears to be brought about by changes in Schwann cells and endoneurial fibroblasts which undergo circumferential elongation, surround groups of axons, and so come to resemble perineurial cells. Morris, Hudson, and Weddell (1972d) suggest that these compartments are organized as a means of re-establishing a constant environment for the regenerating axons. During regeneration, the amount of endoneurial collagen increases, and Schwann cells of all sizes become surrounded by a zone of densely packed collagen fibers (Thomas, 1964b). Around the remnants of the larger myelinated nerve fibers, this new formation of the endoneurium occurs inside the original inner endoneurial sheaths, which are still lined by the persisting basal laminae from Schwann cells previously ensheathing the now degenerated axon. Hence "Schwann tubes" are formed (Thomas, 1964b), and these provide pathways along which the regenerating nerve fibers grow and become oriented.

Chapter XIII

THE MENINGES

The meninges enclosing the central nervous system consist of three layers: the dura mater, the arachnoid mater, and the pia mater (Figure 13-1). The first comprehensive account of these layers was given by Key and Retzius (1876). Frequently the pia and the arachnoid are together termed the leptomeninges, since they are connected by numerous trabeculae that traverse the subarachnoid space between them and their cells have a similar appearance.

The dura mater is a strong and dense membrane. In the vertebral canal it is separated from the inner surface of the periosteum of the vertebrae by an epidural space containing loose connective and fatty tissue with an epidural venous plexus. For the most part, the collagen fibers of the spinal dura run in a longitudinal di-

rection with respect to the length of the spinal cord.

The cranial dura also begins development as two distinct layers: the dura proper and the periosteum of the skull. In the adult, however, these two layers become fully adherent and are together referred to as the cranial dura. Separation between the two layers only occurs in places where the large venous sinuses are located and where the inner layer forms a fold such as the falx cerebri. The outer layer of the cranial dura still functions as a periosteum, for it is a looser tissue than the inner layer and contains many blood vessels. The inner layer of the dura is thinner, and its connective tissue fibers form an almost continuous sheet.

The arachnoid is a thin, net-like membrane

Figure 13-1. **Meninges.**

These pictures are scanning electron micrographs.

The **upper picture** shows the meninges of the spinal cord. The transversely cut face of the spinal cord lies at the bottom of the picture and the pia mater (*PM*) lies directly on its surface. Separating the pia mater from the arachnoid mater (*AM*) is the subarachnoid space (*SS*) which is traversed by arachnoid trabeculae (*arrows*). Also lying in this space is an artery (*A*). Separating the thick dura mater (*DM*) from the arachnoid is a space which is an artifact of preparation.
Spinal cord of young dog. × *200.*

Micrograph by M. W. Cloyd and F. N. Low.

The **lower picture** shows the meninges of the cerebral hemisphere. The cut face of the cerebral cortex is at the bottom of the picture. Lying over it is the thin pia mater (*PM*), which is separated from the arachnoid mater (*AM*) by a narrow subarachnoid space (*SS*) containing a blood vessel (*A*). Two arachnoid trabeculae are apparent on the right (*arrows*). The dura mater (*DM*) is thick and is separated from the arachnoid by an artifactitious subdural space.
Cerebral hemisphere of young dog. × *360.*

Micrograph by D. J. Allen and F. N. Low.

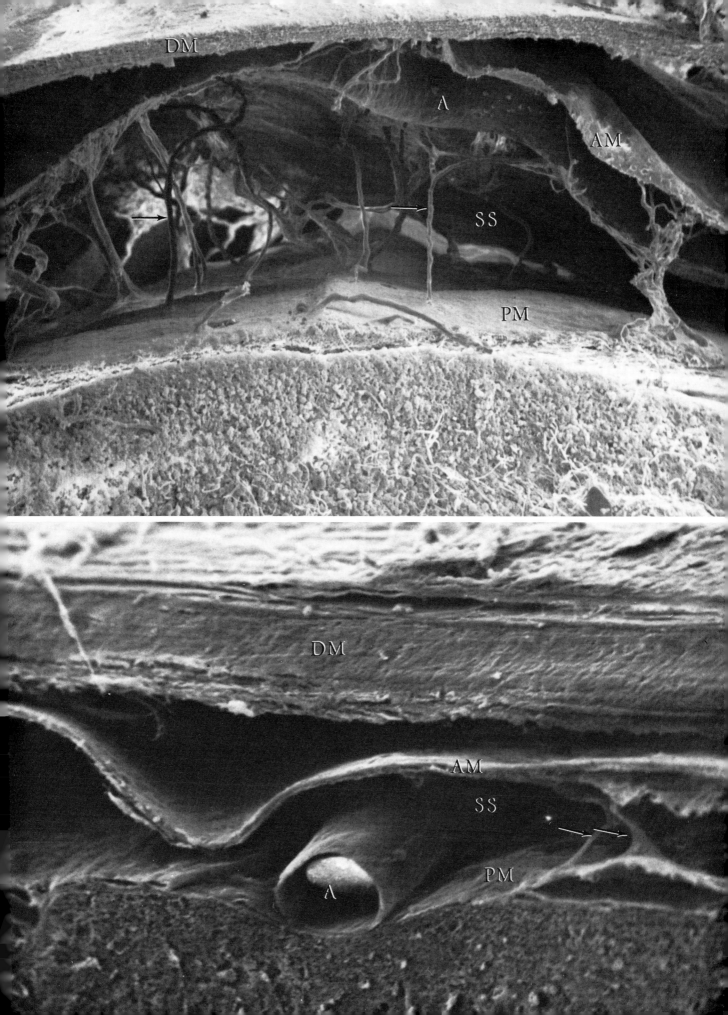

which is devoid of blood vessels, and although its outer surface against the dura is smooth, the inner surface has many threads, or trabeculae, joining it to the pia mater (see Figure 13–1). These trabeculae traverse the subarachnoid space, which contains cerebrospinal fluid. The arachnoid mater passes over the surfaces of small fissures in the surface of the brain and spinal cord, such as the sulci of the cerebral hemispheres, and so it follows the contours of the dura mater. In contrast, the pia closely adheres to the surface of the brain and spinal cord and contains a large number of blood vessels that supply the underlying nervous tissue. The relations between the meningeal layers of the spinal cord have recently been shown in some very attractive scanning electron microscope pictures such as that in Figure 13–1, published by Cloyd and Low (1974).

Both the pia and arachnoid are composed of interlacing bundles of collagen fibers intermixed with some elastic fibers (see Figure 13–3). The fibroblasts forming these connective tissue fibers are flattened cells oriented in the plane of the meninges, and some of them line the fluid-filled subarachnoid space. Between them are fixed macrophages, which like the macrophages of other tissues are capable of being activated to engulf foreign bodies.

The dura and pia are both supplied with nerve fibers, which are often associated with blood vessels. So far as can be ascertained, these nerves belong to the sympathetic system and have their origins from the carotid and vertebral plexuses, as well as from some of the cranial nerves (see Millen and Woollam, 1962). Some of the nerve fibers form sensory endings within the meninges and around blood vessels.

The general form and structure of the meninges have been described by Weed (1932) and by Millen and Woollam (1961 and 1962), and accounts of their fine structure are available in the articles by Pease and Schultz (1958), Andres (1967a), Waggener and Beggs (1967), and Cloyd and Low (1974). Reference to articles dealing with specific portions of the meninges will be included in appropriate places in the following account.

DURA MATER

Dense interlacing bundles of collagen are the most prominent constituent of the dura mater, but elastic fibers and flattened fibroblasts are evident throughout its thickness (Figure 13–2). The fibroblasts have long processes and a conspicuously well-developed rough endoplasmic reticulum surrounding a dense nucleus in which the chromatin is clumped. Blood vessels, lymphatics, and nerve fasciculi also occur toward the middle of the dura, where they are grouped into discrete aggregates (Waggener and Beggs, 1967).

The outer surface of the cranial dura is usually fragmented in electron microscope preparations as a result of its necessary separation from the inside of the skull, and so there are no useful accounts of its fine structure. The spinal dura is more easy to study, however, and Waggener and Beggs (1967) have shown that beyond the inner collagenous matrix there is a perimeter of one or more cellular layers which may be attenuated and so appear as thin overlapping sheets.

The inner border of the dura is also bounded by multiple overlapping and interlocking cellular laminae, in which contiguous plasma membranes display zonulae occludentes and maculae adhaerentes. Andres (1967a) refers to this inner layer of dural cells and their processes as the "subdural neurothelium" and states that this layer is continuous with the perineurial sheaths of peripheral nerves where these are attached to the central nervous system.

Usually an artificial split occurs between the dura and arachnoid maters (Figure 13–1) but when the dural-arachnoid interface is maintained in position (Pease and Schultz, 1958; Andres, 1967a); Waggener and Beggs, 1967), the border between these two meningeal layers is

---

Figure 13–2.   **Dura Mater.**

The dura mater surrounding the optic nerve of the monkey is quite thick and is composed of collagen fibers arranged in layers, so that some fibers are sectioned transversely (Col_1), some obliquely (Col_2), and others longitudinally (Col_3), when they display the typical repeating pattern. Interlaced with these collagen fibers are elastic fibers (*arrows*) which are composed of fine, closely packed filaments (*f*).

These connective tissue fibers are formed by fibroblasts such as the one passing down the left half of the field.

Dura mater of monkey optic nerve. × 20,000.

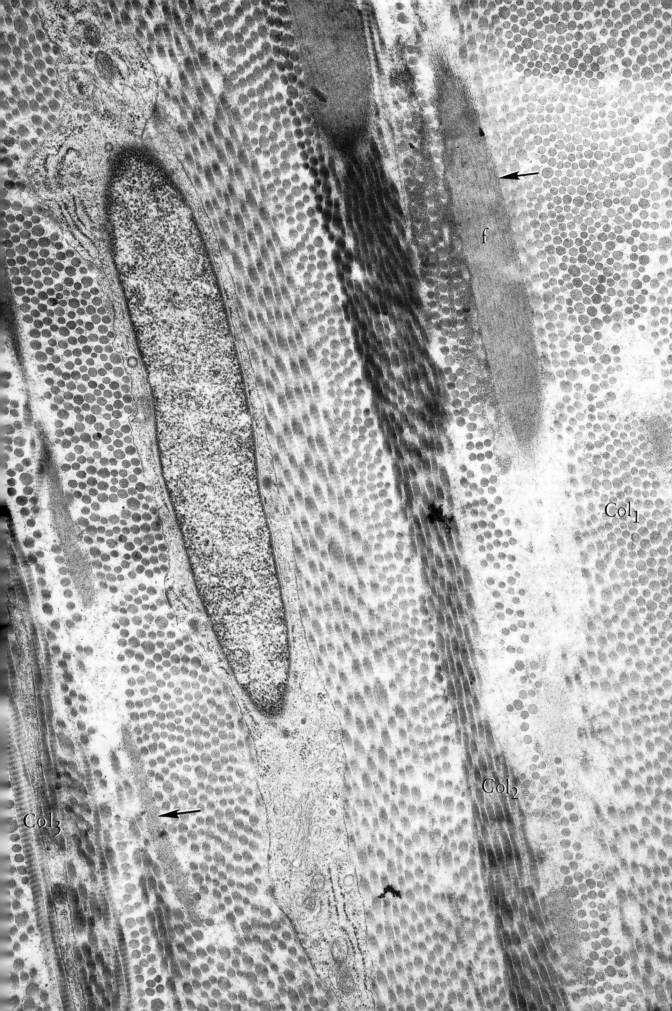

readily identified by the sharp contrast between the electron-dense dural cells and the more lucid arachnoid cells (Figure 13–3). There is also a dense material in the subdural space that makes the interface between the two meningeal layers stand out clearly (Andres, 1967b; Waggener and Beggs, 1967). In some regions the surfaces of these two meningeal layers may be closely apposed to each other, so that there is a gap of only 20 nm between them; elsewhere the separation is greater and in these locations the granular, dense material in the subdural space is more prominent.

In their account of the meninges, Pease and Schultz (1958), following the pattern set by earlier students of the meninges, refer to the cells forming the inner boundary of the dura, that is, the neurothelium of Andres (1967a), as being a mesothelium, and hence similar in form to the cells lining the cavities of the body. While it is true that these cells are flattened and have essentially the form of a squamous epithelium joined together at their edges, Waggener and Beggs (1967) point out that unlike a mesothelium the dural cells do not rest upon a basal lamina and do not have microvilli on their free surfaces facing the potential subdural space.

In a more recent account of the meninges Nabeshima, Reese, Landis, and Brightman (1975) refer to this mesothelium, or neurothelial layer of cells, as the layer of dural border cells. They conclude that the split that forms the so-called subdural space actually occurs within this layer of dural border cells and not between the layer of border cells and the layer of arachnoid to which they are apposed, even though these two layers have no recognizable junctions between them.

ARACHNOID MATER

In contrast to those of the dura, the arachnoid cells in the rat have a lucent cytoplasm and are formed into overlapping tiers intermingled with connective tissue trabeculae (Figure 13–3). The processes of the arachnoid cells rather loosely overlap and interweave in the flat plane of the thickness of the membrane, so that in effect the arachnoid mater can be regarded as being several layers thick. Between the cells, however, are pockets of connective tissue fibers (Andres, 1967b) which run in extracellular tunnels lined intermittently by a fragmented basal lamina (Andres, 1967b; Himango and Low, 1971). The cells of the arachnoid have many mitochondria, and the Golgi apparatus is prominent, lying next to an elongate nucleus displaying clumps of chromatin beneath the nuclear envelope. Within the cytoplasm are ribosomal rosettes and dispersed microfibrils, while lysosomes and lipid droplets are frequently encountered. The plasma membrane is invaginated at intervals to form pinocytotic and coated vesicles (Waggener and Beggs, 1967). In the dog (Figure 13–1) and monkey the arachnoid appears thicker than in the rat, and Shabo and Maxwell (1971) describe it as being composed of outer and inner sheets, each with two to four layers of cells, usually 20 nm apart, which overlap and interdigitate. It should be emphasized, however, that the inner face of the arachnoid mater, the one facing the pia, is more irregular than the one facing the dura (Figure 13–3). Consequently, the arachnoid has a quite variable thickness. Some irregular cell aggregates span the subarachnoid space and become continuous with the pia, while others contribute to the trabeculae (Figure 13–1).

Between the cells of the arachnoid are frequent junctions with the form of zonulae occludentes, zonulae adhaerentes, and maculae adhaerentes (Figure 13–3). The latter seem to be relatively rare in the rat (Waggener and Beggs, 1967), and perhaps more common in the cat (Andres, 1967b) and in monkeys and dogs (Shabo and Maxwell, 1971). Zonulae occludentes are frequently encountered close to the

Figure 13–3.   **Arachnoid Mater.**

In this picture the subarachnoid space *(SS)* is to the left. The arachnoid mater is composed of loosely overlapping cell processes *(X)* joined by intercellular junctions *(arrow)*. Between the cellular processes are tunnels of extracellular space, which may contain collagen *(Col)*. The face of the arachnoid directed toward the dura mater, which was detached in this specimen, has cells with denser cytoplasm than that of the cells on the more loosely arranged surface bordering the subarachnoid space *(SS)*. These darker cells make up part of the subdural neurothelium.
Arachnoid mater above the visual cortex of rat. × 12,500.

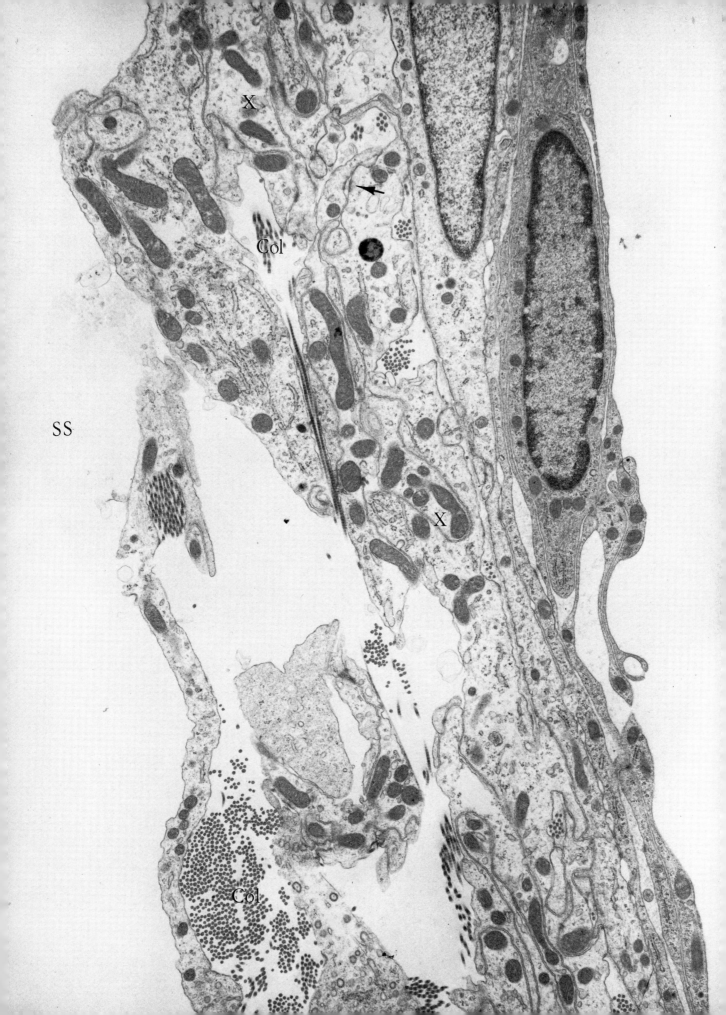

surface of the arachnoid which is exposed to the cerebrospinal fluid, but they may occur wherever two flattened cell processes come into proximity, and so far as Waggener and Beggs (1967) were able to determine, there is no fixed sequence of the different kinds of junctions. Undoubtedly, it is the presence of these junctions between arachnoid cells which allows the arachnoid mater to be an effective physiological barrier separating the cerebrospinal fluid from the surrounding milieu.

This description of the junctions between arachnoid cells forming the physiological barrier has been enlarged upon by Nabeshima, Reese, Landis, and Brightman (1975), who used both sectioned and freeze-fractured preparations. These authors showed that the arachnoid cells close to the inner surface of the dura mater typically have tight junctions, or zonulae occludentes, between them. Between these outer arachnoidal cells and the inner ones, and between the inner arachnoidal cells themselves, gap junctions also exist along with maculae adhaerentes.

PIA MATER

There is considerable variation in the organization of the pia mater in different locations. Histologically, it is composed of flat connective tissue cells which may be separated from the underlying neural tissue by variable amounts of extracellular connective tissue, mainly consisting of loose collagen fibers (Figure 13–4).

Over the spinal cord and the cerebellum of the rat (Waggener and Beggs, 1967) the pia mater is essentially represented by one or more cellular laminae interspersed with collagen fibers. The same is true of the cerebral cortex (Figure 13–4). In appearance the cells cannot be distinguished from those of the arachnoid mater and the cellular trabeculae spanning the subarachnoid space. In general the pial cells tend to overlap each other, although they form a thinner sheet than the arachnoid (Figures 13–3 and 13–4). In many areas this sheet is only one cell thick and may have fenestrations, so that the basal lamina covering the glia limitans is exposed directly to the subarachnoid space (Brightman, 1965b; Morse and Low, 1972a). On the other hand, the pia surrounding the optic chiasm is several cells thick (Morse and Low, 1972a). In scanning electron micrographs of the spinal pia mater, Cloyd and Low (1974) showed that the subarachnoid faces of pial cells have both long and short microvilli as well as blebs. It may be suggested that these processes are filopodia or spikes, concerned with the locomotion of the pial cells over the surfaces of the subarachnoid space (see Miranda, Godman, Deitch, and Tanenbaum, 1974).

On its inner surface the pia approaches the basal lamina of the astrocytic glia limitans surrounding the neural elements of the central nervous system. This boundary is always apparent, since the cells of the pia lack their own basal lamina (Figure 13–4). The space separating the pia from the glia limitans is variable, however, for while the pial cells may be closely approxi-

---

Figure 13–4.   **Pia Mater and Glia Limitans.**

In the **upper picture** the glia limitans (*GL*) that extends diagonally across the figure is composed of the processes of protoplasmic astrocytes. One of these cells (*As*) occupies the center of the field, and other processes emanating from the perikaryon of this cell extend into the adjacent neuropil. The outer face of the glia limitans is covered by a basal lamina (*B*) and beyond this is the thin pia mater (*PM*). On the right is a portion of the wall of an arteriole lying in the subarachnoid space (*SS*). The wall of the vessel has a tunica media which is only one smooth muscle cell (*SM*) thick. This blood vessel is also covered by a thin leptomeningeal layer (*arrows*), which in part appears to be derived from extensions of the cells in the pia mater.

Note that some collagen fibers (*Col*) are present in the subpial space separating the pia mater from the surfaces of the brain and the arteriole.
Visual cortex of rat. × *15,000.*

The **lower picture** shows a process of an astrocyte (*As*) in the glia limitans. Beneath the plasma membrane of the cell are localized densities (*arrows*) that resemble half of a punctum adhaerens (see also Figure 7–6). These probably serve as attachments between the astrocyte process and its basal lamina (*B*). Above the basal lamina is part of the overlying pia mater (*PM*).
Visual cortex of rat. × *30,000.*

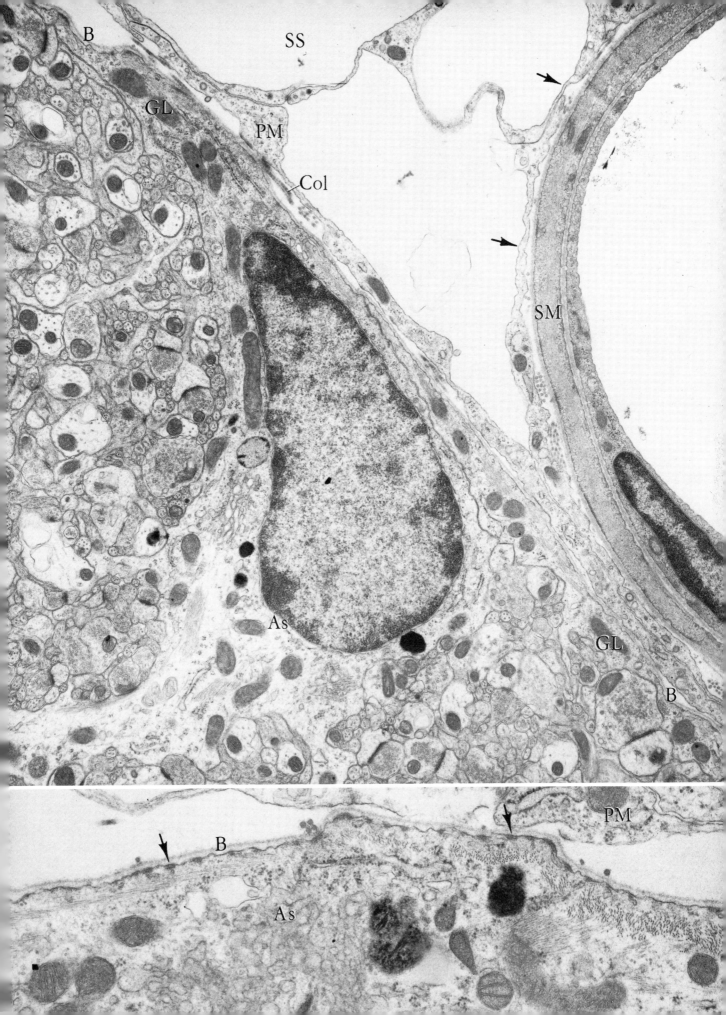

mated to this basal lamina in some places, elsewhere they are separated from it by a significant space which may include collagen fibers.

In the trabeculae the cells of the pia and arachnoid are contiguous and any entity that traverses the subarachnoid space is covered by cells of these leptomeninges (see Cloyd and Low, 1974; Figure 13–4). The leptomeninges ensheath blood vessels penetrating into the central nervous system and follow their subdivisions until they form capillaries (see page 304). Frequently, the leptomeningeal cells also form extensive sheaths around bundles of collagen fibers and around the nerve roots as they cross the subarachnoid space to gain access to, or pass from, the central nervous system.

It should be pointed out that particularly over the surface of the cerebral cortex, the subarachnoid space is not continuously patent. Thus, it may be precluded in sites where the pia and arachnoid come into such close proximity that it is impossible to distinguish between the cells of the pia and those of the overlying arachnoid mater.

In addition to the fibroblastic pial cell another type of cell common in the pia is the macrophage. Indeed, these cells occur throughout the leptomeninges. Macrophages are distinguished from the pial cells by lacking long cytoplasmic processes and by containing membrane-bound inclusions and a varying number of vacuoles in their cytoplasm (see Morse and Low, 1972b). Despite these differences in morphology there is experimental evidence that all of the cells lining the subarachnoid space are potential macrophages (Essick, 1920). In more recent experiments Shabo and Maxwell (1971) showed that if peroxidase is injected into the subarachnoid space, leptomeningeal cells are quick to phagocytose this marker during the first one to four hours. Later, polymorphonuclear leukocytes invade the subarachnoid space and actively phagocytose the peroxidase and sequester it into vacuoles. An essentially similar reaction is evoked by *E. coli*, which is also taken up into membrane-limited vacuoles by invading polymorphonuclear leukocytes and other macrophages (Nelson, Blinzinger, and Hager, 1962).

For an account of the development of the pia-arachnoid membranes in the mouse, reference should be made to the study by McLone and Bondareff (1975). They show that the development of these membranes takes place in three phases. The first phase occurs after the closure of the neural tube, when mesenchyme is interposed between the developing neuroepithelium and the overlying layer of squamous ectoderm. This mesenchyme seems to form the vascular and meningeal elements, and from it blood vessels develop which invade the underlying nervous tissue. By prenatal days 14 to 16 the limits of the subarachnoid space are defined, and the cells of the pia-arachnoid tend to become aligned parallel to the brain surface. Then between prenatal day 17 and birth the meninges become more mature, and the blood vessels in the subarachnoid space become ensheathed by meningeal cells. After birth macrophages appear in the subarachnoid space, smooth muscle cells are added to the walls of the larger blood vessels, and there is a general increase in the amount of collagenous and elastic fibers.

ENTRY OF PERIPHERAL NERVES INTO THE CENTRAL NERVOUS SYSTEM

Where a peripheral nerve is attached to the central nervous system a change occurs in the form of the cellular sheaths of the axons. For a myelinated axon the change takes place at a node of Ranvier. On the peripheral side of this node the myelin is formed by a Schwann cell and on the central side by an oligodendrocyte (Waggener, 1963; Maxwell, Kruger, and Pineda, 1969). Unmyelinated axons also lose their peripheral investment of Schwann cells but remain unsheathed once they enter the central nervous system.

The endoneurium persists between the nerve fibers, as long as they retain their Schwann cells. But as the axons enter the central nervous system they penetrate through a dome-shaped boundary composed of astrocytic processes. At the site of penetration the basal laminae of the Schwann cells in the peripheral nerve become confluent with the basal lamina coating the outsides of the astrocytic processes forming the dome (Maxwell, Kruger, and Pineda, 1969). The situation is also relatively simple in the case of the epineurium, for it becomes confluent with the dura mater as a nerve penetrates the meninges. The question of the relations of the perineurium to the meninges is less clear, and opinions differ. A review of some of the difficulties in interpreting these relations at the transition zone between the peripheral and central nervous system has been presented by Shantha and Bourne (1968). They propose that the epineurium and the outer layers of the perineurium are continuous with the dura, and that the inner, cellular, layers of the perineurium are continuous with the arachnoid and pia.

What is apparent, however, is that as a peripheral nerve pierces the dura mater and loses its epineurium, it enters the subarachnoid space which it must traverse to reach the surface of the brain or spinal cord. The sheath which the nerve carries with it across the subarachnoid space has been called the "root sheath" by Haller and Low (1971), and it is the derivation of this root sheath which is not fully understood.

Haller and Low (1971), Haller, Haller, and Low (1972), Cloyd and Low (1974), and Malloy and Low (1974) have given the most recent accounts of the root sheath. They consider that where the nerve penetrates the meninges the more superficial layers of the perineurium diverge from its surface and join the dura and arachnoid maters, while the inner layers of the perineurium persist as the deeper part of the root sheath. An additional layer of cells, resembling the loose cells lining the subarachnoid space, completes the root sheath by forming a covering outside the persisting portion of the perineurial sheath. The inner layers of the perineurium, which persist as the deeper layers

of the root sheath, apparently terminate as an open-ended tube near the junction of the peripheral and central nervous systems. Continuity between the interstitial space of the endoneurium and the subarachnoid space is established through gaps or fenestrations between pial cells.

This description differs from that given by Andres (1967a), who in a diagram shows the perineurium to be in continuity with the subdural neurothelium (Figure 13–3), which, it may be recalled, is the layer of cells and their processes bounding the inner surface of the dura mater, and which splits to form the subdural space. Consequently, Andres (1967a) considers the nerve roots in the subarachnoid space to be covered by cells derived only from the pia and arachnoid. It would be appropriate to re-evaluate the question by further study, however, since the published pictures of the transition zone area are generally of portions too small for a reader to draw his own conclusions.

Between the ventral and dorsal root is a lateral recess of the subarachnoid space in which Himango and Low (1971) have found conspicuous amounts of cellular debris and numerous free macrophages. Since a communication between the subarachnoid space and the interstitial spaces of peripheral nerves has long been suspected, Himango and Low (1971) consider the possiblity that toxins may enter the subarachnoid space from the periphery through this lateral recesses.

ARACHNOID VILLI

The arachnoid villi are herniations of the arachnoid membrane and subarachnoid tissue into veins and venous sinuses of the dura. Arachnoid granulations are also described in the literature, and the only difference between these and villi seems to be one of size. Granulations are structures visible with the naked eye, while the villi are microscopic. In the following description, the term villus will be employed, although it can be assumed that the account applies equally well to the granulations.

In most mammals, the villi have the form of small bulbs projecting into either the cranial venous sinuses or lateral lacunae of veins entering the sinuses, or into the large spinal extradural veins. Descriptions of the light microscope appearance of the arachnoid villi can be found in

the accounts by Weed (1914), Welch and Friedman (1960), and Millen and Woollam (1962), while their fine structure is considered by Jayatilaka (1965), Alksne and White (1965), Thomas (1966), Andres (1967a), Shabo and Maxwell (1968a), Hayes, McCombs, and Faherty (1971), and Gomez, Potts, and Deonarine (1974). Each villus has a body situated in the lumen of a blood vessel and a neck which is ringed by the dura mater through which the villus protrudes. It is generally agreed that the body of a villus is covered by endothelial cells and that the core of the neck and the body contains arachnoidal tissue within which are interstices communicating with the subarachnoid space. Beyond this, however, there is sharp disagreement between investigators who have examined the fine structure of villi, for two quite disparate views of their structure obtain.

Thus, Alksne and White (1965), Thomas (1966), Andres (1967a), and Shabo and Maxwell (1968a) consider the core of a villus to be composed of a stroma of arachnoidal cells and collagen fibers organized in no particular pattern. This group of authors also believes the endothelial covering of villi to be complete and uninterrupted under normal conditions. Shabo and Maxwell (1968a) state, however, that beneath the endothelial covering of a villus there is a subendothelial space with sparser cells than in the core and a loose stroma consisting primarily of collagen fibers.

In contrast to this interpretation, Welch and Friedman (1960), Jayatilaka (1965), Hayes, McCombs, and Faherty (1971), and Gomez, Potts, and Deonarine (1974) maintain that the core of a villus contains interconnecting tubules which pass through the stroma of collagen, fibroblasts, and arachnoid cells. They show evidence that at the surface of a villus some of the tubules open into the sinus, so that in sections through villi, crypts, representing the venous ends of the tubules, appear as indentations of the surface of a villus. At their other ends the tubules are said to widen and to open into the subarachnoid space which contains the cerebrospinal fluid.

Jayatilaka (1965), who examined sheep, regards the cells lining the walls of the tubules as endothelial and states that there are two types of tubules: those containing cerebrospinal fluid and others (capillaries) which contain blood cells. The capillaries do not open into the venous sinuses, however, and their identity as blood vessels is shown by the fact that they fill with India ink when this marker is injected into the carotid arteries. The larger tubules containing cerebrospinal fluid do not fill under these circumstances, but fill when India ink is injected into the subarachnoid space (Jayatilaka, 1965).

In their article published later than that of Jayatilaka (1965), Shabo and Maxwell (1968a) state that in the monkey they have been unable to find the tubules linking the subarachnoid space with the lumen of the venous sinus. They suggest that some of the structures interpreted as tubules might be wrinkles in the surfaces of the villi and propose that there may be species differences in the form of the villi. There is a clear need to reassess the question of the presence or absence of tubules in the arachnoid villi, although interpretations would have to be supported by experiments using electron-dense markers and by the examination of a number of different species.

So far as the function of the arachnoid villi is concerned, Weed (1914) showed that if potassium ferrocyanide and iron ammonium acetate are injected into the subarachnoid space, and the heads of the animals later fixed in acidified formalin, particles of Prussian blue are encountered both in the cores of the villi and in the venous sinuses into which they project. Weed interpreted this result to indicate that subarachnoid fluid passes into the blood by filtration through the walls of the bodies of the arachnoid villi. In an effort to investigate the situation further, Shabo and Maxwell (1968b) injected peroxidase into the subarachnoid space and examined the distribution of the marker with the electron microscope. They found that the arachnoid cells of the villi, and especially those bordering the subendothelial space, become phagocytic. They suggest that such phagocytic activity is necessary to remove debris from the core of a villus so that it does not become clogged and unable to act as a filter. Shabo and Maxwell make no mention of the marker passing through the walls of the villi.

Just before electron microscope studies of villi were initiated, Welch and Friedman (1960) showed that villi swell up if pressure in the subarachnoid space is increased. Alksne and White (1965), studying the morphological effect of swelling, found that the endothelial cells covering villi become thinner under these conditions but that the junctions between endothelial cells remain intact, despite the stretching involved. It is of interest that vitamin A deficiency, which increases cerebrospinal fluid pressure, also causes villi to swell (Hayes, McCombs, and Faherty, 1971).

Welch and Friedman (1960) further demonstrated that in isolated preparations of villi, fluid passes through the villi in an essentially unidirectional manner, from the subarachnoid space to the venous side. Hence the villi appeared to them to act as valves. These observations were followed by studies in which Welch and Pollay (1961) found that particles injected into the subarachnoid space pass through tubular spaces that run from the bases of the villi and open into the venous sinuses.

As pointed out above, the existence of tubules in villi is supported by Jayatilaka (1965), Hayes, McCombs, and Faherty (1971), and Gomez, Potts, and Deonarine (1974). Jayatilaka (1965) and Gomez, Potts, and Deonarine (1974) performed rather similar experiments to those of

Welch and Pollay (1961). They also found that particulate material injected into the cerebrospinal fluid enters tubules and leaks into the venous sinuses. The proposal put forward as a result of these observations is that villi act as valves which are normally open since the pressure of the cerebrospinal fluid exceeds that of the venous blood. In this condition the villi remain turgid and the tubules patent, allowing cerebrospinal fluid to pass into the blood. Conversely, if the venous pressure is the higher, the villi should collapse so that the tubules flatten and become sealed, allowing no blood to enter the cerebrospinal fluid. As further evidence for the valve-like action of the arachnoid villi, Welch and Friedman (1960) point out that if the cerebrospinal fluid pressure is reduced by removal of samples for diagnostic purposes, no blood enters the cerebrospinal fluid. Fluid may also pass both between endothelial cells and across endothelial cells by pinocytosis.

A recent scanning electron microscope study by Gomez and Potts (1974) has been concerned with the arachnoid granulations in sheep. The granulations were fixed, as the pressure difference between the subarachnoid space and the superior sagittal sinus was maintained at increasingly higher values. When the pressure difference was increased, the granulations became larger and less collapsed. Microvilli covering the endothelial cells on the surface of the granulations decreased in number and size, indicating that the cells stretched. Areas of apposition between adjacent endothelial cells became more irregular, and the sites of emergence of the tubules at the surface of the granulations became more obvious. Gomez and Potts (1974) consider that these changes support their previous conclusions that cerebrospinal fluid may pass out through the tubules into the sinus, as well as between the endothelial cells.

In surveying the literature, it seems that both the existence and the absence of tubules are well documented in the various studies. Consequently, we can express no opinion about which view is correct and assume that some of the differences in results can be attributed to variations among species. Only further careful study will resolve the problem.

REFERENCES

Adamo, N. J., and Daigneault, E. A. 1973a. Ultrastructural features of neurons and nerve fibres in the spiral ganglia of cats. *J. Neurocytol.* 2:91–103.

Adamo, N. J., and Daigneault, E. A. 1973b. Ultrastructural morphology of Schwann cell–neuronal relationships in the spiral ganglia of cats. *Am. J. Anat.* 138:73–78.

Adrian, E. K., and Williams, M. G. 1973. Cell proliferation in injured spinal cord. An electron microscope study. *J. Comp. Neurol.* 151:1–24.

Agduhr, E. 1932. Choroid plexus and ependyma. In: *Cytology and Cellular Pathology of the Nervous System*, Vol. 2. W. Penfield, Ed. New York, Paul B. Hoeber, pp. 537–573.

Aghajanian, G. K., and Bloom, F. E. 1966. Electron microscopic autoradiography of rat hypothalamus after intraventricular H³-norepinephrine. *Science* 153:308–310.

Aghajanian, G. K., and Bloom, F. E. 1967. The formation of synaptic junctions in developing rat brain: A quantitative electron microscopic study. *Brain Res.* 6:716–727.

Aker, F. D. 1972. A study of hematic barriers in peripheral nerves of albino rabbits. *Anat. Rec.* 174:21–37.

Akert, K., Cuénod, M., and Moor, H. 1971. Further observations on the enlargement of synaptic vesicles in degenerating optic nerve terminals of the avian tectum. *Brain Res.* 25:255–263.

Akert, K., Moor, H., Pfenninger, K., and Sandri, C. 1969. Contributions of new impregnation methods and freeze etching to the problems of synaptic fine structure. In: *Progress in Brain Research*, Vol. 31, *Mechanisms of Synaptic Transmission*. K. Akert and P. G. Waser, Eds. Amsterdam, Elsevier, pp. 223–240.

Akert, K., and Pfenninger, K. 1969. Synaptic fine structure and neuronal dynamics. In: *Symposium of the International Society for Cell Biology*, Vol. 8, *Cellular Dynamics of the Neuron*. S. H. Barondes, Ed. New York, Academic Press, pp. 245–260.

Akert, K., Pfenninger, K., and Sandri, C. 1967. The fine structure of synapses in the subfornical organ of the cat. *Z. Zellforsch. Mikrosk. Anat.* 81:537–556.

Akert, K., Pfenninger, K., Sandri, C., and Moor, H. 1972. Freeze etching and cytochemistry of vesicles and membrane complexes in synapses of the central nervous system. In: *Structure and Function of Synapses*. G. D. Pappas and D. P. Purpura, Eds. New York, Raven Press, pp. 67–86.

Alksne, J. F., and White, L. E. 1965. Electron-microscope study of the effects of increased intracranial pressure on the arachnoid villus. *J. Neurosurg.* 22:481–488.

Allen, D., and Low, F. N. 1973. The ependymal surface of the lateral ventricle of the dog as revealed by scanning electron microscopy. *Am. J. Anat.* 173:483–489.

Allen, R. A. 1965. Isolated cilia in inner retinal neurons and in retinal pigment epithelium. *J. Ultrastruct. Res.* 12:730–747.

Allt, G. 1972. An ultrastructural analysis of remyelination following segmental demyelination. *Acta Neuropathol. (Berl.)* 22:333–344.

Alnaes, E., and Rahamimoff, R. 1975. On the role of mitochondria in transmitter release from motor nerve terminals. *J. Physiol. (Lond.)* 248:285–306.

Altman, J. 1966. Autoradiographic and histological studies of postnatal neurogenesis. II. A longitudinal investigation of the kinetics, migration and transformation of cells incorporating tritiated thymidine in infant rats, with special reference to postnatal neurogenesis in some brain regions. *J. Comp. Neurol.* 128:431–473.

Altman, J. 1967. Postnatal growth and differentiation of the mammalian brain, with implications for a morphological theory of memory. In: *The Neurosciences*, G. C. Quarten, T. Melnechuk, and F. O.

345

Schmitt, Eds. New York, Rockefeller University Press, pp. 723–743.

Altman, J. 1971. Coated vesicles and synaptogenesis. A developmental study in the cerebellar cortex of the rat. *Brain Res.* 30:311–322.

Alzheimer, A. 1904. Histologische Studien zur Differenzialdiagnose der progressiven Paralyse. *Histol. Histopathol. Arb. Grosshirnrinde* 1:18–314.

Andersen, P., and Eccles, J. C. 1965. Locating and identifying postsynaptic inhibitory synapses by the correlation of physiological and histological data. *Symp. Biol. Hung.* 5:219–242.

Andersen, P., Eccles, J. C., and Voorhoeve, P. E. 1963. Inhibitory synapses on somas of Purkinje cells in the cerebellum. *Nature (Lond.)* 199:655–656.

Anderson, R. G. W. 1972. The three-dimensional structure of the basal body from the rhesus monkey oviduct. *J. Cell Biol.* 54:246–265.

Anderson, T. F. 1951. Techniques for the preservation of three dimensional structure in preparing specimens for the electron microscope. *Trans. N.Y. Acad. Sci. Ser. II* 13:130–134.

Anderson, W. A., Weissman, A., and Ellis, R. A. 1966. A comparative study of microtubules in some vertebrate and invertebrate cells. *Z. Zellforsch. Mikrosk. Anat.* 71:1–13.

Andersson-Cedergren, E. L. C. 1959. Ultrastructure of motor end plate and sarcoplasmic components of mouse skeletal muscle fiber as revealed by three-dimensional reconstructions from serial sections. *J. Ultrastruct. Res.* Suppl. 1, pp. 1–191.

Andres, K. H. 1961. Untersuchungen über den Feinbau von Spinalganglien. *Z. Zellforsch. Mikrosk. Anat.* 55:1–48.

Andres, K. H. 1964. Mikropinozytose im Zentralnervensystem. *Z. Zellforsch. Mikrosk. Anat.* 64:63–73.

Andres, K. H. 1965a. Der Feinbau des Bulbus olfactorius der Ratte unter besonderer Berücksichtigung der synaptischen Verbindungen. *Z. Zellforsch. Mikrosk. Anat.* 65:530–561.

Andres, K. H. 1965b. Über die Feinstruktur besonderer Einrichtungen in markhaltigen Nervenfasern des Kleinhirns der Ratte. *Z. Zellforsch. Mikrosk. Anat.* 65:701–712.

Andres, K. H. 1966. Der Feinbau der Regio olfactoria von Makrosmatikern. *Z. Zellforsch. Mikrosk. Anat.* 69:140–154.

Andres, K. H. 1967a. Über die Feinstruktur der Arachnoidea und Dura mater von Mammalia. *Z. Zellforsch. Mikrosk. Anat.* 79:272–295.

Andres, K. H. 1967b. Zur Feinstruktur der Arachnoidalzotten bei Mammalia. *Z. Zellforsch. Mikrosk. Anat.* 82:92–109.

Andres, K. H. 1970. Anatomy and ultrastructure of the olfactory bulb in fish, amphibia, reptiles, birds and mammals. In: *CIBA Foundation Symposium on Taste and Smell in Vertebrates.* G. E. W. Wolstenholme and J. Knight, Eds. London, Churchill, pp. 117–194.

Andrews, J. M., and Sekhon, S. S. 1969. Varieties of intranuclear filamentous aggregates in cerebral neurons. *Bull. Los Angeles Neurol Soc.* 34:163–174.

Angeletti, P. U., Levi-Montalcini, R., and Caramia, F. 1971. Ultrastructural changes in sympathetic neurons of newborn and adult mice treated with nerve growth factor. *J. Ultrastruct. Res.* 36:24–36.

Angevine, J. B. 1965. Time of neuron origin in the hippocampal region. An autoradiographic study in the mouse. *Exp. Neurol.* 2(Suppl):1–70.

Angevine, J. B. 1970. Critical cellular events in the shaping of neural centers. In: *The Neurosciences Second Study Program.* F. O. Schmitt, Ed. New York, Rockefeller University Press, pp. 62–72.

Apáthy, S. 1897. Das leitende Element des Nervensystems und seine topographischen Beziehungen zu den Zellen. *Mittheil. Zool. Station Neapel* 12:495–748.

Ariëns-Kappers, J. 1953. Beitrag zur experimentellen Untersuchung von Funktion und Herkunft der Kolmerschen Zellen des Plexus choroideus beim Axolotl und Meerschweinchen. *Z. Anat. Entwicklungsgesch.* 117:1–19.

Ariëns-Kappers, J. 1958. Structural and functional changes in the telencephalic choroid plexus during human ontogenesis. In: *Ciba Foundation Symposium, Cerebrospinal Fluid.* G. E. W. Wolstenholme and C. M. O'Conner, Eds. Boston, Little, Brown and Co., pp. 3–31.

Armstrong, D. M., and Schild, R. F. 1970. A quantitative study of the Purkinje cells in the cerebellum of the albino rat. *J. Comp. Neurol.* 139:449–456.

Arnold, G., and Holtzman, E. 1975. Peroxisomes in rat sympathetic ganglia and adrenal medulla. *Brain Res.* 83:509–515.

Arnold, W. 1970. On peculiar neuronal cells in the ependyma of the canalis centralis in the salamander. *Z. Zellforsch. Mikrosk. Anat.* 105:176–187.

Arstila, A. U., and Hopsu, V. K. 1964. Studies on the rat pineal gland. I. Ultrastructure. *Ann. Acad. Sci. Fenn. (Med.)* 113:1–21.

Arvidsson, B., Kristensson, K., and Olsson, Y. 1973. Vascular permeability to fluorescent protein tracer in trigeminal nerve and Gasserian ganglion. *Acta Neuropathol.* 26:199–205.

Asada, Y., and Bennett, M. V. L. 1971. Experimental alteration of coupling resistance at an electrotonic synapse. *J. Cell Biol.* 49:159–172.

Asbury, A. K. 1973. Renaut bodies. A forgotten endoneurial structure. *J. Neuropathol. Exp. Neurol.* 32:334–343.

Auerbach, L. 1898. Nervenendigung in Centralorganen. *Neurol. Centralbl.* 17:445–454.

Bairati, A. 1958. Fibrillar structure of astrocytes. In: *Biology of Neuroglia.* W. F. Windle, Ed. Springfield, Ill., Charles C Thomas, pp. 66–72.

Bak, I. J., and Choi, W. B. 1974. Electron microscopic investigation of synaptic organization of the trochlear nucleus in cat. I. Normal ultrastructure. *Cell Tissue Res.* 150:409–423.

Bak, I. J., Hassler, R., and Kim, J. S. 1969. Differential monoamine depletion by oxypertine in nerve terminals. Granulated synaptic vesicles in relation to depletion of norepinephrine, dopamine and serotonin. *Z. Zellforsch. Mikrosk. Anat. 101:*448–462.

Bakay, L. 1956. *Blood Brain Barrier.* Springfield, Ill., Charles C Thomas.

Baker, P. C. 1965. Fine structure and morphogenic movements in the gastrula of the treefrog, *Hyla regilla. J. Cell Biol. 24:*95–116.

Baker, P. C., and Schroeder, T. E. 1967. Cytoplasmic filaments and morphogenetic movements in the amphibian neural tube. *Dev. Biol. 15:*432–450.

Baker, R., and Llinás, R. 1970. Electrotonic coupling between neurons in the mesencephalic root of the Vth nerve in the rat. *Biophys. J. 10:*64a.

Balazs, R., Brooksbank, B. W. L., Davison, A. N., Eayrs, J. T., and Wilson, D. A. 1969. The effect of neonatal thyroidectomy on myelination in the rat brain. *Brain Res. 15:*219–232.

Banker, G., Churchill, L., and Cotman, C. W. 1974. Proteins of the postsynaptic density. *J. Cell Biol. 63:*456–465.

Banks, P., Mayor, D., and Mraz, P. 1973. Cytochalasin B and the intra-axonal movement of noradrenaline storage vesicles. *Brain Res. 49:*417–421.

Bär, T., and Wolff, J. R. 1972. The formation of capillary basement membranes during internal vascularization of the rat's cerebral cortex. *Z. Zellforsch. Mikrosk. Anat. 133:*231–248.

Bär, T., and Wolff, J. R. 1973. Quantitative Beziehungen zwischen der Verzweigungsdichte und Länge von Capillaren im Neocortex der Ratte während der postnatalen Entwicklung. *Z. Anat. Entwicklungsgesch. 141:*207–221.

Barer, R., Heller, H., and Lederis, K. 1963. The isolation, identification and properties of the hormonal granules of the neurohypophysis. *Proc. R. Soc. Ser. B 158:*388–416.

Bargmann, W. 1966. Neurosecretion. *Int. Rev. Cytol 19:*183–201.

Bargmann, W., and Lindner, E. 1964. Über den Feinbau des Nebennierenmarkes des Igels (*Erinaceus europaeus* L.). *Z. Zellforsch. Mikrosk. Anat. 64:*868–912.

Barker, L. F. 1899. *The Nervous System and Its Constituent Neurones.* New York, Appleton.

Barnes, B. G. 1961. Ciliated secretory cells in the pars distalis of the mouse hypophysis. *J. Ultrastruct. Res. 5:*453–467.

Barnicot, N. A. 1966. A note on the structure of spindle fibers. *J. Cell Sci. 1:*217–222.

Barón, M., and Gallego, A. 1972. The relation of the microglia with the pericytes in the cat cerebral cortex. *Z. Zellforsch. Mikrosk. Anat. 128:*42–57.

Barondes, S. H. 1967. Axoplasmic transport: A report of an NRP work session. *Neurosci. Res. Prog. Bull. 5(4):*307–419.

Barr, M. L. 1966. The significance of the sex chromatin. *Int. Rev. Cytol. 19:*35–95.

Barr, M. L., Bertram, L. F., and Lindsay, H. A. 1950. The morphology of the nerve cell nucleus, according to sex. *Anat. Rec. 107:*283–297.

Barrett, J. N., and Crill, W. E. 1974. Influence of dendritic location and membrane properties on the effectiveness of synapses on cat motoneurones. *J. Physiol. (Lond.) 293:*325–345.

Barron, K. D., Chiang, T. Y., Daniels, A. C., and Doolin, P. F. 1971. Subcellular accompaniments of axon reaction in cervical motoneurons of the cat. In: *Progress in Neuropathology*, Vol. 1. H. M. Zimmermann, Ed. New York, Grune and Stratton, pp. 255–280.

Barron, K. D., Doolin, P. F., and Oldershaw, J. B. 1967. Ultrastructural observations on retrograde atrophy of lateral geniculate body. I. Neuronal alterations. *J. Neuropathol. Exp. Neurol. 26:*300–326.

Bartelmez, G. W., and Hoerr, N. L. 1933. The vestibular club endings in Ameiurus. Further evidence on the morphology of the synapse. *J. Comp. Neurol. 57:*401–428.

Beams, H. W., and Kessel, R. G. 1968. The Golgi apparatus: structure and function. *Int. Rev. Cytol. 23:*209–276.

Bennett, G., Leblond, C. P., and Haddad, A. 1974. Migration of glycoprotein from the Golgi apparatus to the surface of various cell types as shown by radioautography after labeled fucose injection into rats. *J. Cell Biol. 60:*258–284.

Bennett, L. L., Simpson, L., and Skipper, H. E. 1960. On the metabolic stability of nucleic acids in mitotically inactive adult tissues labeled during embryonic development. *Biochim. Biophys. Acta 42:*237–243.

Bennett, M. V. L. 1970. Comparative physiology: electric organs. *Annu. Rev. Physiol. 32:*471–528.

Bennett, M. V. L. 1971. Electric organs. In: *Fish Physiology*, Vol. 5. J. S. Hoar and D. J. Randall, Eds. New York, Academic Press, pp. 347–491.

Bennett, M. V. L. 1972a. A comparison of electrically and chemically mediated transmission. In: *Structure and Function of Synapses*. G. D. Pappas and D. P. Purpura, Eds. New York, Raven Press, pp. 221–256.

Bennett, M. V. L. 1972b. Electrical versus chemical transmissions. In: *Research Publication of the A. R. N. M. D.*, Vol. 50, *Neurotransmitters*. Baltimore, Williams & Wilkins, pp. 58–89.

Bennett, M. V. L. 1973. Function of electrotonic junctions in embryonic and adult tissues. *Fed. Proc. 32:*65–75.

Bennett, M. V. L. 1974. Flexibility and rigidity in electrotonically coupled systems. In: *Synaptic Transmission and Neuronal Interaction*. M. V. L. Bennett, Ed. New York, Raven Press, pp. 153–178.

Bennett, M. V. L., Aljure, G., Nakajima, Y., and Pappas, G. D. 1963. Electrotonic junctions between teleost spinal neurons: electrophysiology and ultrastructure. *Science 141:*262–264.

Bennett, M. V. L., and Dunham, P. B. 1970. Sucrose permeability of junctional membrane at an electrotonic synapse. *Biophys. J. 10:*117a.

Bennett, M. V. L., Dunham, P. B., and Pappas, G. D. 1967. Ion fluxes through a "tight junction." *J. Gen. Physiol. 50:*1094.

Bennett, M. V. L., Nakajima, Y., and Pappas, G. D. 1967a. Physiology and ultrastructure of electrotonic junctions. I. Supramedullary neurons. *J. Neurophysiol. 30*:161–179.

Bennett, M. V. L., Nakajima, Y., and Pappas, G. D. 1967b. Physiology and ultrastructure of electrotonic junction. III. Giant electromotor neurons of *Malapterurus electricus. J. Neurophysiol. 30*:209–235.

Bennett, M. V. L., Pappas, G. D., Aljure, E., and Nakajima, Y. 1967. Physiology and ultrastructure of electrotonic junctions. II. Spinal and medullary electromotor nuclei in mormyrid fish. *J. Neurophysiol. 30*:180–208.

Bennett, M. V. L., Pappas, G. D., Giménez, M., and Nakajima, Y. 1967. Physiology and ultrastructure of electrotonic junctions. IV. Medullary electromotor nuclei in gymnotid fish. *J. Neurophysiol. 30*:236–300.

Bensley, R. R., and Gersh, I. 1933. Studies on cell structure by the freezing-drying method. III. The distribution in cells of the basophil substances, in particular the Nissl substance of the nerve cell. *Anat. Rec. 57*:369–385.

Bergeron, J. J. M., Ehrenreich, J. H., Siekevitz, P., and Palade, G. E. 1973. Golgi fractions prepared from rat liver homogenates. II. Biochemical characterization. *J. Cell Biol. 59*:73–88.

Bering, E. A. 1962. Circulation of the cerebrospinal fluid. *J. Neurosurg. 19*:405–413.

Berner, A., Torvik, A., and Stenwig, A. E. 1973. Origin of macrophages in traumatic lesions and Wallerian degeneration in peripheral nerves. *Acta Neuropathol. (Berl.) 25*:228–236.

Bernhard, W., and Granboulan, H. 1968. Electron microscopy of the nucleolus in vertebrate cells. In: *Ultrastructure in Biological Systems*, Vol. 3, *The Nucleus*. A. J. Dalton and F. Haguenau, Eds. New York, Academic Press, pp. 81–149.

Bernstein, J. J. 1966. Relationship of cortico-spinal tract growth to age and body weight in the rat. *J. Comp. Neurol. 127*:207–218.

Berthold, C. H. 1968. Ultrastructure of the node-paranode region of mature feline ventral lumbar spinal root fibers. *Acta Soc. Med. Upsal. 73*:37–73.

Berthold, C. H. 1973a. Histochemistry of postnatally developing feline spinal roots. II. Occurrence of acid phosphatase activity as studied by light and electron microscopical methods. *Neurobiology 3*:291–310.

Berthold, C. H. 1973b. Local "demyelination" in developing feline nerve fibres. *Neurobiology 3*:339–352.

Bethe, A. 1897–1898. Das Nervensystem von *Carcinus maenas*. Ein anatomisch-physiologischer Versuch. *Archiv Mikroskop. Anat. 50*:460–546, 589–639 (1897); *51*:382–452 (1898).

Bethe, A. 1900. Ueber die Neurofibrillen in den Ganglienzellen von Wirbelthieren und ihre Beziehungen zu den Golginetzen. *Arch. Mikroskop. Anat. 55*:513–558.

Bethe, A. 1904. Der heutige Stand der Neurontheorie. *Dtsch. Med. Wochenschr. 30*:1201–1204.

Bevan, S., Miledi, R., and Grampp, W. 1973. Induced transmitter release from Schwann cells and its suppression by actinomycin D. *Nature [New Biol.] 241*:85–86.

Bidder, F. H. 1847. *Zur Lehre von dem Verhältniss der Ganglienkörper zu den Nervenfasern.* Leipzig, Breitkopf and Haertel.

Billings, S. M., and Swartz, F. J. 1969. DNA content of Mauthner cell nuclei in *Xenopus laevis:* a spectrophotometric study. *Z. Anat. Entwicklungsgesch. 129*:14–23.

Billings-Gagliardi, S., Webster, H. deF., and O'Connell, M. F. 1974. *In vivo* and electron microscopic observations on Schwann cells in developing tadpole nerve fibers. *Am. J. Anat. 141*:375–392.

Birks, R. I. 1966. The fine structure of motor nerve endings at frog myoneural junction. *Ann. N.Y. Acad. Sci. 135*:8–19.

Birks, R. I. 1974. The relationship of transmitter release and storage to fine structure in a sympathetic ganglion. *J. Neurocytol. 3*:133–160.

Birks, R. I., Huxley, H. E., and Katz, B. 1960. The fine structure of the neuromuscular junction of the frog. *J. Physiol. (Lond.) 150*:134–144.

Birks, R. I., Mackey, M. C., and Weldon, P. R. 1972. Organelle formation from pinocytotic elements in neurites of cultured sympathetic ganglion. *J. Neurocytol. 1*:311–340.

Bischoff, A., and Moor, H. 1967a. Ultrastructural differences between the myelin sheaths of peripheral nerve fibers and CNS white matter. *Z. Zellforsch. Mikrosk. Anat. 81*:303–310.

Bischoff, A., and Moor, H. 1967b. The ultrastructure of the "difference factor" in the myelin. *Z. Zellforsch. Mikrosk. Anat. 81*:571–580.

Biscoe, T. J., Caddy, K., Pallot, D., Pehrson, M., and Stirling, C. A. 1974. The neurological lesion in the dystrophic mouse. *Brain Res. 76*:534–536.

Bittner, G. D., and Kennedy, D. 1970. Quantitative aspects of transmitter release. *J. Cell Biol. 47*:585–592.

Blackstad, T. W. 1967. Cortical grey matter. A correlation of light and electron microscopic data. In: *The Neuron*. H. Hydén, Ed. Amsterdam, Elsevier, pp. 49–118.

Blackstad, T. W. 1970. Electron microscopy of Golgi preparations. In: *Contemporary Research Methods in Neuroanatomy*. W. J. H. Nauta and S. O. E. Ebbesson, Eds. New York, Springer-Verlag, pp. 186–216.

Blackstad, T. W., and Dahl, H. A. 1961. Quantitative evaluation of structures in contact with neuronal somata. *Acta Morphol. Neerl. Scand. 4*:329–343.

Blakemore, W. F. 1969a. The ultrastructure of the subependymal plate in the rat. *J. Anat. 104*:423–433.

Blakemore, W. F. 1969b. Schmidt-Lantermann incisures in the central nervous system. *J. Ultrastruct. Res. 29*:496–498.

Blakemore, W. F. 1972. Microglial reaction following

thermal necrosis of the rat cortex: An electron microscope study. *Acta Neuropathol.* 21:11–22.

Blakemore, W. F., and Jolly, R. D. 1972. The subependymal plate and associated ependyma in the dog. An ultrastructural study. *J. Neurocytol.* 1:69–84.

Blank, W. F., Bunge, M. B., and Bunge, R. P. 1974. The sensitivity of the myelin sheath, particularly the Schwann cell-axolemmal junction, to lowered calcium levels in cultured sensory ganglia. *Brain Res.* 67:503–518.

Bleier, R. 1971. The relations of ependyma to neurons and capillaries in the hypothalamus: A Golgi-Cox study. *J. Comp. Neurol.* 142:439–464.

Blinzinger, K., and Kreutzberg, G. 1968. Displacement of synaptic terminals from regenerating motoneurons by microglial cells. *Z. Zellforsch. Mikrosk. Anat.* 85:145–157.

Bloom, F. E. 1970. Correlating structure and function of synaptic ultrastructure. In: *The Neurosciences. Second Study Program.* F. O. Schmitt, Ed. New York, The Rockefeller University Press, pp. 729–746.

Bloom, F. E. 1972. The formation of synaptic junctions in developing rat brain. In: *Structure and Function of Synapses.* G. D. Pappas and D. P. Purpura, Eds. New York, Raven Press, pp. 101–120.

Bloom, F. E. 1973. Ultrastructural identification of catecholamine-containing central synaptic terminals. *J. Histochem. Cytochem.* 21:333–348.

Bloom, F. E., and Aghajanian, G. K. 1966. Cytochemistry of synapses: Selective staining for electron microscopy. *Science* 154:1575–1577.

Bloom, F. E., and Aghajanian, G. K. 1968a. An electron microscopic analysis of large granular synaptic vesicles of the brain in relation to monoamine content. *J. Pharmacol. Exp. Ther.* 159:261–273.

Bloom, F. E., and Aghajanian, G. K. 1968b. An osmiophilic substance in brain synaptic vesicles not associated with catecholamine content. *Experientia* 24:1225–1227.

Bloom, F. E., and Aghajanian, G. K. 1968c. Fine structural cytochemical analysis of the staining of synaptic junctions with phosphotungstic acid. *J. Ultrastruct. Res.* 22:361–375.

Bloom, F. E., and Barrnett, R. J. 1966. Fine structural localization of noradrenaline in vesicles of autonomic nerve endings. *Nature (Lond.)* 210:599–601.

Bloom, F. E., and Giarman, N. J. 1968. Physiologic and pharmacologic considerations of biogenic amines in the nervous system. *Annu. Rev. Pharmacol.* 8:229–258.

Bloom, R. E., Hoffer, B. J., Siggins, G. R., Barker, J. L., and Nicoll, R. A. 1972. Effects of serotonin on central neurons: microiontophoretic administration. *Fed. Proc.* 31:97–106.

Bloom, F. E., Iversen, L. L., and Schmitt, F. O. 1970. Macromolecules in synaptic function. *Neurosci. Res. Prog. Bull.* 8:325–455.

Blunt, M. J., Baldwin, F., and Wendell-Smith, C. P. 1972. Gliogenesis and myelination in kitten optic nerve. *Z. Zellforsch. Mikrosk. Anat.* 124:293–310.

Bodian, D. 1937. The structure of the vertebrate synapse. A study of the axon endings on Mauthner's cell and neighboring centers in the goldfish. *J. Comp. Neurol.* 68:117–145.

Bodian, D. 1942. Cytological aspects of synaptic function. *Physiol. Rev.* 22:146–169.

Bodian, D. 1962. The generalized vertebrate neuron. *Science* 137:323–326.

Bodian, D. 1964. An electron microscopic study of the monkey spinal cord. *Bull. Johns Hopkins Hosp.* 114:13–119.

Bodian, D. 1966a. Synaptic types on spinal motoneurons: An electron microscopic study. *Bull. Johns Hopkins Hosp.* 119:16–45.

Bodian, D. 1966b. Development of fine structure of spinal cord in monkey fetuses. I. The motoneuron neuropil at the time of onset of reflex activity. *Bull. Johns Hopkins Hosp.* 119:129–149.

Bodian, D. 1966c. Electron microscopy: Two major synaptic types on spinal motoneurons. *Science* 151:1093–1094.

Bodian, D. 1970a. An electron microscope characterization of classes of synaptic vesicles by means of controlled aldehyde fixation. *J. Cell Biol.* 44:115–124.

Bodian, D. 1970b. A model of synaptic and behavioral ontogeny. In: *The Neurosciences. Second Study Program.* F. O. Schmitt, Ed. New York, The Rockefeller University Press, pp. 129–140.

Bodian, D. 1972. Synaptic diversity and characterization by electron microscopy. In: *Structure and Function of Synapses.* G. D. Pappas and D. P. Purpura, Eds. New York, Raven Press, pp. 45–65.

Bodian, D. 1975. Origin of specific synaptic types in the motoneuron neuropil of the monkey. *J. Comp. Neurol.* 159:225–244.

Bodian, D., Melby, E. C., and Taylor, N. 1968. Development of fine structure of spinal cord in monkey fetuses. II. Pre-reflex period to period of long intersegmental reflexes. *J. Comp. Neurol.* 133:113–166.

Bodian, D., and Mellors, R. C. 1945. The regenerative cycle of motoneurons, with special reference to phosphatase activity. *J. Exp. Med.* 81:469–488.

Bodian, D., and Taylor, N. 1963. Synapse arising at central node of Ranvier, and note on fixation of the central nervous system. *Science* 139:330–332.

Bohan, T. P., Boyne, A. F., Guth, P. S., Narayan, Y., and Williams, T. H. 1973. Electron-dense particle in cholinergic synaptic vesicles. *Nature (Lond.)* 244:32.

Bohr, V., and Møllgård, K. 1974. Tight junctions in human fetal choroid plexus visualized by freeze-etching. *Brain Res.* 81:314–318.

Bondareff, W. 1957. Genesis of intracellular pigment in the spinal ganglia of senile rats: An electron microscope study. *J. Gerontol.* 12:364–369.

Bondareff, W. 1966. Localization of α-methylnorepinephrine in sympathetic fibers of the pineal body. *Exp. Neurol.* 16:131–135.

Bondareff, W. 1967. An intercellular substance in rat cerebral cortex: Submicroscopic distribution of ruthenium red. *Anat. Rec.* 157:527–535.

Bondareff, W., and McLone, D. G. 1973. The extreme glial limiting membrane in *Macaca:* Ultrastructure of a laminated glioepithelium. *Am. J. Anat. 136:*277–296.

Bondareff, W., and Sjöstrand, J. 1969. Cytochemistry of synaptosomes. *Exp. Neurol 24:*450–458.

Bondy, S. C., and Modsen, C. J. 1973. Axoplasmic transport of RNA. *J. Neurobiol. 4:*535–542.

Bone, Q., and Denton, E. J. 1971. The osmotic effects of electron microscope fixatives. *J. Cell Biol. 49:*571–581.

Boquist, L. 1969. Intranuclear rods in pancreatic islet beta cells. *J. Cell Biol. 43:*377–381.

Booz, K. H., and Desaga, U. 1973. Sub- und interependymale Basalmembranlabyrinthe am Ventrikelsystem und Zentralkanal der weissen Ratte. *Verh. Anat. Ges. 67:*609–612.

Boulder Committee. 1970. Embryonic vertebrate central nervous system. Revised terminology. *Anat. Rec. 166:*257–261.

Bowers, B. 1964. Coated vesicles in the pericardial cells of the aphid (*Myzus persicae* Sulz). *Protoplasma 59:*351–367.

Boycott, B. B., Gray, E. G., and Guillery, R. W. 1961. Synaptic structure and its alteration with environmental temperature: a study by light and electron microscopy of the central nervous system of lizards. *Proc. R. Soc. Ser. B. 154:*151–172.

Bozler, E. 1927. Untersuchungen über des Nervensystem der Coelenteraten. I. Kontinuität oder Kontakt zwischen den Nervenzellen? *Z. Zellforsch. Mikrosk. Anat. 5:*244–262.

Bradley, W. G., and Asbury, A. K. 1970. Duration of synthesis phase in neurilemma cells in mouse sciatic nerve during degeneration. *Exp. Neurol. 26:*275–282.

Brandes, D. 1965. Observations on the apparent mode of formation of 'pure' lysosomes. *J. Ultrastruct. Res. 12:*63–80.

Branton, D. 1966. Fracture faces of frozen membranes. *Proc. Natl. Acad. Sci. U.S.A. 55:*1048–1056.

Branton, D. 1967. Fracture faces of frozen myelin. *Exp. Cell Res. 45:*703–707.

Brattgård, S.-O., Edström, J. E., and Hydén, H. 1957. The chemical changes in regenerating neurons. *J. Neurochem. 1:*316–325.

Brattgård, S.-O., Edström, J. E., and Hydén, H. 1958. The productive capacity of the neuron in retrograde reaction. *Exp. Cell Res. Suppl. 5:*185–200.

Brawer, J. W. 1971. The role of the arcuate nucleus in the brain-pituitary-gonad axis. *J. Comp. Neurol. 143:*411–446.

Brawer, J. R. 1972. The fine structure of the ependymal tanycytes at the level of the arcuate nucleus. *J. Comp. Neurol. 145:*25–42.

Brawer, J. R., Lin, P. S., and Sonnenschein, C. 1974. Morphological plasticity in the wall of the third ventricle during the estrous cycle in the rat: A scanning electron microscopic study. *Anat. Rec. 179:*481–489.

Brawer, J. R., Morest, D. K., and Kane, E. C. 1974.

The neuronal architecture of the cochlear nucleus of the cat. *J. Comp. Neurol. 155:*251–300.

Bray, D. 1973. Branching patterns of individual sympathetic neurons in culture. *J. Cell Biol. 56:*702–712.

Bray, D., and Bunge, M. B. 1973. The growth cone in neuritic extensions. In: *Locomotion of Tissue Cells.* Ciba Foundation Symposium 14. Amsterdam, Elsevier Excerpta Medica, North Holland, pp. 195–209.

Brierley, J. B. 1957. The blood-brain barrier: structural aspects. In: *Metabolism of the Nervous System.* D. Richter, Ed. New York, Pergamon Press, pp. 121–135.

Brightman, M. W. 1962. An electron microscopic study of ferritin uptake from the cerebral ventricles of rats. *Anat. Rec. 142:*219.

Brightman, M. W. 1965a. The distribution within the brain of ferritin injected into cerebrospinal fluid compartments. I. Ependymal distribution. *J. Cell Biol. 26:*99–123.

Brightman, M. W. 1965b. The distribution within the brain of ferritin injected into cerebrospinal fluid compartments. II. Parenchymal distribution. *Am. J. Anat. 117:*193–219.

Brightman, M. W. 1967. Intracerebral movement of proteins injected into blood and cerebrospinal fluid. *Anat. Rec. 157:*219.

Brightman, M. E. 1968. The intracerebral movement of proteins injected into blood and cerebrospinal fluid of mice. In: *Progress in Brain Research,* Vol. 29, *Brain Barrier Systems.* A. Lajtha and D. H. Ford, Eds. Amsterdam, Elsevier, pp. 19–37.

Brightman, M. W., Hori, M., Rapoport, S. I., Reese, T. S., and Westergaard, E. 1974. Osmotic opening of tight junctions in cerebral endothelium. *J. Comp. Neurol. 152:*317–326.

Brightman, M. W., Klatzo, I., Olsson, Y., and Reese, T. S. 1970. The blood-brain barrier to proteins under normal and pathological conditions. *J. Neurol. Sci. 10:*215–239.

Brightman, M. W., and Palay, S. L. 1963. The fine structure of ependyma in the brain of the rat. *J. Cell Biol. 19:*415–439.

Brightman, M. W., and Reese, T. S. 1967. Astrocytic and ependymal junctions in the mouse brain. *J. Cell Biol. 35:*16A–17A.

Brightman, M. W., and Reese, T. S. 1969. Junctions between intimately apposed cell membranes in the vertebrate brain. *J. Cell Biol. 40:*648–677.

Brightman, M. W., Reese, T. S., Olsson, Y., and Klatzo, I. 1971. Morphologic aspects of the blood-brain barrier to peroxidase in elasmobranchs. *Progr. Neuropathol. 1:*146–161.

Bruni, J. E., Montemurro, D. G., Clattenburg, R. E., and Singh, R. P. 1972. A scanning electron microscopic study of the ependymal surface of the third ventricle of the rabbit, rat, mouse and human brain. *Anat. Rec. 174:*407–420.

Bruni, J. E., Montemurro, D. G., Clattenburg, R. E., and Singh, R. P. 1973. Scanning electron microscopy of the ependymal surface of the third ventricle after silver nitrate staining. *Brain Res.* *61*:207–216.

Budd, G. C., and Salpeter, M. M. 1969. The distribution of labeled norepinephrine within sympathetic nerve terminals studied with electron microscopic radioautography. *J. Cell Biol. 41*:21–32.

Bullock, T. H., and Horridge, G. A. 1965. *Structure and Function in the Nervous Systems of Invertebrates.* San Francisco, Freeman.

Bullock, T. H., and Quarton, G. C. 1966. Simple systems for the study of learning mechanisms. Report of an NRP work session. *NRP Bull. 4*:105–233.

Bunge, M. B. 1973. Fine structure of nerve fibers and growth cones of isolated sympathetic neurons in cultures. *J. Cell Biol. 56*:713–735.

Bunge, M. B., Bunge, R. P., and Pappas, G. D. 1962. Electron microscopic demonstration of connections between glia and myelin sheaths in the developing mammalian central nervous system. *J. Cell Biol. 12*:448–453.

Bunge, M. B., Bunge, R. P., Peterson, E. R., and Murray, M. R. 1967. A light and electron microscope study of long-term organized cultures of rat dorsal root ganglia. *J. Cell Biol. 32*:439–466.

Bunge, M. B., Bunge, R. P., and Ris, H. 1961. Ultrastructural study of remyelination in an experimental lesion in adult cat spinal cord. *J. Biophys. Biochem. Cytol. 10*:67–94.

Bunge, R. P. 1968. Glial cells and the central myelin sheath. *Physiol. Rev. 48*:197–251.

Bunge, R. P., Bunge, M. B., and Peterson, E. R. 1965. An electron microscope study of cultured rat spinal cord. *J. Cell Biol. 24*:163–191.

Bunge, R. P., Bunge, M. B., and Ris, H. 1960. Electron microscopic study of demyelination in an experimentally induced lesion in adult cat spinal cord. *J. Biophys. Biochem. Cytol. 7*:685–696.

Bunge, R. P., and Glass, P. M. 1965. Some observations on myelin-glial relationships and on the etiology of the cerebrospinal fluid exchange lesion. *Ann. N.Y. Acad. Sci. 122*:15–28.

Bunt, A. H. 1971. Enzymatic digestion of synaptic ribbons in amphibian retinal photoreceptors. *Brain Res. 25*:571–577.

Burkel, W. E. 1967. The histological fine structure of perineurium. *Anat. Rec. 158*:177–190.

Burnside, B. 1971. Microtubules and microfilaments in newt neurulation. *Dev. Biol. 26*:416–441.

Burton, P. R., and Fernandez, H. L. 1973. Delineation by lanthanum staining of filamentous elements associated with the surfaces of axonal microtubules. *J. Cell Sci. 12*:567–583.

Buttlar-Brentano, K. von 1954. Zur Lebensgeschichte des Nucleus basalis, tuberomammillaris, supraopticus, und paraventricularis unter normalen und pathogenen Bedingungen. *J. Hirnforsch. 1*:337–419.

Byers, M. R. 1970. Chromatolysis in a pair of identifiable metathoracic neurons in the cockroach *Diploptera punctata. Tissue Cell 2*:255–279.

Byers, M. R. 1974. Structural correlates of rapid axonal transport: Evidence that microtubules may not be directly involved. *Brain Res. 75*:97–113.

Cajal, S. R. 1888a. Estructura de los centros nerviosos de las aves. *Rev. Trimestr. Histol. No. 1* (May):1–10.

Cajal, S. R. 1888b. Sobre las fibras nerviosas de la capa molecular del cerebelo. *Rev. Trimestr. Histol. No. 2*(August):33–41.

Cajal, S. R. 1894. Croonian lecture. La fine structure des centres nerveux. *Proc. R. Soc. 55*:444–468.

Cajal, S. R. 1896. Estructura del protoplasma nervioso. *Rev. Trimestr. Micrográfica 1*:1–30.

Cajal, S. R. 1899. Estudios sobre la corteza cerebral humana. *Rev. Trimestr. Micrográfica 4*:1–63 and 117–200.

Cajal, S. R. 1904. Variations morphologiques du réticule nerveux d'invertébrés et de vertébrés soumis à l'action de conditions naturelles. *Trab. Lab. Invest. Biol. Univ. Madr. 3*:311–322.

Cajal, S. R. 1906. The structure and connexions of neurons. In: *Nobel Lectures: Physiology or Medicine, 1901–1921.* Amsterdam, Elsevier, 1967, pp. 220–253.

Cajal, S. R. 1909–1911. *Histologie du Système Nerveux de l'Homme et des Vertébrés,* Vols. I and II. Paris, Maloine. Reprinted Madrid, Consejo Superior de Investigaciones Cientificas, 1952.

Cajal, S. R. 1913. Sobre un nuevo proceder de impregnación de la neuroglia y sus resultados en los centros nerviosos del hombre y animales. *Trab. Lab. Invest. Biol. Univ. Madr. 11*:219–237.

Cajal, S. R. 1916. El proceder del oro-sublimado para la coloración de la neuroglia. *Trab. Lab. Invest. Biol. Univ. Madr. 14*:155–162.

Cajal, S. R. 1928. *Degeneration and Regeneration of the Nervous System,* Vol. 2. R. M. May, Trans. and Ed., reprinted New York, Hafner, 1959, p. 459.

Cajal, S. R. 1929. Études sur la neurogenèse de quelques vertébrés. Madrid. Trans. into English by L. Guth, as *Studies on Vertebrate Neurogenesis.* Springfield, Ill., Charles C Thomas, 1960.

Cajal, S. R. 1934. Les preuves objectives de l'unité anatomique des cellules nerveuses. *Trab. Lab. Invest. Biol. Univ. Madr. 29*:1–137. Trans. from the Spanish into English by M. U. Purkiss and C. A. Fox, as *Neuron Theory or Reticular Theory? Objective Evidence of the Anatomical Unity of Nerve Cells.* Madrid, Consejo Superior de Investigaciones Cientificas, 1954.

Caley, D. W. 1967. Ultrastructural differences between central and peripheral myelin sheath formation in the rat. *Anat. Rec. 157*:223.

Caley, D. W., and Butler, A. B. 1974. Formation of central and peripheral myelin sheaths in the rat: an electron microscopic study. *Am. J. Anat. 140*:339–348.

Caley, D. W., and Maxwell, D. S. 1968. An electron microscope study of the neuroglia during postnatal development of the rat cerebrum. *J. Comp. Neurol. 133*:45–69.

Caley, D. W., and Maxwell, D. S. 1970. Development

of the blood vessels and extracellular spaces during postnatal maturation of rat cerebral cortex. *J. Comp. Neurol. 138*:31–48.

Cammermeyer, J. 1965a. I. Juxtavascular karyokinesis and microglia cell proliferation during retrograde reaction in the mouse facial nucleus. *Ergeb. Anat. Entwicklungsgesch. 38*:1–22.

Cammermeyer, J. 1965b. VI. Histiocytes, juxtavascular mitotic cells and microglia cells during retrograde changes in the facial nucleus of rabbits of varying age. *Ergeb. Anat. Entwicklungsgesch. 38*:195–229.

Cammermeyer, J. 1965c. The hypependymal microglia cell. *Z. Anat. Entwicklungsgesch. 124*:543–561.

Cammermeyer, J. 1966. Morphologic distinctions between oligodendrocytes and microglia cells in the rabbit cerebral cortex. *Am. J. Anat. 118*:227–247.

Cammermeyer, J. 1970. The life history of the microglial cell: a light microscopic study. In: *Neurosciences Research*, Vol. 3. S. Ehrenpreis and O. C. Solnitzky, Eds. New York, Academic Press, pp. 44–130.

Cantino, O., and Mugnaini, E. 1975. The structural basis for electrotonic coupling in the avian ciliary ganglion. A study with thin sectioning and freeze-fracturing. *J. Neurocytol. 4*:505–536.

Carlsen, F., Knappeis, G. G., and Behse, F. 1974. Schwann cell length in unmyelinated fibres of human sural nerve. *J. Anat. 117*:463–467.

Carpenter, S. J., McCarthy, L. E., and Borison, H. L. 1970. Electron microscopic study of the epiplexus (Kolmer) cells of the cat choroid plexus. *Z. Zellforsch. Mikrosk. Anat. 110*:471–486.

Case, N. M. 1959. Hemosiderin granules in the choroid plexus. *J. Biophys. Biochem. Cytol. 6*:527–530.

Caspar, D. L. D., and Kirschner, D. A. 1971. Myelin membrane structure at 10Å resolution. *Nature [New Biol.] 231*:46–52.

Castel, M., Sahar, A., and Erlij, D. 1974. The movement of lanthanum across diffusion barriers in the choroid plexus of the cat. *Brain Res. 67*:178–184.

Cathcart, R. S., and Worthington, W. C. 1964. Ciliary movement in the rat cerebral ventricles: clearing action and direction of current. *J. Neuropathol. Exp. Neurol. 23*:609–618.

Causey, G. 1960. *The Cell of Schwann.* Edinburgh, E. & S. Livingstone, Ltd.

Causey, G., and Barton, A. A. 1959. The cellular content of the endoneurium of peripheral nerve. *Brain 82*:594–598.

Ceccarelli, B., Clementi, F., and Mantegazza, P. 1971. Synaptic transmission in the superior cervical ganglion of the cat after reinnervation by vagus fibers. *J. Physiol. (Lond.) 216*:87–98.

Ceccarelli, B., Hurlbut, W. P., and Mauro, A. 1972. Depletion of vesicles from frog neuromuscular junctions by prolonged tetanic stimulation. *J. Cell Biol. 54*:30–38.

Ceccarelli, B., Hurlbut, W. P., and Mauro, A. 1973. Turnover of transmitter and synaptic vesicles at the frog neuromuscular junction. *J. Cell Biol. 57*:499–524.

Cérvos-Navarro, J. 1960. Elektronenmikroskopische Untersuchungen an Spinalganglien. II. Satellitenzellen. *Arch. Psychiatr. Nervenkr. Z. Gesamte. Neurol. Psychiatr. 200*:267–283.

Chalcroft, J. A., and Bullivant, S. 1970. An interpretation of the liver cell membranes and junction structure based on observations of freeze-fracture replicas of both sides of the fracture. *J. Cell Biol. 47*:49–60.

Chamberlain, J. G. 1973. Analysis of developing ependymal and choroidal surfaces in rat brains using scanning electron microscopy. *Dev. Biol. 31*:22–30.

Chamberlain, J. G. 1974. Scanning electron microscopy of epiplexus cells (macrophages) in the fetal rat brain. *Am. J. Anat. 139*:443–447.

Chambers, R. 1949. Micrurgical studies on protoplasm. *Biol. Rev. 24*:246–265.

Chandler, R. L., and Willis, R. 1966. An intranuclear fibrillar lattice in neurons. *J. Cell Sci. 1*:283–286.

Chan-Palay, V. 1972. The tripartite structure of the undercoat in initial segments of Purkinje cell axons. *Z. Anat. Entwicklungsgesch. 139*:1–10.

Chan-Palay, V. 1973a. A light microscope study of the cytology and organization of neurons in the simple mammalian nucleus lateralis: Columns and swirls. *Z. Anat. Entwicklungsgesch. 141*:125–150.

Chan-Palay, V. 1973b. Cytology and organization in the nucleus lateralis of the cerebellum: The projections of neurons and their processes into afferent axon bundles. *Z. Anat. Entwicklungsgesch. 141*:151–159.

Chan-Palay, V. 1973c. The cytology of neurons and their dendrites in the simple mammalian nucleus lateralis. An electron microscope study. *Z. Anat. Entwicklungsgesch. 141*:289–317.

Chan-Palay, V. 1973d. Afferent axons and their relations with neurons in the nucleus lateralis of the cerebellum: A light microscopic study. *Z. Anat. Entwicklungsgesch. 142*:1–21.

Chan-Palay, V. 1973e. Neuronal plasticity in the cerebellar cortex and lateral nucleus. *Z. Anat. Entwicklungsgesch. 142*:23–35.

Chan-Palay, V. 1973f. Axon terminals of the intrinsic neurons in the nucleus lateralis of the cerebellum. An electron microscope study. *Z. Anat. Entwicklungsgesch. 142*:187–206.

Chan-Palay, V. 1973g. On certain fluorescent axon terminals containing granular synaptic vesicles in the cerebellar nucleus lateralis. *Z. Anat. Entwicklungsgesch. 142*:239–258.

Chan-Palay, V. 1973h. A brief note on the chemical nature of the precipitate within nerve fibers after the rapid Golgi reaction: Selected area diffraction in high voltage electron microscopy. *Z. Anat. Entwicklungsgesch. 139*:115–117.

Chan-Palay, V. 1975. On the identification of CAT$_2$ serotonin axons in the mammalian cerebellum. The roles of large granular, small, and granular alveolate vesicles in transmitter storage, discharge, and reuptake: An hypothesis. In: *SIF Cells. Structure and Function of the Small Intensely Fluorescent Sympathetic Cells.* O. Eranko, Ed. Washington, D.C., U.S. Government Printing Office.

Chan-Palay, V., and Palay, S. L. 1970. Interrelations of basket cell axons and climbing fibers in the cerebellar cortex of the rat. *Z. Anat. Entwicklungsgesch. 132:*191–227.

Chan-Palay, V., and Palay, S. L. 1972a. High voltage electron microscopy of rapid Golgi preparations. Neurons and their processes in the cerebellar cortex of monkey and rat. *Z. Anat. Entwicklungsgesch. 137:*125–152.

Chan-Palay, V., and Palay, S. L. 1972b. The form of velate astrocytes in the cerebellar cortex of monkey and rat: High voltage electron microscopy of rapid Golgi preparations. *Z. Anat. Entwicklungsgesch. 138:*1–19.

Chan-Palay, V., Palay, S. L., and Billings-Gagliardi, S. M. 1974. Meynert cells in the primate visual cortex. *J. Neurocytol. 3:*631–658.

Charlton, B. T., and Gray, E. G. 1965. Electron microscopy of specialized synaptic contacts suggesting possible electrical transmission in frog spinal cord. *J. Physiol. (Lond.) 179:*2P–4P.

Charlton, B. T., and Gray, E. G. 1966. Comparative electron microscopy of synapses in the vertebrate spinal cord. *J. Cell Sci. 1:*67–80.

Chason, J. G., and Pearse, A. G. E. 1961. Phenazine methosulfate and nicotinamide in the histochemical demonstration of dehydrogenases in rat brain. *J. Neurochem. 6:*259–266.

Chiba, T. 1973. Electron microscopic and histochemical studies on the synaptic vesicles in mouse vas deferens and atrium after 5-hydroxydopamine administration. *Anat. Rec. 176:*35–48.

Christensen, B. N. 1973. Procion brown: An intracellular dye for light and electron microscopy. *Science 182:*1255–1256.

Church, R. L., Tanzer, M. L., and Pfeiffer, S. E. 1973. Collagen and procollagen production by a clonal line of Schwann cells. *Proc. Natl. Acad. Sci. U.S.A. 70:*1943–1946.

Citkowitz, E., and Holtzman, E. 1973. Peroxisomes in dorsal root ganglia. *J. Histochem. Cytochem. 21:*34–41.

Clark, A. W., Hurlbut, W. P., and Mauro, A. 1972. Changes in the fine structure of the neuromuscular junction of the frog caused by black widow spider venom. *J. Cell Biol. 52:*1–14.

Clark, E., and O'Malley, C. D. 1968. *The Human Brain and Spinal Cord. A Historical Study Illustrated By Writings from Antiquity to the Twentieth Century.* Berkeley, University of California Press.

Claude, A. 1970. Growth and differentiation of cytoplasmic membranes in the course of lipoprotein granule synthesis in the hepatic cell. I. Elaboration of elements of the Golgi complex. *J. Cell Biol. 47:*745–766.

Clementi, F., and Morini, D. 1972. The surface fine

structure of the walls of the cerebral ventricles and choroid plexus in cat. *Z. Zellforsch. Mikrosk. Anat. 123:*82–95.

Clos, J., and Legrand, J. 1970. Influence de la déficience thyroidienne et de la sous-alimentation sur la croissance et la myélinisation des fibres nerveuses du nerf sciatique chez le jeune rat blanc. Étude au microscope électronique. *Brain Res. 22:*285–297.

Cloyd, M. W., and Low, F. N. 1974. Scanning electron microscopy of the subarachnoid space in the dog. I. Spinal cord levels. *J. Comp. Neurol. 153:*325–368.

Coates, P. W. 1973a. Supraependymal cells in the recess of the monkey third ventricle. *Am. J. Anat. 136:*533–539.

Coates, P. W. 1973b. Supraependymal cells: light and transmission electron microscopy extends scanning electron microscopic demonstration. *Brain Res. 57:*502–507.

Cobb, S. 1932. The cerebrospinal blood vessels. In: *Cytology and Cellular Pathology of the Nervous System*, Vol. 2. W. Penfield, Ed. New York, Hoeber, pp. 577–610.

Coggeshall, R. E. 1967. A light and electron microscope study of the abdominal ganglion of *Aplysia californica. J. Neurophysiol. 30:*1263–1287.

Coggeshall, R. E., Yaksta, B. A., and Swartz, F. J. 1970. A cytophotometric analysis of the DNA in the nucleus of the giant cell, R-2, in *Aplysia. Chromosoma 32:*205–212.

Cohen, J., Dutton, G. R., Wilkin, G. P., Wilson, J. E., and Balázs, R. 1974. A preparation of viable cell perikarya from developing rat cerebellum with preservation of a high degree of morphological integrity. *J. Neurochem. 23:*899–901.

Cohen, J., Mareš, V., and Lodin, Z. 1973. DNA content of purified preparations of mouse Purkinje neurons isolated by a velocity sedimentation technique. *J. Neurochem. 20:*651–657.

Cohen, L. B. 1973. Changes in neuron structure during action potential propagation and synaptic transmission. *Physiol. Rev. 53:*373–418.

Cohen, L. B., Keynes, R. D., and Hille, B. 1968. Light scattering and birefringence changes during nerve activity. *Nature (Lond.) 218:*438–441.

Cohen, M. J., and Jacklet, J. W. 1965. Neurons of insects: RNA changes during injury and regeneration. *Science 148:*1237–1239.

Collin, J.-P. 1971. Differentiation and regression of the cells of the sensory line in the epiphysis cerebri. In: *The Pineal Gland.* A Ciba Foundation Symposium. G. E. W. Wolstenholme and J. Knight, Eds. Edinburgh, Churchill Livingstone, pp. 79–120.

Colonnier, M. 1965. On the nature of intranuclear rods. *J. Cell Biol. 25:*646–653.

Colonnier, M. 1968. Synaptic patterns on different cell types in the different laminae of the cat visual cortex. An electron microscope study. *Brain Res. 9:*268–287.

Colonnier, M., and Guillery, R. W. 1964. Synaptic organization in the lateral geniculate nucleus of the monkey. *Z. Zellforsch. Mikrosk. Anat. 62*:333–355.

Connell, C. J., and Mercer, K. L. 1974. Freeze-fractured appearance of the capillary endothelium in the cerebral cortex of mouse brain. *Am. J. Anat. 140*:595–600.

Conradi, S. 1969a. Ultrastructure and distribution of neuronal and glial elements on the motoneuron surface in the lumbosacral spinal cord of the adult cat. *Acta Physiol. Scand. Suppl. 332*:5–48.

Conradi, S. 1969b. Ultrastructure and distribution of neuronal and glial elements on the surface of the proximal part of a motoneuron dendrite as analysed by serial sections. *Acta Physiol. Scand. Suppl. 332*:49–64.

Conradi, S. 1969c. Observations on the ultrastructure of the axon hillock and initial axon segment of lumbosacral motoneurons in the cat. *Acta Physiol. Scand. Suppl. 332*:65–84.

Conradi, S., and Skoglund, S. 1969a. Observations on the ultrastructure and distribution of neuronal and glial elements on the motoneuron surface in the lumbosacral spinal cord of the cat during postnatal development. *Acta Physiol. Scand. Suppl. 333*:5–52.

Conradi, S., and Skoglund, S. 1969b. Observations on the ultrastructure of the initial motoraxon segment and dorsal root boutons on the motoneurons in the lumbosacral spinal cord of the cat during postnatal development. *Acta Physiol. Scand. Suppl. 333*:53–76.

Cook, R. D., and Wiśniewski, H. M. 1973. The role of oligodendroglia and astroglia in Wallerian degeneration of the optic nerve. *Brain Res. 61*:191–206.

Cotman, C. W., Banker, G., Churchill, L., and Taylor, D. 1974. Isolation of postsynaptic densities from rat brain. *J. Cell Biol. 63*:441–455.

Cotman, C. W., and Taylor, D. 1972. Isolation and structural studies on synaptic complexes from rat brain. *J. Cell Biol. 55*:696–711.

Coupland, R. E. 1962. Nerve endings on chromaffin cells in the rat adrenal medulla. *Nature (Lond.) 194*:310–312.

Couteaux, R. 1955. Localization of cholinesterases at neuromuscular junctions. *Int. Rev. Cytol. 4*:335–375.

Couteaux, R. 1960. Motor end plate structure. In: *The Structure and Function of Muscle*, Vol. 1. G. H. Bourne, Ed. New York, Academic Press, pp. 337–380.

Couteaux, R. 1961. Principaux critères morphologiques et cytochimiques utilisables aujourd'hui pour définir les divers types de synapses. *Actual. Neurophysiol.*, 3ᵉ série:145–173.

Couteaux, R. 1963. The differentiation of synaptic areas. *Proc. R. Soc. Ser. B 158*:457–480.

Cowan, W. M., Gottlieb, D. I., Hendrickson, A. E., Price, J. L., and Woolsey, T. A. 1972. The autoradiographic demonstration of axonal connections in the central nervous system. *Brain Res. 37*:21–51.

Cragg, B. G. 1967. The density of synapses and neurones in the motor and visual areas of the cerebral cortex. *J. Anat. 101*:639–654.

Cragg, B. G. 1969. Structural changes in naive retinal synapses detectable within minutes of first exposure to daylight. *Brain Res. 15*:79–96.

Cragg, B. G., and Thomas, P. K. 1957. The relationships between conduction velocity and the diameter and internodal length of peripheral nerve fibres. *J. Physiol. (Lond.) 136*:606–614.

Cravioto, H. 1965. The role of Schwann cells in the development of human peripheral nerves. An electron microscope study. *J. Ultrastruct. Res. 12*:634–651.

Cserr, H. F. 1971. Physiology of the choroid plexus. *Physiol. Rev. 51*:312–367.

Cuénod, M., Sandri, C., and Akert, K. 1972. Enlarged synaptic vesicles in optic nerve terminals induced by intraocular injection of colchicine. *Brain Res. 39*:285–296.

Cull, R. E. 1974. Role of nerve-muscle contact in maintaining synaptic connections. *Exp. Brain Res. 20*:307–310.

Cull, R. E. 1975. Effect of sensory nerve division on the afferent synapses of axotomised motor neurones. *Exp. Brain Res. 22*:421–425.

Cummins, J., and Hydén, H. 1962. Adenosine triphosphate levels and adenosine triphosphatases in neurons, glia and neuronal membranes of the vestibular nucleus. *Biochim. Biophys. Acta 60*:271–283.

Curtis, D. R. 1969. The pharmacology of spinal postsynaptic inhibition. In: *Progress in Brain Research*, Vol. 31, *Mechanisms of Synaptic Transmission*. K. Akert and P. G. Waser, Eds. Amsterdam, Elsevier, pp. 171–189.

Cushing, H. 1914. Studies on the cerebrospinal fluid. I. Introduction. *J. Med. Res. 26*:1–19.

Dahl, E. 1970. The fine structure of nuclear inclusions. *J. Anat. 106*:255–262.

Dahl, E. 1973a. The innervation of the cerebral arteries. *J. Anat. 115*:53–63.

Dahl, E. 1973b. The fine structure of intracerebral vessels. *Z. Zellforsch. Mikrosk. Anat. 145*:577–586.

Dahl, H. A. 1963. Fine structure of cilia in rat cerebral cortex. *Z. Zellforsch. Mikrosk. Anat. 60*:369–386.

Dahlström, A., and Füxe, K. 1964. Evidence for the existence of monoamine containing neurons in the central nervous system. I. Demonstration of monoamines in the cell bodies of brain stem neurons. *Acta Physiol. Scand. Suppl. 232*:1–78.

Dale, H. H., Feldberg, W., and Vogt, M. 1936. Release of acetylcholine at voluntary nerve endings. *J. Physiol. (Lond.) 86*:353–380.

Dalton, A. J., and Haguenau, F., Eds. 1968. *Ultrastructure in Biological Systems*, Vol. 3, *The Nucleus*. New York, Academic Press.

Dalton, M. M., Hommes, O. R., and Leblond, C. P. 1968. Correlation of glial proliferation with age in the mouse brain. *J. Comp. Neurol. 134*:397–400.

Dandy, W. E. 1919. Experimental hydrocephalus. *Ann. Surg. 70*:129–142.

Daniels, M. P. 1973. Fine structural changes in neurons and nerve fibers associated with colchicine inhibition of nerve fiber formation in vitro. *J. Cell Biol. 58*:463–470.

David, G. F. X., Herbert, J., and Wright, G. D. S. 1973. The ultrastructure of the pineal gland in the ferret. *J. Anat. 115*:79–97.

Davis, D. A., Lloyd, B. J., and Milhorat, T. 1973. A comparative ultrastructural study of the choroid plexuses of the immature pig. *Anat. Rec. 176*:443–454.

Davison, A. N. 1968. Myelination. In: *Fortschritte der Pädologie*. Vol. II. F. Linneweh, Ed. Berlin, Springer-Verlag, pp. 65–87.

Davison, A. N. 1970. The biochemistry of the myelin sheath. In: *Myelination*. A. N. Davison and A. Peters, Eds. Springfield, Ill., Charles C Thomas, pp. 80–161.

Davison, P. F. 1970. Axoplasmic transport. Physical and chemical aspects. In: *The Neurosciences. Second Study Program*. F. O. Schmitt, Ed. New York, The Rockefeller University Press, pp. 851–857.

Davison, P. F., and Huneeus, F. C. 1970. Fibrillar proteins from squid axons. II. Microtubule protein. *J. Molec. Biol. 52*:429–439.

Davison, P. F., and Winslow, B. 1974. The protein subunit of calf brain neurofilament. *J. Neurobiol. 5*:119–133.

Davson, H. 1967. *Physiology of the Cerebrospinal Fluid*. Boston, Little, Brown and Co.

Davson, H. 1972. The blood-brain barrier. In: *The Structure and Function of Nervous Tissue*, Vol. IV. G. H. Bourne, Ed. New York, Academic Press, pp. 323–445.

de Duve, C. 1963. The lysosome concept. In: *Lysosomes*. A. V. S. de Reuck and M. P. Cameron, Eds. Boston, Little, Brown and Co., pp. 1–31.

Deitch, A. D., and Moses, M. J. 1957. The Nissl substance of living and fixed spinal ganglion cells. II. An ultraviolet absorption study. *J. Biophys. Biochem. Cytol. 3*:449–456.

Deitch, A. D., and Murray, M. R. 1956. The Nissl substance of living and fixed spinal ganglion cells. I. A phase contrast study. *J. Biophys. Biochem. Cytol. 2*:433–444.

Deiters, O. 1865. *Untersuchungen über Gehirn und Rückenmark*. Braunschweig, Vieweg.

del Castillo, J., and Katz, B. 1954. Quantal components of the end plate potential. *J. Physiol. (Lond.) 124*:560–573.

del Castillo, J., and Katz, B. 1955. On localization of acetylcholine receptors. *J. Physiol. (Lond.) 128*:157–181.

Del Cerro, M. P., and Snider, R. S. 1968. Studies in the developing cerebellum. Ultrastructure of growth cones. *J. Comp. Neurol. 133*:341–362.

De Lemos, C., and Pick, J. 1966. The fine structure of thoracic sympathetic neurons in the adult rat. *Z. Zellforsch. Mikrosk. Anat. 71*:189–206.

Dellmann, H.-D. 1973. Degeneration and regeneration of neurosecretory systems. *Int. Rev. Cytol. 36*:215–315.

De Lorenzo, A. J. 1957. Electron microscopic observations of the olfactory mucosa and olfactory nerve. *J. Biophys. Biochem. Cytol. 3*:839–850.

De Lorenzo, A. J. 1960. The fine structure of synapses in the ciliary ganglion of the chick. *J. Biophys. Biochem. Cytol. 7*:31–36.

De Lorenzo, A. J. 1961. Electron microscopy of the cerebral cortex. I. The ultrastructure and histochemistry of synaptic junctions. *Bull. Johns Hopkins Hosp. 108*:258–279.

De Lorenzo, A. J. 1966. Electron microscopy: Tight junctions in synapses of the chick ciliary ganglion. *Science 152*:76–78.

Dempsey, E. W. 1973. Neural and vascular ultrastructure of the area postrema in the rat. *J. Comp. Neurol. 150*:177–200.

Dempsey, E. W., and Wislocki, G. B. 1955. An electron microscopic study of the blood-brain barrier in the rat, employing silver nitrate as a vital stain. *J. Biophys. Biochem. Cytol. 1*:245–256.

Dennison, M. E. 1971. Electron stereoscopy as a means of classifying synaptic vesicles. *J. Cell Sci. 8*:525–539.

Dermietzel, R. 1974a. Junctions in the central nervous system of the cat. I. Membrane fusion in central myelin. *Cell Tiss. Res. 148*:565–576.

Dermietzel, R. 1974b. Junctions in the central nervous system of the cat. II. A contribution to the tertiary structure of the axonal-glial junctions in the paranodal region of the node of Ranvier. *Cell Tiss. Res. 148*:577–586.

De Robertis, E. 1956a. Submicroscopic changes of the synapse after nerve section in the acoustic ganglion of the guinea pig. An electron microscope study. *J. Biophys. Biochem. Cytol. 2*:503–512.

De Robertis, E. 1956b. Morphogenesis of the retinal rods. An electron microscope study. *J. Biophys. Biochem. Cytol. 2(Suppl.)*:209–218.

De Robertis, E. 1958. Submicroscopic morphology and function of the synapse. *Exp. Cell Res.* Suppl. 5, pp. 347–369.

De Robertis, E. 1959. Submicroscopic morphology of the synapse. *Int. Rev. Cytol. 8*:61–96.

De Robertis, E. 1962. Fine structure of synapses in the CNS. In: *Proceedings, IV. International Congress of Neuropathology* (Munich 1961), Vol. 2: *Electronmicroscopy and Biology*. H. Jacob, Ed. Stuttgart, Thieme, pp. 35–38.

De Robertis, E. 1966. Synaptic complexes and synaptic vesicles as structural and biochemical units of the central nervous system. In: *Nerve as a Tissue*. K. Rodahl and B. Issekutz, Jr., Eds. New York, Hoeber, pp. 88–115.

De Robertis, E. 1967. Ultrastructure and cytochemistry of the synaptic region. *Science 156*:907–914.

De Robertis, E., and Bennett, H. S. 1954. Submicroscopic vesicular component in the synapse. *Fed. Proc. 13*:35.

De Robertis, E., and Bennett, H. S. 1955. Some features of the submicroscopic morphology of synapses in frog and earthworm. *J. Biophys. Biochem. Cytol.* 1:47–58.

De Robertis, E., and Gerschenfeld, H. M. 1961. Submicroscopic morphology and function of glial cells. *Int. Rev. Neurobiol.* 3:1–65.

De Robertis, E., and Pellegrino de Iraldi, A. 1961. Plurivesicular secretory processes and nerve endings in the pineal gland of the rat. *J. Biophys. Biochem. Cytol.* 10:361–372.

De Robertis, E., Pellegrino de Iraldi, A., Rodriguez de Lores Arnaiz, G., and Salganicoff, L. 1961. Electron microscope observations on nerve endings isolated from rat brain. *Anat. Rec.* 139:220–221.

De Robertis, E., Pellegrino de Iraldi, A., Rodriguez de Lores Arnaiz, G., and Zieher, L. M. 1965. Synaptic vesicles from the rat hypothalamus. Isolation and norepinephrine content. *Life Sci.* 4:193–201.

De Robertis, E., Rodriguez de Lores Arnaiz, G., Salganicoff, L., Pellegrino de Iraldi, A., and Zieher, L. M. 1963. Isolation of synaptic vesicles and structural organization of the acetylcholine system within brain nerve endings. *J. Neurochem.* 10:225–235.

De Robertis, E., and Vaz Ferreira, A. 1957. Submicroscopic changes of the nerve endings in the adrenal medulla after stimulation of the splanchnic nerve. *J. Biophys. Biochem. Cytol.* 3:611–614.

Descarries, L., and Droz, B. 1970. Intraneural distribution of exogenous norepinephrine in the central nervous system of the rat. *J. Cell Biol.* 44:385–399.

Desclin, J. C. 1974. Histological evidence supporting the inferior olive as the major source of cerebellar climbing fibers in the rat. *Brain Res.* 77:365–384.

Desclin, J. C., and Escubi, J. 1974. Effects of 3-acetylpyridine on the central nervous system of the rat, as demonstrated by silver methods. *Brain Res.* 77:349–364.

de-Thé, G. 1964. Cytoplasmic microtubules in different animal cells. *J. Cell Biol.* 23:265–275.

Dewey, M. M., and Barr, L. 1964. A study of the structure and distribution of the nexus. *J. Cell Biol.* 23:553–585.

Diamond, J., Gray, E. G., and Yasargil, G. M. 1969. The function of dendritic spines: An hypotheses. *J. Physiol.* 202:116P.

Diamond, J., Gray, E. G., and Yasargil, G. M. 1970. The function of the dendritic spine: An hypothesis. In: *Excitatory Synaptic Mechanisms.* P. Andersen and J. K. S. Jansen, Eds. Oslo, Universitetsforlaget, pp. 213–222.

Dixon, A. D. 1963. The ultrastructure of nerve fibers in the trigeminal ganglion of the rat. *J. Ultrastruct. Res.* 8:107–121.

Dixon, J. S. 1966. The fine structure of parasympathetic nerve cells in the otic ganglia of the rabbit. *Anat. Rec.* 156:239–251.

Dixon, J. S. 1970. Nuclear bodies in normal and chromatolytic sympathetic neurons. *Anat. Rec.* 168:179–186.

Dobbing, J. 1961. The blood-brain barrier. *Physiol. Rev.* 41:130–188.

Dogiel, A. S. 1908. *Der Bau der Spinalganglien des Menschen und der Säugetiere.* Jena, Fischer.

Dohrmann, G. L. 1970. The choroid plexus: A historical review. *Brain Res.* 18:197–218.

Doinikow, B. 1913. Histologische und histopathologische Untersuchungen am peripheren Nervensystem mittels vitaler Färbung. *Folia Neuro-biol.* 7:731.

Donahue, S., and Pappas, G. D. 1961. The fine structure of capillaries in the cerebral cortex of the rat at various stages of development. *Am. J. Anat.* 108:331–338.

Donelli, G., D'Uva, D., and Paoletti, L. 1975. Ultrastructure of gliosomes in ependymal cells of the lizard. *J. Ultrastruct. Res.* 50:253–263.

Doolin, P. F., Barron, K. D., and Kwak, S. 1967. Ultrastructural and histochemical analysis of cytoplasmic laminar bodies in lateral geniculate neurons of adult cat. *Am. J. Anat.* 121:601–622.

Dowling, J. E. 1968. Synaptic organization of the frog retina: an electron microscopic analysis comparing the retinas of frogs and primates. *Proc. R. Soc. Ser. B.* 170:205–228.

Dowling, J. E. 1970. Organization of vertebrate retinas. *Invest. Ophthalmol.* 9:655–690.

Dowling, J. E., and Boycott, B. B. 1966. Organization of the primate retina: electron microscopy. *Proc. R. Soc. Ser. B.* 166:80–111.

Dreifuss, J. J., Akert, K., Sandri, C., and Moor, H. 1973. The fine structure of freeze-fractured neurosecretory nerve endings in the neurohypophysis. *Brain Res.* 62:367–372.

Droz, B. 1971. Synthèse et transfert des protéines cellulaires dans les neurones ganglionnaires. Étude radiographique quantitative en microscopie électronique. *J. Microscopie.* 6:201–228.

Droz, B. 1973. Renewal of synaptic proteins. *Brain Res.* 62:383–394.

Droz, B., and Koenig, H. L. 1970. Localization of protein metabolism in neurons. In: *Protein Metabolism of the Nervous System.* A. Lajtha, Ed. New York, Plenum Press, pp. 93–106.

Droz, B., Koenig, H. L., and Di Giamberardino, L. 1973. Axonal migration of protein and glycoprotein to nerve endings. I. Radioautographic analysis of the renewal of protein in nerve endings of chick ciliary ganglion after intracerebral injection of (^{3}H) lysine. *Brain Res.* 60:93–127.

Droz, B., Koenig, H. L., and Rambourg, A. 1974. Transport intracytoplasmique de macromolécules et réticulum endoplasmique lisse: cas du flux axonal rapide. *J. Microscopie.* 20:45a.

Duckett, S., and Scott, T. 1972. Glycogen in human fetal sciatic nerve. *Rev. Can. Biol.* 31:147–151.

Duncan, D. 1934. A relation between axon diameter and myelination determined by measurement of myelinated spinal root fibers. *J. Comp. Neurol.* 60:437–472.

Duncan, D., Morales, R., and Benignus, V. A. 1970. Shapes and sizes of synaptic vesicles in the cerebellum of the Syrian hamster—cortex and deep nuclei. *Anat. Rec. 168*:1–8.

Duncan, D., Nall, D., and Morales, R. 1960. Observations on the fine structure of old age pigment. *J. Geront. 15*:366–372.

Duncan, D., Williams, V., and Morales, R. 1963. Centrioles and cilia-like structures in spinal gray matter. *Tex. Rep. Biol. Med. 21*:185–187.

Düring, M. v. 1967. Über die Feinstruktur der motorischen Endplatte von höheren Wirbeltieren. *Z. Zellforsch. Mikrosk. Anat. 81*:74–90.

Duvernoy, H., and Koritké, J. G. 1965. Contribution à l'étude de l'angioarchitectonie des organes circumventriculaires. *Arch. Biol. (Liège) 75*:849–904.

Ebner, F. F., and Colonnier, M. 1975. Synaptic patterns in the visual cortex of turtle: An electron microscopic study. *J. Comp. Neurol. 160*:51–80.

Eccles, J. C. 1961. The mechanism of synaptic transmission. *Ergeb. Physiol. 51*:299–430.

Eccles, J. C. 1964. *The Physiology of Synapses.* Berlin, Springer-Verlag.

Eccles, J., Ito, M., and Szentágothai, J. 1967. *The Cerebellum As a Neuronal Machine.* New York, Springer-Verlag.

Eccles, J. C., Llinás, R., and Sasaki, K. 1966a. The inhibitory interneurones within the cerebellar cortex. *Exp. Brain Res. 1*:1–16.

Eccles, J. C., Llinás, R., and Sasaki, K. 1966b. The excitatory synaptic action of climbing fibers on the Purkinje cells of the cerebellum. *J. Physiol. (Lond.) 182*:268–296.

Eccleston, D., Thoa, N. B., and Axelrod, J. 1968. Inhibition by drugs of the accumulation, *in vitro,* of 5-hydroxytryptamine in guinea pig vas deferens. *Nature (Lond.) 217*:846–847.

Echandía, R., Ramirez, B. U., and Fernandez, H. L. 1973. Studies on the mechanism of inhibition of axoplasmic transport of neuronal organelles. *J. Neurocytol. 2*:149–156.

Edidin, M. 1974. Two dimensional diffusion in membranes. In: *Transport at the Cellular Level.* M. A. Sleigh and D. H. Jennings, Eds. S.E.B. Symposia XXVIII. London, Cambridge University Press, pp. 1–14.

Edström, A., and Mattsson, H. 1972. Fast axonal transport in vitro in the sciatic system of the frog. *J. Neurochem. 19*:205–222.

Edvinsson, L., Nielsen, K. C., Owman, C. H., and West, K. A. 1974. Adrenergic innervation of the mammalian choroid plexus. *Am. J. Anat. 139*:299–308.

Ehrenreich, J. H., Bergeron, J. J. M., Siekevitz, P., and Palade, G. E. 1973. Golgi fractions prepared from rat liver. I. Isolation procedure and morphological characterization. *J. Cell Biol. 59*:45–72.

Elfvin, L.-G. 1958. The ultrastructure of unmyelinated fibers in the splenic nerve of the cat. *J. Ultrastruct. Res. 1*:428–454.

Elfvin, L.-G. 1961. The ultrastructure of the nodes of Ranvier in cat sympathetic nerve fibers. *J. Ultrastruct. Res. 5*:374–387.

Elfvin, L.-G. 1963. The ultrastructure of the superior cervical sympathetic ganglion of the cat. II. The structure of the preganglionic end fibers and the synapses as studied by serial sections. *J. Ultrastruct Res. 8*:441–476.

Elfvin, L.-G. 1968. The structure and composition of motor, sensory and autonomic nerves and fibers. In: *The Structure and Function of Nervous Tissue,* Vol. 1. G. H. Bourne, Ed. New York, Academic Press, pp. 325–377.

England, J. M., Kadin, M. E., and Goldstein, M. N. 1973. The effect of vincristine sulphate on the axoplasmic flow of proteins in cultured sympathetic neurons. *J. Cell Sci. 12*:549–565.

Engström, A., and Finean, J. B. 1958. *Biological Ultrastructure.* New York, Academic Press.

Engström, H. 1958. On the double innervation of the sensory epithelia of the inner ear. *Acta Otolaryngol. 49*:109–118.

Erikson, H. P. 1974. Microtubule surface lattice and subunit structure and observations on reassembly. *J. Cell Biol. 60*:153–167.

Essick, C. R. 1920. Formation of macrophages by the cells lining the subarachnoid cavity in response to the stimulus of particulate matter. *Carnegie Contrib. Embryol.* No. 42, pp. 379–389.

Essner, E., and Novikoff, A. B. 1960. Human hepatocellular pigments and lysosomes. *J. Ultrastruct. Res. 3*:374–391.

Evans, M. J., and Finean, J. B. 1965. The lipid composition of myelin from brain and peripheral nerve. *J. Neurochem. 12*:729–734.

Everly, J. L., Brady, R. O., and Quarles, R. H. 1973. Evidence that the major protein in rat sciatic nerve myelin is a glycoprotein. *J. Neurochem. 21*:329–334.

Fabergé, A. C. 1973. Direct demonstration of eightfold symmetry in nuclear pores. *Z. Zellforsch. Mikrosk. Anat. 136*:183–190.

Fabergé, A. C. 1974. The nuclear pore complex: its free existence and an hypothesis as to its origin. *Cell Tiss. Res. 151*:403–415.

Fambrough, D. M., and Hartzell, H. C. 1972. Acetylcholine receptors: number and distribution at neuromuscular junctions in rat diaphragm. *Science 176*:189–191.

Famiglietti, E. V. 1970. Dendro-dendritic synapses in the lateral geniculate nucleus of the cat. *Brain Res. 20*:181–191.

Famiglietti, E. V., and Peters, A. 1972. The synaptic glomerulus and the intrinsic neuron in the dorsal lateral geniculate nucleus of the cat. *J. Comp. Neurol. 144*:285–334.

Farquhar, M. G., Bergeron, J. J. M., and Palade, G. E. 1974. Cytochemistry of Golgi fractions prepared from rat liver. *J. Cell Biol. 60*:8–25.

Farquhar, M. G., and Hartmann, J. F. 1957. Neuroglial structure and relationships as revealed by electron microscopy. *J. Neuropathol. Exp. Neurol. 16*:18–39.

Farquhar, M. G., and Palade, G. E. 1963. Junctional complexes in various epithelia. *J. Cell Biol. 17*:375–412.

Fatt, P., and Katz, B. 1950. Some observations on biological noise. *Nature (Lond.)* 166:597–598.

Favard, P., and Carasso, N. 1973. The preparation and observation of thick biological sections in the high voltage electron microscope. *J. Microscopy* 97:59–81.

Fawcett, D. W. 1961. Cilia and flagella. In: *The Cell*, Vol. 2. J. Brachet and A. E. Mirsky, Eds. New York, Academic Press, pp. 217–297.

Fawcett, D. W. 1963. Comparative observations on the fine structure of blood capillaries. In: *The Peripheral Blood Vessels*. J. L. Orbison and D. E. Smith, Eds. Baltimore, Williams & Wilkins, pp. 17–44.

Fawcett, D. W. 1966a. *The Cell: Its Organelles and Inclusions*. Philadelphia, W. B. Saunders Co.

Fawcett, D. W. 1966b. On the occurrence of a fibrous lamina on the inner aspect of the nuclear envelope in certain cells of vertebrates. *Am. J. Anat.* 119:129–146.

Fawcett, D. W., and Porter, K. R. 1954. A study of the fine structure of ciliated epithelia. *J. Morphol.* 94:221–281.

Feder, N. 1971. Microperoxidase: An ultrastructural tracer of low molecular weight. *J. Cell Biol.* 51:339–343.

Feder, N., Reese, T. S., and Brightman, M. W. 1969. Microperoxidase, a new tracer of low molecular weight. A study of the interstitial compartments of the mouse brain. *J. Cell Biol.* 43:35A.

Fehér, O., Joó, F., and Halász, N. 1972. Effect of stimulation on the number of synaptic vesicles in nerve fibres and terminals of the cerebral cortex in the cat. *Brain Res.* 47:37–48.

Feldman, M. L., and Peters, A. 1972. Intranuclear rods and sheets in rat cochlear nucleus. *J. Neurocytol.* 1:109–127.

Fernandez, H. L., Huneeus, F. C., and Davison, P. F. 1970. Studies on the mechanism of axoplasmic transport in the crayfish cord. *J. Neurobiol.* 1:395–409.

Fernandez, H. L., and Samson, F. E. 1973. Axoplasmic transport: Differential inhibition by cytochalasin-B. *J. Neurobiol.* 4:201–206.

Fernández-Morán, H. 1950a. Electron microscope observations on the structure of the myelinated nerve fiber sheath. *Exp. Cell Res.* 1:143–149.

Fernández-Morán, H. 1950b. Sheath and axon structures in the internode portion of vertebrate myelinated nerve fibres. *Exp. Cell Res.* 1:309–340.

Fernández-Morán, H. 1954. The submicroscopic structure of nerve fibres. *Progr. Biophysics* 4:112–147.

Fernández-Morán, H. 1967. Membrane ultrastructure in nerve cells. In: *Neurosciences*. G. C. Quarton, T. Melnechuk, and F. O. Schmitt, Eds. New York, Rockefeller University Press, pp. 281–304.

Fernández-Morán, H., and Finean, J. B. 1957. Electron microscope and low-angle x-ray diffraction studies of the nerve myelin sheath. *J. Biophys. Biochem. Cytol.* 3:725–748.

Fernández-Morán, H., Oda, T., Blair, P. V., and Green, D. E. 1964. A macromolecular repeating unit of mitochondrial structure and function. *J. Cell Biol.* 22:63–100.

Ferraro, A., and Davidoff, L. M. 1928. The reaction of the oligodendroglia to injury of the brain. *Arch. Pathol.* 6:1030–1053.

Fieandt, H. 1910. Eine neue Methode zur Darstellung des Gliagewebes nebst Beiträgen zur Kenntnis des Baues und der Anordnung der Neuroglia des Hundehirns. *Arch. Mikroskop. Anat.* 76:125–209.

Field, E. J., and Peat, A. 1971. Intranuclear inclusions in neurones and glia: a study in the aging mouse. *Gerontologia* 17:129–138.

Fifková, E. 1970. The effects of monocular deprivation on the synaptic contacts of the visual cortex. *J. Neurobiol.* 1:285–294.

Finean, J. B. 1958. X-ray diffraction studies of the myelin sheath in peripheral and central nerve fibres. *Exp. Cell Res.* Suppl. 5, pp. 18–32.

Finean, J. B. 1960. Electron microscope and x-ray diffraction studies of the effects of dehydration on the structure of nerve myelin. II. Optic nerve. *J. Biophys. Biochem. Cytol.* 8:31–37.

Finean, J. B. 1961. X-ray diffraction and electron microscope studies of nerve myelin. In: *Electron Microscopy in Anatomy*. J. D. Boyd, F. R. Johnson, and J. D. Lever, Eds. London, Arnold, pp. 114–125.

Finean, J. B., Hawthorne, H. N., and Patterson, J. D. E. 1957. Structural and chemical differences between optic and sciatic nerve myelins. *J. Neurochem.* 1:256–259.

Fink, R. P., and Heimer, L. 1967. Two methods for selective silver impregnation of degenerative axons and their synaptic endings in the central nervous system. *Brain Res.* 4:369–374.

Fisher, K. S. 1972. A somato-somatic synapse between amacrine and bipolar cells in the cat retina. *Brain Res.* 43:587–590.

Fleischer, B., Fleischer, S., and Ozawa, H. 1969. Isolation and characterization of Golgi membranes from bovine liver. *J. Cell Biol.* 43:59–79.

Fleischhauer, K. 1972. Ependyma and subependymal layer. In: *The Structure and Function of Nervous Tissue*. Vol. VI. G. H. Bourne, Ed. New York, Academic Press, pp. 1–46.

Fleischhauer, K. 1974. On different patterns of dendritic bundling in the cerebral cortex of the cat. *Z. Anat. Entwicklungsgesch.* 143:115–126.

Fleischhauer, K., Petsche, H., and Wittkowski, W. 1972. Vertical bundles of dendrites in the neocortex. *Z. Anat. Entwicklungsgesch.* 136:213–223.

Fleischhauer, K., and Wartenberg, H. 1967. Elektronenmikroskopische Untersuchungen über das Wachstum der Nervenfasern und über das Auftreten von Markscheiden im Corpus callosum der Katze. *Z. Zellforsch Mikrosk. Anat.* 83:568–581.

Flickinger, C. J. 1969. Fenestrated cisternae in the Golgi apparatus of the epididymis. *Anat. Rec.* 163:39–53.

Florey, H. 1966. The endothelial cell. *Br. Med. J.* 2:487–490.

Florkin, M. 1960. *Naissance et Déviation de la*

Théorie Cellulaire dans l'Oeuvre de Théodore Schwann. Paris, Hermann.

Follenius, E. 1970. Organisation scalariforme du réticulum endoplasmique dans certains processus nerveux de l'hypothalamus de *Gasterosteus aculeatus* L. *Z. Zellforsch. Mikrosk. Anat.* 106:61–68.

Foster, M., and Sherrington, C. S. 1897. *A Text Book of Physiology, Part III: The Central Nervous System,* 7th ed. London, Macmillan.

Fox, C. A., Andrade, A. N., Qui, I. J. L. and Rafols, J. A. 1974. The primate globus pallidus. A Golgi and electron microscopic study. *J. Hirnforsch.* 15:75–93.

Fraher, J. P. 1972. A quantitative study of anterior root fibres during early myelination. *J. Anat.* 112:99–124.

Fraher, J. P. 1973. A quantitative study of anterior root fibres during early myelination. II. Longitudinal variation in sheath thickness and axon circumference. *J. Anat.* 115:421–444.

Franke, W. W. 1974a. Nuclear envelopes. Structure and biochemistry of the nuclear envelope. *Phil. Trans. R. Soc. Ser. B.* 268:67–93.

Franke, W. W. 1974b. Structure, biochemistry, and functions of the nuclear envelope. *Int. Rev. Cytol. Suppl.* 4:71–236.

Franke, W. W., and Scheer, U. 1970. The ultrastructure of the nuclear envelope of amphibian oocytes: a reinvestigation. II. The immature oocyte and dynamic aspects. *J. Ultrastruct. Res.* 30:317–327.

Franke, W. W., and Scheer, U. 1974. Pathways of nucleocytoplasmic translocation of ribonucleoproteins. In: *Transport at the Cellular Level.* M. A. Sleigh and D. H. Jennings, Eds. S.E.B. Symposia XXVIII. London, Cambridge University Press, pp. 249–282.

Fraser, H., Smith, W., and Gray, E. W. 1970. Ultrastructural morphology of cytoplasmic inclusions within neurons of ageing mice. *J. Neurol. Sci.* 11:123–128.

Frederickson, R. G., and Low, F. N. 1969. Blood vessels and tissue space associated with the brain of the rat. *Am. J. Anat.* 125:123–146.

Fregerslev, S., Blackstad, T. W., Fredens, K., and Holm, M. J. 1971. Golgi potassium-dichromate silver nitrate impregnation. Nature of the precipitate studied by X-ray powder diffraction methods. *Histochemie* 25:63–71.

Friede, R. L. 1965. Enzyme histochemistry of neuroglia. In: *Progress in Brain Research,* Vol. 15, *Biology of Neuroglia.* E. D. P. De Robertis and R. Carrea, Eds. Amsterdam, Elsevier, pp. 35–47.

Friede, R. L. 1967. Incorporation patterns of tritiated thymidine following cutting of the sciatic nerve in rats. *J. Neuropathol. Exp. Neurol.* 26:134–135.

Friede, R. L. 1972. Control of myelin formation by axon caliber (with a model of the control mechanism). *J. Comp. Neurol.* 144:233–252.

Friede, R. L., and Miyagishi, T. 1972. Adjustment of the myelin sheath to changes in axon caliber. *Anat. Rec.* 172:1–14.

Friede, R. L., and Pax, R. A. 1961. Mitochondria and mitochondrial enzymes. A comparative study of localization in the cat's brain stem. *Histochemie* 2:186–191.

Friede, R. L., and Samorajski, T. 1967. Relation between the number of myelin lamellae and axon circumference in fibers of vagus and sciatic nerves of mice. *J. Comp. Neurol.* 130:223–231.

Friede, R. L., and Samorajski, T. 1968. Myelin formation in the sciatic nerve of the rat. A quantitative electron microscopic, histochemical and radioactive study. *J. Neuropathol. Exp. Neurol.* 27:546–571.

Friede, R. L., and Samorajski, T. 1969. The clefts of Schmidt-Lantermann: a quantitative electron microscopic study of their structure in developing and adult sciatic nerves of the rat. *Anat. Rec.* 165:89–102.

Friede, R. L., and Samorajski, T. 1970. Axon caliber related to neurofilaments and microtubules in sciatic nerve fibers of rats and mice. *Anat. Rec.* 167:379–388.

Friede, R. L., and Seitelberger, F., Eds. 1971. *Symposium on Pathology of Axons and Axonal Flow.* Berlin, Springer-Verlag.

Friedemann, U. 1942. Blood-brain barrier. *Physiol. Rev.* 22:125–145.

Friend, D. S. 1969. Cytochemical staining of multivesicular body and Golgi vesicles. *J. Cell Biol.* 41:269–279.

Friend, D. S., and Farquhar, M. G. 1967. Functions of coated vesicles during protein absorption in the rat vas deferens. *J. Cell Biol.* 35:357–376.

Friend, D. S., and Gilula, N. B. 1972. Variations in tight and gap junctions in mammalian tissues. *J. Cell Biol.* 53:758–776.

Friend, D. S., and Murray, M. J. 1965. Osmium impregnation of the Golgi apparatus. *Am. J. Anat.* 117:135–149.

Frisch, D. 1969. A photographic reinforcement analysis of neurotubules and cytoplasmic membranes. *J. Ultrastruct. Res.* 29:357–72.

Fujita, S. 1963. The matrix cell and cytogenesis in the developing central nervous system. *J. Comp. Neurol.* 120:37–42.

Fujita, S. 1965. An autoradiographic study on the origin and fate of the sub-pial glioblast in the embryonic chick spinal cord. *J. Comp. Neurol.* 124:51–60.

Fujita, S. 1973. Genesis of glioblasts in the human spinal cord as revealed by Feulgen cytophotometry. *J. Comp. Neurol.* 151:25–34.

Fujita, S. 1974. DNA constancy in neurons of the human cerebellum and spinal cord as revealed by Feulgen cytophotometry and cytofluorometry. *J. Comp. Neurol.* 155:195–202.

Fujita, S., Hattori, T., Fukuda, M., and Kitamura, T. 1974. DNA contents in Purkinje cells and inner granule neurons in the developing rat cerebellum. *Dev. Growth Differ.* 16:205–211.

Fukami, Y. 1969. Two types of synaptic bulb in snake and frog spinal cord. The effects of fixation. *Brain Res.* 14:137–145.

Furshpan, E. J. 1964. "Electrical transmission" at an excitatory synapse in a vertebrate brain. *Science* 144:878–880.

Furshpan, E. J., and Potter, D. D. 1959. Transmission at the giant motor synapses of the crayfish. *J. Physiol. (Lond.)* 145:289–325.

Furukawa, T., and Furshpan, E. J. 1963. Two inhibitory mechanisms in the Mauthner neurons of goldfish. *J. Neurophysiol.* 26:140–176.

Fuxe, K., Hökfelt, T., and Nilsson, O. 1965. A fluorescence and electronmicroscopic study on certain brain regions rich in monoamine terminals. *Am. J. Anat.* 117:33–46.

Fuxe, K., Hökfelt, T., Nilsson, O., and Reinius, S. 1966. A fluorescence and electronmicroscopic study on central monoamine cells. *Anat. Rec.* 155:33–40.

Gambetti, P., and Gonatas, N. K. 1967. Fibrils and lattice-like intranuclear structures in nuclei of neurons. *Riv. Patol. Nerv. Ment.* 88:188–196.

Gamble, H. J. 1964. Comparative electron-microscopic observations on the connective tissues of a peripheral nerve and a spinal nerve root in the rat. *J. Anat.* 98:17–25.

Gamble, H. J. 1966. Further electron microscope studies of human foetal peripheral nerves. *J. Anat.* 100:487–502.

Gamble, H. J., and Breathnach, A. S. 1965. An electron-microscope study of human foetal peripheral nerves. *J. Anat.* 99:573–584.

Gamble, H. J., and Eames, R. A. 1964. An electron microscope study of the connective tissues of human peripheral nerve. *J. Anat.* 98:655–663.

Ganong, W. F. 1972. Evidence for a central nonadrenergic system that inhibits ACTH secretion. In: *Brain-Endocrine Interaction. Median Eminence: Structure and Function.* K. M. Knigge, D. E. Scott, and A. Weindl, Eds. Basel, Karger, pp. 254–266.

Gasser, H. S. 1952. Discussion of a paper by B. Frankenhaeuser. In: *Cold Spring Harbor Symposia on Quantitative Biology*, Vol. 17, *The Neuron.* K. B. Warren, Ed. Cold Spring Harbor, New York, The Biological Laboratory, pp. 32–36.

Gasser, H. S. 1955. Properties of dorsal root unmedullated fibers on two sides of the ganglion. *J. Gen. Physiol.* 38:709–728.

Gasser, H. S. 1956. Olfactory nerve fibers. *J. Gen. Physiol.* 39:473–496.

Geffen, L. B., and Livett, B. G. 1971. Synaptic vesicles in sympathetic neurons. *Physiol. Rev.* 51:98–157.

Gentschev, T. and Sotelo, C. 1973. Degenerative patterns in the ventral cochlear nucleus of the rat after primary deafferentation. An ultrastructural study. *Brain Res.* 62:37–60.

Geren, B. B. 1954. The formation from the Schwann cell surface of myelin in the peripheral nerves of chick embryos. *Exp. Cell Res.* 7:558–562.

Gerlach, J. 1858. *Mikroskopische Studien aus dem Gebiete der menschlichen Morphologie.* Erlangen, Enke.

Gerlach, J. 1872. The spinal cord. In: *Manual of Human and Comparative Histology*, Vol. 2. S. Stricker, Ed., trans. from German by H. Power. London, The New Sydenham Society, pp. 327–366.

Giacobini, E. 1964. Metabolic relations between glia and neurons studied in single cells. In: *Morphological and Biochemical Correlates of Neural Activity.* M. M. Cohen and R. S. Snider, Eds. New York, Hoeber, pp. 15–38.

Gillette, R., and Pomeranz, B. 1973. Neuron geometry and circuitry via the electron microscope: Intracellular staining with osmiophilic polymer. *Science* 182:1256–1258.

Gilmore, S. A. 1971. Neuroglial population in the spinal white matter of neonatal and early postnatal rats: An autoradiographic study of numbers of neuroglia and changes in their proliferative activity. *Anat. Rec.* 171:283–292.

Giorgi, P. P., Karlsson, J. O., Sjöstrand, J., and Field, E. J. 1973. Axonal flow and myelin protein in the optic pathway. *Nature [New Biol.]* 244:121–124.

Gitlin, G. and Singer, M. 1974. Myelin movements in mature mammalian peripheral nerve fibers. *J. Morphol.* 143:167–186.

Glees, P. 1955. *Neuroglia, Morphology and Function.* Springfield, Ill., Charles C Thomas.

Glees, P., and Gopinath, G. 1973. Age changes in the centrally and peripherally located sensory neurons in rat. *Z. Zellforsch. Mikrosk. Anat.* 141:285–298.

Globus, A., and Scheibel, A. B. 1966. Loss of dendritic spines as an index of presynaptic terminal patterns. *Nature (Lond.)* 212:463–465.

Globus, A., and Scheibel, A. B. 1967a. Synaptic loci on visual cortical neurons of the rabbit. The specific afferent radiation. *Exp. Neurol.* 18:116–131.

Globus, A., and Scheibel, A. B. 1967b. The effects of visual deprivation on cortical neurons: A Golgi study. *Exp. Neurol.* 19:331–345.

Globus, A., and Scheibel, A. B. 1967c. Synaptic loci on parietal cortical neurons: Terminations of corpus callosum fibers. *Science* 156:1127–1129.

Globus, J. H., and Kuhlenbeck, H. 1944. The subependymal cell plate (matrix) and its relationship to brain tumors of the ependymal type. *J. Neuropathol. Exp. Neurol.* 3:1–35.

Gobel, S. 1971. Axo-axonic septate junctions in the basket formations of the cat cerebellar cortex. J. Cell Biol. 51:328–332.

Gobel, S. 1974. Synaptic organization of the substantia gelatinosa glomeruli in the spinal trigeminal nucleus of the adult cat. *J. Neurocytol.* 3:219–243.

Gobel, S., and Dubner, R. 1969. Fine structural studies of the main sensory trigeminal nucleus in the cat and rat. *J. Comp. Neurol.* 137:459–494.

Golgi, C. 1873. Sulla sostanza grigia del cervello. *Gazz. Med. Lombarda* 6:244–246.

Golgi, C. 1874. Sulla fina anatomia del cervelletto umano. Lecture, Istituto Lombardo di Sci. e Lett. 8 Jan. 1874. Chap. V In: *Opera Omnia*, Vol. I: *Istologia normale.* 1870–1883, pp. 99–111, Milan, Ulrico Hoepli, 1903.

Golgi, C. 1882–1885. Sulla fine anatomia degli organi

centrali del sistema nervoso. *Riv. Sper. Freniat. Med. Leg.* 8:165–195, 361–391 (1882–1883); 9:1–17, 161–192, 385–402 (1883); *11*:72–123, 193–220 (1885). Recherches sur l'histologie des centres nerveux. *Arch. Ital. Biol.* 3:285–317 (1883); 4:92–123 (1883). Sur l'anatomie microscopique des organes centraux du système nerveux. *Arch. Ital. Biol.* 7:15–47 (1886). Beitrag zur feineren Anatomie der Centralorgane des Nervensystems. In: *Untersuchungen über den feineren Bau des centralen und peripherischen Nervensystems.* A compilation of papers by C. Golgi, Trans. from Italian by R. Teuscher. Jena, Fischer, pp. 1–34, 1894.

Golgi, C. 1891. La rete nervosa diffusa degli organi centrali del sistemo nervosa: Suo significato fisiologico. *Rendiconti R. Ist. Lombardo Sci. Lett.,* Ser. 2, 24:595–656. Le reseau nerveux diffus des centres du système nerveux; ses attributs physiologiques; méthode suivie dans les recherches histologiques. *Arch. Ital. Biol.* 15:434–463 (1891). Das diffuse nervöse Netz der Centralorgane des Nervensystems. In: *Untersuchungen uber den feineren Bau des centralen und peripherischen Nervensystems.* A compilation of papers by C. Golgi. Trans. from Italian by R. Teuscher. Jena, Fisher, 1894, pp. 245–260.

Golgi, C. 1898a. Sur la structure des cellules nerveuses. *Arch. Ital. Biol.* 30:60–71.

Golgi, C. 1898b. Sur la structure des cellules nerveuses des ganglions spinaux. *Arch. Ital. Biol.* 30:278–286.

Golgi, C. 1899. De nouveau sur la structure des cellules nerveuses des ganglions spinaux. *Arch. Ital. Biol.* 31:273–280.

Golgi, C. 1906. The neuron doctrine – Theory and facts. In: *Nobel Lectures: Physiology or Medicine, 1901–1921.* Amsterdam, Elsevier, 1967, pp. 189–217.

Gomez, D. G., and Potts, D. G. 1974. The surface characteristics of arachnoid granulations. *Arch. Neurol.* 31:88–93.

Gomez, D. G., Potts, G., and Deonarine, V. 1974. Arachnoid granulations of the sheep. Structural and ultrastructural changes with varying pressure differences. *Arch. Neurol.* 30:169–175.

Gonatas, N. K. 1967. Axonic and synaptic lesions in neuropsychiatric disorders. *Nature (Lond.)* 214:352–355.

Gonatas, N. K., and Gambetti, P. 1970. The pathology of the synapse in Alzheimer's disease. In: *Ciba Foundation Symposium on Alzheimer's Disease and Related Conditions.* G. E. Wolstenholme and M. O'Connor, Eds. London, Churchill, pp. 169–183.

Gonatas, N. K., and Goldensohn, E. S. 1965. Unusual neocortical presynaptic terminals in a patient with convulsions, mental retardation and cortical blindness: an electron microscopic study. *J. Neuropathol. Exp. Neurol.* 24:539–562.

Goodenough, D. A., and Gilula, N. B. 1974. The splitting of hepatocyte gap junctions and zonulae occludentes with hypertonic disaccharides. *J. Cell Biol. 61:575–590.*

Goodenough, D. A., and Revel, J. P. 1970. A fine structure analysis of intercellular junctions in the mouse liver. *J. Cell Biol.* 45:272–290.

Gottlieb, D. I., and Cowan, W. M. 1972. On the distribution of axonal terminals containing spheroidal and flattened synaptic vesicles in the hippocampus and dentate gyrus of the rat and cat. *Z. Zellforsch. Mikrosk. Anat.* 129:413–429.

Grafstein, B. 1969. Axonal transport: Communication between soma and synapse. In: *Advances in Biochemical Psychopharmacology*, Vol. 1. E. Costa and P. Greengaard, Eds. New York, Raven Press, pp. 11–25.

Grafstein, B., McEwen, B. S., and Shelanski, M. 1970. Axonal transport of neurotubule protein. *Nature (Lond.)* 227:289–290.

Graham, R. C., Jr., and Karnovsky, M. J. 1966. The early stages of absorption of injected horseradish peroxidase in the proximal tubules of mouse kidney: ultrastructural cytochemistry by a new technique. *J. Histochem. Cytochem.* 14:291–302.

Gray, E. G. 1959. Axo-somatic and axo-dendritic synapses of the cerebral cortex: An electron microscope study. *J. Anat.* 93:420–433.

Gray, E. G. 1960. Regular organisation of material in certain mitochondria of neuroglia of lizard brain. *J. Biophys. Biochem. Cytol.* 8:282–285.

Gray, E. G. 1961a. Ultra-structure of synapses of the cerebral cortex and of certain specialisations of neuroglial membranes. In: *Electron Microscopy in Anatomy.* J. D. Boyd, F. R. Johnson, and J. D. Lever, Eds. London, Arnold, pp. 54–73.

Gray, E. G. 1961b. The granule cells, mossy synapses and Purkinje spine synapses of the cerebellum: Light and electron microscope observations. *J. Anat.* 95:345–356.

Gray, E. G. 1962. A morphological basis for presynaptic inhibition? *Nature (Lond.)* 193:82–83.

Gray, E. G. 1963. Electron microscopy of presynaptic organelles of the spinal cord. *J. Anat.* 97:101–106.

Gray, E. G. 1964. Tissue of the central nervous system. In: *Electron Microscopic Anatomy.* S. M. Kurtz, Ed. New York, Academic Press, pp. 369–417.

Gray, E. G. 1966. Problems of interpreting the fine structure of vertebrate and invertebrate synapses. *Int. Rev. Gen. Exp. Zool.* 2:139–170.

Gray, E. G. 1969a. Electron Microscopy of excitatory and inhibitory synapses: a brief review. In: *Progress in Brain Research*, Vol. 31, *Mechanisms of Synaptic Transmission.* K. Akert and P. G. Waser, Eds. Amsterdam, Elsevier, pp. 141–155.

Gray, E. G. 1969b. Round and flat synaptic vesicles in the fish central nervous system. *Symp. Int. Soc. Cell Biol.* 8:211–227.

Gray, E. G. 1970. The fine structure of nerve. *Comp. Biochem. Physiol.* 36:419–448.

Gray, E. G. 1972. Are the coats of coated vesicles artefacts? *J. Neurocytol.* 1:363–382.

Gray, E. G. 1973. The cytonet, plain and coated vesicles, reticulosomes, multivesicular bodies, and nuclear pores. *Brain Res.* 62:329–335.

Gray, E. G. 1975. Presynaptic microtubules and their

association with synaptic vesicles. *Proc. R. Soc. Lond. Ser. B. 190*:369–372.

Gray, E. G. 1976. Problems in understanding synaptic substructure. *Progr. Brain Res.* (in press).

Gray, E. G., and Guillery, R. W. 1961. The basis for silver staining of synapses of the mammalian spinal cord: A light and electron microscope study. *J. Physiol. (Lond.) 157*:581–588.

Gray, E. G., and Guillery, R. W. 1963a. On nuclear structure in the ventral nerve cord of the leech *Hirudo medicinalis. Z. Zellforsch. Mikrosk. Anat. 59*:738–745.

Gray, E. G., and Guillery, R. W. 1963b. A note on the dendritic spine apparatus. *J. Anat. 97*:389–392.

Gray, E. G., and Guillery, R. W. 1966. Synaptic morphology in the normal and degenerating nervous system. *Int. Rev. Cytol. 19*:111–182.

Gray, E. G., and Paula-Barbosa, M. 1974. Dense particles within synaptic vesicles fixed with acid-aldehyde. *J. Neurocytol. 3*:487–496.

Gray, E. G., and Pease, H. L. 1971. On understanding the organisation of the retinal receptor synapses. *Brain Res. 35*:1–15.

Gray, E. G., and Whittaker, V. P. 1962. The isolation of nerve endings from brain: an electron microscopic study of cell fragments derived by homogenization and centrifugation. *J. Anat. 96*:79–88.

Gray, E. G., and Willis, R. A. 1970. On synaptic vesicles, complex vesicles and dense projections. *Brain Res. 24*:149–168.

Graybiel, A. M., and Devor, M. 1974. A microelectrophoretic delivery technique for use with horseradish peroxidase. *Brain Res. 68*:167–173.

Green, J. D., and Van Breemen, V. I. 1955. Electron microscopy of the pituitary and observations on neurosecretion. *Am. J. Anat. 97*:177–227.

Grillo, M. A. 1966. Electron microscopy of sympathetic tissues. *Pharmacol. Rev. 18*:387–399.

Grillo, M. A. 1970. Cytoplasmic inclusions resembling nucleoli in sympathetic neurons of adult rats. *J. Cell Biol. 45*:100–117.

Grillo, M. A., and Palay, S. L. 1962. Granule-containing vesicles in the autonomic nervous system. In: *Electron Microscopy, Proceedings of the Fifth International Congress for Electron Microscopy, 1962.* S. S. Breese, Jr., Ed. New York, Academic Press, Vol. 2, p. U-1.

Grillo, M. A., and Palay, S. L. 1963. Ciliated Schwann cells in the autonomic nervous system of the adult rat. *J. Cell Biol. 16*:430–436.

Grimstone, A. V., and Klug, A. 1966. Observations on the substructure of flagellar fibres. *J. Cell Sci. 1*:351–362.

Grinnell, A. D. 1966. A study of the interaction between motoneurons in the frog spinal cord. *J. Physiol. (Lond.) 182*:612–648.

Grinnell, A. D., and Miledi, R. 1965. Unpublished observations, quoted in Gray, E. G., and Guillery, R. W. (1966). *Int. Rev. Cytol. 19*:111–182.

Guillery, R. W. 1967. A light and electron microscopical study of neurofibrils and neurofilaments at neuro-neuronal junctions in the dorsal lateral geniculate nucleus of the cat. *Am. J. Anat. 120*:583–604.

Guillery, R. W. 1969. The organization of synaptic interconnections in the laminae of the dorsal lateral geniculate nucleus of the cat. *Z. Zellforsch. Mikrosk. Anat. 96*:1–38.

Guillery, R. W. 1970. Light- and electron-microscopical studies of normal and degenerating axons. In: *Contemporary Research Methods in Neuroanatomy.* W. J. H. Nauta and S. O. E. Ebbesson, Eds. New York, Springer-Verlag, pp. 77–105.

Guillery, R. W., and Colonnier, M. 1970. Synaptic patterns in the dorsal lateral geniculate nucleus of the monkey. *Z. Zellforsch. Mikrosk. Anat. 103*:90–108.

Güldner, F.-H. and Wolff, J. R. 1974. Dendro-dendritic synapses in the suprachiasmatic nucleus of the rat hypothalamus. *J. Neurocytol. 3*:245–250.

Ha, H. 1970. Axonal bifurcation in the dorsal root ganglion of the cat: a light and electron microscopic study. *J. Comp. Neurol. 140*:227–240.

Hager, H. 1961. Ergebnisse der Elektronenmikroskopie am zentralen, peripheren and vegetativen Nervensystem. *Ergeb. Biol. 24*:106–154.

Hajdu, F., Somogyi, G., and Tömböl, T. 1974. Neuronal and synaptic arrangement in the lateralis posterior-pulvinar complex of the thalamus in the cat. *Brain Res. 73*:89–104.

Hall, S. M. 1973. Some aspects of remyelination after demyelination produced by the intraneural injection of lysophosphatidyl choline. *J. Cell Sci. 13*:461–478.

Hall, S. M., and Williams, P. L. 1970. Some observations on the "incisures" of Schmidt and Lanterman. *J. Cell Sci. 6*:767–792.

Hall, S. M., and Williams, P. L. 1971. The distribution of electron-dense tracers in peripheral nerve fibers. *J. Cell Sci. 8*:541–555.

Haller, F. R., Haller, A. C., and Low, F. N. 1972. The fine structure of cellular layers and connective tissue space at spinal root attachments in the rat. *Am. J. Anat. 133*:109–124.

Haller, F. R., and Low, F. N. 1971. The fine structure of the peripheral nerve root sheath in the subarachnoid space in the rat and other laboratory animals. *Am. J. Anat. 131*:1–20.

Hama, K. 1961. Some observations on the fine structure of the giant fibers of the crayfishes (*Cambarus virilus* and *Cambarus clarkii*) with special reference to the submicroscopic organization of the synapses. *Anat. Rec. 141*:275–293.

Hama, K. 1965. Some observations of the fine structure of the lateral line organ of the Japanese sea eel, *Lyncozymba nystromi. J. Cell Biol. 24*:193–210.

Hama, K. 1969. A study of the fine structure of the saccular macula of the goldfish. *Z. Zellforsch. Mikrosk. Anat. 94*:155–171.

Hamberger, A. 1963. Difference between isolated neuronal and vascular glia with respect to respiratory activity. *Acta Physiol. Scand. 58*(Suppl. 203):1–58.

Hamberger, A., Hansson, H., and Sjöstrand, J. 1970.

Surface structure of isolated neurons. Detachment of nerve terminals during axon regeneration. *J. Cell Biol.* 47:319–331.

Hamburger, V. 1975. Cell death in the development of the lateral motor column of the chick embryo. *J. Comp. Neurol.* 160:535–546.

Hamlyn, L. H. 1962. The fine structure of the mossy fibre endings in the hippocampus of the rabbit. *J. Anat.* 96:112–120.

Hámori, J., and Szentágothai, J. 1965. The Purkinje cell baskets: ultrastructure of an inhibitory synapse. *Acta Biol. Acad. Sci. Hung.* 15:465–479.

Hámori, J., and Szentágothai, J. 1968. Identification of synapses formed in the cerebellar cortex by Purkinje axon collaterals: an electron microscope study. *Exp. Brain Res.* 5:118–128.

Hannah, R. S., and Nathaniel, E. J. H. 1974. The postnatal development of blood vessels in the substantia gelatinosa of rat cervical cord. An ultrastructural study. *Anat. Rec.* 178:691–710.

Hannover, A. 1844. *Recherches Microscopiques sur le Système Nerveux.* Copenhagen, Philipsen.

Hansson, H.-A., and Sjöstrand, J. 1971. Ultrastructural effects of colchicine on the hypoglossal and dorsal vagal neurons of the rabbit. *Brain Res.* 35:379–396.

Harding, B. N. 1971. Dendro-dendritic synapses including reciprocal synapses in the ventro-lateral nucleus of the monkey thalamus. *Brain Res.* 34:181–185.

Harkin, J. C. 1964. A series of desmosomal attachments in the Schwann cell sheath of myelinated mammalian nerves. *Z. Zellforsch. Mikrosk. Anat.* 64:189–195.

Harkin, J. C. 1965. Localization of the cellular site of collagen synthesis in peripheral nerves by electron microscopic autoradiography using H^3-proline. Proceedings, Fifth International Congress of Neuropathology. *Excerpta Med. Int. Congr. Ser.* 100:861–863.

Harrison, R. G. 1907. Observations on the living developing nerve fiber. *Anat. Rec.* 1:116–118.

Harrison, R. G. 1910. The outgrowth of the nerve fibers as a mode of protoplasmic movement. *J. Exp. Zool.* 9:787–846.

Harrison, R. G. 1924. Neuroblast versus sheath cell in the development of peripheral nerves. *J. Comp. Neurol.* 37:123–203.

Hartmann, J. F. 1951. Electron microscopy of myelin sheath in sections of spinal cord. *Exp. Cell Res.* 2:126–132.

Hartmann, J. F. 1953. An electron optical study of sections of central nervous system. *J. Comp. Neurol.* 99:201–249.

Hartmann, J. F. 1962. Identification of neuroglia in electron micrographs of normal nerve tissue. In: *Proceedings, IV. International Congress of Neuropathology* (Munich 1961), Vol. 2: *Electron-microscopy and Biology.* H. Jacob, Ed. Stuttgart, Thieme, pp. 32–35.

Hasan, M., and Glees, P. 1972. Genesis and possible dissolution of neuronal lipofuscin. *Gerontologia* 18:217–236.

Hashimoto, P. H. 1969. Electron microscopic study of gliosome formation in postnatal development of spinal cord in the cat. *J. Comp. Neurol.* 137:251–266.

Haug, H. 1971. Die Membrana limitans gliae superficialis der Sehrinde der Katze. *Z. Zellforsch. Mikrosk. Anat.* 115:79–87.

Hay, E. D. 1968. Structure and function of the nucleolus in developing cells. In: *Ultrastructure in Biological Systems.* Vol. 3, *The Nucleus.* A. J. Dalton and F. Haguenau, Eds. New York, Academic Press, pp. 1–79.

Hayes, K. C., McCombs, H. L., and Faherty, T. P. 1971. The fine structure of vitamin A deficiency. II. Arachnoid granulations and CSF pressure. *Brain* 94:213–224.

Hebb, C. 1970. CNS at the cellular level: identity of transmitter agents. *Annu. Rev. Physiol.* 32:165–192.

Hedley-Whyte, E. T., and Meuser, C. S. 1971. The effect of undernutrition on myelination of rat sciatic nerve. *Lab. Invest.* 24:156–161.

Hedley-Whyte, E. T., Rawlins, F. A., Salpeter, M. M., and Uzman, B. G. 1969. Distribution of cholesterol-1,2-H^3 during maturation of mouse peripheral nerve. *Lab. Invest.* 21:536–547.

Heimer, L. 1970. Bridging the gap between light and electron microscopy in the experimental tracing of fiber connections. In: *Contemporary Research Methods in Neuroanatomy.* W. J. H. Nauta and S. O. E. Ebbesson, Eds. New York, Springer-Verlag, pp. 162–172.

Heimer, L., and Peters, A. 1968. An electron microscope study of a silver stain for degenerating boutons. *Brain Res.* 8:337–346.

Held, H. 1897. Beiträge zur Structur der Nervenzellen und ihrer Fortsätze. Part II. *Arch. Anat. Physiol., Anat. Abt.,* pp. 204–293; and Part III. *Arch. Anat. Physiol., Anat. Abt.* (Suppl. for 1897), pp. 273–312.

Held, H. 1909. *Die Entwicklung des Nervengewebes bei den Wirbeltieren.* Leipzig, Barth.

Helmholtz, H. 1842. *De Fabrica Systematis Nervosi Evertebratorum.* Berlin, Typis Nietackianis.

Hendelman, W. J., and Bunge, R. P. 1969. Radioautographic studies of choline incorporation into peripheral nerve myelin. *J. Cell Biol* 40:190–208.

Henrikson, C. K., and Vaughn, J. E. 1974. Fine structural relationships between neurites and radial glial processes in developing mouse spinal cord. *J. Neurocytol.* 3:659–675.

Herman, C. J., and Lapham, L. W. 1968. DNA content of neurons in the cat hippocampus. *Science* 160:537.

Herman, M. M., and Ralston, H. J. 1970. Laminated cytoplasmic bodies and annulate lamellae in cat ventrobasal and posterior thalamus. *Anat. Rec.* 167:183–196.

Herndon, R. M. 1963. The fine structure of the Purkinje cell. *J. Cell Biol.* 18:167–180.

Herndon, R. M. 1964. The fine structure of the rat cerebellum. II. The stellate neurons, granule cells, and glia. *J. Cell Biol.* 23:277–293.

Herschkowitz, N., Vassella, F., and Bischoff, A. 1971. Myelin differences in the central and peripheral nervous systems in the "jimpy" mouse. *J. Neurochem. 18*:1361–1363.

Hess, A. 1955. The fine structure of young and old spinal ganglia. *Anat. Rec. 123*:399–423.

Hess, A. 1965. Developmental changes in the structure of the synapse on the myelinated cell bodies of the chicken ciliary ganglion. *J. Cell Biol. 25*:1–19.

Hess, A., and Young, J. Z. 1949. Correlation of internodal length and fibre diameter in the central nervous system. *Nature (Lond.) 164*:490–491.

Hess, A., and Young, J. Z. 1952. The nodes of Ranvier. *Proc. R. Soc. Ser. B 140*:301–320.

Heuser, J. E., and Miledi, R. 1971. Effect of lanthanum ions on function and structure of frog neuromuscular junctions. *Proc. R. Soc. Ser. B 179*:247–260.

Heuser, J. E., and Reese, T. S. 1972. Stimulation induced uptake and release of peroxidase from synaptic vesicles in frog neuromuscular junctions. *Anat. Rec. 172*:329–330.

Heuser, J. E., and Reese, T. S. 1973. Evidence for recycling of synaptic vesicle membrane during transmitter release at the frog neuromuscular junction. *J. Cell Biol. 57*:315–344.

Heuser, J. E., and Reese, T. S. 1974. Morphology of synaptic vesicle discharge and reformation at the frog neuromuscular junction. In: *Synaptic Transmission and Neuronal Interaction.* M. V. L. Bennett Ed. New York, Raven Press, pp. 59–77.

Heuser, J. E., Reese, T. S., and Landis, D. M. D. 1974. Functional changes in frog neuromuscular junctions studied with freeze-fracture. *J. Neurocytol. 3*:109–131.

Hild, W. 1957. Myelogenesis in cultures of mammalian central nervous tissue. *Z. Zellforsch. Mikrosk. Anat. 46*:71–95.

Hild, W. 1959. Myelin formation in cultures of mammalian central nervous tissue. In: *The Biology of Myelin.* S. R. Korey, Ed. New York, Hoeber, pp. 188–200.

Hildebrand, C. 1971a. Ultrastructural and light-microscopic studies of the nodal region on large myelinated fibers of the adult feline spinal cord white matter. *Acta Physiol. Scand. Suppl. 364*:43–80.

Hildebrand, C. 1971b. Ultrastructural and light-microscopic studies of the developing feline spinal cord white matter. I. The nodes of Ranvier. *Acta Physiol. Scand. Suppl. 364*:81–109.

Hildebrand, C. 1971c. Ultrastructural and light-microscopic studies of the developing feline spinal cord white matter. II. Cell death and myelin sheath disintegration in the early postnatal period. *Acta Physiol. Scand. Suppl. 364*:109–144.

Hildebrand, C. 1972. Evidence for a correlation between myelin period and number of myelin lamellae in fibers of the feline spinal cord white matter. *J. Neurocytol. 1*:223–232.

Hillman, D. E., and Llinás, R. 1974. Calcium-containing electron-dense structures in the axons of the squid giant synapse. *J. Cell Biol. 61*:146–155.

Himango, W. A., and Low, F. N. 1971. The fine structure of a lateral recess of the subarachnoid space in the rat. *Anat. Rec. 171*:1–20.

Hinds, J. W. 1970. Reciprocal and serial dendro-dendritic synapses in the glomerular layer of the rat olfactory bulb. *Brain Res. 17*:530–534.

Hinds, J. W. 1972. Early neuron differentiation in the mouse olfactory bulb. II. Electron microscopy. *J. Comp. Neurol. 146*:253–276.

Hinds, J. W., and Hinds, P. L. 1972. Reconstruction of dendritic growth cones in neonatal mouse olfactory bulb. *J. Neurocytol. 1*:169–187.

Hinds, J. W., and Hinds, P. L. 1974. Early ganglion cell differentiation in the mouse retina: An electron microscopic analysis utilizing serial sections. *Dev. Biol. 37*:381–416.

Hinds, J. W., and Ruffett, T. L. 1973. Mitral cell development in the mouse olfactory bulb: reorientation of the perikaryon and maturation of the axon initial segment. *J. Comp. Neurol. 151*:281–305.

Hinkley, R. E. 1973. Axonal microtubules and associated filaments stained by Alcian blue. *J. Cell Sci. 13*:753–761.

Hinojosa, R. 1973. Synaptic ultrastructure in the tangential nucleus of the goldfish (*Carassius auratus*). *Am. J. Anat. 137*:159–186.

Hinojosa, R., and Robertson, J. D. 1967. Ultrastructure of the spoon type synaptic endings in the nucleus vestibularis tangentialis of the chick. *J. Cell Biol. 34*:421–430.

Hinrichsen, C. F. L., and Larramendi, L. M. H. 1968. Synapses and cluster formation in the mouse mesencephalic fifth nucleus. *Brain Res. 7*:296–299.

Hinrichsen, C. F. L., and Larramendi, L. M. H. 1970. The trigeminal mesencephalic nucleus. II. Electron microscopy. *Am. J. Anat. 127*:303–320.

Hirano, A. 1968. A confirmation of the oligodendroglial origin of myelin in the adult rat. *J. Cell Biol. 38*:637–640.

Hirano, A., Becker, N. H., and Zimmerman, H. M. 1969. Isolation of the periaxonal space of the central myelinated fiber with regard to diffusion of peroxidase. *J. Histochem. Cytochem. 17*:512–516.

Hirano, A., and Dembitzer, H. M. 1967. A structural analysis of the myelin sheath in the central nervous system. *J. Cell Biol. 34*:555–567.

Hirano, A., and Dembitzer, H. M. 1969. The transverse bands as a means of access to the periaxonal space of the central myelinated nerve fiber. *J. Ultrastruct. Res. 28*:141–149.

Hirano, A., Levine, S., and Zimmerman, H. M. 1968. Remyelination in the central nervous system after cyanide intoxication. *J. Neuropathol. Exp. Neurol. 27*:234–245.

Hirano, A., and Zimmerman, H. M. 1967. Some new observations on the normal rat ependymal cell. *Anat. Rec. 158*:293–302.

Hirano, A., Zimmerman, H. M., and Levine, S. 1966. Myelin in the central nervous system as observed in experimentally induced edema in the rat. *J. Cell Biol.* 31:397–411.

Hirata, Y. 1966. Occurrence of cylindrical synaptic vesicles in the central nervous system perfused with buffered formalin solution prior to OsO₄-fixation. *Arch. Histol. Jap.* 26:269–279.

Hirose, G., and Bass, N. H. 1973. Maturation of oligodendroglia and myelinogenesis in rat optic nerve: a quantitative histochemical study. *J. Comp. Neurol.* 152:201–210.

Hiscoe, H. B. 1947. The distribution of nodes and incisures in normal and regenerating nerve fibers. *Anat. Rec.* 99:447–476.

Hoerr, N. L. 1936. Cytological studies by the Altmann-Gersh freezing-drying method. III. The preexistence of neurofibrillae and their disposition in the nerve fiber. *Anat. Rec.* 66:81–90.

Hofer, H. O. 1968. The phenomenon of neurosecretion. In: *The Structure and Function of Nervous Tissue*, Vol. 1. G. H. Bourne, Ed. New York, Academic Press, pp. 461–517.

Hökfelt, T. 1966. The effect of reserpine on the intraneuronal vesicles of the rat vas deferens. *Experientia* 22:56–57.

Hökfelt, T. 1967a. The possible ultrastructural identification of tubero-infundibular dopamine-containing nerve endings in the median eminence of the rat. *Brain Res.* 5:121–123.

Hökfelt, T. 1967b. On the ultrastructural localization of noradrenaline in the central nervous system. *Z. Zellforsch. Mikrosk. Anat.* 79:110–117.

Hökfelt, T. 1968. *In vitro* studies on central and peripheral monoamine neurons at the ultrastructural level. *Z. Zellforsch. Mikrosk. Anat.* 91:1–74.

Holmgren, E. 1900. Weitere Mitteilungen über die "Saftkanälchen" der Nervenzellen. *Anat. Anz.* 18:290–296.

Holz, A., and Weber, W. 1970. Periodische auftretende Querstrukturen in Nervenfasern des Bulbus olfactorius des Eltrize *Phoxinus laevis*. *Experientia* 26:1349–1350.

Holtzman, E. 1971. Cytochemical studies of protein transport in the nervous system. *Phil. Trans. R. Soc. Ser. B.* 261:407–421.

Holtzman, E., and Novikoff, A. B. 1965. Lysosomes in the rat sciatic nerve following crush. *J. Cell Biol.* 27:651–669.

Holtzman, E., Novikoff, A. B., and Villaverde, H. 1967. Lysosomes and GERL in normal and chromatolytic neurons of rat ganglion nodosum. *J. Cell Biol.* 33:419–435.

Holtzman, E., and Peterson, E. R. 1969. Uptake of protein by mammalian neurons. *J. Cell Biol.* 40:863–869.

Holtzman, E., Teichberg, S., Abrahams, S. J., Citkowitz, E., Crain, S. M., Kawai, N., and Peterson, E. R. 1973. Notes on synaptic vesicles and related structures, endoplasmic reticulum, lysosomes, and peroxisomes in nervous tissue and the adrenal medulla. *J. Histochem. Cytochem.* 21:349–385.

Hommes, O. R., and Leblond, C. P. 1967. Mitotic division of neuroglia in the normal adult rat. *J. Comp. Neurol.* 129:269–278.

Honjin, R. 1959. Electron microscopic studies on the myelinated nerve fibers in the central nervous system. *Acta Anat. Nippon.* 34:43–44 (in Japanese).

Honjin, R., and Changus, G. W. 1964. Electron microscopy of nerve fibers. VIII. Again on the radial component in the myelin sheath. *Okajimas Folia Anat. Jap.* 39:251–261.

Honjin, R., Kosaka, T., Takano, I., and Hiramatsu, K. 1963. Electron microscopy of nerve fibers. VII. On the electron dense radial component in the laminated myelin sheath. *Okajimas Folia Anat. Jap.* 39:39–53.

Hopsu, V. K., and Arstila, A. U. 1965. An apparent somato-somatic synaptic structure in the pineal gland of the rat. *Exp. Cell Res.* 37:484–487.

Horstmann, E. 1954. Die Faserglia des Selachiergehirns. *Z. Zellforsch. Mikrosk. Anat.* 39:588–617.

Hoyosa, Y., and Fujita, T. 1973. Scanning electron microscope observations of intraventricular macrophages (Kolmer cells) in the rat brain. *Arch. Histol. Jap.* 35:133–140.

Hubbard, J. I., and Kwanbunbumpen, S. 1968. Evidence for the vesicle hypothesis. *J. Physiol. (Lond.)* 194:407–420.

Huneeus, F. C., and Davison, P. F. 1970. Fibrillar proteins from squid axons. I. Neurofilament protein. *J. Mol. Biol.* 52:415–428.

Huxley, R. E. 1973. Axonal microtubules and associated filaments stained by Alcian blue. *J. Cell Sci.* 13:753–761.

Hydén, H. 1959. Biochemical changes in glial cells and nerve cells at varying activity. In: *Proceedings of the Fourth International Congress of Biochemistry*, Vol. 3, *Symposium III, Biochemistry of the Central Nervous System*. F. Brücke, Ed. Oxford, Pergamon Press, pp. 64–88.

Hydén, H. 1962. A molecular basis of neuron-glia interaction. In: *Macromolecular Specificity and Biological Memory*. F. O. Schmitt, Ed. Cambridge, Mass., M.I.T. Press, pp. 55–69.

Hydén, H. 1967. Dynamic aspects of the neuron-glia relationship, a study with micro-chemical methods. In: *The Neuron*. H. Hydén, Ed. Amsterdam, Elsevier, pp. 179–219.

Hydén, H., and Egyházi, E. 1963. Glial RNA changes during a learning experiment in rats. *Proc. Natl. Acad. Sci. U.S.A.* 49:618–624.

Hydén, H., and Lange, P. W. 1970. Protein changes in nerve cells related to learning and conditioning. In: *The Neurosciences Second Study Program*. F. O. Schmitt, Ed. New York, The Rockefeller University Press, pp. 278–289.

Hydén, H., and Pigon, A. 1960. A cytophysiological study of the functional relationship between oligodendroglial cells and nerve cells of Deiters' nucleus. *J. Neurochem.* 6:57–72.

Ishii, S., Thomas, P., and Nakamura, T. 1973. Morphometric classification of the neurosecretory granules in the rat pars nervosa. *Z. Zellforsch. Mikrosk. Anat.* 146:463–471.

Iversen, L. L., and Bloom, F. E. 1972. Studies of the uptake of ³H-GABA and ³H-glycine in slices and homogenates of rat brain and spinal cord by electron microscope autoradiography. *Brain Res.* 41:131–143.

Jacobson, S. 1967. Dimensions of the dendritic spine in the sensorimotor cortex of the rat, cat, squirrel monkey and man. *J. Comp. Neurol.* 129:49–58.

James, K. A. C., Bray, J. J., Morgan, J. G., and Austin, L. 1970. The effects of colchicine on the transport of axonal proteins in the chicken. *Biochem. J.* 117:767–771.

Jande, S. S. 1966. Fine structure of lateral line organs in frog tadpoles. *J. Ultrastruct. Res.* 15:496–509.

Jayatilaka, A. D. P. 1965. An electron microscopic study of sheep arachnoid granulations. *J. Anat.* 99:635–649.

Johnson, J. E., and Miquel, J. 1974. Fine structural changes in the lateral vestibular nucleus of aging rats. *Mech. Ageing Dev.* 3:203–224.

Johnston, M. C. 1966. A radioautographic study of the migration and fate of cranial neural crest cells in the chick embryo. *Anat. Rec.* 156:143–156.

Johnston, M. C., Bhakdinaronk, A., and Reid, Y. C. 1973. An expanded role of the neural crest in oral and pharyngeal development. In: *Fourth Symposium on Oral Sensation and Perception.* J. F. Bosma, Ed. Washington, D.C., U.S. Government Printing Office, pp. 37–52.

Johnston, M. C., and Hazelton, R. D. 1972. Embryonic origins of facial structures related to oral sensory and motor functions. In: *Third Symposium on Oral Sensation and Perception.* James F. Bosma, Ed. Springfield, Ill., Charles C Thomas, pp. 76–97.

Johnston, M. C., and Listgarten, M. A. 1972. The migration, interaction and early differentiation of oro-facial tissues. In: *Developmental Aspects of Oral Biology.* H. S. Slavkin and L. A. Bavetta, Eds. New York, Academic Press, pp. 55–80.

Jones, D. S. 1973. Some factors affecting the PTA staining of synaptic junctions. A preliminary comparison of PTA stained junctions in various regions of the CNS. *Z. Zellforsch. Mikrosk. Anat.* 143:301–312.

Jones, E. G. 1970. On the mode of entry of blood vessels into the cerebral cortex. *J. Anat.* 106:507–520.

Jones, E. G., and Leavitt, R. Y. 1973. Demonstration of thalamo-cortical connectivity in the cat somatosensory system by retrograde axonal transport of horseradish peroxidase. *Brain Res.* 63:414–418.

Jones, E. G., and Leavitt, R. Y. 1974. Retrograde axonal transport and the demonstration of nonspecific projections to the cerebral cortex and striatum from thalamic intralaminar nuclei in the rat, cat and monkey. *J. Comp. Neurol.* 154:349–378.

Jones, E. G., and Powell, T. P. S. 1969a. Electron

microscopy of synaptic glomeruli in the thalamic relay nuclei of the cat. *Proc. R. Soc. Ser. B* 172:153–171.

Jones, E. G., and Powell, T. P. S. 1969b. Morphological variations in the dendritic spines of the neocortex. *J. Cell Sci.* 5:509–529.

Jones, E. G., and Powell, T. P. S. 1969c. Synapses on the axon hillocks and initial segments of pyramidal cell axons in the cerebral cortex. *J. Cell Sci.* 5:495–507.

Jones, E. G., and Powell, T. P. S. 1970a. Electron microscopy of the somatic sensory cortex of the cat. I. Cell types and synaptic organization. *Phil. Trans. R. Soc. Ser. B.* 257:1–11.

Jones, E. G., and Powell, T. P. S. 1970b. Electron microscopy of the somatic sensory cortex of the cat. II. The fine structure of layers I and II. *Phil. Trans. R. Soc. Ser. B.* 257:13–21.

Jones, E. G., and Powell, T. P. S. 1970c. Electron microscopy of the somatic sensory cortex of the cat. III. The fine structure of layers III to VI. *Phil. Trans. R. Soc. Ser. B.* 257:23–28.

Jones, E. G., and Powell, T. P. S. 1970d. An electron microscopic study of terminal degeneration in the neocortex of the cat. *Phil. Trans. R. Soc. Ser. B.* 257:29–43.

Jones, E. G., and Powell, T. P. S. 1970e. An electron microscopic study of the laminar pattern and mode of termination of afferent fiber pathways in the somatic sensory cortex of the cat. *Phil. Trans. R. Soc. Ser. B.* 257:45–62.

Jones, S. F., and Kwanbunbumpen, S. 1968. On the role of synaptic vesicles in transmitter release. *Life Sci.* 7:1251–1255.

Joó, F., and Csillik, B. 1966. Topographic correlation between the hemato-encephalic barrier and the cholinesterase activity of brain capillaries. *Exp. Brain Res.* 1:147–151.

Kadota, K., and Kadota, T. 1973a. Isolation of coated vesicles, plain synaptic vesicles and fine particles from synaptosomes of guinea pig whole brain. *J. Elect. Microsc.* 22:91–98.

Kadota, K., and Kadota, T. 1973b. Isolation of coated vesicles, plain synaptic vesicles, and flocculent material from a crude synaptosome fraction of guinea pig whole brain. *J. Cell Biol.* 58:135–151.

Kagawa, Y., and Racker, E. 1966. Partial resolution of the enzymes catalyzing oxidative phosphorylation. X. Correlation of morphology and function in submitochondrial particles. *J. Biol. Chem.* 241:2475–2482.

Kaiserman-Abramof, I. R., and Palay, S. L. 1969. Fine structural studies of the cerebellar cortex in a mormyrid fish. In: *Neurobiology of Cerebellar Evolution and Development.* R. Llinás, Ed. Chicago, American Medical Association, pp. 171–205.

Kaiserman-Abramof, I. R., and Peters, A. 1972. Some aspects of the morphology of Betz cells in the cerebral cortex of the cat. *Brain Res.* 43:527–546.

Kamiya, H.-O., Kadota, K., and Kadota, T. 1974. Distribution of choline and acetylcholine in coated vesicles and plain synaptic vesicles. *Brain Res.* 76:367–370.

Kanaseki, T., and Kadota, K. 1969. The "vesicle in a basket." A morphological study of the coated vesicle isolated from the nerve endings of the guinea pig brain with special reference to the mechanism of membrane movements. *J. Cell Biol.* 42:202–220.

Kane, E. C. 1974. Patterns of degeneration in the caudal cochlear nucleus of the cat after cortical ablation. *Anat. Rec.* 179:67–92.

Karlsson, J. O., and Sjöstrand, J. 1969. The effect of colchicine on the axonal transport of protein in the optic nerve and tract of the rabbit. *Brain Res.* 13:617–619.

Karlsson, U. 1966a. Comparison of the myelin period of peripheral and central origin by electron microscopy. *J. Ultrastruct. Res.* 15:451–468.

Karlsson, U. 1966b. Three-dimensional studies of neurons in the lateral geniculate nucleus of the rat. I. Organelle organization in the perikaryon and its proximal branches. *J. Ultrastruct. Res.* 16:429–481.

Karlsson, U. 1966c. Three-dimensional studies of neurons in the lateral geniculate nucleus of the rat. II. Environment of perikarya and proximal parts of their branches. *J. Ultrastruct. Res.* 16:482–504.

Karnovsky, M. J. 1965. A formaldehyde-glutaraldehyde fixative of high osmolality for use in electron microscopy. *J. Cell Biol.* 27:137A.

Karnovsky, M. J. 1971. Use of ferrocyanide-reduced osmium tetroxide in electron microscopy. *Abstracts of Papers, Eleventh Annual Meeting of the American Society for Cell Biology*, p. 146.

Kartenbeck, J., Zentgraf, H., Scheer, U., and Franke, W. W. 1971. The nuclear envelope in freeze-etching. *Ergeb. Anat. Entwicklungsgesch.* 45:1–55.

Kater, W. B., and Nicholson, C. 1973. *Intracellular Staining in Neurobiology.* New York, Springer-Verlag.

Katz, B. 1966. *Nerve, Muscle, and Synapse.* New York, McGraw-Hill.

Katz, B., and Miledi, R. 1965. The effect of calcium on acetylcholine release from motor nerve terminals. *Proc. R. Soc. Ser. B.* 161:496–503.

Katz, B., and Miledi, R. 1967a. A study of synaptic transmission in the absence of nerve impulses. *J. Physiol. (Lond.)* 192:407–436.

Katz, B., and Miledi, R. 1967b. The release of acetylcholine from nerve endings by graded electric pulses. *Proc. R. Soc., Ser. B* 167:23–38.

Kawana, E., Akert, K., and Bruppacher, H. 1971. Enlargement of synaptic vesicles as an early sign of terminal degeneration in the rat caudate nucleus. *J. Comp. Neurol.* 142:297–308.

Kawana, E., Akert, K., and Sandri, C. 1969. Zinc iodide-osmium tetroxide impregnation of nerve terminals in the spinal cord. *Brain Res.* 16:325–331.

Kawana, E., Sandri, C., and Akert, K. 1971. Ultrastruc-

ture of growth cones in the cerebellar cortex of the neonatal rat and cat. *Z. Zellforsch. Mikrosk. Anat.* 115:284–298.

Kellerth, J.-O. 1973. Intracellular staining of cat spinal motoneurons with procion yellow for ultrastructural studies. *Brain Res.* 50:415–418.

Kelly, J. P., and Van Essen, D. C. 1974. Cell structure and function in the visual cortex of the cat. *J. Physiol. (Lond.)* 238:515–547.

Kerjaschki, D., and Stockinger, L. 1970. Zur Struktur und Funktion des Perineuriums. *Z. Zellforsch. Mikrosk. Anat.* 110:386–400.

Kerns, J. M., and Hinsman, E. J. 1973a. Neuroglial response to sciatic neurectomy. I. Light microscopy and autoradiography. *J. Comp. Neurol.* 151:237–254.

Kerns, J. M., and Hinsman, E. J. 1973b. Neuroglial response to sciatic neurectomy. II. Electron microscopy. *J. Comp. Neurol.* 151:255–280.

Kerns, J. M., and Peters, A. 1974. Ultrastructure of a large ventro-lateral dendritic bundle in the rat ventral horn. *J. Neurocytol.* 3:533–555.

Kety, S. S., and Samson, F. E. 1967. Neural properties of the biogenic amines: A report of an NRP work session. *Neurosci. Res. Progr. Bull.* 5:1–119.

Key, A. H., and Retzius, G. 1876. *Studien in der Anatomie des Nervensystems und des Bindegewebes.* Stockholm, Samson and Wallin.

Keynes, R. D. 1970. Evidence for structural changes during nerve activity and their relation to the conduction mechanism. In: *The Neurosciences. Second Study Program.* F. O. Schmitt, Ed. New York, The Rockefeller University Press, pp. 707–714.

Khattab, F. I. 1966. Synaptic contacts at nodes of Ranvier in central nervous tissue. *Anat. Rec.* 156:91–97.

Kidd, M. 1962. Electron microscopy of the inner plexiform layer of the retina in the cat and the pigeon. *J. Anat.* 96:179–187.

Kim, S. U., Masurovsky, E. G., Benitez, H. H., and Murray, M. R. 1970. Histochemical studies of the intranuclear rodlet in neurons of chicken sympathetic and sensory ganglia. *Histochemie* 24:33–40.

King, J. S. 1968. A light and electron microscopic study of perineuronal glial cells and processes in the rabbit neocortex. *Anat. Rec.* 161:111–124.

King, J. S., and Schwyn, R. C. 1970. The fine structure of neuroglial cells and pericytes in the primate red nucleus and substantia nigra. *Z Zellforsch. Mikrosk. Anat.* 106:309–321.

Kirkpatrick, J. B. 1968. Chromatolysis in the hypoglossal nucleus of the rat: an electron microscopic analysis. *J. Comp. Neurol.* 132:189–211.

Kirkpatrick, J. B., Hyams, L., Thomas, V. L., and Howley, P. M. 1970. Purification of intact microtubules from brain. *J. Cell Biol.* 47:384–394.

Kitamura, T., Hattori, H., and Fujita, S. 1972. Autoradiographic studies on histogenesis of brain macrophages in the mouse. *J. Neuropathol. Exp. Neurol.* 31:502–518.

Klemm, H. 1970. Das Perineurium als Diffusionsbarriere gegenüber Peroxydase bei epi- und endoneuraler Applikation. *Z. Zellforsch. Mikrosk. Anat. 108*:431–445.

Klinkerfuss, G. N. 1964. An electron microscopic study of the ependymal glia of the lateral ventricle of the cat. *Am. J. Anat. 115*:71–100.

Knigge, K. M., and Scott, D. E. 1970. Structure and function of the median eminence. *Am. J. Anat. 129*:223–244.

Knigge, K. M., Scott, D. E., and Weindl, A., Eds. 1972. *Brain-Endocrine Interaction. Median Eminence: Structure and Function.* Munich, Basel, S. Karger.

Knobler, R. L., and Stempak, J. G. 1973. Serial section analysis of myelin development in the central nervous system of the albino rat: An electron microscopical study of early axonal ensheathment. In: *Progress in Brain Research. Neurobiological Aspects of Maturation and Aging.* Vol. 40. D. H. Ford, Ed. Amsterdam, Elsevier Press, pp. 407–423.

Knobler, R. L., Stempak, J. G., and Laurencin, M. 1974. Oligodendroglial ensheathment of axons during myelination in the developing rat central nervous system. A serial section electron microscopical study. *J. Ultrastruct. Res. 49*:34–49.

Knowles, F. 1972. Ependyma of the third ventricle in relation to pituitary function. In: *Progress in Brain Research*, Vol. 38, *Topics in Neuroendocrinology.* J. A. Kappers and J. P. Schadé, Eds. Amsterdam, Elsevier, pp. 255–270.

Knowles, F., and Anand-Kumar, T. C. 1967. Structural changes, related to reproduction, in the hypothalamus and in the pars tuberalis of the rhesus monkey. Part I. The hypothalamus. Part II. The pars tuberalis. *Phil. Trans. R. Soc. Ser. B 256*:357–375.

Kobayashi, H., Matsui, T., and Ishii, S. 1970. Functional electron microscopy of the hypothalamic median eminence. *Int. Rev. Cytol. 29*:281–381.

Kobayashi, H., Wada, M., Uemura, H., and Ueck, M. 1972. Uptake of peroxidase from the third ventricle by ependymal cells of the median eminence. *Z. Zellforsch. Mikrosk. Anat. 127*:545–551.

Kobayashi, T., Kobayashi, T., Yamamoto, K., and Kaibara, M. 1967. Electron microscopic observation on the hypothalamo-hypophyseal system in the rat. II. Ultrafine structure of the median eminence and of the nerve cells of the arcuate nucleus. *Endocrinol. Jap. 14*:158–167.

Koenig, H. 1964. RNA metabolism in the nervous system: Some RNA-dependent functions of neurons and glia. In: *Morphological and Biochemical Correlates of Neural Activity.* M. M. Cohen and R. S. Snider, Eds. New York, Hoeber, pp. 39–56.

Koenig, H. L., di Giamberardino, L., and Bennett, G. 1973. Renewal of proteins and glycoproteins of synaptic constituents by means of axonal transport. *Brain Res. 62*:413–417.

Kohno, K. 1964. Neurotubules contained within the dendrite and axon of Purkinje cell of frog. *Bull. Tokyo Med. Dent. Univ. 11*:411–442.

Kohno, K. 1970. Symmetrical axo-axonic synapses in the axon cap of the goldfish Mauthner cell. *Brain Res. 23*:255–258.

Kohno, K., Chan-Palay, V., and Palay, S. L. 1975. Cytoplasmic inclusions of neurons in the monkey visual cortex. *J. Anat. Embryol. 147*:117–125.

Kohno, K., Nakai, Y., and Yamada, H. 1972. Synaptic contacts from nodes of Ranvier in the granular layer of the frog cerebellum. *J. Neurocytol. 1*:255–262.

Kolb, H., and Famiglietti, E. V. 1974. Rod and cone pathways in the inner plexiform layer of cat retina. *Science 186*:47–49.

Kölliker, A. 1844. Die Selbständigkeit und Abhängigkeit des sympathischen Nervensystems, durch anatomische Beobachtungen bewiesen. Zürich, Meyer und Zeller.

Kolmer, W. 1921. Uber eine eigenartige Beziehung von Wanderzellen zu den Choroidealplexus des Gehirns der Wirbeltiere. *Anat. Anz. 54*:15–19.

Konigsmark, B. W., and Sidman, R. L. 1963. Origin of brain macrophages in the mouse. *J. Neuropathol. Exp. Neurol. 22*:643–676.

Korneliussen, H. 1972a. Ultrastructure of normal and stimulated motor end plates, with comments on the origin and fate of synaptic vesicles. *Z. Zellforsch. Mikrosk. Anat. 130*:28–57.

Korneliussen, H. 1972b. Elongated profiles of synaptic vesicles in motor end plates. Morphological effects of fixative variations. *J. Neurocytol. 1*:279–296.

Kornguth, S. E., and Scott, G. 1972. The role of climbing fibers in the formation of Purkinje cell dendrites. *J. Comp. Neurol. 146*:61–82.

Kozlowski, G. P., Scott, D. E., and Krobisch-Dudley, G. 1973. Scanning electron microscopy of the lateral ventricles of sheep. *Am. J. Anat. 135*:561–566.

Kozlowski, G. P., Scott, D. E., and Murphy, J. A. 1972. Scanning electron microscopy of the lateral ventricles of the sheep. *Am. J. Anat. 135*:561–566.

Kraus-Ruppert, R., Laissue, J., Bürki, H., and Odartchenko, N. 1973. Proliferation and turnover of glial cells in the forebrain of young adult mice as studied by repeated injections of ^{3}H-thymidine over a prolonged period of time. *J. Comp. Neurol. 148*:211–216.

Kreutzberg, G. W. 1969. Neuronal dynamics and axonal flow. IV. Blockage of intra-axonal enzyme transport by colchicine. *Proc. Natl. Acad. Sci. U.S.A. 62*:722–728.

Kreutzberg, G. W., and Schubert, P. 1974. Neuronal activity and axonal flow. In: *Central Nervous System; Studies on Metabolic Regulation and Function. International Symposium on Metabolic Regulation and Functional Activity in the Central Nervous System, St. Vincent, Italy, 1972.* E. Genazzani and H. Herken, eds. Berlin, Springer-Verlag, pp. 84–93.

Kreutzberg, G. W., Schubert, P., Tóth, L., and Rieske, E. 1973. Intradendritic transport to postsynaptic sites. *Brain Res. 62*:399–404.

Kreutzberg, G. W., and Tóth, L. 1974. Dendritic secretion: a way for the neuron to communicate with the vasculature. *Naturwissenschaften 61*:37–39.

Krisch, B. 1974. Different populations of granules and their distribution in the hypothalamo-neurohypophysial tract of the rat under various experimental conditions. 1. Neurohypophysis, nucleus supraopticus and nucleus paraventricularis. *Cell Tiss. Res. 151*:117–140.

Krishnan, N., and Singer, M. 1973. Penetration of peroxidase into peripheral nerve fibers. *Am. J. Anat. 136*:1–14.

Kristensson, K. 1970. Transport of fluorescent protein tracer in peripheral nerves. *Acta Neuropathol. (Berl.) 16*:293–300.

Kristensson, K., and Olsson, Y. 1971a. Retrograde axonal transport of protein. *Brain Res. 29*:363–365.

Kristensson, K., and Olsson, Y. 1971b. Uptake and retrograde axonal transport of peroxidase in hypoglossal neurons. *Acta Neuropathol. (Berl.) 19*:1–9.

Kristensson, K., and Olsson, Y. 1971c. The perineurium as a diffusion barrier to protein tracers. Differences between mature and immature animals. *Acta Neuropathol. (Berl.) 17*:127–138.

Kristensson, K., and Olsson, Y. 1973. Diffusion pathways and retrograde axonal transport of protein tracers in peripheral nerves. In: *Progress in Neurobiology*, Vol. 1, Part 2. G. A. Kerkut and J. W. Phillis, Eds. New York, Pergamon Press, pp. 85–109.

Kristensson, K., Olsson, Y., and Sjöstrand, J. 1971. Axonal uptake and retrograde transport of exogenous proteins in the hypoglossal nerve. *Brain Res. 32*:399–406.

Krnjevic, K. 1974. Chemical nature of synaptic transmission in vertebrates. *Physiol. Rev. 54*:418–540.

Kruger, L., and Maxwell, D. S. 1966. Electron microscopy of oligodendrocytes in normal rat cerebrum. *Am. J. Anat. 118*:411–435.

Kruger, L., and Maxwell, D. S. 1967. Comparative fine structure of vertebrate neuroglia: teleosts and reptiles. *J. Comp. Neurol. 129*:115–142.

Kruger, L., and Maxwell, D. S. 1969. Cytoplasmic laminar bodies in the striate cortex. *J. Ultrastruct. Res. 26*:387–390.

Kuffler, S. W., and Nicholls, J. G. 1966. The physiology of neuroglial cells. *Ergeb. Physiol. 57*:1–90.

Kuypers, H. G. J. M., Koevit, J., and Groen-Klevant, A. C. 1974. Retrograde axonal transport of horseradish peroxidase in rat's forebrain. *Brain Res. 67*:211–218.

Laatsch, R. H., and Cowan, W. M. 1966a. Electron microscope studies of the dentate gyrus of the rat. I. Normal structure with reference to synaptic organization. *J. Comp. Neurol. 128*:359–396.

Laatsch, R. H., and Cowan, W. M. 1966b. A structural specialization at nodes of Ranvier in the central nervous system. *Nature (Lond.) 210*:757–758.

Lafontaine, J. -G. 1968. Structural components of the nucleus in mitotic plant cells. In: *Ultrastructure in Biological Systems*, Vol. 3, The Nucleus. A. J.

Dalton and F. Haguenau, Eds. New York, Academic Press, pp. 151–196.

Laidlaw, G. F. 1930. Silver staining of the endoneural fibres of the cerebrospinal nerves. *Am. J. Pathol. 6*:435–444.

Lampert, P. W. 1965. Demyelination and remyelination in experimental allergic encephalomyelitis. Further electron microscope observations. *J. Neuropathol. Exp. Neurol. 24*:371–385.

Lampert, P. W. 1968. Fine structural changes of myelin sheaths in the central nervous system. In: *The Structure and Function of Nervous Tissue*, Vol. I. G. H. Bourne, Ed. New York, Academic Press, pp. 187–204.

Landis, D. M. D., and Reese, T. S. 1974a. Arrays of particles in freeze-fractured astrocytic membranes. *J. Cell Biol. 60*:316–320.

Landis, D. M. D., and Reese, T. S. 1974b. Differences in membrane structure between excitatory and inhibitory synapses in the cerebellar cortex. *J. Comp. Neurol. 155*:93–126.

Landis, D. M. D., Reese, T. S., and Raviola, E. 1974. Differences in membrane structure between excitatory and inhibitory components of the reciprocal synapse in the olfactory bulb. *J. Comp. Neurol. 155*:67–92.

Landon, D. N., and Langley, O. K. 1971. The local chemical environment of nodes of Ranvier: a study of cation binding. *J. Anat. 108*:419–432.

Lane, N. J. 1968. Distribution of phosphatases in the Golgi region and associated structures of the thoracic ganglionic neurons in the grasshopper, *Melanopus differentialis. J. Cell Biol. 37*:89–104.

Lane, N. J., and Treherne, J. E. 1970. Lanthanum staining of neurotubules in axons from cockroach ganglia. *J. Cell Sci. 7*:217–231.

Lange, W., and Halata, Z. 1972. Die Ultrastruktur der Kapillaren der Kleinhirnrinde und das perikapilläre Gewebe. *Z. Zellforsch. Mikrosk. Anat. 128*:83–99.

Langley, O. K., and Landon, D. N. 1968. A light and electron histochemical approach to the node of Ranvier and myelin of peripheral nerve fibres. *J. Histochem. Cytochem. 15*:722–731.

Langman, J. 1968. Histogenesis of the central nervous system. In: *The Structure and Function of Nervous Tissue*, Vol. I. G. H. Bourne, Ed. New York, Academic Press, pp. 33–65.

Lanterman, A. J. 1877. Ueber den feineren Bau der markhaltigen Nervenfasern. *Arch. Mikrosk. Anat. Entwicklungsmech. 13*:1–8.

Lapham, L. W. 1965. The tetraploid DNA content of normal human Purkinje cells and its development during the perinatal period. A quantitative cytochemical study. Proceedings, Fifth International Congress of Neuropathology. *Excerpta Med. Int. Congr. Ser. 100*:445–449.

Lapham, L. W. 1968. Tetraploid DNA content of Purkinje neurons of human cerebellar cortex. *Science 159*:310–312.

Larramendi, L. M. H., Fickenscher, L., and Lemkey-

Johnston, N. 1967. Synaptic vesicles of inhibitory and excitatory terminals in the cerebellum. *Science* 156:967–969.

Larramendi, L. M. H., and Victor, T. 1967. Synapses on the Purkinje cell spines in the mouse. An electron microscope study. *Brain Res.* 5:15–30.

Lascelles, R. G., and Thomas, P. K. 1966. Changes due to age in internodal length in the sural nerve in man. *J. Neurol. Neurosurg. Psychiatr.* 29: 40–44.

Lasek, R. J. 1968. Axoplasmic transport in cat dorsal root ganglion cells: as studied with [³H]-L-leucine. *Brain Res.* 7:360–377.

Lasek, R. J. 1970. Protein transport in neurons. *Int. Rev. Neurobiol.* 13:289–321.

Lasek, R. J., and Dower, W. J. 1971. *Aplysia californica:* Analysis of nuclear DNA in individual nuclei of giant neurons. *Science* 172:278–280.

Lauder, J. M., and Bloom, F. E. 1975. Ontogeny of monoamine neurons in the locus coeruleus, raphe nuclei and substantia nigra of the rat. II. Synaptogenesis. *J. Comp. Neurol.* 163:251–264.

La Vail, J. H., and La Vail, M. M. 1972. Retrograde axonal transport in the central nervous system. *Science* 176:1416–1417.

La Vail, J. H., and La Vail, M. M. 1974. The retrograde intraaxonal transport of horseradish peroxidase in the chick visual system: A light and electron microscopic study. *J. Comp. Neurol.* 157:303–357.

La Vail, J. H., Winston, K. R., and Tish, A. 1973. A method based on retrograde transport of protein for identification of cell bodies of origin of axons terminating in the CNS. *Brain Res.* 58:470–477.

LaVelle, A. 1956. Nucleolar and Nissl substance development in nerve cells. *J. Comp. Neurol.* 104:175–205.

Le Beux, Y. J. 1971. An ultrastructural study of the neurosecretory cells of the medial vascular prechiasmatic gland, the preoptic recess and the anterior part of the suprachiasmatic area. I. Cytoplasmic inclusions resembling nucleoli. *Z. Zellforsch. Mikrosk. Anat.* 114:404–440.

Le Beux, Y. J. 1972a. An ultrastructural study of a cytoplasmic filamentous body, termed nematosome, in the neurons of the rat and cat substantia nigra. The association of nematosomes with the other cytoplasmic organelles in the neuron. *Z. Zellforsch. Mikrosk. Anat.* 133:289–325.

Le Beux, Y. J. 1972b. Subsurface cisterns and lamellar bodies: particular forms of the endoplasmic reticulum in the neurons. *Z. Zellforsch. Mikrosk. Anat.* 133:327–352.

Le Beux, Y. J. 1973. An ultrastructural study of the synaptic densities, nematosomes, neurotubules, neurofilaments and of a further three-dimensional filamentous network as disclosed by the E-PTA staining procedure. *Z. Zellforsch. Mikrosk. Anat.* 143:239–272.

Le Beux, Y. J., Langelier, P., and Poirier, L. J. 1971. Further ultrastructural data on the cytoplasmic nucleolus resembling bodies or nematosomes.

Their relationship with the subsynaptic web and a cytoplasmic filamentous network. *Z. Zellforsch. Mikrosk. Anat.* 118:147–155.

Ledbetter, M. C., and Porter, K. R. 1963. A "microtubule" in plant cell fine structure. *J. Cell Biol.* 19:239–250.

Lederis, K. 1965. An electron microscopical study of the human neurohypophysis. *Z. Zellforsch. Mikrosk. Anat.* 85:847–868.

Lehninger, A. L. 1967. Cell organelles: the mitochondrion. In: *The Neurosciences.* G. C. Quarton, T. Melnechuk, and F. O. Schmitt, Eds. New York, Rockefeller University Press, pp. 91–100.

Lehninger, A. L. 1968. The neuronal membrane. *Proc. Natl. Acad. Sci. U.S.A.* 60:1069–1080.

Lemkey-Johnston, N., and Larramendi, L. M. H. 1968a. Morphological characteristics of mouse stellate and basket cells and their neuroglial envelope: An electron microscope study. *J. Comp. Neurol.* 134:39–72.

Lemkey-Johnston, N., and Larramendi, L. M. H. 1968b. Types and distribution of synapses upon basket and stellate cells of the mouse cerebellum: An electron microscopic study. *J. Comp. Neurol.* 134:73–112.

Lenn, N. J., and Reese, T. S. 1966. The fine structure of nerve endings in the nucleus of the trapezoid body and the ventral cochlear nucleus. *Am. J. Anat.* 118:375–389.

Lentz, R. D., and Lapham, L. W. 1970. Postnatal development of tetraploid DNA content in rat Purkinje cells: A quantitative cytochemical study. *J. Neuropathol. Exp. Neurol.* 29:43–56.

Lentz, T. L. 1969. Development of the neuromuscular junction. 1. Cytological and cytochemical studies on the neuromuscular junction of differentiating muscle in the regenerating limb of the newt *Triturus. J. Cell Biol.* 42:431–443.

Leonhardt, H. 1966. Über ependymale Tanycyten des III Ventrikels beim Kaninchen in elektronenmikroskopischer Betrachtung. *Z. Zellforsch. Mikrosk. Anat.* 74:1–11.

Leonhardt, H. 1967a. Über die Blutkapillaren und perivaskulären Strukturen der Area Postrema des Kaninchens und über ihr Verhalten im Pentamethylentetrazol-("Carbiazol")-Kampf. *Z. Zellforsch. Mikrosk. Anat.* 76:511–524.

Leonhardt, H. 1967b. Zur Frage einer intraventrikulären Neurosekretion. Eine bisher unbekannte nervöse Struktur im IV. Ventrikel des Kaninchens. *Z. Zellforsch. Mikrosk. Anat.* 79:172–184.

Leonhardt, H. 1968. Intraventrikuläre markhaltige Nervenfasern nahe des Apertura lateralis ventriculi quarti des Kaninchengehirns. *Z. Zellforsch. Mikrosk. Anat.* 84:1–8.

Leonhardt, H. 1970. Subependymale Basalmembranlabyrinthe im Hinterhorn des Seitenventrikels des Kaninchengehirns. Zur Frage des Liquorabflusses. *Z. Zellforsch. Mikrosk. Anat.* 105:595–604.

Leonhardt, H., and Backhus-Roth, A. 1969. Synapsenartige Kontakte zwischen intraventrikularen Axonendigungen und freien Oberflächer von Ependymzellen des Kaninchengehirns. *Z. Zellforsch. Mikrosk. Anat.* 97:369–376.

Leonhardt, H., and Lindemann, B. 1973a. Surface morphology of the subfornical organ in the rabbit's brain. *Z. Zellforsch. Mikrosk. Anat.* 146:243–260.

Leonhardt, H., and Lindemann, B. 1973b. Über ein supraependymales Nervenzell-, Axon- und Gliazellsystem. Eine raster- und transmissions elektronenmikroskopische Untersuchung an IV Ventrikel (Apertura lateralis) des Kaninchengehirns. *Z. Zellforsch. Mikrosk. Anat.* 139:185–302.

Leonhardt, H., and Lindner, E. 1967. Marklose Nervenfaseren im III. und IV. Ventrikel des Kaninchen- und Katzengehirns. *Z. Zellforsch. Mikrosk. Anat.* 78:1–18.

Leonhardt, H., and Prien, H. 1968. Eine weitere Art intraventrikularer Kolbenformiger Axonendingungen aus dem IV. Ventrikel des Kaninchengehirns. *Z. Zellforsch. Mikrosk. Anat.* 92:394–399.

LeVay, S. 1971. On the neurons and synapses of the lateral geniculate nucleus of the monkey and the effects of eye enucleation. *Z. Zellforsch. Mikrosk. Anat.* 113:396–419.

LeVay, S. 1973. Synaptic patterns in the visual cortex of the cat and monkey. Electron microscopy of Golgi preparations. *J. Comp. Neurol.* 150:53–85.

Levi, G. 1916. Sull'origine delle reti nervose nelle colture di tessuti. *Rendiconti R. Accad. Lincei, Cl. Sci. Fis. Mat. Nat.* 25:Ser. 5a.

Levine, Y. K. 1972. Physical studies of membrane structure. In: *Progress in Biophysics and Molecular Biology*, Vol. 24. J. A. V. Butler and D. Noble, Eds. Oxford, Pergamon Press, pp. 1–74.

Lewis, P. D. 1968a. A quantitative study of cell proliferation in the subependymal layer of the adult rat brain. *Exp. Neurol.* 20:203–207.

Lewis, P. D. 1968b. The fate of the subependymal cell in the adult rat brain, with a note on the origins of microglia. *Brain* 91:721–736.

Lieberman, A. R. 1968. The connective tissue elements of the mammalian nodose ganglion. An electron microscope study. *Z. Zellforsch. Mikrosk. Anat.* 89:95–111.

Lieberman, A. R. 1971a. Microtubule associated smooth endoplasmic reticulum in the frog's brain. *Z. Zellforsch. Mikrosk. Anat.* 116:564–577.

Lieberman, A. R. 1971b. The axon reaction. A review of the principal features of perikaryal responses to axon injury. *Int. Rev. Neurobiol.* 14:49–124.

Lieberman, A. R. 1973. Neurons with presynaptic perikarya and presynaptic dendrites in the rat lateral geniculate nucleus. *Brain Res.* 59:35–59.

Lieberman, A. R. 1974a. Comments on the fine structural organization of the dorsal lateral geniculate nucleus of the mouse. *Z. Anat. Entwicklungsgesch.* 145:261–267.

Lieberman, A. R. 1974b. Some factors affecting retrograde neuronal responses to axonal lesions. In: *Essays on the Nervous System.* R. Bellairs and E.

G. Gray, Eds. London, Oxford University Press, pp. 71–105.

Lieberman, A. R., Špaček, J., and Webster, K. E. 1971. Unusual organelles in rat thalamic neurons. *J. Anat.* 109:365.

Lieberman, A. R., and Webster, K. E. 1972. Presynaptic dendrites and a distinctive class of synaptic vesicle in the rat dorsal lateral geniculate body. *Brain Res.* 42:196–200.

Lieberman, A. R., and Webster, K. E. 1974. Aspects of the synaptic organization of intrinsic neurons in the dorsal lateral geniculate nucleus. An ultrastructural study of the normal and of the experimentally deafferented nucleus in the rat. *J. Neurocytol.* 3:677–710.

Lieberman, A. R., Webster, K. E., Špaček, J. 1972. Multiple myelinated branches from nodes of Ranvier in the central nervous system. *Brain Res.* 44:652–655.

Livingston, R. B. 1949. Cerebrospinal fluid. In: *A Textbook of Physiology.* J. F. Fulton, Ed. Philadelphia, W. B. Saunders Co., pp. 908–916.

Livingston, R. B., Pfenninger, K., Moor, H., and Akert, K. 1973. Specialized paranodal and interparanodal glial-axonal junctions in the peripheral and central nervous system: a freeze-etching study. *Brain Res.* 58:1–24.

Llinás, R., Baker, R., and Sotelo, C. 1974. Electrotonic coupling between neurons in cat inferior olive. *Brain Res.* 67:560–571.

Llinás, R., and Hillman, D. E. 1969. Physiological and morphological organization of the cerebellar circuits in various vertebrates. In: *Neurobiology of Cerebellar Evolution and Development.* R. Llinás, Ed. Chicago, AMA-ERF Institute for Biomedical Research, pp. 43–73.

Lloret, I. L. P., and Saavedra, J. P. 1975. Enlargement of synaptic vesicles in degenerating nerve endings: a comparison between cat and monkey. *J. Neurocytol.* 4:1–6.

Löfgren, F. 1959. The infundibular recess, a component of the hypothalamic-adenohypophyseal system. *Acta Morphol. Neerl. Scand.* 3:55–78.

Lorez, H. P., and Richards, J. G. 1973. Distribution of indolealkylamine nerve terminals in the ventricles of the rat brain. *Z. Zellforsch. Mikrosk. Anat.* 144:511–522.

Lovas, B. 1971. Tubular networks in the terminal endings of the visual receptor cells in the human, the monkey, the cat and the dog. *Z. Zellforsch. Mikrosk. Anat.* 121:341–357.

Lowenstein, W. R., and Kanno, Y. 1964. Studies on an epithelial (gland) cell junction. I. Modifications of surface membrane permeability. *J. Cell Biol.* 22:565–586.

Lubínska, L. 1958. "Intercalated" internodes in nerve fibres. *Nature (Lond.)* 181:957–958.

Lubínska, L. 1961. Sedentary and migratory states of Schwann cells. *Exp. Cell Res. Suppl.* 8:74–90.

Lubínska, L. 1975. On axoplasmic flow. *Int. Rev. Neurobiol.* 17:241–296.

Lubínska, L., and Niemierko, S. 1971. Velocity and

intensity of bidirectional migration of acetylcholinesterase in transected nerves. *Brain Res.* 27:329–342.

Luft, J. H. 1971. Ruthenium red and violet. II. Fine structural localization in animal tissues. *Anat. Rec.* 171:369–416.

Lund, J. S., and Lund, R. D. 1972. The effects of varying periods of visual deprivation on synaptogenesis in the superior colliculus of the rat. *Brain Res.* 42:21–32.

Lund, R. D. 1969. Synaptic patterns of the superficial layers of the superior colliculus of the rat. *J. Comp. Neurol.* 135:179–208.

Lund, R. D. 1972. Synaptic patterns in the superficial layer of the superior colliculus of the monkey, *Macaca mulatta. Exp. Brain Res.* 15:194–211.

Lund, R. D., and Westrum, L. E. 1966. Synaptic vesicle differences after primary formalin fixation. *J. Physiol. (Lond.)* 185:7P–9P.

Lynch, G., Gall, C., Mensah, P., and Cotman, C. W. 1974. Horseradish peroxidase histochemistry: a new method for tracing efferent projections in the central nervous system. *Brain Res.* 65:373–380.

Machen, T. E., Erlij, D. and Wooding, F. B. P. 1972. Permeable junctional complexes. The movement of lanthanum across rabbit gall-bladder and intestine. *J. Cell Biol.* 54:302–312.

Maciewicz, R. J. 1974. Afferents to the lateral suprasylvian gyrus of the cat traced with horseradish peroxidase. *Brain Res.* 78:139–143.

Magalhães, M. M. 1967. Intranuclear bodies in cells of rabbit and rat retina. *Exp. Cell Res.* 47:628–632.

Majorossy, K., Réthelyi, M., and Szentágothai, J. 1965. The large glomerular synapse of the pulvinar. *J. Hirnforsch.* 7:415–432.

Malloy, J. J., and Low, F. N. 1974. Scanning electron microscopy of the subarachnoid space in the dog. II. Spinal nerve exits. *J. Comp. Neurol.* 157:87–107.

Malmgren, L. T., and Brink, J. J. 1975. Permeability barriers to cytochrome-C in nerves of adult and immature rats. *Anat. Rec.* 181:755–766.

Mann, D. M. A., and Yates, P. O. 1973. Polyploidy in the human nervous system. I. The DNA content of neurons and glia of the cerebellum. *J. Neurol. Sci.* 18:183–196.

Mann, D. M. A., and Yates, P. O. 1974. Lipoprotein pigments—Their relationship to aging in the human nervous system. I. The lipofuscin content of nerve cells. *Brain* 97:481–488.

Mannen, H. 1966. Contribution to the quantitative study of the nervous tissue. A new method for measurement of the volume and surface area of neurons. *J. Comp. Neurol.* 126:75–89.

Manuelidis, L., and Manuelidis, E. E. 1972. The proliferation and differentiation of glial cells *in vitro. J. Neuropathol. Exp. Neurol.* 31:193 (abstract).

Manuelidis, L., and Manuelidis, E. E. 1974. On the DNA content of cerebellar Purkinje cells *in vivo* and *in vitro. Exp. Neurol.* 43:192–206.

Marcarian, H. Q., and Smith, R. D. 1968. A quantita-

tive study on the vasa nervorum in the ulnar nerve of cats. *Anat. Rec.* 161:105–110.

Marchbanks, R. M. 1969. Biochemical organization of cholinergic nerve terminals in the cerebral cortex. In: *Symposium of the International Society for Cell Biology,* Vol. 8, *Cellular Dynamics of the Neuron.* S. H. Barondes, Ed. New York, Academic Press, pp. 115–135.

Marchbanks, R. M. 1975. The subcellular origin of the acetylcholine released at synapses. *Int. J. Biochem.* 6:303–312.

Marchesi, V. T., and Barrnett, R. J. 1964. The localization of nucleosidephosphatase activity in different types of small blood vessels. *J. Ultrastruct. Res.* 10:103–115.

Mareš, V., Lodin, Z., and Šácha, J. 1973. A cytochemical and autoradiographic study of nuclear DNA in mouse Purkinje cells. *Brain Res.* 53:273–289.

Mareš, V., Schultze, B., and Maurer, W. 1974. Stability of DNA in Purkinje cell nuclei of the mouse. An autoradiographic study. *J. Cell Biol.* 63:665–674.

Marinesco, G. 1909. *La Cellule Nerveuse.* Vols. I and II. Paris, Doin.

Marin-Padilla, M. 1967. Number and distribution of the apical dendritic spines of the layer V pyramidal cells in man. *J. Comp. Neurol.* 131:475–490.

Marin-Padilla, M. 1974. Structural organization of the cerebral cortex (motor area) in human chromosomal aberrations. A Golgi study. 1. D_1 (13–15) trisomy, Patau syndrome. *Brain Res.* 66:375–391.

Martin, A. R., and Miledi, R. 1975. A presynaptic complex in the giant synapse of the squid. *J. Neurocytol.* 4:121–129.

Martin, A. R., and Pilar, G. 1963a. Dual mode of synaptic transmission in the avian ciliary ganglion. *J. Physiol. (Lond.)* 168:443–463.

Martin, A. R., and Pilar, G. 1963b. Transmission through the ciliary ganglion of the chick. *J. Physiol. (Lond.)* 168:464–475.

Martin, A. R., and Pilar, G. 1964. An analysis of electrical coupling at synapses in the avian ciliary ganglion. *J. Physiol. (Lond.)* 171:454–475.

Martin, J. R., and Webster, H. deF. 1973. Mitotic Schwann cells in developing nerve: their changes in shape, fine structure and axon relationships. *Dev. Biol.* 32:417–431.

Marx, R., Graf, E., and Wesemann, W. 1973. Histochemical and biochemical demonstration of sialic acid and sulphate in vesicles and membranes isolated from nerve endings of rat brain. *J. Cell Sci.* 13:237–255.

Massing, W., and Fleischhauer, K. 1973. Further observations on vertical bundles of dendrites in the cerebral cortex of the rabbit. *Z. Anat. Entwicklungsgesch.* 141:115–123.

Masurovsky, E. B., Benitez, H. H., Kim, S.-U., and Murray, M. R. 1968. Development and nature of intranuclear rodlets and associated bodies in chicken sympathetic neurons. *J. Cell Biol.* 39:86A–87A.

Masurovsky, E. B., Benitez, H. H., Kim, S.-U., and

Murray, M. R. 1970. Origin, development, and nature of intranuclear rodlets and associated bodies in chicken sympathetic neurons. *J. Cell Biol. 44*:172–191.

Mathieu, A. M., and Colonnier, M. 1968. Electron microscopic observations in the molecular layer of the cat cerebellar cortex after section of the parallel fibers. *Anat. Rec. 160*:391 (abstract).

Matthews, M. A. 1968. An electron microscopic study of the relationship between axon diameter and the initiation of myelin production in the peripheral nervous system. *Anat. Rec. 161*:337–351.

Matthews, M. A., and Duncan, D. 1971. A quantitative study of the morphological changes accompanying the initiation and progress of myelin production in the dorsal funiculus of the rat spinal cord. *J. Comp. Neurol. 142*:1–22.

Matthews, M. A., and Kruger, L. 1973a. Electron microscopy of non-neuronal cellular changes accompanying neural degeneration in thalamic nuclei of the rabbit. I. Reactive hematogenous and perivascular elements within the basal lamina. *J. Comp. Neurol. 148*:285:312.

Matthews, M. A., and Kruger, L. 1973b. Electron microscopy of non-neuronal cellular changes accompanying neural degeneration in thalamic nuclei of the rabbit. II. Reactive elements within the neuropil. *J. Comp. Neurol. 148*:313–346.

Matthews, M. R., and Nash, J. R. G. 1970. An efferent synapse from a small granule-containing cell to a principal neurone in the superior cervical ganglion. *J. Physiol. (Lond.) 210*:11P–13P.

Matthews, M. R., and Raisman, G. 1969. The ultrastructure and somatic efferent synapses of small granule-containing cells in the superior cervical ganglion. *J. Anat. 105*:255–282.

Matthews, M. R., and Raisman, G. 1972. A light and electron microscopic study of the cellular response to axonal injury in the superior cervical ganglion of the rat. *Proc. R. Soc. Ser. B 181*:43–79.

Maturana, H. R. 1960. The fine anatomy of the optic nerve of Anurans—an electron microscope study. *J. Biophys. Biochem. Cytol. 7*:107–120.

Matus, A. I., and Dennison, M. E. 1971. Autoradiographic localization of tritiated glycine at 'flat vesicle' synapses in spinal cord. *Brain Res. 32*:195–197.

Matus, A. I., Walters, B. B., and Mughal, S. 1975. Immunohistochemical demonstration of tubulin associated with microtubules and synaptic junctions in mammalian brain. *J. Neurocytol. 4*:733–744.

Maul, G. G., Price, J. W., and Lieberman, M. W. 1971. Formation and distribution of nuclear pore complexes in interphase. *J. Cell Biol. 51*:405–418.

Maxwell, D. S., and Kruger, L. 1965a. The fine structure of astrocytes in the cerebral cortex and their response to focal injury produced by heavy ionizing particles. *J. Cell Biol. 25*(No. 2, Part 2):141–157.

Maxwell, D. S., and Kruger, L. 1965b. Small blood vessels and the origin of phagocytes in the rat cerebral cortex following heavy particle irradiation. *Exp. Neurol. 12*:33–54.

Maxwell, D. S., Kruger, L., and Pineda, A. 1969. The trigeminal nerve root with special reference to the central-peripheral transition zone: an electron microscope study in the Macaque. *Anat. Rec. 164*:113–126.

Maxwell, D. S., and Pease, D. C. 1956. The electron microscopy of the choroid plexus. *J. Biophys. Biochem. Cytol. 2*:467–476.

Maynard, E. A., Schultz, R. L., and Pease, D. C. 1957. Electron microscopy of the vascular bed of rat cerebral cortex. *Am. J. Anat. 100*:409–433.

McDonald, D. M., and Mitchell, R. A. 1975. The innervation of glomus cells, ganglion cells and blood vessels in the rat carotid body: a quantitative ultrastructural analysis. *J. Neurocytol. 4*:177–230.

McDonald, D. M., and Rasmussen, G. L. 1971. Ultrastructural characteristics of synaptic endings in the cochlear nucleus having acetylcholinesterase activity. *Brain Res. 28*:1–18.

McDonald, W. J., and Ohlrich, G. D. 1971. Quantitative anatomical measurements on simple isolated fibres from the cat spinal cord. *J. Anat. 110*:191–202.

McEwen, B. S., Forman, D. S., and Grafstein, B. 1971. Components of fast and slow axonal transport in the goldfish optic nerve. *J. Neurobiol. 2*:361–377.

McFarland, D. E., and Friede, R. L. 1971. Number of fibers per sheath cell and internodal length in cat cranial nerves. *J. Anat. 109*:169–176.

McIntosh, J. R., Ogata, E. S., and Landis, S. C. 1973. The axostyle of *Saccinobacalus*. I. Structure of the organism and its microtubule bundle. *J. Cell Biol. 56*:304–323.

McLaughlin, B. J., Wood, J. G., Saito, K., Barber, R., Roberts, E., and Wu, J. -Y. 1974. Fine structural localization of glutamic acid decarboxylase in adult and developing cerebellum in rodents. *Anat. Rec. 178*:407–408.

McLaughlin, B. J., Wood, J. G., Saito, K., Barber, R., Vaughn, J. E., Roberts, E., and Wu, J. -Y. 1974. The fine structural localization of glutamate decarboxylase in synaptic terminals of rodent cerebellum. *Brain Res. 76*:377–391.

McLone, D. G., and Bondareff, W. 1975. Developmental morphology of the subarachnoid space and contiguous structures in the mouse. *Am. J. Anat. 142*:273–294.

McMahan, U. J. 1967. Fine structure of synapses in the dorsal nucleus of the lateral geniculate body in normal and blinded rats. *Z. Zellforsch. Mikrosk. Anat. 76*:116–146.

McMahan, U. J., Spitzer, N. C., and Peper, K. 1972. Visual identification of nerve terminals in living isolated skeletal muscle. *Proc. R. Soc. Ser. B. 181*:421–430.

McNutt, N. S., and Weinstein, R. S. 1970. The ultrastructure of the nexus. A correlated thin-section and freeze-cleave study. *J. Cell Biol. 47*:666–688.

Merker, G. 1970. Fasergliastruktur der dorsalen Wand

des Aquaeductus cerebri bei einigen Primaten. Z. *Zellforsch. Mikrosk. Anat.* 107:564–585.

Metuzals, J. 1960. Ultrastructure of myelinated nerve fibers and nodes of Ranvier in the central nervous system of the frog. In: *The Proceedings of the European Regional Conference on Electron Microscopy,* Delft 1960. A. L. Houwink and B. J. Spit, Eds. Delft, Nederlandse Vereniging voor Electronenmicroscopie, Vol. 2, pp. 799–802.

Metuzals, J. 1963. Ultrastructure of myelinated nerve fibers in the central nervous system of the frog. *J. Ultrastruct. Res.* 8:30–47.

Metuzals, J. 1965. Ultrastructure of the nodes of Ranvier and their surrounding structures in the central nervous system. *Z. Zellforsch. Mikrosk. Anat.* 65:719–759.

Metuzals, J., and Mushynski, W. E. 1974. Electron microscope and experimental investigations of the neurofilamentous network in Deiters' neurons. Relationship with the cell surface and nuclear pores. *J. Cell Biol.* 61:701–722.

Mezler, R. M., Pappas, G. D., and Bennett, M. V. L. 1972. Morphological demonstration of electrotonic coupling of neurons by way of presynaptic fibers. *Brain Res.* 37:412–415.

Mezler, R. M., Pappas, G. D., and Bennett, M. V. L. 1974. Morphology of the electromotor system in the spinal cord of the electric eel, *Electrophorus electricus. J. Neurocytol.* 3:251–261.

Miale, I. L., and Sidman, R. L. 1961. An autoradiographic analysis of histogenesis in the mouse cerebellum. *Exp. Neurol.* 4:277–296.

Milhaud, M., and Pappas, G. D. 1966a. Post-synaptic bodies in the habenula and interpeduncular nuclei of the cat. *J. Cell Biol.* 30:437–441.

Milhaud, M., and Pappas, G. D. 1966b. The fine structure of neurons and synapses of the habenula of the cat with special reference to sub-junctional bodies. *Brain Res.* 3:158–173.

Milhaud, M., and Pappas, G. D. 1968. Cilia formation in the adult cat brain after pargyline treatment. *J. Cell Biol.* 37:599–609.

Millen, J. W., and Rogers, G. E. 1956. An electron microscopic study of the choroid plexus in the rabbit. *J. Biophys. Biochem. Cytol.* 2:407–415.

Millen, J. W., and Woollam, D. H. M. 1961. On the nature of the pia mater. *Brain* 84:514–520.

Millen, J. W., and Woollam, D. H. M. 1962. *The Anatomy of the Cerebrospinal Fluid.* London, Oxford University Press.

Millhouse, O. E. 1971. A Golgi study of third ventricle tanycytes in the adult rodent brain. *Z. Zellforsch. Mikrosk. Anat.* 121:1–13.

Millhouse, O. E. 1972. Light and electron microscope studies of the ventricular wall. *Z. Zellforsch. Mikrosk. Anat.* 127:149–174.

Miranda, A. F., Godman, G. C., Deitch, A. D., and Tanenbaum, S. W. 1974. Action of cytochalasin D on cells of established lines. I. Early events. *J. Cell Biol.* 61:481–500.

Miyagishi, T., Takahata, M., and Lizuka, R. 1967. Electron microscopic studies on the lipopigments

in the cerebral cortex nerve cells of senile and vitamin E deficient rats. *Acta Neuropathol.* 9:7–17.

Moe, H., Rostgaard, J., and Behnke, O. 1965. On the morphology and origin of virgin lysosomes in the intestinal epithelium of rat. *J. Ultrastruct. Res.* 12:396–403.

Mokrasch, L. C., Bear, R. S., and Schmitt, F. O. 1971. Myelin. A report based on an NRP work session. *Neurosci. Res. Progr. Bull.* 9:440–598.

Mollenhauer, H. H., and Whaley, W. G. 1963. An observation on the functioning of the Golgi apparatus. *J. Cell Biol.* 17:222–225.

Monneron, A., and Bernhard, W. 1969. Fine structural organization of the interphase nucleus in some mammalian cells. *J. Ultrastruct. Res.* 27:266–288.

Moore, K. L., and Barr, M. L. 1953. Morphology of the nerve cell nucleus in mammals, with special reference to the sex chromatin. *J. Comp. Neurol.* 98:213–231.

Morales, R., and Duncan, D. 1966. Multilaminated bodies and other unusual configurations of endoplasmic reticulum in the cerebellum of the cat. An electron microscopic study. *J. Ultrastruct. Res.* 15:480–489.

Morales, R., and Duncan, D. 1971. Prismatic and other unusual arrays of mitochondrial cristae in astrocytes of cats and hamsters. *Anat. Rec.* 171:545–551.

Morales, R., Duncan, D., and Rehmet, R. 1964. A distinctive laminated cytoplasmic body in the lateral geniculate body neurons of the cat. *J. Ultrastruct. Res.* 10:116–123.

Morest, D. K. 1965. The laminar structure of the medial geniculate body of the cat. *J. Anat.* 99:143–160.

Morest, D. K. 1969a. The differentiation of cerebral dendrites: a study of the post-migratory neuroblast in the medial nucleus of the trapezoid body. *Z. Anat. Entwicklungsgesch.* 133:216–246.

Morest, D. K. 1969b. The growth of dendrites in the mammalian brain. *Z. Anat. Entwicklungsgesch.* 128:290–317.

Morest, D. K. 1970. Electron microscopic study of the synaptic organization in the geniculate body of the cat. *Anat. Rec.* 166:351.

Morest, D. K. 1971. Dendrodendritic synapses of cells that have axons: the fine structure of the Golgi type II cell in the medial geniculate body of the cat. *Z. Anat. Entwicklungsgesch.* 133:216–246.

Mori, S. 1966. Some observations on the fine structure of the corpus striatum of the rat brain. *Z. Zellforsch. Mikrosk. Anat.* 70:461–488.

Mori, S., and Leblond, C. P. 1969a. Identification of microglia in light and electron microscopy. *J. Comp. Neurol.* 135:57–80.

Mori, S., and Leblond, C. P. 1969b. Electron microscopic features and proliferation of astrocytes in the corpus callosum of the rat. *J. Comp. Neurol.* 137:197–226.

Mori, S., and Leblond, C. P. 1970. Electron microscopic identification of three classes of oligodendrocytes and a preliminary study of their proliferative activity in the corpus callosum of young rats. *J. Comp. Neurol.* 139:1–30.

Morris, J. H., Hudson, A. R., and Weddell, G. 1972a. A study of degeneration and regeneration in the divided rat sciatic nerve based on electron microscopy. I. The traumatic degeneration of myelin in the proximal stump of the divided nerve. *Z. Zellforsch. Mikrosk. Anat.* 124:76–102.

Morris, J. H., Hudson, A. R., and Weddell, G. 1972b. A study of degeneration and regeneration in the divided rat sciatic nerve based on electron microscopy. II. The development of the "regenerating unit." *Z. Zellforsch. Mikrosk. Anat.* 124:103–130.

Morris, J. H., Hudson, A. R., and Weddell, G. 1972c. A study of degeneration and regeneration in the divided rat sciatic nerve based on electron microscopy. III. Changes in the axons of the proximal stump. *Z. Zellforsch. Mikrosk. Anat.* 124:131–164.

Morris, J. H., Hudson, A. R., and Weddell, G. 1972d. A study of degeneration and regeneration in the divided rat sciatic nerve based on electron microscopy. IV. Changes in fascicular microtopography, perineurium and endoneurial fibroblasts. *Z. Zellforsch. Mikrosk. Anat.* 124:165–203.

Morrison, L. R. 1931. The role of oligodendroglia in myelinogenesis. *Trans. Am. Neurol. Assoc.* 57:444–450.

Morse, D. E., and Low, F. N. 1972a. The fine structure of the pia mater of the rat. *Am. J. Anat.* 133:349–368.

Morse, D. E., and Low, F. N. 1972b. The fine structure of subarachnoid macrophages in the rat. *Anat. Rec.* 174:469–476.

Mountford, S. 1963. Effects of light and dark adaptation on the vesicle populations of receptor-bipolar synapses. *J. Ultrastruct. Res.* 9:403–418.

Mugnaini, E. 1964. Helical filaments in astrocytic mitochondria of the corpus striatum in the rat. *J. Cell Biol.* 23:173–182.

Mugnaini, E. 1965. "Dark cells" in electron micrographs from the central nervous system of vertebrates. *J. Ultrastruct. Res.* 12:235–236.

Mugnaini, E. 1967. On the occurrence of filamentous rodlets in neurons and glia cells of *Myxine glutinosa* (L.). *Sarsi* 29:221–232.

Mugnaini, E. 1970. The relation between cytogenesis and the formation of different types of synaptic contact. *Brain Res.* 17:169–179.

Mugnaini, E. 1972. The histology and cytology of the cerebellar cortex. In: *The Comparative Anatomy and Histology of the Cerebellum: The Human Cerebellum, Cerebellar Connections and Cerebellar Cortex.* O. Larsell and J. Jansen, Eds. Minneapolis, University of Minnesota Press, pp. 201–262.

Mugnaini, E., and Schnapp, B. 1974. Possible role of zonula occludens of the myelin sheath in demyelinating conditions. *Nature (Lond.)* 251:725–727.

Mugnaini, E., and Walberg, F. 1964. Ultrastructure of neuroglia. *Ergeb. Anat. Entwicklungsgesch.* 37:194–236.

Mugnaini, E., Walberg, F., and Hauglie-Hanssen, E. 1967. Observations on the fine structure of the lateral vestibular nucleus (Deiters' nucleus) in the cat. *Exp. Brain Res.* 4:146–186.

Muir, A. R., and Peters, A. 1962. Quintuple layered membrane junctions at terminal bars between endothelial cells. *J. Cell Biol.* 12:443–448.

Mungai, J. M. 1967. Dendritic patterns in the somatic sensory cortex of the cat. *J. Anat.* 101:403–418.

Munro, H. N., Roel, L., and Wurtman, R. J. 1973. Inhibition of brain protein synthesis by doses of L-Dopa that disaggregate brain polysomes. *J. Neural Transm.* 34:321–323.

Murray, M. R. 1959. Factors bearing on myelin formation in vitro. In: *The Biology of Myelin.* S. R. Korey, Ed. New York, Hoeber, pp. 201–221.

Murray, M. R. 1965. Nervous Tissue *in vitro.* In: *Cells and Tissues in Culture,* Vol. 2. E. N. Willmer, Ed. New York, Academic Press, pp. 373–456.

Murray, M. R., and Herrmann, A. 1968. Passive movements of Schmidt-Lantermann clefts during continuous observation *in vitro. J. Cell Biol.* 39:149a.

Nabeshima, S., Reese, T. S., Landis, D. M. D., and Brightman, M. W. 1975. Junctions in the meninges and marginal glia. *J. Comp. Neurol.* 164:127–170.

Nageotte, J. 1910. Phénomènes de sécrétion dans le protoplasma des cellules névrogliques de la substance grise. *C. R. Soc. Biol. Paris* 68:1068–1069.

Nageotte, J. 1932. Sheaths of the peripheral nerves. Nerve degeneration and regeneration. In: *Cytology and Cellular Pathology of the Nervous System.* W. Penfield, Ed. New York, Hoeber, pp. 189–240.

Nakajima, Y. 1974. Fine structure of the synaptic endings on the Mauthner cell of the goldfish. *J. Comp. Neurol.* 156:375–402.

Nanda, B. S., and Getty, K. 1973. Occurrence of aging pigment (lipofuscin) in the nuclei and cortices of the canine brain. *Exp. Gerontol.* 8:1–17.

Nandy, K. 1968. Further studies on the effects of centrophenoxine on the lipofuscin pigment in the neurons of senile guinea pigs. *J. Gerontol.* 23:82–92.

Nandy, K. 1971. Properties of neuronal lipofuscin pigment in mice. *Acta Neuropathol.* 19:25–32.

Nandy, K., and Bourne, G. 1966. Effects of centrophenoxine on the lipofuscin pigment in neurons of senile guinea pig. *Nature (Lond.)* 210:313–314.

Napolitano, L., LeBaron, F., and Scaletti, J. 1967. Preservation of myelin lamellar structure in the absence of lipid: A correlated chemical and morphological study. *J. Cell Biol.* 34:817–826.

Napolitano, L. M., and Scallen, T. J. 1969. Observations on the fine structure of peripheral nerve myelin. *Anat. Rec.* 163:1–6.

Nathaniel, E. J. H., and Nathaniel, D. R. 1966. Fine structure of the neurons of the posterior horn in the rat spinal cord. *Anat. Rec.* 155:629–641.

Nathaniel, E. J. H., and Pease, D. C. 1963. Collagen and basement membrane formation by Schwann cells during nerve regeneration. *J. Ultrastruct. Res.* 9:550–560.

Nauta, H. J. W., Kaiserman-Abramof, I. R., and Lasek, R. J. 1975. Electron microscopic observations of horseradish peroxidase transported from the caudoputamen to the substantia nigra in the rat: possible involvement of the agranular reticulum. *Brain Res.* 85:373–384.

Nauta, H. J. W., Pritz, M. B., and Lasek, R. J. 1974. Afferents to the rat caudoputamen studied with horseradish peroxidase. An evaluation of a retrograde neuroanatomical research method. *Brain Res.* 67:219–238.

Neal, M. J., and Iversen, L. L. 1972. Autoradiographic localization of ³H-GABA in rat retina. *Nature (New Biology)* 235:217–218.

Nelson, E., Blinzinger, K., and Hager, H. 1962. Ultrastructural observations on phagocytosis of bacteria in experimental *(E. coli)* meningitis. *J. Neuropathol. Exp. Neurol.* 21:155–169.

Netsky, M. G., and Shuangshoti, S. 1970. Studies on the choroid plexus. In: *Neurosciences Research*, Vol. 3. S. Ehrenpreis and O. C. Solnitzky, Eds. New York, Academic Press, pp. 131–173.

Neutra, M., and Leblond, C. P. 1966a. Synthesis of the carbohydrate of mucus in the Golgi complex as shown by electron microscope radioautography of goblet cells from rats injected with glucose-H³. *J. Cell Biol.* 30:119–136.

Neutra, M., and Leblond, C. P. 1966b. Radioautographic comparison of the uptake of galactose-H³ and glucose-H³ in the Golgi region of various cells secreting glycoprotein or mucopolysaccharides. *J. Cell Biol.* 30:137–150.

Nickel, E., and Potter, L. T. 1970. Synaptic vesicles in freeze-etched electric tissue of Torpedo. *Brain Res.* 23:95–100.

Nissl, F. 1892. Über die Veränderungen der Ganglienzellen am Facialiskern des Kaninchens nach Ausreissung der Nerven. *Allg. Z. Psychiatr.* 48:197–198.

Nissl, F. 1894. Über die soganannten Granula der Nervenzellen. *Neurol. Zentralb.* 13:676–685 and 781–789.

Nissl, F. 1899. Ueber einige Beziehungen zwischen Nervenzellenerkrankungen und gliösen Erscheinungen bei verschiedenen Psychosen. *Arch. Psychiatr.* 32:656–676.

Nissl, F. 1903. *Die Neuronlehre und ihre Anhänger.* Jena, Fischer.

Noack, W., Dumitrescu, L., and Schweichel, J. U. 1972. Scanning and electron microscopical investigations of the surface of the lateral ventricles in the cat. *Brain Res.* 46:121–129.

Norton, W. T. 1972. Myelin. In: *Basic Neurochemistry.* R. W. Albers, G. J. Siegel, R. Katzman, and B. W. Agranoff, Eds. Boston, Little, Brown and Co., pp. 365–386.

Nosal, G., and Radouco-Thomas, C. 1971. Ultrastructural study of the differentiation and development of the nerve cell; the "nucleus-ribosome" system.

In: *Advances in Cytopharmacology.* Vol. I. *First International Symposium on Cell Biology and Cytopharmacology.* New York, Raven Press, pp. 433–456.

Novikoff, A. B. 1967a. Enzyme localization and ultrastructure of neurons. In: *The Neuron.* H. Hydén, Ed. Amsterdam, Elsevier, pp. 255–318.

Novikoff, A. B. 1967b. Lysosomes in nerve cells. In: *The Neuron.* H. Hydén, Ed. Amsterdam, Elsevier, pp. 319–377.

Novikoff, A. B., Essner, E., and Quintana, N. 1964. Golgi apparatus and lysosomes. *Fed. Proc.* 23:1010–1022.

Novikoff, A. B., and Goldfischer, S. 1961. Nucleosidediphosphatase activity in the Golgi apparatus and its usefulness for cytological studies. *Proc. Natl. Acad. Sci. U.S.A.* 47:802–810.

Novikoff, A. B., and Shin, W.-Y. 1964. The endoplasmic reticulum in the Golgi zone and its relations to microbodies, Golgi apparatus and autophagic vacuoles in rat liver cells. *J. Microscopie* 3:187–206.

Novikoff, P. M., Novikoff, A. B., Quintana, N., and Hauw, J. J. 1971. Golgi apparatus, GERL, and lysosomes of neurons in rat dorsal root ganglion, studies by thick section and thin section cytochemistry. *J. Cell Biol.* 50:859–886.

Ochoa, J. 1971. The sural nerve of the human fetus: electron microscope observations and counts of axons. *J. Anat.* 108:231–245.

Ochs, S. 1971. Characteristics and a model for fast axoplasmic transport in nerve. *J. Neurobiol.* 2:331–345.

Ochs, S. 1972. Rate of fast axoplasmic transport in mammalian nerve fibres. *J. Physiol. (Lond.)* 227:627–645.

O'Connor, T. M., and Wyttenbach, C. R. 1974. Cell death in the embryonic chick spinal cord. *J. Cell Biol.* 60:448–459.

Oemichen, M., Grüninger, H., Saebich, R., and Narita, Y. 1973. Mikroglia und Pericyten als Transformationsformen der Blut-Monocyten mit erhaltener Proliferations fähigkeit. *Acta Neuropathol.* 23:200–218.

Ogden, T. E. 1966. Intraretinal slow potentials evoked by brain stimulation in the primate. *J. Neurophysiol.* 29:898–908.

Olsson, Y. 1968. Topographical differences in the vascular permeability of the peripheral nervous system. *Acta Neuropathol. (Berl.)* 10:26–33.

Olsson, Y. 1971. Studies on vascular permeability in peripheral nerves. IV. Distribution of intravenously injected protein tracers in the peripheral nervous system of various species. *Acta. Neuropathol. (Berl.)* 17:114–126.

Olsson, Y., and Reese, T. S. 1971. Permeability of vasa nervorum and perineurium in mouse sciatic nerve studied by fluorescence and electron microscopy. *J. Neuropathol. Exp. Neurol.* 30:105–119.

Ondo, J. G., Mical, R. S., and Porter, J. C. 1972. Passage of radioactive substances from CSF to hypophyseal portal blood. *Endocrinology* 91:1239–1246.

Orosz, A., Hamori, J., Falus, A., Madarasz, E., Lakos, I., and Adam, G. 1973. Specific antibody-fragments against the postsynaptic web. *Nature [New Biol.]* 245:18–19.

Oschman, J. L., Hall, T. A., Peters, P. D., and Wall, B. J. 1974. Association of calcium with membranes of squid giant axon. Ultrastructure and microprobe analysis. *J. Cell Biol.* 61:156–165.

Oschman, J. L., Wall, B. J., and Gupta, B. L. 1974. Cellular basis of water transport. In: *Transport at the Cellular Level.* M. A. Sleigh and D. H. Jennings, Eds. S.E.B. Symposia XXVIII. London, Cambridge University Press, pp. 305–350.

Oseroff, A. R., Robbins, P. W., and Burger, M. M. 1973. The cell surface membrane: Biochemical aspects and biophysical probes. *Annu. Rev. Biochem.* 42:647–682.

Osinchak, J. 1964. Electron microscopic localization of acid phosphatase and thiamine pyrophosphatase activity in hypothalamic neurosecretory cells of the rat. *J. Cell Biol.* 21:35–47.

Padykula, H. A., and Gauthier, G. T. 1970. The ultrastructure of the neuromuscular junctions of mammalian red, white and intermediate skeletal muscle fibers. *J. Cell Biol.* 46:27–41.

Palade, G. E. 1953. An electron microscope study of the mitochondrial structure. *J. Histochem. Cytochem.* 1:188–211.

Palade, G. E., and Palay, S. L. 1954. Electron microscope observations of interneuronal and neuromuscular synapses. *Anat. Rec.* 118:335–336.

Palay, S. L. 1955. An electron microscope study of the neurohypophysis in normal, hydrated and dehydrated rats. *Anat. Rec.* 121:348.

Palay, S. L. 1956a. Structure and function in the neuron. In: *Progress in Neurobiology. I. Neurochemistry.* S. Korey and J. I. Nurnberger, Eds. New York, Hoeber, pp. 64–82.

Palay, S. L. 1956b. Synapses in the central nervous system. *J. Biophys. Biochem. Cytol.* 2(Suppl.):193–202.

Palay, S. L. 1957. The fine structure of the neurohypophysis. In: *Progress in Neurobiology,* Vol. 2, *Ultrastructure and Cellular Chemistry of Neural Tissue.* H. Waelsch, Ed. New York, Hoeber, pp. 31–44.

Palay, S. L. 1958a. The morphology of secretion. In: *Frontiers of Cytology.* S. L. Palay, Ed. New Haven, Yale University Press, pp. 305–342.

Palay, S. L. 1958b. The morphology of synapses in the central nervous system. *Exp. Cell Res. Suppl. 5,* pp. 275–293.

Palay, S. L. 1960a. On the appearance of absorbed fat droplets in the nuclear envelope. *J. Biophys. Biochem. Cytol.* 7:391–392.

Palay, S. L. 1960b. The fine structure of secretory neurons in the preoptic nucleus of the goldfish *(Carassius auratus). Anat. Rec.* 138:417–443.

Palay, S. L. 1961a. Structural peculiarities of the neurosecretory cells in the preoptic nucleus of the goldfish. *Carassius auratus. Anat. Rec.* 139:262.

Palay, S. L. 1961b. The electron microscopy of the glomeruli cerebellosi. In: *Cytology of Nervous Tissue, Proceedings of the Anatomical Society of Great Britain and Ireland.* London, Taylor and Francis, pp. 82–84.

Palay, S. L. 1963a. Multivesicular bodies in Purkinje cells of the rat's cerebellum. *J. Cell Biol.* 19:54A–55A.

Palay, S. L. 1963b. Alveolate vesicles in Purkinje cells of the rat's cerebellum. *J. Cell Biol.* 19:89A–90A.

Palay, S. L. 1964. The structural basis for neural action. In: *Brain Function*, Vol. 2, *RNA and Brain Function; Memory and Learning.* M. A. B. Brazier, Ed. Berkeley, University of California Press, pp. 69–108.

Palay, S. L. 1966. The role of neuroglia in the organization of the central nervous system. In: *Nerve As a Tissue.* K. Rodahl and B. Issekutz, Jr., Eds. New York, Hoeber, pp. 3–10.

Palay, S. L. 1967. Principles of cellular organization in the nervous system. In: *The Neurosciences.* G. C. Quarton, T. Melnechuk, and F. O. Schmitt, Eds. New York, Rockefeller University Press, pp. 24–31.

Palay, S. L., Billings-Gagliardi, S. M., and Chan-Palay, V. 1974. Neuronal perikarya with dispersed, single ribosomes in the visual cortex of *Macaca mulatta. J. Cell Biol.* 63:1074–1089.

Palay, S. L., and Chan-Palay, V. 1973. High voltage electron microscopy of the central nervous system in Golgi preparations. *J. Microscopy* 97:41–47.

Palay, S. L., and Chan-Palay, V. 1974. *Cerebellar Cortex, Cytology and Organization.* New York, Springer-Verlag.

Palay, S. L., McGee-Russell, S. M., Gordon, S., and Grillo, M. A. 1962. Fixation of neural tissues for electron microscopy by perfusion with solutions of osmium tetroxide. *J. Cell Biol.* 12:385–410.

Palay, S. L., and Palade, G. E. 1955. The fine structure of neurons. *J. Biophys. Biochem. Cytol.* 1:69–88.

Palay, S. L., Sotelo, C., Peters, A., and Orkand, P. M. 1968. The axon hillock and the initial segment. *J. Cell Biol.* 38:193–201.

Palkovits, M., Magyar, P., and Szentágothai, J. 1971. Quantitative histological analysis of the cerebellar cortex in the cat. I. Number and arrangement in space of the Purkinje cells. *Brain Res.* 32:1–13.

Pannese, E. 1960. Observations on the morphology, submicroscopic structure and biological properties of satellite cells (s.c.) in sensory ganglia of mammals. *Z. Zellforsch. Mikrosk. Anat.* 52:567–597.

Pannese, E. 1963. Investigation on the ultrastructural changes of the spinal ganglion neurons in the course of axon regeneration and cell hypertrophy. I. Changes during axon regeneration. *Z. Zellforsch. Mikrosk. Anat.* 60:711–740.

Pannese, E. 1969. Unusual membrane-particle complexes in nerve cells of the spinal ganglia. *J. Ultrastruct. Res.* 29:334–342.

Pannese, E., Bianchi, R., Calligaris, B., Ventura, R., and Weibel, E. R. 1972. Quantitative relationships between nerve and satellite cells in spinal ganglia. An electron microscopical study. I. Mammals. *Brain Res.* 46:215–234.

Pappas, G. D. 1966. Electron microscopy of neuronal junctions involved in transmission in the central nervous system. In: *Nerve As a Tissue.* K. Rodahl and B. Issekutz, Jr., Eds. New York, Hoeber, pp. 49–87.

Pappas, G. D., Asada, Y., and Bennett, M. V. L. 1971. Morphological correlates of increased coupling resistance at an electrotonic synapse. *J. Cell Biol.* 49:173–188.

Pappas, G. D., and Bennett, M. V. L. 1966. Specialized junctions involved in electrical transmission between neurons. *Ann. N.Y. Acad. Sci.* 137:495–508.

Pappas, G. D., Cohen, E. B., and Purpura, D. P. 1966. Fine structure of synaptic and nonsynaptic neuronal relations in the thalamus of the cat. In: *The Thalamus.* D. P. Purpura and M. D. Yahr, Eds. New York, Columbia University Press, pp. 47–75.

Pappas, G. D., and Purpura, D. P. 1961. Fine structure of dendrites in the superficial neocortical neuropil. *Exp. Neurol.* 4:507–530.

Pappas, G. D., and Tennyson, V. M. 1962. An electron microscopic study of the passage of colloidal particles from the blood vessels of the ciliary processes and choroid plexus of the rabbit. *J. Cell. Biol.* 15:227–240.

Pappas, G. D., and Waxman, S. G. 1972. Synaptic fine structure—morphological correlations of chemical and electrotonic transmission. In: *Structure and Function of Synapses.* G. D. Pappas and D. P. Purpura, Eds. New York, Raven Press, pp. 1–43.

Pappenheimer, J. R., Heisey, S. R., and Jordan, E. F. 1961. Active transport of diodrast and phenolsulfonphthalein from cerebrospinal fluid to blood. *Am. J. Physiol.* 200:1–10.

Parnavelas, J. G., Lynch, G., Brecha, N., Cotman, C. W., and Globus, A. 1974. Spine loss and regrowth in hippocampus following deafferentation. *Nature* 248:71–73.

Patek, P. R. 1944. The perivascular spaces of the mammalian brain. *Anat. Rec.* 88:1–24.

Paterson, J. A., Privat, A., Ling, A., and Leblond, C. P. 1973. Investigation of glial cells in semi-thin sections. III. Transformation of subependymal cells into glial cells, as shown by radioautography after ³H-thymidine injection into the lateral ventricle of the brain of young rats. *J. Comp. Neurol.* 149:83–102.

Payton, B. W., Bennett, M. V. L., and Pappas, G. D. 1969. Permeability and structure of junctional membranes at an electrotonic synapse. *Science* 166:1641–1643.

Peachey, L. D. 1964. Electron microscopic observa-
tions on the accumulation of divalent cations in intramitochondrial granules. *J. Cell Biol.* 20:95–111.

Pease, D. C. 1955. Nodes of Ranvier in the central nervous system. *J. Comp. Neurol.* 103:11–15.

Pease, D. C. 1963. The ultrastructure of flagellar fibrils. *J. Cell Biol.* 18:313–326.

Pease, D. C. 1973. Glycol methacrylate copolymerized with glutaraldehyde and urea as an embedment retaining lipids. *J. Ultrastruct. Res.* 45:124–148.

Pease, D. C., and Molinari, S. 1960. Electron microscopy of muscular arteries; pial vessels of the cat and monkey. *J. Ultrastruct. Res.* 3:447–468.

Pease, D. C., and Schultz, R. L. 1958. Electron microscopy of rat cranial meninges. *Am. J. Anat.* 102:301–321.

Pellegrino de Iraldi, A., and Etcheverry, G. J. 1967. Ultrastructural changes in the nerve endings of the median eminence after nialamide-DOPA administration. *Brain Res.* 6:614–618.

Pellegrino de Iraldi, A., Farini Duggan, H., and De Robertis, E. 1963. Adrenergic synaptic vesicles in the anterior hypothalamus of the rat. *Anat. Rec.* 145:521–531.

Penfield, W. 1924. Oligodendroglia and its relation to classical neuroglia. *Brain* 47:430–452.

Penfield, W. 1932. Neuroglia: normal and pathological. In: *Cytology and Cellular Pathology of the Nervous System,* Vol 2. W. Penfield, Ed. New York, Hoeber, pp. 421–479.

Peper, K., Dreyer, F., Sandri, C., Akert, K., and Moor, H. 1974. Structure and ultrastructure of the frog motor endplate. *Cell Tiss. Res.* 149:437–455.

Peracchia, C. 1970. A system of parallel septa in crayfish nerve fibers. *J. Cell Biol.* 44:125–133.

Peracchia, C. 1973a. Low resistance junctions in crayfish. I. Two arrays of globules in junctional membranes. *J. Cell Biol.* 57:54–65.

Peracchia, C. 1973b. Low resistance junctions in crayfish. II. Structural details and further evidence for intercellular channels by freeze-fracture and negative staining. *J. Cell Biol.* 57:66–76.

Peracchia, C., and Robertson, J. D. 1971. Increase in osmiophilia of axonal membranes of crayfish as a result of electrical stimulation, asphyxia, or treatment with reducing agents. *J. Cell Biol.* 51:223–239.

Perdue, J. F. 1973. The distribution, ultrastructure, and chemistry of microfilaments in cultured chick embryo fibroblasts. *J. Cell Biol.* 58:265–283.

Périer, O., and de Harven, E. 1961. Electron microscope observations on myelinated tissue cultures of mammalian cerebellum. In: *Cytology of Nervous Tissue, Proceedings of the Anatomical Society of Great Britain and Ireland.* London, Taylor and Francis, pp. 78–81.

Perri, V., Sacchi, O., Raviola, E., and Raviola, G. 1972. Evaluation of the number and distribution of synaptic vesicles at cholinergic nerve-endings after sustained stimulation. *Brain Res.* 39:526–529.

Peters, A. 1960a. The structure of myelin sheaths in the central nervous system of *Xenopus laevis* (Daudin). *J. Biophys. Biochem. Cytol. 7*:121–126.

Peters, A. 1960b. The formation and structure of myelin sheaths in the central nervous system. *J. Biophys. Biochem. Cytol. 8*:431–446.

Peters, A. 1961a. The development of peripheral nerves in *Xenopus laevis*. In: *Electron Microscopy in Anatomy*. J. D. Boyd, F. R. Johnson, and J. D. Lever, Eds. London, Arnold, pp. 142–159.

Peters, A. 1961b. A radial component of central myelin sheaths. *J. Biophys. Biochem. Cytol. 11*:733–735.

Peters, A. 1962a. Myelinogenesis in the central nervous system. In: *Proceedings, IV. International Congress of Neuropathology* (Munich 1961), Vol. 2: *Electronmicroscopy and Biology*. H. Jacob, Ed. Stuttgart, Thieme, pp. 50–54.

Peters, A. 1962b. Plasma membrane contacts in the central nervous system. *J. Anat. 96*:237–248.

Peters, A. 1964a. Further observations on the structure of myelin sheaths in the central nervous system. *J. Cell Biol. 20*:281–296.

Peters, A. 1964b. Observations on the connexions between myelin sheaths and glial cells in the optic nerves of young rats. *J. Anat. 98*:125–134.

Peters, A. 1966. The node of Ranvier in the central nervous system. *Q. J. Exp. Physiol. 51*:229–236.

Peters, A. 1967. Microtubules and neurofilaments within axons of the rat's central nervous system. *J. Cell Biol. 35*:102A.

Peters, A. 1968. The morphology of axons of the central nervous system. In: *The Structure and Function of Nervous Tissue*, Vol. I. G. H. Bourne, Ed. New York, Academic Press, pp. 141–186.

Peters, A. 1971. Stellate cells in the rat parietal cortex. *J. Comp. Neurol. 141*:345–374.

Peters, A. 1974. The surface fine structure of the choroid plexus and ependymal lining of the rat lateral ventricle. *J. Neurocytol. 3*:99–108.

Peters, A., and Feldman, M. F. 1973. The cortical plate and molecular layer of the late rat fetus. *Z. Anat. Entwicklungsgesch. 141*:3–37.

Peters, A., and Kaiserman-Abramof, I. R. 1969. The small pyramidal neuron of the rat cerebral cortex. The synapses upon dendritic spines. *Z. Zellforsch. Mikrosk. Anat. 100*:487–506.

Peters, A., and Kaiserman-Abramof, I. R. 1970. The small pyramidal neuron of the rat cerebral cortex. The perikaryon, dendrites and spines. *Am. J. Anat. 127*:321–356.

Peters, A., and Muir, A. R. 1959. The relationship between axons and Schwann cells during development of peripheral nerves in the rat. *Q. J. Exp. Physiol. 44*:117–130.

Peters, A., and Palay, S. L. 1965. An electron microscope study of the distribution and patterns of astroglial processes in the central nervous system. *J. Anat. 99*:419.

Peters, A., and Palay, S. L. 1966. The morphology of laminae A and A₁ of the dorsal nucleus of the lateral geniculate body of the cat. *J. Anat. 100*:451–486.

Peters, A., Palay, S. L., and Webster, H. deF. 1970. *Fine Structure of the Nervous System*. New York, Harper & Row.

Peters, A., Proskauer, C. C., and Kaiserman-Abramof, I. R. 1968. The small pyramidal neuron of the rat cerebral cortex: the axon hillock and initial segment. *J. Cell Biol. 39*:604–619.

Peters, A., and Vaughn, J. E. 1967. Microtubules and filaments in the axons and astrocytes of early postnatal rat optic nerves. *J. Cell Biol. 32*:113–119.

Peters, A., and Vaughn, J. E. 1970. Morphology and development of the myelin sheath. In: *Myelination*. A. N. Davison and A. Peters, Eds. Springfield, Ill., Charles C Thomas, pp. 3–79.

Peters, A., and Walsh, T. M. 1972. A study of the organization of apical dendrites in the somatic sensory cortex of the rat. *J. Comp. Neurol. 144*:253–268.

Peterson, E. R., and Murray, M. R. 1965. Patterns of peripheral demyelination *in vitro*. *Ann. N.Y. Acad. Sci. 122*:39–50.

Peterson, R. G., and Pease, D. C. 1972. Myelin embedded in polymerized glutaraldehyde-urea. *J. Ultrastruct. Res. 41*:115–132.

Pevzner, L. Z. 1965. Topochemical aspects of nucleic acid and protein metabolism within the neuron-neuroglia unit of the superior cervical ganglion. *J. Neurochem. 12*:993–1002.

Peyronnard, J.-M., Aguayo, A. J., and Bray, G. M. 1973. Schwann cell internuclear distances in normal and regenerating unmyelinated nerve fibers. *Arch. Neurol. 29*:56–59.

Pfenninger, K. H. 1971a. The cytochemistry of synaptic densities. I. An analysis of the bismuth iodide impregnation method. *J. Ultrastruct. Res. 34*:103–122.

Pfenninger, K. H. 1971b. The cytochemistry of synaptic densities. II. Proteinaceous components and the mechanism of synaptic connectivity. *J. Ultrastruct. Res. 35*:451–475.

Pfenninger, K. 1973. Synaptic morphology and cytochemistry. *Progr. Histochem. Cytochem. 5*:1–86.

Pfenninger, K. H., Akert, K., Moor, H., and Sandri, C. 1972. The fine structure of freeze-fractured presynaptic membranes. *J. Neurocytol. 1*:129–149.

Pfenninger, K. H., and Bunge, R. P. 1974. Freeze-fracturing of nerve growth cones and young fibers. A study of developing plasma membrane. *J. Cell Biol. 63*:180–196.

Pfenninger, K. H., and Rovainen, C. M. 1974. Stimulation- and calcium-dependence of vesicle attachment sites in the presynaptic membrane; a freeze-cleavage study on the lamprey spinal cord. *Brain Res. 72*:1–23.

Pfenninger, K. H., Sandri, C., Akert, K., and Engster, C. 1969. Contribution to the problem of structural organization of the presynaptic area. *Brain Res. 12*:10–18.

Phelps, C. H. 1972a. The development of gliovascular relationships in the rat spinal cord. An electron microscopic study. *Z. Zellforsch. Mikrosk. Anat. 128*:555–562.

Phelps, C. H. 1972b. Barbiturate-induced glycogen accumulation in brain: An electron microscopic study. *Brain Res.* 39:225–234.

Phillips, D. D., Hibbs, R. G., Ellison, P., and Shapiro, H. 1972. An electron microscopic study of central and peripheral nodes of Ranvier. *J. Anat.* 111:229–238.

Picken, L. 1960. *The Organization of Cells.* New York, Oxford University Press.

Pinching, A. J. 1970. Synaptic connexions in the glomerular layer of the olfactory bulb. *J. Physiol. (Lond.)* 210:14P–15P.

Pinching, A. J. 1971. Myelinated dendritic segments in the monkey olfactory bulb. *Brain Res.* 29:133–138.

Pinching, A. J., and Powell, T. P. S. 1971a. The neuropil of the glomeruli of the olfactory bulb. *J. Cell Sci.* 9:347–378.

Pinching, A. J., and Powell, T. P. S. 1971b. The neuropil of the periglomerular region of the olfactory bulb. *J. Cell Sci.* 9:379–409.

Pineda, A., Maxwell, D. S., and Kruger, L. 1967. The fine structure of neurons and satellite cells in the trigeminal ganglion of cat and monkey. *Am. J. Anat.* 121:461–487.

Pinner, B., and Campbell, J. B. 1965. Alkaline phosphatase activity of incisures and nodes during degeneration and regeneration of peripheral nerve fibers. *Exp. Neurol.* 12:159–172.

Pitman, R. M., Tweedle, C. D., and Cohen, M. J. 1972. Branching of central neurons: Intracellular cobalt injection for light and electron microscopy. *Science* 176:412–414.

Plenk, H. 1927. Über Argyrophile Fasern (Gitterfasern) und ihre Bildungszellen. *Ergeb. Anat. Entwicklungsgesch.* 27:302–412.

Politoff, A., Pappas, G. D., and Bennett, M. V. L. 1974. Cobalt ions cross an electrotonic synapse if cytoplasmic concentration is low. *Brain Res.* 76:343–346.

Politoff, A. L., Rose, S., and Pappas, G. D. 1974. The calcium binding sites of synaptic vesicles of the frog sartorius neuromuscular junction. *J. Cell Biol.* 61:818–823.

Pollard, T. D., Shelton, E., Weihung, R. R., and Korn, E. D. 1970. Ultrastructural characterization of F-actin isolated from *Acanthamoeba castellarii* and identification of cytoplasmic filaments as F-actin by reaction with rabbit heavy meromysin. *J. Molec. Biol.* 50:91–97.

Pollen, D. A. 1973. Focal epilepsy and the neuroglial impairment hypothesis. In: *Epilepsy. Its Phenomena in Man.* M. A. Brazier, Ed. New York, Academic Press, pp. 29–35.

Pomerat, C. M., Hendelman, W. J., Raiborn, C. W., and Massey, J. F. 1967. Dynamic activities of nervous tissue *in vitro.* In: *The Neuron.* H. Hydén, Ed. Amsterdam, Elsevier, pp. 119–178.

Porter, K. R. 1953. Observations on a submicroscopic basophilic component of cytoplasm. *J. Exp. Med.* 97:727–750.

Porter, K. R. 1966. Cytoplasmic microtubules and

their function. In: *Principles of Biomolecular Organization.* G. E. W. Wolstenholme and M. O'Connor, Eds. London, Churchill, pp. 308–345.

Porter, W. W., Barnard, L. A., and Chiu, J. H. 1973. The ultrastructural localization and quantitation of cholinergic receptors at the mouse motor endplates. *J. Membrane Biol.* 14:383–402.

Potter, H. D. 1971. The distribution of neurofibrils coextensive with microtubules and neurofilaments in dendrites and axons of the tectum, cerebellum, and pallium of the frog. *J. Comp. Neurol.* 143:385–410.

Potter, H. D. 1973. Alterations in neurofibrillar rings in the lizard brain during cold acclimation. *J. Neurocytol.* 2:29–45.

Potter, H. D., and Hafner, G. S. 1974. Sequence of changes in neurofibrils (neurofilaments) induced in synaptic regions of bullfrogs by environmental temperature changes. *J. Comp. Neurol.* 155:409–424.

Price, D. S. 1972. The response of amphibian glial cells to axon transection. *J. Neuropathol. Exp. Neurol.* 31:267–277.

Price, D. L., and Porter, K. R. 1972. The response of ventral horn neurons to axonal transection. *J. Cell Biol.* 53:24–37.

Price, J. L. 1968. The termination of centrifugal fibres in the olfactory bulb. *Brain Res.* 7:483–486.

Price, J. L., and Powell, T. P. S. 1970a. The synaptology of the granule cells of the olfactory bulb. *J. Cell Sci.* 7:125–156.

Price, J. L., and Powell, T. P. S. 1970b. The mitral and short axon cells of the olfactory bulb. *J. Cell Sci.* 7:631–651.

Privat, A. 1970. Sur l'origine des divers types de névroglie chez le rat. Proc. 6th Int. Congr. Neuropathol. Paris, pp. 447–448, Masson, Paris.

Privat, A., and Leblond, C. P. 1972. The subependymal layer and neighboring region in the brain of the young rat. *J. Comp. Neurol.* 146:277–302.

Pruijs, W. M. 1927. Ueber Mikroglia, ihre Herkunft, Funktion und ihr Verhältnis zu anderen Gliaelementen. *Z. Ges. Neurol. Psychiatr.* 108:298–331.

Purkinje, J. 1836. Ueber Flimmerbewegungen in Gehirn. *Müller's Arch. Anat. Physiol.* 3:289–290.

Purpura, D. P. 1974. Dendritic spines, "dysgenesis," and mental retardation. *Science* 186:1126–1128.

Purves, D., and McMahan, U. J. 1972. The distribution of synapses on a physiologically identified motor neuron in the central nervous system of the leech: an electron microscopic study after the injection of the fluorescent dye procion yellow. *J. Cell. Biol.* 55:205–220.

Purves, D., and McMahan, U. J. 1973. Procion yellow as a marker for electron microscopic examination of functionally identified nerve cells. In: *Intracellular Staining in Neurobiology.* S. B. Kater and C. Nicholson, Eds. New York, Springer-Verlag, pp. 71–82.

Pysh, J. J., and Wiley, R. G. 1974. Synaptic vesicle depletion and recovery in the cat sympathetic ganglia electrically stimulated *in vivo:* Evidence for transmitter secretion by exocytosis. *J. Cell Biol.* 60:356–374.

Quarles, R. H., Everly, J. L., and Brady, R. O. 1973. Evidence for the close association of a glycoprotein with myelin in rat brain. *J. Neurochem.* 21:1177–1191.

Quilliam, T. A., and Sato, M. 1955. The distribution of myelin on nerve fibres from Pacinian corpuscles. *J. Physiol. (Lond.)* 129:167–176.

Quinton, P. M., Wright, E. M., and Tormey, J. McD. 1973. Localization of sodium pumps in the choroid plexus epithelium. *J. Cell Biol.* 58:724–730.

Radouco-Thomas, C., Nosal, G., and Radouco-Thomas, S. 1971. The nuclear-ribosomal system during neuronal differentiation and development. In: *Chemistry and Brain Development.* R. Paoletti and A. N. Davison, Eds. New York, Plenum Press, pp. 291–308.

Rafols, J. A., and Valverde, E. 1973. The structure of the dorsal lateral geniculate nucleus in the mouse. A Golgi and electron microscopic study. *J. Comp. Neurol.* 150:303–332.

Raine, C., Ghetti, B., and Shelanski, M. L. 1971. On the association between microtubules and mitochondria within axons. *Brain Res.* 34:389–393.

Raisman, G. and Matthews, M. R. 1972. Degeneration and regeneration of synapses. In: *The Structure and Function of Nervous Tissue,* Vol. 5. G. H. Bourne, Ed. New York, Academic Press, pp. 61–104.

Rakic, P. 1972a. Mode of cell migration to the superficial layers of fetal monkey neocortex. *J. Comp. Neurol.* 145:61–84.

Rakic, P. 1972b. Extrinsic cytological determinants of basket and stellate cell dendritic pattern in the cerebellar molecular layer. *J. Comp. Neurol.* 146:335–354.

Rakic, P. 1973. Kinetics of the proliferation and the latency between final division and onset of differentiation of the cerebellar stellate and basket cells. *J. Comp. Neurol.* 147:523–546.

Rakic, P., and Sidman, R. L. 1973a. Sequence of developmental abnormalities leading to granule cell deficit in cerebellar cortex of weaver mutant mice. *J. Comp. Neurol.* 152:103–132.

Rakic, P., and Sidman, R. L. 1973b. Organization of cerebellar cortex secondary to deficit of granule cells in weaver mutant mice. *J. Comp. Neurol.* 152:133–162.

Rall, W. 1970a. Dendritic neuron theory and dendrodendritic synapses in a simple cortical system. In: *The Neurosciences: Second Study Program.* F. O. Schmitt, Ed. New York, Rockefeller University Press. pp. 552–565.

Rall, W. 1970b. Cable properties of dendrites and effects of synaptic location. In: *Excitatory Synaptic Mechanisms.* P. Andersen and J. K. S. Jansen, Eds. Oslo, Universitetsforlaget, pp. 175–187.

Rall, W., and Rinzel, J. 1973. Branch input resistance and steady attenuation for input to one branch of a dendritic neuron model. *Biophys. J.* 13:648–688.

Rall, W., and Shepherd, G. M. 1968. Theoretical reconstruction of field potentials and dendrodendritic synaptic interactions in olfactory bulb. *J. Neurophysiol.* 31:884–915.

Rall, W., Shepherd, G. M., Reese, T. S., and Brightman, M. W. 1966. Dendrodendritic synaptic pathway for inhibition in the olfactory bulb. *Exp. Neurol.* 14:44–56.

Ralston, H. J. 1965. The organization of the substantia gelatinosa Rolandi in the cat lumbosacral spinal cord. *Z. Zellforsch. Mikrosk. Anat.* 67:1–23.

Ralston, H. J. 1968. The fine structure of neurons in the dorsal horn of the cat spinal cord. *J. Comp. Neurol.* 132:275–302.

Ralston, H. J. 1969. The synaptic organization of the lemniscal projections to the ventro-basal thalamus of the cat. *Brain Res. 14* 99–116.

Ralston, H. J. 1971. Evidence for presynaptic dendrites and a proposal for their mechanism of action. *Nature (Lond.)* 230:585–587.

Ralston, H. J., and Herman, M. M. 1969. The fine structure of neurons and synapses in the ventrobasal thalamus of the cat. *Brain Res.* 14:77–97.

Ralston, H. J., and Sharp, P. V. 1973. The identification of thalamocortical relay cells in the adult cat by means of retrograde axonal transport of horseradish peroxidase. *Brain Res.* 62:273–278.

Rambourg, A., Hernandez, W., and Leblond, C. P. 1969. Detection of complex carbohydrates in the Golgi apparatus of rat cells. *J. Cell Biol.* 40:395–414.

Rambourg, A., and Leblond, C. P. 1967. Electron microscope observations on the carbohydrate rich cell coat present at the surface of cells in the rat. *J. Cell Biol.* 32:27–54.

Rambourg, A., Marraud, A., and Chretien, M. 1973. Tri-dimensional structure of the forming face of the Golgi apparatus as seen in the high voltage electron microscope after osmium impregnation of the small nerve cells in the semilunar ganglion of the trigeminal nerve. *J. Microscopy* 97:49–57.

Ramón-Moliner, E. 1958. A study on neuroglia. The problem of transitional forms. *J. Comp. Neurol.* 110:157–171.

Ramón-Moliner, E. 1968. The morphology of dendrites. In: *The Structure and Function of Nervous Tissue,* Vol. I. G. H. Bourne, Ed. New York, Academic Press, pp. 205–267.

Ramón-Moliner, E. 1974. The locus coeruleus of cat. III. Light and electron microscopic studies. *Cell Tiss. Res.* 149:205–221.

Ramón-Moliner, E., and Ferrari, J. 1972. Electron microscopy of previously identified cells and processes within the central nervous system. *J. Neurocytol.* 1:85–100.

Ramsey, H. J. 1965. Fine structure of the surface of the cerebral cortex of human brain. *J. Cell Biol.* 26:323–333.

Ranish, N., and Ochs, S. 1972. Fast axoplasmic transport of acetylcholinesterase in mammalian nerve fibres. *J. Neurochem.* 19:2641–2650.

Ranvier, M. L. 1878. *Leçons Sur L'Histologie du Système Nerveux.* Paris, F. Savy.

Rascol, M., and Izard, J. 1972. La jonction cortico-pie-mérienne et la pénétration des vaisseaux dans le cortex cérébral chez l'homme. Structure et ultra-structure. *Z. Zellforsch. Mikrosk. Anat. 123*:337–355.

Rash, J. E., and Ellisman, M. H. 1974. Studies of excitable membranes. I. Macromolecular specializations of the neuromuscular junction and the nonjunctional sarcolemma. *J. Cell Biol. 63*:567–586.

Rash, J. E., Ellisman, M. H., and Staehelin, L. A. 1973. Freeze-cleaved neuromuscular junctions: macromolecular architecture of postsynaptic membranes of normal vs. denervated muscle. *J. Cell Biol. 59*:280A.

Raviola, E., and Gilula, N. B. 1973. Gap junctions between photoreceptor cells in the vertebrate retina. *Proc. Natl. Acad. Sci. U.S.A. 70*:1677–1681.

Raviola, G., and Raviola, E. 1967. Light and electron microscopic observations on the inner plexiform layer of the rabbit retina. *Am. J. Anat. 120*:403–425.

Rawlins, F. A. 1973. A time-sequence autoradiographic study of the in vivo incorporation of (1,2-^{3}H) cholesterol into peripheral nerve myelin. *J. Cell Biol. 58*:42–53.

Rawlins, F. A., and Uzman, B. G. 1970a. Retardation of peripheral nerve myelination in mice treated with inhibitors of cholesterol biosynthesis. A quantitative electron microscopic study. *J. Cell Biol. 47*:505–517.

Rawlins, F. A., and Uzman, B. G. 1970b. Effect of AY-9944, a cholesterol biosynthesis inhibitor on peripheral nerve myelination. *Lab. Invest. 23*:184–189.

Reale, E., Luciano, L., and Spitznas, M. 1975. Zonulae occludentes of the myelin lamellae in the nerve fibre layer of the retina and in the optic nerve of the rabbit: a demonstration by the freeze-fracture method. *J. Neurocytol. 4*:131–140.

Reese, T. S., Bennett, M. V. L., and Feder, N. 1971. Cell-to-cell movement of peroxidases injected into the septate axon of crayfish. *Anat. Rec. 169*:409.

Reese, T. S., and Brightman, M. W. 1965. Electron microscopic studies on the rat olfactory bulb. *Anat. Rec. 151*:492.

Reese, T. S., and Brightman, M. W. 1968. Similarity in structure and permeability to peroxidase of epithelia overlying fenestrated cerebral capillaries. *Anat. Rec. 160*:414.

Reese, T. S., and Brightman, M. W. 1970. Olfactory surface and central olfactory connections in some vertebrates. In: *CIBA Foundation Symposium on Taste and Smell in Vertebrates*. G. E. W. Wolstenholme and J. Knight, Eds. London, Churchill, pp. 115–149.

Reese, T. S., and Karnovsky, M. J. 1967. Fine structural localization of a blood-brain barrier to exogenous peroxidase. *J. Cell Biol. 34*:207–217.

Reese, T. S., and Shepherd, G. M. 1972. Dendro-dendritic synapses in the central nervous system. In: *Structure and Function of Synapses*. G. D.

Pappas and D. P. Purpura, Eds. New York, Raven Press, pp. 121–136.

Reger, J. F. 1958. The fine structure of neuromuscular synapses of gastrocnemii from mouse and frog. *Anat. Rec. 130*:7–24.

Reier, P. J., Froelich, J. S., Sawchak, J. A., and Hughes, A. F. W. 1974. Maturation of nonmyelinated fiber bundles in a strain of dwarf (Snell's) mice. *Anat. Rec. 178*:103–118.

Reier, P. J., and Webster, H. deF. 1974. Regeneration and remyelination of *Xenopus* tadpole optic nerve fibres following transection or crush. *J. Neurocytol. 3*:591–618.

Remak, R. 1838. *Observationes Anatomicae et Microscopicae de Systematis Nervosi Structura*. Berlin, Reimer.

Remak, R. 1841. Anatomische Beobachtungen über das Gehirn, das Rückenmark und die Nervenwurzeln. *Müller's Arch.* pp. 506–522.

Renaut, J. 1881a. Recherche sur quelque points particulier d'histologie des nerfs. *Arch. Physiol. (Paris) 8*:180–190.

Renaut, J. 1881b. Système hyalin de soutenement des centres nerveux et de quelques organes des sens. *Arch. Physiol. (Paris) 8*:846–859.

Réthelyi, M., and Szentágothai, J. 1969. The large synaptic complexes of the substantia gelatinosa. *Exp. Brain Res. 7*:258–274.

Revel, J.-P., and Hamilton, D. W. 1969. The double nature of the intermediate dense line in the peripheral nerve myelin. *Anat. Rec. 163*:7–16.

Revel, J.-P., and Karnovsky, M. J. 1967. Hexagonal array of subunits in intercellular junctions of the mouse heart and liver. *J. Cell Biol. 33*:C7–C12.

Rhodin, J. A. G. 1962. Fine structure of vascular walls in mammals with special reference to smooth muscle component. *Physiol. Rev. 42*:43–81.

Rhodin, J. A. G. 1968. Ultrastructure of mammalian venous capillaries, venules and small collecting veins. *J. Ultrastruct. Res. 25*:452–500.

Richards, J. G., Lorez, H. P., and Tranzer, J. P. 1973. Indolealkylamine nerve terminals in cerebral ventricles: Identification by electron microscopy and fluorescence histochemistry. *Brain Res. 57*:277–288.

Richardson, K. C. 1960. Studies on the structure of autonomic nerves in the small intestine, correlating the silver-impregnated image in light microscopy with the permanganate-fixed ultrastructure in electron microscopy. *J. Anat. 94*:457–472.

Richardson, K. C. 1962. The fine structure of autonomic nerve endings in smooth muscle of the rat vas deferens. *J. Anat. 96*:427–442.

Richardson, K. C. 1964. The fine structure of the albino rabbit iris with special reference to the identification of adrenergic and cholinergic nerves and nerve endings in its intrinsic muscles. *Am. J. Anat. 114*:173–205.

Richardson, K. C. 1968. Cholinergic and adrenergic axons in methylene blue-stained rat iris: An electronmicroscopical study. *Life Sci. 7*:599–604.

Rinne, U. K. 1966. Ultrastructure of the median eminence of the rat. *Z. Zellforsch. Mikrosk. Anat.* 74:98–122.

del Rio Hortega, P. 1919. El "tercer elemento" de los centros nerviosos. *Bol. Soc. Espan. Biol.* 9:69–120.

del Rio Hortega, P. 1921. Estudios sobre la neuroglia. La glía de escasas radiaciones (oligodendroglia). *Bol. Real Soc. Espan. Hist. Nat.* 21:63–92.

del Rio Hortega, P. 1928. Tercera aportacion al conocimiento morfologico e interpretacion functional de la oligodendroglia. *Mem. Real Soc. Espan. Hist. Nat.* 14:5–122.

del Rio Hortega, P. 1932. Microglia. In: *Cytology and Cellular Pathology of the Nervous System,* Vol. 2. W. Penfield, Ed. New York, Hoeber, pp. 483–534.

Robertson, F. 1900. A microscopic demonstration of the normal and pathological histology of mesoglia cells. *J. Ment. Sci.* 46:724.

Robertson, J. D. 1953. Ultrastructure of two invertebrate synapses. *Proc. Soc. Exp. Biol. Med.* 82:219–223.

Robertson, J. D. 1955a. The ultrastructure of adult vertebrate peripheral myelinated nerve fibers in relation to myelinogenesis. *J. Biophys. Biochem. Cytol.* 1:271–278.

Robertson, J. D. 1955b. Recent electron microscope observations on the ultrastructure of the crayfish median-to-motor giant synapse. *Exp. Cell Res.* 8:226–229.

Robertson, J. D. 1956. The ultrastructure of a reptilian myoneural junction. *J. Biophys. Biochem. Cytol.* 2:381–395.

Robertson, J. D. 1957. New observations on the ultrastructure of the membranes of frog peripheral nerve fibers. *J. Biophys. Biochem. Cytol.* 3:1043–1048.

Robertson, J. D. 1958a. The ultrastructure of Schmidt-Lantermann clefts and related shearing defects of the myelin sheath. *J. Biophys. Biochem. Cytol.* 4:39–46.

Robertson, J. D. 1958b. Structural alterations in nerve fibers produced by hypotonic and hypertonic solutions. *J. Biophys. Biochem. Cytol.* 4:349–364.

Robertson, J. D. 1959a. The ultrastructure of cell membranes and their derivatives. In: *Biochemical Society Symposia,* Vol. 16, *The Structure and Function of Subcellular Components.* E. M. Crook, Ed. Cambridge, England, Cambridge University Press, pp. 3–43.

Robertson, J. D. 1959b. Preliminary observations on the ultrastructure of nodes of Ranvier. *Z. Zellforsch. Mikrosk. Anat.* 50:553–560.

Robertson, J. D. 1960a. Electron microscopy of the motor end-plate and the neuromuscular spindle. *Am. J. Phys. Med.* 39:1–43.

Robertson, J. D. 1960b. The molecular structure and contact relationships of cell membranes. *Progr. Biophys.* 10:343–418.

Robertson, J. D. 1961. The unit membrane. In: *Electron Microscopy in Anatomy.* J. D. Boyd, F. R. Johnson, and J. D. Lever, Eds. London, Arnold, pp. 74–99.

Robertson, J. D. 1963. The occurrence of subunit pattern in the unit membranes of club endings in Mauthner cell synapses in goldfish brains. *J. Cell Biol.* 19:201–221.

Robertson, J. D. 1964. Unit membranes: A review with recent new studies of experimental alterations and a new subunit structure in synaptic membranes. In: *Cellular Membranes in Development.* M. Locke, Ed. New York, Academic Press, 1–81.

Robertson, J. D. 1965. The synapse: morphological and chemical correlates of function: A report of an NRP work session. *Neurosci. Res. Progr. Bull.* 3:1–79.

Robertson, J. D. 1966. Current problems of unit membrane structure and contact relationships. In: *Nerve As a Tissue.* K. Rodahl and B. Issekutz, Jr., Eds. New York, Hoeber, pp. 11–48.

Robertson, J. D., Bodenheimer, T. S., and Stage, D. E. 1963. The ultrastructure of Mauthner cell synapses and nodes in goldfish brains. *J. Cell Biol.* 19:159–199.

Rodríguez-Echandía, E. L., and Piezzi, R. S. 1968. Microtubules in the nerve fibers of the toad *Bufo arenarum* Hensel. Effect of low temperature on the sciatic nerve. *J. Cell Biol.* 39:491–497.

Rodríguez-Echandía, E. L., Piezzi, R. S., and Rodríguez, E. M. 1968. Dense-core microtubules in neurons and gliocytes of the toad *Bufo arenarum* Hensel. *Am. J. Anat.* 122:157–168.

Rodríguez-Echandía, E. L., Ramirez, B. U., and Fernandez, H. L. 1973. Studies on the mechanism of inhibition of axoplasmic transport of neuronal organelles. *J. Neurocytol.* 2:149–156.

Rohr, V. U. 1966. Zum Feinbau der Subfornikal-Organs der Katze. I. Der Gefäss-Apparat. *Z. Zellforsch. Mikrosk. Anat.* 73:246–271.

Rohrschneider, I., Schinko, I., and Wetzstein, R. 1972. Der Feinbau der Area postrema der Maus. *Z. Zellforsch. Mikrosk. Anat.* 123:251–276.

Rosenbluth, J. 1962a. The fine structure of acoustic ganglia in the rat. *J. Cell Biol.* 12:329–359.

Rosenbluth, J. 1962b. Subsurface cisterns and their relationship to the neuronal plasma membrane. *J. Cell Biol.* 13:405–421.

Rosenbluth, J. 1963. Contrast between osmium-fixed and permanganate-fixed toad spinal ganglia. *J. Cell Biol.* 16:143–157.

Rosenbluth, J. 1966. Redundant myelin sheaths and other ultrastructural features of the toad cerebellum. *J. Cell Biol.* 28:73–93.

Rosenbluth, J. 1973. Postjunctional membrane specialization at cholinergic myoneural junctions in the leech. *J. Comp. Neurol.* 151:399–406.

Rosenbluth, J. 1974. Substructure of amphibian motor end plate. Evidence for a granular component projecting from the outer surface of the receptive membrane. *J. Cell Biol.* 62:755–766.

Rosenbluth, J., and Palay, S. L. 1961. The fine structure of nerve cell bodies and their myelin sheaths in the eighth nerve ganglion of the goldfish. *J. Biophys. Biochem. Cytol.* 9:853–877.

Rosenbluth, J., and Wissig, S. L. 1964. The distribution of exogenous ferritin in toad spinal ganglia and the mechanism of its uptake by neurons. *J. Cell Biol.* 23:307–325.

Ross, L. L. 1964. Peripheral nervous tissue. In: *Electron Microscopic Anatomy*. S. M. Kurtz, Ed. New York, Academic Press, pp. 341–367.

Ross, L. L., Bornstein, M. B., and Lehrer, G. M. 1962. Electron microscopic observations of rat and mouse cerebellum in tissue culture. *J. Cell Biol.* 14:19–30.

Rossi, A., and Palombi, F. 1969. A neurofibrillar body in the perikarya of nervus terminalis ganglion cells in teleosts. *Z. Zellforsch. Mikrosk. Anat.* 93:395–403.

Roth, T. F., and Porter, K. R. 1964. Yolk protein uptake in the oocyte of the mosquito *Aedes aegypti* L. *J. Cell Biol.* 20:313–332.

Rovainen, C. M. 1974a. Synaptic interactions of identified nerve cells in the spinal cord of the sea lamprey. *J. Comp. Neurol.* 154:189–206.

Rovainen, C. M. 1974b. Synaptic interactions of reticulospinal neurons and nerve cells in the spinal cord of the sea lamprey. *J. Comp. Neurol.* 154:207–223.

Rozsa, G., Morgan, C., Szent-Györgyi, A., and Wyckoff, R. W. G. 1950. The electron microscopy of myelinated nerve. *Biochim. Biophys. Acta* 6:13–27.

Rustioni, A., and Sotelo, C. 1974. Synaptic organization of the nucleus gracilis of the cat. Experimental identification of dorsal root fibers and cortical afferents. *J. Comp. Neurol.* 155:441–468.

Rydberg, E. 1932. Cerebral injury in newborn children consequent on birth trauma; with an inquiry into the normal and pathological anatomy of the neuroglia. *Acta Pathol. Microbiol. Scand.* Suppl. 10.

Sabatini, D. D., Bensch, K., and Barrnett, R. J. 1963. Cytochemistry and electron microscopy: The preservation of cellular ultrastructure and enzymatic activity by aldehyde fixation. *J. Cell Biol.* 17:19–58.

Sabri, M. J., and Ochs, S. 1973. Characterization of fast and slow transported proteins in dorsal root and sciatic nerve of cat. *J. Neurobiol.* 4:145–165.

Sachs, H. 1963. Studies on the intracellular distribution of vasopressin. *J. Neurochem.* 10:289–297.

Saito, A., and Zacks, S. I. 1969. Ultrastructure of Schwann and perineural sheaths at the mouse neuromuscular junction. *Anat. Rec.* 164:379–390.

Saito, K. 1972. The initial segment of DSCT (dorsal spinocerebellar tract) neurons in the cat. *J. Electron Microsc.* 21:325–326.

Saito, K. 1974. The synaptology and cytology of the Clarke cell in nucleus dorsalis of the cat: an electron microscopic study. *J. Neurocytol.* 3:179–197.

Saito, K., Barber, R., Wu, J.-Y., Matsuda, T., Roberts, E., and Vaughn, J. E. 1974. Immunohistochemical localization of glutamate decarboxylase in rat cerebellum. *Proc. Natl. Acad. Sci. U.S.A.* 71:269–273.

Salpeter, M. M., McHenry, F. A., and Feng, H. H. 1974. Myoneural junctions in the extraocular muscles of the mouse. *Anat. Rec.* 179:201–224.

Samarasinghe, D. D. 1965. The innervation of the cerebral arteries in the rat. An electron microscope study. *J. Anat.* 99:815–828.

Samorajski, T., Friede, R. L., and Reimer, P. R. 1970. Hypomyelination in the quaking mouse. A model for the analysis of disturbed myelin formation. *J. Neuropathol. Exp. Neurol.* 29:507–523.

Samorajski, T., Keefe, J. R., and Ordy, J. M. 1964. Intracellular localization of lipofuscin age pigments in the nervous system. *J. Gerontol.* 19:262–276.

Samorajski, T., Ordy, J. M., and Keefe, J. R. 1965. The fine structure of lipofuscin age pigment in the nervous system of aged mice. *J. Cell Biol.* 26:779–795.

Sandborn, E. B. 1966. Electron microscopy of the neuron membrane systems and filaments. *Can. J. Physiol. Pharmacol.* 44:329–338.

Sandborn, E. B., LeBuis, J.-J., and Bois, P. 1966. Cytoplasmic microtubules in blood platelets. *Blood* 27:247–252.

Sandborn, E. B., Szeberenyi, A., Messier, P.-E., and Bois, P. 1965. A new membrane model derived from a study of filaments, microtubules and membranes. *Rev. Can. Biol.* 24:243–276.

Sandri, C., Akert, K., Livingston, R. B., and Moor, H. 1972. Particle aggregations at specialized sites in freeze-etched postsynaptic membranes. *Brain Res.* 41:1–16.

Sandritter, W., Nováková, V., Pilny, J., and Kiefer, G. 1967. Cytophotometrische Messungen des Nukleinsäure- und Proteingehaltes von Ganglienzellen der Ratte während der postnatalen Entwicklung und im Alter. *Z. Zellforsch. Mikrosk. Anat.* 80:145–152.

Santolaya, R. C. 1973. Nucleolus-like bodies in the neuronal cytoplasm of the mouse arcuate nucleus. *Z. Zellforsch. Mikrosk. Anat.* 146:319–328.

Santolaya, R. C., and Rodríguez-Echandía, E. L. 1968. The surface of the choroid plexus cells under normal and experimental conditions. *Z. Zellforsch. Mikrosk. Anat.* 92:43–51.

Satir, P., and Gilula, N. B. 1970. The cell junction in a lamellibranch gill ciliated epithelium. Localization of pyroantimonate precipitate. *J. Cell Biol.* 47:468–487.

Schadé, J. P., and Caveness, W. F. 1968. Alterations in dendritic organization. *Brain Res.* 7:59–86.

Schechter, J., and Weiner, R. 1972. Ultrastructural changes in the ependymal lining of the median eminence following the intraventricular administration of catecholamine. *Anat. Rec.* 172:643–650.

Scheer, U. 1970. The ultrastructure of the nuclear envelope of amphibian oocytes: a reinvestigation. III. Actinomycin-induced decrease in central granules within the pores. *J. Cell Biol.* 45:445–449.

Scheer, U. 1972. The ultrastructure of the nuclear envelope of amphibian oocytes. IV. On the chemical nature of the nuclear pore complex material. *Z. Zellforsch. Mikrosk. Anat.* 127:127–148.

Scheibel, M. E., Davies, T. L., Lindsay, R. D., and

Scheibel, A. B. 1974. Basilar dendrite bundles of giant pyramidal cells. *Exp. Neurol.* 42:307–319.

Scheibel, M. E., and Scheibel, A. B. 1955. The inferior olive. A Golgi study. *J. Comp. Neurol.* 102:77–131.

Scheibel, M. E., and Scheibel, A. B. 1968a. On the nature of dendritic spines – report of a workshop. *Commun. Behav. Biol. Part A* 1:231–265.

Scheibel, M. E., and Scheibel, A. B. 1968b. Terminal axonal patterns in cat spinal cord. II. The dorsal horn. *Brain Res.* 9:32–58.

Scheibel, M. E., and Scheibel, A. B. 1970. Organization of spinal motoneuron dendrites in bundles. *Exp. Neurol.* 28:106–112.

Scheibel, M. E., and Scheibel, A. B. 1973a. Dendrite bundles as sites for central programs: an hypothesis. *Int. J. Neurosci.* 6:195–202.

Scheibel, M. E., and Scheibel, A. B. 1973b. Dendrite bundles in the ventral commissure of cat spinal cord. *Exp. Neurol.* 39:482–488.

Schlaepfer, W. W., and Bunge, R. P. 1973. Effects of calcium ion concentration on the degeneration of amputated axons in tissue culture. *J. Cell Biol.* 59:456–470.

Schlaepfer, W. W., and Myers, F. K. 1973. Relationship of myelin internode elongation and growth in the rat sural nerve. *J. Comp. Neurol.* 147:255–266.

Schleiden, M. J. 1838. Beiträge zur Phytogenesis. *Müller's Arch.* pp. 137–176, trans. by H. Smith, as "Contributions to phytogenesis." In: *Microscopical Researches into the Accordance in the Structure and Growth of Animals and Plants*. T. Schwann. London, Sydenham Society, 1847, pp. 231–263.

Schlüter, G. 1973. Ultrastructural observations on cell necrosis during formation of the neural tube in mouse embryos. *Z. Anat. Entwicklungsgesch.* 141:251–264.

Schmidt, H. D. 1874. On the construction of the dark or double-bordered nerve fibre. *Mon. Microsc. J. (Lond.)* 11:200–221.

Schmitt, F. O. 1968. The molecular biology of neuronal fibrous proteins. *Neurosci. Res. Progr. Bull.* 6:119–144.

Schmitt, F. O., and Bear, R. S. 1939. The ultrastructure of the nerve axon sheath. *Biol. Rev.* 14:27–50.

Schmitt, F. O., Bear, R. S., and Palmer, K. J. 1941. X-ray diffraction studies on the structure of the nerve myelin sheath. *J. Cell Comp. Physiol.* 18:31–41.

Schmitt, F. O., and Davison, P. F. 1961. Biologie moléculaire des neurofilaments. *Actual. Neurophysiol.* 3ᵉ *Sér.*:355–369.

Schmitt, F. O., and Geschwind, N. 1957. The axon surface. *Progr. Biophys.* 8:165–215.

Schmitt, F. O., and Samson, F. E. 1968. Neuronal fibrous proteins. *Neurosci. Res. Progr. Bull.* 6:113–219.

Schmitt, F. O., Schneider, D. M., and Crothers, D. M., Eds. 1975. *Functional Linkage in Biomolecular Systems*. New York, Raven Press.

Schnaitman, C., and Greenawalt, J. W. 1968. Enzymatic properties of the inner and outer membranes of rat liver mitochondria. *J. Cell Biol.* 38:158–175.

Schnapp, B., and Mugnaini, E. 1975. The myelin sheath: Electron microscopic studies with thin sections and freeze-fracture. In: *Golgi Centennial Symposium: Perspectives in Neurobiology*. M. Santini, Ed. New York, Raven Press, pp. 209–233.

Schonbach, J., Schonbach, C., and Cuénod, M. 1971. Rapid phase of axoplasmic flow and synaptic proteins: An electron microscopical autoradiographic study. *J. Comp. Neurol.* 141:485–497.

Schonbach, J., Schonbach, C., and Cuénod, M. 1973. Distribution of transported proteins in the slow phase of axoplasmic flow. An electron microscopical autoradiographic study. *J. Comp. Neurol.* 152:1–16.

Schoultz, T. W., and Swett, J. E. 1972. The fine structure of the Golgi tendon organ. *J. Neurocytol.* 1:1–26.

Schultz, R. L. 1964. Macroglial identification in electron micrographs. *J. Comp. Neurol.* 122:281–295.

Schultz, R. L., and Karlsson, U. 1966. Spine apparatus occurrence during different fixation procedures. *J. Ultrastruct. Res.* 14:268–276.

Schultz, R. L., Maynard, E. A., and Pease, D. C. 1957. Electron microscopy of neurons and neuroglia of cerebral cortex and corpus callosum. *Am. J. Anat.* 100:369–407.

Schultz, R. L., and Pease, D. C. 1959. Cicatrix formation in rat cerebral cortex as revealed by electron microscopy. *Am. J. Pathol.* 35:1017–1041.

Schultze, H. 1878. Axencylinder and Ganglienzelle. Mikroskopische Studien über die Structur der Nervenfaser und Nervenzelle bei Wirbelthieren. *Arch. Anat. Physiol. Anat. Abt.* 1:259–287.

Schultze, M. 1861. Ueber Muskelkörperchen und das, was man eine Zelle zu nennen habe. *Müller's Arch.*, pp. 1–27.

Schwann, T. 1839. *Mikroskopische Untersuchungen über die Uebereinstimmung in der Struktur und dem Wachstum der Thiere und Pflanzen*. Berlin, Sander'sche Buchhandlung. Trans. by H. Smith, as Microscopical Researches into the Accordance in the Structure and Growth of Animals and Plants. London, Sydenham Society, 1847.

Schwyn, R. C. 1967. An autoradiographic study of satellite cells in autonomic ganglia. *Am. J. Anat.* 121:727–739.

Scott, D. E., and Knigge, K. M. 1970. Ultrastructural changes in the median eminence of the rat following deafferentation of the basal hypothalamus. *Z. Zellforsch. Mikrosk. Anat.* 105:1–32.

Scott, D. E., Kozlowski, G. P., and Dudley, G. K. 1973. A comparative ultrastructural analysis of the third cerebral ventricle of the North American Mink (*Mustela vison*). *Anat. Rec.* 175:155–168.

Scott, D. E., Kozlowski, G. P., Paull, W. K., Ramalingen, S., and Krobisch-Dudley, G. 1973. Scanning electron microscopy of the human cerebral ventricular system. II. The fourth ventricle. *Z. Zellforsch. Mikrosk. Anat.* 139:61–68.

Scott, D. E., Kozlowski, G. P., and Sheridan, M. N.

1974. Scanning electron microscopy in the ultrastructural analysis of the mammalian cerebral ventricular system. *Int. Rev. Cytol.* 37:349–388.

Scott, D. E., Paull, W. K., and Dudley, G. K. 1972. A comparative scanning electron microscopic analysis of the human cerebral ventricular system. I. The third ventricle. *Z. Zellforsch. Mikrosk. Anat.* 132:203–215.

Scott, G. L., and Guillery, R. W. 1974. Studies with the high voltage electron microscope of normal, degenerating and Golgi impregnated neuronal processes. *J. Neurocytol.* 3:567–590.

Seïte, R. 1970. Étude ultrastructurale de divers types d'inclusions nucléaires dans les neurones sympathiques du chat. *J. Ultrastruct. Res.* 30:152–165.

Seïte, R., Escaig, J., and Couineau, S. 1971. Microfilaments et microtubules nucléaires et organisation ultrastructurale des bâtonnets intranucléaires des neurones sympathiques. *J. Ultrastruct. Res.* 37: 449–478.

Seïte, R., and Mei, N. 1971. Influence de la stimulation electrique sur la fréquence des bâtonnets intranucléaires des neurones sympathiques. Étude quantitative en microscopie electronique. *C. R. Hebd. Acad. Sci. (Paris)* 272:3352–3355.

Seïte, R., Mei, N., and Couineau, S. 1971. Modification quantitative des bâtonnets intranucléaires des neurones sympathiques sous l'influence de la stimulation electrique. *Brain Res.* 34:277–290.

Seïte, R., Mei, N., and Vuillet-Luciani, J. 1973. Effects of electrical stimulation on nuclear microfilaments and microtubules of sympathetic neurons submitted to cycloheximide. *Brain Res.* 50:419–423.

Sekhon, S. S., and Maxwell, D. S. 1974. Ultrastructural changes in neurons of the spinal anterior horn of aging mice with particular reference to the accumulation of lipofuscin pigment. *J. Neurocytol.* 3:59–72.

Sétáló, G., and Székely, G. 1967. The presence of membrane specializations indicative of somatodendritic synaptic junctions in the optic tectum of the frog. *Exp. Brain Res.* 4:237–242.

Shabo, A. L., and Maxwell, D. S. 1968a. The morphology of the arachnoid villi: a light and electron microscopic study in the monkey. *J. Neurosurg.* 29:451–463.

Shabo, A. L., and Maxwell, D. S. 1968b. Electron microscopic observations on the fate of particulate matter in the cerebrospinal fluid. *J. Neurosurg.* 29:464–474.

Shabo, A. L., and Maxwell, D. S. 1971. The subarachnoid space following the introduction of a foreign protein: an electron microscopic study with peroxidase. *J. Neuropathol. Exp. Neurol.* 30:506–524.

Shantha, T. R., and Bourne, G. H. 1968. The perineural epithelium—A new concept. In: *The Structure and Function of Nervous Tissue*, Vol. 4. G. H. Bourne, Ed. New York, Academic Press, pp. 447–511.

Shelanski, M. L. 1973. Chemistry of the filaments and tubules of brain. *J. Histochem. Cytochem.* 21:529–539.

Shelanski, M. L., Albert, S., Devries, G. H., and Norton, W. T. 1971. Isolation of filaments from brain. *Science* 174:1242–1245.

Shelanski, M. L., and Feit, H. 1972. Filaments and tubules in the nervous system. In: *The Structure and Function of Nervous Tissue*, Vol. 6. G. H. Bourne, Ed. New York, Academic Press, pp. 47–80.

Shelanski, M. L., and Taylor, E. W. 1967. Isolation of a protein subunit from microtubules. *J. Cell Biol.* 34:549–554.

Shelanski, M. L., and Taylor, E. W. 1968. Properties of the protein subunit of central-pair and outer-doublet microtubules of sea urchin flagella. *J. Cell Biol.* 38:304–315.

Shepherd, G. M. 1972. The neuron doctrine: a revision of functional concepts. *Yale J. Biol. Med.* 45:584–599.

Shepherd, G. M. 1974. *The Synaptic Organization of the Brain. An Introduction.* New York, Oxford University Press.

Shofer, R. J., Pappas, G. D., and Purpura, D. P. 1964. Radiation-induced changes in morphological and physiological properties of immature cerebellar cortex. In: *Response of the Nervous System to Ionizing Radiation.* T. J. Haley and R. S. Snider, Eds. Boston, Little, Brown and Co., pp. 476–508.

Shuangshoti, S., and Netsky, M. G. 1966. Histogenesis of choroid plexus in man. *Am. J. Anat.* 118:283–316.

Sidman, R. L. 1970a. Autoradiographic methods and principles for study of the nervous system with thymidine-H³. In: *Contemporary Research Techniques of Neuroanatomy.* S. O. E. Ebbesson and W. J. H. Nauta, Eds. New York, Springer-Verlag, pp. 252–274.

Sidman, R. L. 1970b. Cell proliferation, migration, and interaction in the developing mammalian central nervous system. In: *The Neurosciences: Second Study Program.* F. O. Schmitt, Ed. New York, Rockefeller University Press, pp. 100–107.

Sidman, R. L. 1974. Cell-cell recognition in the developing central nervous system. In: *The Neurosciences: Third Study Program.* F. O. Schmitt and F. G. Worden, Eds. Cambridge, Mass., M. I. T. Press, pp. 743–758.

Sidman, R. L., and Rakic, P. 1973. Neuronal migration, with special reference to developing human brain: a review. *Brain Res.* 62:1–35.

Siegesmund, K. A. 1968. The fine structure of subsurface cisterns. *Anat. Rec.* 162:187–196.

Siegesmund, K. A., Dutta, C. R., and Fox, C. A. 1964. The ultrastructure of the intranuclear rodlet in certain nerve cells. *J. Anat.* 98:93–97.

Silveira, M., and Porter, K. R. 1964. The spermatozoids of flatworms and their microtubular systems. *Protoplasma* 59:240–265.

Simionescu, M., Simionescu, N., and Palade, G. E.

1975. Segmental differentiations of cell junctions in the vascular endothelium. The microvasculature. *J. Cell Biol.* 67:863–885.

Simpson, F. O., and Devine, C. E. 1966. The fine structure of autonomic neuromuscular contacts in arterioles of sheep renal cortex. *J. Anat.* 100:127–137.

Singer, M., and Bryant, S. V. 1969. Movements in the myelin Schwann sheath of the vertebrate axon. *Nature* 221:1148–1150.

Singer, M., and Green, M. R. 1968. Autoradiographic studies of uridine incorporation in peripheral nerve of the newt, *Triturus. J. Morphol.* 124:321–344.

Singer, M., and Salpeter, M. M. 1966. The transport of ³H-l-histidine through the Schwann and myelin sheath into the axon, including a reevaluation of myelin function. *J. Morphol.* 120:281–315.

Singer, S. J., and Nicholson, G. 1972. The fluid mosaic model of the structure of cell membranes. *Science* 175:720–731.

Singer, S. J., and Rothfield, L. I. 1973. Synthesis and turnover of cell membranes. *Neurosci. Res. Progr. Bull.* 11:1–86.

Sjöstrand, F. S. 1950. Electron-microscopic demonstration of a membrane structure isolated from nerve tissue. *Nature (Lond.)* 165:482–483.

Sjöstrand, F. S. 1953. The lamellated structure of the nerve myelin sheath as revealed by high resolution electron microscopy. *Experientia* 9:68–69.

Sjöstrand, F. S. 1958. Ultrastructure of retinal rod synapses of the guinea pig eye as revealed by three-dimensional reconstructions from serial sections. *J. Ultrastruct. Res.* 2:122–170.

Sjöstrand, F. S. 1961. Electron microscopy of the retina. In: *The Structure of the Eye.* G. K. Smelser, Ed. New York, Academic Press, pp. 1–28.

Sjöstrand, F. S. 1963a. A new ultrastructural element of the membranes in mitochondria and of some cytoplasmic membranes. *J. Ultrastruct. Res.* 9:340–361.

Sjöstrand, F. S. 1963b. The structure and formation of the myelin sheath. In: *Mechanisms of Demyelination.* A. S. Rose and C. M. Pearson, Eds. New York, McGraw-Hill Book Co., pp. 1–43.

Sjöstrand, F. S., and Rhodin, J. 1953. The ultrastructure of the proximal convoluted tubules of the mouse kidney as revealed by high resolution electron microscopy. *Exp. Cell Res.* 4:426–456.

Skoff, R. P., and Hamburger, V. 1974. Fine structure of dendritic and axonal growth cones in embryonic chick spinal cord. *J. Comp. Neurol.* 153:107–148.

Slautterback, D. B. 1963. Cytoplasmic microtubules. I. Hydra. *J. Cell Biol.* 18:367–388.

Sloper, J. C. 1966. Hypothalamic neurosecretion. The validity of the concept of neurosecretion and its physiological and pathological implications. *Br. Med. Bull.* 22:209–215.

Sloper, J. J. 1971. Dendro-dendritic synapses in the primate motor cortex. *Brain Res.* 34:186–192.

Sloper, J. J. 1972. Gap junctions between dendrites in the primate cortex. *Brain Res.* 44:641–646.

Sloper, J. J., and Powell, T. P. S. 1973. Observations in the axon initial segment and other structures in the neocortex using conventional staining and ethanolic phosphotungstic acid. *Brain Res.* 50:163–169.

Smart, I., and Leblond, C. P. 1961. Evidence for division and transformations of neuroglia cells in the mouse brain, as derived from radioautography after injection of thymidine-H³. *J. Comp. Neurol.* 116:349–367.

Smith, C. A., and Sjöstrand, F. S. 1961a. A synaptic structure in the hair cells of the guinea pig cochlea. *J. Ultrastruct. Res.* 5:184–192.

Smith, C. A., and Sjöstrand, F. S. 1961b. Structure of the nerve endings on the external hair cells of the guinea pig cochlea as studied by serial sections. *J. Ultrastruct. Res.* 5:523–556.

Smith, D. S., Järlfors, U., and Beránek, R. 1970. The organization of synaptic axoplasm in the lamprey (*Petromyzon marinus*) central nervous system. *J. Cell Biol.* 46:199–219.

Smith, D. S., and Treherne, J. E. 1963. Functional aspects of the organization of the insect nervous system. In: *Advances in Insect Physiology,* Vol. I. J. W. L. Beament, J. E. Treherne, and V. B. Wigglesworth, Eds. New York, Academic Press, pp. 401–484.

Smith, J. M., O'Leary, J. L., Harris, A. B., and Gay, A. J. 1964. Ultrastructural features of the lateral geniculate nucleus of the cat. *J. Comp. Neurol.* 123:357–377.

Sorokin, S. P. 1968. Reconstructions of centriole formation and ciliogenesis in mammalian lungs. *J. Cell Sci.* 3:207–230.

Sotelo, C. 1968. Permanence of postsynaptic specializations in the frog sympathetic ganglion cells after denervation. *Exp. Brain Res.* 6:294–305.

Sotelo, C. 1969. Ultrastructural aspects of the cerebellar cortex of the frog. In: *Neurobiology of Cerebellar Evolution and Development.* R. Llinás, Ed. Chicago, American Medical Association, pp. 327–371.

Sotelo, C. 1971a. General features of the synaptic organization in the central nervous system. In: *Advances in Experimental Medicine and Biology,* Vol. 13, *Chemistry and Brain Development.* R. Paoletti and A. N. Davison, Eds. New York, Plenum Press, pp. 239–280.

Sotelo, C. 1971b. The fine structural localization of norepinephrine-³H in the substantia nigra and area postrema of the rat. An autoradiographic study. *J. Ultrastruct. Res.* 36:824–841.

Sotelo, C. 1973. Permanence and fate of paramembranous synaptic specializations in "mutants" and experimental animals. *Brain Res.* 62:345–351.

Sotelo, C., and Angaut, P. 1973. The fine structure of the cerebellar central nuclei in the cat. I. Neurons and neuroglial cells. *Exp. Brain Res.* 16:410–430.

Sotelo, C., and Changeux, J.-P. 1974. Transsynaptic

degeneration "en cascade" in the cerebellar cortex of staggerer mutant mice. *Brain Res.* 67:519–526.

Sotelo, C., Hillman, D. E., Zamora, A. J., and Llinás, R. 1975. Climbing fiber deafferentation: its action on Purkinje cell dendritic spines. *Brain Res.* 98:574–581.

Sotelo, C., and Llinás, R. 1972. Specialized membrane junctions between neurons in the vertebrate cerebellar cortex. *J. Cell Biol.* 53:271–289.

Sotelo, C., Llinás, R., and Baker, R. 1974. Structural study of inferior olivary nucleus of the cat: Morphological correlates of electrotonic coupling. *J. Neurophysiol.* 37:541–559.

Sotelo, C., and Palay, S. L. 1967. Synapses avec des contacts étroits (tight junctions) dans le noyau vestibulaire latéral du rat. *J. Microscopie* 6:83a.

Sotelo, C., and Palay, S. L. 1968. The fine structure of the lateral vestibular nucleus in the rat. I. Neurons and neuroglial cells. *J. Cell Biol.* 36:151–179.

Sotelo, C., and Palay, S. L. 1970. The fine structure of the lateral vestibular nucleus in the rat. II. Synaptic organization. *Brain Res.* 18:93–115.

Sotelo, C., and Palay, S. L. 1971. Altered axons and axon terminals in the lateral vestibular nucleus of the rat. Possible example of axonal remodelling. *Lab. Invest.* 25:653–671.

Sotelo, C., and Riche, D. 1974. The smooth endoplasmic reticulum and the retrograde and fast orthograde transport of horseradish peroxidase in the nigro-striato-nigral loop. *Anat. Embryol.* 146:209–218.

Špaček, J. 1971. Three-dimensional reconstruction of astroglia and oligodendroglia cells. *Z. Zellforsch. Mikrosk. Anat.* 112:430–442.

Špaček, J., and Lieberman, A. R. 1974. Ultrastructure and three-dimensional organization of synaptic glomeruli in rat somatosensory thalamus. *J. Anat.* 117:487–516.

Speidel, C. C. 1964. In vitro studies of myelinated nerve fibers. *Int. Rev. Cytol.* 16:173–231.

Spencer, P. S., Raine, C., and Wiśniewski, H. 1973. Axon diameter and myelin thickness—unusual relationships in dorsal root ganglia. *Anat. Rec.* 176:225–244.

Spooner, B. S., Yamada, K. M., and Wessells, N. K. 1971. Microfilaments and cell locomotion. *J. Cell Biol.* 49:595–613.

Stell, W. K. 1965. Correlation of retinal cytoarchitecture and ultrastructure in Golgi preparations. *Anat. Rec.* 153:389–397.

Stelly, N., Stevens, B. J., and André, J. 1970. Étude cytochimique de la lamelle dense de l'enveloppe nucléaire. *J. Microscopie* 9:1015–1028.

Stelzner, D. J. 1971. The relation between synaptic vesicles, Golgi apparatus, and smooth endoplasmic reticulum: A developmental study using zinc iodide-osmium technique. *Z. Zellforsch. Mikrosk. Anat.* 120:332–345.

Stempak, J. G., and Knobler, R. L. 1972. Bidirectionality in the tongue processes of the oligodendroglial cell investment of axons in the albino rat. *Am. J. Anat.* 135:287–292.

Stensaas, L. J., and Gilson, B. C. 1972. Ependymal and subependymal cells in the caudatopallial junction in the lateral ventricle of the neonatal rabbit. *Z. Zellforsch. Mikrosk. Anat.* 132:297–322.

Stensaas, L. J., and Stensaas, S. S. 1968. Astrocytic neuroglial cells, oligodendrocytes and microliacytes in the spinal cord of the toad. II. Electron microscopy. *Z. Zellforsch. Mikrosk. Anat.* 86:184–213.

Stensaas, S. S., Edwards, E. Q., and Stensaas, L. J. 1972. An experimental study of hyperchromatic nerve cells in the cerebral cortex. *Exp. Neurol.* 36:472–487.

Stenwig, A. E. 1972. The origin of brain macrophages in traumatic lesions, Wallerian degeneration, and retrograde degeneration. *J. Neuropathol. Exp. Neurol.* 31:696–704.

Sterling, P. 1970. A light and electron microscopic study of the superficial gray of the cat superior colliculus. *Anat. Rec.* 166:383.

Stirling, C. A. 1975a. Abnormalities in Schwann cell sheaths in spinal nerve roots of dystrophic mice. *J. Anat.* 119:169–180.

Stirling, C. A. 1975b. Experimentally induced myelination of amyelinated axons in dystrophic mice. *Brain Res.* 87:130–135.

Streit, P., Akert, K., Sandri, C., Livingston, R. B., and Moor, H. 1972. Dynamic ultrastructure of presynaptic membranes at nerve terminals in the spinal cord of rats. Anesthetized and unanesthetized preparations compared. *Brain Res.* 48:11–26.

Stretton, A. O. W., and Kravitz, E. A. 1968. Neuronal geometry: determination with a technique of intracellular dye injection. *Science* 162:132–134.

Stretton, A. O. W., and Kravitz, E. A. 1973. Intracellular dye injection: The selection of Procion yellow and its application in preliminary studies of neuronal geometry in the lobster nervous system. In: *Intracellular Staining in Neurobiology*. S. B. Kater and C. Nicholson, Eds. New York, Springer-Verlag, pp. 21–40.

Strong, L. H. 1961. The first appearance of vessels within the spinal cord of the mammal: their developing patterns as far as partial formation of the dorsal septum. *Acta Anat.* 44:80–108.

Strong, L. H. 1964. The early embryonic pattern of internal vascularization of the mammalian cerebral cortex. *J. Comp. Neurol.* 123:121–138.

Stubblefield, E. 1973. The structure of mammalian chromosomes. *Int. Rev. Cytol.* 35:1–60.

Sturrock, R. R. 1974. Histogenesis of the anterior limb of the anterior commissure of the mouse brain. III. An electron microscope study of gliogenesis. *J. Anat.* 117:37–54.

Sumner, B. E. H. 1975. A quantitative analysis of the responses of presynaptic boutons to postsynaptic motor neuron axotomy. *Exp. Neurol.* 46:605–615.

Sutherland, S. 1965. The connective tissues of peripheral nerves. *Brain* 88:841–854.

Swift, H. W. 1962. Nucleic acids and cell morphology

in Dipteran salivary glands. In: *The Molecular Control of Cellular Activity*. J. M. Allen, Ed. New York, McGraw-Hill Book Co., pp. 73–125.

Szamier, R. B. 1974. Enzymatic digestion of presynaptic structures in electroreceptors of elasmobranchs. *Am. J. Anat. 139*:567–574.

Szebro, Z. 1965. The ultrastructure of gliosomes in the brains of amphibia. *J. Cell Biol. 26*:313–322.

Szentágothai, J. 1963. The structure of the synapse in the lateral geniculate body. *Acta Anat. 55*:166–185.

Szentágothai, J. 1970. Glomerular synapses, complex synaptic arrangements and their operational significance. In: *The Neurosciences. Second Study Program*. F. O. Schmitt, Ed. New York, The Rockefeller University Press, pp. 427–443.

Szentágothai, J., Hámori, J., and Tömböl, T. 1966. Degeneration and electron microscope analysis of the synaptic glomeruli in the lateral geniculate body. *Exp. Brain Res. 2*:283–301.

Takahashi, K., and Hama, K. 1965. Some observations on the fine structure of the synaptic area in the ciliary ganglion of the chick. *Z. Zellforsch. Mikrosk. Anat. 67*:174–184.

Takeichi, M. 1967. The fine structure of ependymal cells. Part II: An electron microscopic study of the soft-shelled turtle paraventricular organ, with special reference to the fine structure of ependymal cells and so-called albuminous substance. *Z. Zellforsch. Mikrosk. Anat. 76*:471–485.

Tani, E., and Ametani, T. 1970. Substructure of microtubules in brain nerve cells as revealed by ruthenium red. *J. Cell Biol. 46*:159–165.

Tani, E., and Ametani, T. 1971. Extracellular distribution of ruthenium red positive substance in the cerebral cortex. *J. Ultrastruct. Res. 34*:1–14.

Tani, E., Ikeda, K., and Nishiura, M. 1973. Freeze-etching images of central myelinated nerve fibers. *J. Neurocytol. 2*:305–314.

Tani, E., Nishiura, M., and Higashi, N. 1973. Freeze-fracture studies of gap junctions of normal and neoplastic astrocytes. *Acta Neuropathol. 26*:127–138.

Tarlov, I. M. 1937. Structure of the nerve root. I. Nature of the junction between the central and the peripheral nervous system. *Arch. Surg. (Chicago) 37*:555–583.

Tasaki, I., Carnay, L., Sandlin, R., and Watanabe, A. 1969. Fluorescence changes during conduction in nerves stained with acridine orange. *Science 163*:683–685.

Taxi, J. 1961. Étude de l'ultrastructure des zones synaptiques dans les ganglions sympathiques de la Grenouille. *C. R. Acad. Sci. (Paris) 252*:174–176.

Taxi, J. 1964. Étude de certaines synapses interneuronales du système nerveux autonome. *Acta Neuroveg. (Wien) 26*:360–370.

Taxi, J., and Droz, B. 1966. Étude de l'incorporation de noradrénaline-³H (NA-³H) et de 5-hydroxytryptophane-³H (5HTP-³H) dans les fibres nerveuses du canal déférens et de l'intestin. *C. R. Acad. Sci. [D] 263*:1237–1240.

Tello, J. F. 1904. Las neurofibrillas en los vertebrados inferiores. *Trab. Lab. Invest. Biol. Univ. Madrid 3*:113–1151.

Tennyson, V. M. 1970. The fine structure of the axon and growth cone of the dorsal root neuroblast of the rabbit embryo. *J. Cell Biol. 44*:62–79.

Tennyson, V. M., and Pappas, G. D. 1961. Electron microscope studies of the developing telencephalic choroid plexus in normal and hydrocephalic rabbits. In: *Disorders of the Developing Nervous System*. W. Fields and M. Desmond, Eds. Springfield, Ill., Charles C Thomas, pp. 267–318.

Tennyson, V. M., and Pappas, G. D. 1962. An electron microscope study of ependymal cells of the fetal, early postnatal and adult rabbit. *Z. Zellforsch. Mikrosk. Anat. 56*:595–618.

Tennyson, V. M., and Pappas, G. D. 1964. Fine structure of the developing telencephalic and myelencephalic choroid plexus in the rabbit. *J. Comp. Neurol. 123*:379–412.

Tennyson, V. M., and Pappas, G. D. 1968. The fine structure of the choroid plexus; adult and developmental stages. In: *Progress in Brain Research*, Vol. 29, *Brain Barrier Systems*. A. Lajtha and D. H. Ford, Eds. Amsterdam, Elsevier, pp. 63–85.

Terry, R. D. 1963. The fine structure of neurofibrillary tangles in Alzheimer's disease. *J. Neuropathol. Exp. Neurol. 22*:629–642.

Terry, R. D., and Peña, C. 1965. Experimental production of neurofibrillary degeneration. II. Electron microscopy, phosphatase histochemistry, and electron probe analysis. *J. Neuropathol. Exp. Neurol. 24*:200–210.

Terry, R. D., and Weiss, M. 1963. Studies in Tay-Sachs disease. II. Ultrastructure of the cerebrum. *J. Neuropathol. Exp. Neurol. 22*:18–55.

Terry, R. D., and Wiśniewski, H. 1968. Fibrous constituents in some pathological states. *Neurosci. Res. Progr. Bull. 6*:184–187.

Thomas, E., and Pearse, A. G. E. 1961. The fine localization of dehydrogenases in the nervous system. *Histochemie 2*:266–282.

Thomas, P. K. 1955. Growth changes in the myelin sheath of peripheral nerve fibres. *Proc. R. Soc. Ser. B 143*:380–391.

Thomas, P. K. 1956. Growth changes in the diameter of peripheral nerve fibres in fishes. *J. Anat. 90*:5–14.

Thomas, P. K. 1963. The connective tissue of peripheral nerve: an electron microscope study. *J. Anat. 97*:35–44.

Thomas, P. K. 1964a. Changes in the endoneurial sheaths of peripheral myelinated nerve fibers during Wallerian degeneration. *J. Anat. 98*:175–182.

Thomas, P. K. 1964b. The deposition of collagen in relation to Schwann cell basement membrane during peripheral nerve regeneration. *J. Cell Biol. 23*:375–382.

Thomas, P. K., and Jones, D. G. 1967. The cellular response to nerve injury. 2. Regeneration of the perineurium after nerve section. *J. Anat. 101*:45–55.

Thomas, P. K., and Young, J. Z. 1949. Internode lengths in the nerves of fishes. *J. Anat.* 83:336–350.

Thureson-Klein, A. 1972. Giant mitochondria in Schwann cells of bovine splenic nerve. *Tissue Cell* 4:519–524.

Tilney, L. G. 1971. How microtubule patterns are generated. The relative importance of nucleation and bridging of microtubules in the formation of the axoneme of *Raphidiophrys*. *J. Cell Biol.* 51:837–854.

Tilney, L. G., Bryan, J., Bush, D. J., Fujiwara, K., Mooseker, M. S., Murphy, D. B., and Snyder, D. H. 1973. Microtubules: Evidence for 13 protofilaments. *J. Cell Biol.* 59:267–275.

Tilney, L. G., Hiramoto, Y., and Marsland, D. 1966. Studies on the microtubules in heliozoa. III. A pressure analysis of the role of these structures in the formation and maintenance of the axopodia of *Actinosphaerium nucleofilum* (Barrett). *J. Cell Biol.* 29:77–95.

Tilney, L. G., and Porter, K. R. 1967. Studies on the microtubules of *Heliozoa*. II. The effect of low temperature on these structures in the formation and maintenance of the axopodia. *J. Cell Biol.* 34:327–343.

Tokuyasu, K., and Yamada, E. 1959. The fine structure of the retina studied with the electron microscope. IV. Morphogenesis of outer segments of retinal rods. *J. Biophys. Biochem. Cytol.* 6:225–230.

Torack, R. L., and Barrnett, R. J. 1964. The fine structural localization of nucleoside phosphatase activity in the blood-brain barrier. *J. Neuropathol. Exp. Neurol.* 23:46–59.

Torvik, A. 1972. Phagocytosis of nerve cells during retrograde degeneration. An electron microscopic study. *J. Neuropathol. Exp. Neurol.* 31:132–146.

Torvik, A., and Skjörten, F. 1971. Electron microscopic observations on nerve cell regeneration and degeneration after axon lesions. *Acta Neuropathol.* 17:248–264.

Torvik, A., and Söreide, A. J. 1972. Nerve cell regeneration after axon lesions in newborn rabbits. Light and electron microscopic study. *J. Neuropathol. Exp. Neurol.* 31:683–695.

Toth, S. E. 1968. The origin of lipofuscin age pigment. *Exp. Gerontol.* 3:19–30.

Tranzer, J. P., Thoenen, H., Snipes, R. L., and Richards, J. G. 1969. Recent developments on the ultrastructural aspects of adrenergic nerve endings in various experimental conditions. In: *Progress in Brain Research*, Vol. 31, *Mechanisms of Synaptic Transmission.* K. Akert and P. G. Waser, Eds. Amsterdam, Elsevier, pp. 33–46.

Turner, P. T., and and Harris, A. B. 1974. Ultrastructure of exogenous peroxidase in cerebral cortex. *Brain Res.* 74:305–326.

Tusques, J., and Pradal, G. 1968. Inclusion d'aspect filamenteux, dans le noyau des cellules argyrophiles de la muqueuse gastrique du lapin mise en évidence en microscopie électronique. *C. R. Hebd. Acad. Sci. (Paris)* 267:1738–1741.

Uchizono, K. 1965. Characteristics of excitatory and inhibitory synapses in the central nervous system of the cat. *Nature (Lond.)* 207:642–643.

Uchizono, K. 1967. Inhibitory synapses on the stretch receptor neurone of the crayfish. *Nature (Lond.)* 214:833–834.

Uchizono, K. 1968. Axon identification in the cerebellar cortex of the cat. *Arch. Histol. Jap.* 29:399–424.

Uchizono, K. 1969. Synaptic organization of the mammalian cerebellum. In: *Neurobiology of Cerebellar Evolution and Development.* R. Llinás, Ed. Chicago, AMA-ERF Institute for Biomedical Research, pp. 549–581.

Uchizono, K. 1973. Structural and chemical considerations of the presynaptic inhibitory synapses. *Proc. Jap. Acad.* 49:569–574.

Uzman, B. G. 1964. The spiral configuration of myelin lamellae. *J. Ultrastruct. Res.* 11:208–212.

Uzman, B. G., and Nogueira-Graf, G. 1957. Electron microscope studies of the formation of nodes of Ranvier in mouse sciatic nerves. *J. Biophys. Biochem. Cytol.* 3:589–598.

Uzman, B. G., and Villegas, G. M. 1960. A comparison of nodes of Ranvier in sciatic nerves with node-like structures in optic nerves of the mouse. *J. Biophys. Biochem. Cytol.* 7:761–762.

Valdivia, O. 1971. Methods of fixation and the morphology of synaptic vesicles. *J. Comp. Neurol.* 142:257–274.

Valentin, G. G. 1836. Über den Verlauf und die letzten Ende der Nerven. *Nova Acta phys. med. Acad. caes. Leopold-Carol. Natl. Curiosorum, Breslau* 18:51–240.

Valverde, F. 1966. The pyramidal tract in rodents. A study of its relations with the posterior column nuclei, dorsolateral reticular formation of the medulla oblongata, and cervical spinal cord. *Z. Zellforsch. Mikrosk. Anat.* 71:297–363.

Valverde, F. 1967. Apical dendritic spines of the visual cortex and light deprivation in the mouse. *Exp. Brain Res.* 3:337–352.

Valverde, F. 1968. Structural changes in the area striata of the mouse after enucleation. *Exp. Brain Res.* 5:274–292.

Valverde, F. 1971. Rate and extent of recovery from dark rearing in the visual cortex of the mouse. *Brain Res.* 33:1–11.

Valverde, F., and Ruiz-Marcos, A. 1969. Dendritic spines in the visual cortex of the mouse: Introduction to a mathematical model. *Exp. Brain Res.* 8:269–283.

Van Breemen, V. L., and Clemente, C. D. 1955. Silver deposition in the central nervous system and the hematoencephalic barrier studied with the electron microscope. *J. Biophys. Biochem. Cytol.* 1:161–165.

van der Loos, H. 1963. Fine structure of synapses in the cerebral cortex. *Z. Zellforsch. Mikrosk. Anat.* 60:815–825.

van der Loos, H. 1964. Similarities and dissimilarities in submicroscopical morphology of interneuronal contact sites of presumably different functional character. In: *Progress in Brain Research*, Vol. 6, *Topics in Basic Neurology*. W. Bargmann and J. P. Schadé, Eds. Amsterdam, Elsevier, pp. 43–58.

van der Loos, H. 1967. The history of the neuron. In: *The Neuron*. H. Hydén, Ed. Amsterdam, Elsevier, pp. 1–47.

Van Orden, L. S., Bensch, K. G., and Giarman, N. J. 1967. Histochemical and functional relationships of catecholamines in adrenergic nerve endings. II. Extravesicular norepinephrine. *J. Pharmacol. Exp. Ther. 155*:428–439.

Van Orden, L. S., Bloom, F. E., Barrnett, R. J., and Giarman, N. J. 1966. Histochemical and functional relationships of catecholamines in adrenergic nerve endings. I. Participation of granular vesicles. *J. Pharmacol. Exp. Ther. 154*:185–199.

Varkonyi, T., Domokos, H., Maurer, M., Zoltan, O. T., Csillik, B., and Földi, M. 1970. Die Wirkung von DL-Kavain und Magnesium-Orotat auf die feinstrukturellen neuropathologischen Veränderungen der experimentellen lymphogenen Enzephalopathie. *Z. Gerontol. 3*:254–260.

Vaughan, D. W., and Peters, A. 1973. A three dimensional study of layer I of the rat parietal cortex. *J. Comp. Neurol. 149*:355–370.

Vaughan, D. W., and Peters, A. 1974. Neuroglial cells in the cerebral cortex of rats from young adulthood to old age: an electron microscope study. *J. Neurocytol. 3*:405–429.

Vaughn, J. E. 1967. Undifferentiated neuroglial cells in adult rat optic nerve. *J. Cell Biol. 35*:136A–137A.

Vaughn, J. E. 1969. An electron microscopic analysis of gliogenesis in rat optic nerves. *Z. Zellforsch. Mikrosk. Anat. 94*:293–324.

Vaughn, J. E., and Grieshaber, J. A. 1972. An electron microscopic investigation of glycogen and mitochondria in developing and adult rat spinal cord neuropil. *J. Neurocytol. 1*:397–412.

Vaughn, J. E., Henrikson, C. K., and Grieshaber, J. A. 1974. A quantitative study of synapses on motor neuron dendritic growth cones in developing mouse spinal cord. *J. Cell Biol. 60*:664–672.

Vaughn, J. E., Hinds, P. L., and Skoff, R. P. 1970. Electron microscopic studies of Wallerian degeneration in rat optic nerves. I. The multipotential glia. *J. Comp. Neurol. 140*:175–206.

Vaughn, J. E., and Pease, D. C. 1967. Electron microscopy of classically stained astrocytes. *J. Comp. Neurol. 131*:143–153.

Vaughn, J. E., and Pease, D. C. 1970. Electron microscopic studies of Wallerian degeneration in rat optic nerves. II. Astrocytes, oligodendrocytes and adventitial cells. *J. Comp. Neurol. 140*:207–226.

Vaughn, J. E., and Peters, A. 1967. Electron microscopy of the early postnatal development of fibrous astrocytes. *Am. J. Anat. 121*:131–152.

Vaughn, J. E., and Peters, A. 1968. A third neuroglial cell type. An electron microscope study. *J. Comp. Neurol. 133*:269–288.

Vaughn, J. E., and Peters, A. 1971. The morphology and development of neuroglial cells. In: *Cellular Aspects of Neural Growth and Differentiation*. D. C. Pease, Ed. Berkeley, University of California Press, pp. 103–134.

Verworn, M. 1899. *General Physiology, An Outline of the Science of Life*. Trans. from the second German edition by F. S. Lee. London, Macmillan.

Vigh-Teichmann, I., Vigh, B., and Koritsanszky, S. 1970. Liquorkontaktneurone im Nucleus lateralis tuberis von Fischen. *Z. Zellforsch. Mikrosk. Anat. 105*:325–338.

Virchow, R. 1846. Ueber das granulierte Ansehen der Wandungen der Gehirnventrikel. *Allg. Z. Psychiatr. 3*:424–450.

Virchow, R. 1860. *Cellular Pathology*. Trans. from the second German edition by F. Chance. London, Churchill.

Vizoso, A. D., and Young, J. Z. 1948. Internode length and fibre diameter in developing and regenerating nerves. *J. Anat. 82*:110–134.

Vollrath, L., and Huss, H. 1973. The synaptic ribbons of the guinea pig pineal gland under normal and experimental conditions. *Z. Zellforsch. Mikrosk. Anat. 139*:417–429.

Wachtel, A. W., and Szamier, R. B. 1966. Special cutaneous organs of fish: The tuberous organ of *Eigenmannia*. *J. Morphol. 119*:51–80.

Wade, J. B., and Karnovsky, M. J. 1974. The structure of the zonula occludens. A single fibril model based on freeze-fracture. *J. Cell Biol. 60*:168–180.

Waggener, J. D. 1963. The ultrastructure of the glial–Schwann cell junction of the rat. *Anat. Rec. 145*:296.

Waggener, J. D. 1964. Electron microscopic studies of brain-barrier mechanisms. *J. Neuropathol. Exp. Neurol. 23*:174.

Waggener, J. D., and Beggs, J. 1967. The membranous coverings of neural tissues: An electron microscopy study. *J. Neuropathol. Exp. Neurol. 26*:412–426.

Waggener, J. D., Bunn, S. M., and Beggs, J. 1965. The diffusion of ferritin within the peripheral nerve sheath: An electron microscopy study. *J. Neuropathol. Exp. Neurol. 24*:430–443.

Wagner, R. 1847. *Neue Untersuchungen über den Bau und die Endigung der Nerven und die Struktur der Ganglien*. Leipzig, Voss.

Waksman, B. H. 1961. Experimental study of diphtheritic polyneuritis in the rabbit and guinea pig. III. The blood-nerve barrier in the rabbit. *J. Neuropathol. Exp. Neurol. 20*:35–77.

Walberg, F. 1963. An electron microscopic study of the inferior olive of the cat. *J. Comp. Neurol. 120*:1–17.

Walberg, F. 1964. Further electron microscopical investigations of the inferior olive of the cat. In: *Progress in Brain Research*, Vol. 6, *Topics in Basic Neurology*. W. Bargmann and J. P. Schadé, Eds. Amsterdam, Elsevier, pp. 59–75.

Walberg, F. 1965a. A special type of synaptic vesicles in *boutons* in the inferior olive. J. Ultrastruct. Res. 12:237.

Walberg, F. 1965b. Axoaxonic contacts in the cuneate

nucleus, probable basis for presynaptic depolarization. *Exp. Neurol.* 13:218–231.

Walberg, F. 1966a. The fine structure of the cuneate nucleus in normal cats and following interruption of afferent fibers. *Exp. Brain Res.* 2:107–128.

Walberg, F. 1966b. Elongated vesicles in terminal boutons of the central nervous system, a result of aldehyde fixation. *Acta Anat.* 65:224–235.

Waldeyer, W. 1891. Ueber einige neuere Forschungen im Gebiete der Anatomie des Central-nervensystems. *Dtsch. Med. Wochenschr.* 17:1213–1218, 1244–1246, 1267–1269, 1287–1289, 1331–1332, and 1352–1356.

Waller, A. V. 1850. Experiments on the section of the glossopharyngeal and hypoglossal nerves of the frog, and observations of the alterations produced thereby in the structure of their primitive fibres. *Phil. Trans. R. Soc.* 140:423–429.

Waller, A. V. 1852a. Examen des altérations qui ont lieu dans les filets d'origine du nerf pneumogastrique et des nerfs rachidiens, par suite de la section de ces nerfs au-dessus de leur ganglions. *C. R. Hebd. Séanc. Acad. Sci. (Paris)* 34:842–847.

Waller, A. V. 1852b. Septième mémoire sur le système nerveux. *C. R. Hebd. Séanc. Acad. Sci. (Paris)* 35:301–306.

Waller, A. V. 1852c. Huitième mémoire sur le système nerveux. *C. R. Hebd. Séanc. Acad. Sci. (Paris)* 35:561–564.

Walters, B. B., and Matus, A. I. 1975. Tubulin in postsynaptic junctional lattice. *Nature (Lond.)* 257:496–498.

Warner, J. R., Knopf, P. M. and Rich, A. 1963. A multiple ribosomal structure in protein synthesis. *Proc. Natl. Acad. Sci. U.S.A.* 49:122–129.

Warr, W. B. 1973. Localization of olivocochlear neurons by means of retrograde axonal transport of horseradish peroxidase. *Anat. Rec.* 175:464.

Watson, M. L. 1955. The nuclear envelope: its structure and relation to cytoplasmic membranes. *J. Biophys. Biochem. Cytol.* 1:257–270.

Watson, W. E. 1965. An autoradiographic study of the incorporation of nucleic-acid precursors by neurons and glia during nerve regeneration. *J. Physiol. (Lond.)* 180:741–753.

Watson, W. E. 1968. Observations on the nucleolar and total cell body nucleic acid of injured nerve cells. *J. Physiol. (Lond.)* 196:655–676.

Waxman, S. G. 1972. Regional differentiation of the axon: a review with special reference to the concept of the multiplex neuron. *Brain Res.* 47:269–288.

Waxman, S. G. 1974. Ultrastructural differentiation of the axon membrane at synaptic and nonsynaptic central nodes of Ranvier. *Brain Res.* 65:338–342.

Waxman, S. G., Kriebel, M. E., Bennett, M. V. L., and Pappas, G. D. 1968. Fine structural basis of synaptic activity in oculomotor nuclei of the spiny boxfish. *J. Cell Biol.* 39:140a.

Waxman, S. G., and Pappas, G. D. 1969. Pinocytosis at postsynaptic membranes: electron microscopic evidence. *Brain Res.* 14:240–244.

Waxman, S. G., and Pappas, G. D. 1970. Synaptic organization of the oculomotor nucleus: a comparative electron microscope study. *Biol. Bull.* 139:442.

Waxman, S. G., Pappas, G. D., and Bennett, M. V. L. 1972. Morphological correlates of functional differentiation of nodes of Ranvier along single nerve fibers in the neurogenic electric organ of the Knife-fish *Sternarchus*. *J. Cell Biol.* 53:210–224.

Webster, H. deF. 1962. Transient, focal accumulation of axonal mitochondria during the early stages of Wallerian degeneration. *J. Cell Biol.* 12:361–383.

Webster, H. deF. 1964. Some ultrastructural features of segmental demyelination and myelin regeneration in peripheral nerve. In: *Progress in Brain Research*, Vol. 13, *Mechanisms of Neural Regeneration*. M. Singer and J. P. Schadé, Eds. Amsterdam, Elsevier, pp. 151–174.

Webster, H. deF. 1965. The relationship between Schmidt-Lantermann incisures and myelin segmentation during Wallerian degeneration. *Ann. N.Y. Acad. Sci.* 122:29–38.

Webster, H. deF. 1971. The geometry of peripheral myelin sheaths during their formation and growth in rat sciatic nerves. *J. Cell Biol.* 48:348–367.

Webster, H. deF. 1975. Development of peripheral myelinated and unmyelinated nerve fibers. In: *Peripheral Neuropathy*. P. J. Dyck, P. K. Thomas, and E. H. Lambert, Eds. Philadelphia, W. B. Saunders Co., pp. 37–61.

Webster, H. deF., and Ames, A. 1965. Reversible and irreversible changes in the fine structure of nervous tissue during oxygen and glucose deprivation. *J. Cell Biol.* 26:885–909.

Webster, H. deF., and Billings, S. M. 1972. Myelinated nerve fibers in *Xenopus* tadpoles: In vivo observations and fine structure. *J. Neuropathol. Exp. Neurol.* 31:102–112.

Webster, H. deF., Martin, J. R., and O'Connell, M. F. 1973. The relationships between interphase Schwann cells and axons before myelination: a quantitative electron microscopic study. *Dev. Biol.* 32:401–416.

Webster, H. deF., and O'Connell, M. F. 1970. Myelin formation in peripheral nerves. A morphological reappraisal and its neuropathological significance. *VIe Congrès International de Neuropathologie*. Comptes Rendus, Masson et Cie, Paris, pp. 579–588.

Webster, H. deF., and Spiro, D. 1960. Phase and electron microscopic studies of experimental demyelination. I. Variations in myelin sheath contour in normal guinea pig sciatic nerve. *J. Neuropathol. Exp. Neurol.* 19:42–69.

Webster, H. deF., Spiro, D., Waksman, B., and Adams, R. D. 1961. Phase and electron microscopic studies of experimental demyelination. II. Schwann cell changes in guinea pig sciatic nerves during experimental diphtheritic neuritis. *J. Neuropathol. Exp. Neurol.* 20:5–34.

Weed, L. H. 1914. Studies on cerebrospinal fluid. No.

3. The pathways of escape from the subarachnoid space, with particular reference to arachnoid villi. *J. Med. Res. 31*:51–91.

Weed, L. H. 1932. The Meninges, with special reference to the cell coverings of the leptomeninges. In: *Cytology and Cellular Pathology of the Nervous System.* Vol. 2. W. Penfield, Ed. New York, Hoeber, pp. 611–634.

Weigert, F. 1895. Beiträge zur Kenntnis der normalen menschlichen Neuroglia. Frankfurt am Main, Weisbrod.

Weindl, A. 1973. Neuroendocrine aspects of circumventricular organs. In: *Frontiers in Neuroendocrinology, 1973.* W. F. Ganong and L. Martini, Eds. New York, Oxford University Press, pp. 3–32.

Weinstein, H., Malamed, S., and Sachs, H. 1961. Isolation of vasopressin-containing granules from the neurohypophysis of the dog. *Biochim. Biophys. Acta 50*:386–389.

Weinstock, A., and Leblond, C. P. 1971. Elaboration of the matrix glycoprotein of enamel by the secretory ameloblasts of the rat incisor as revealed by radioautography and galactose-^{3}H injection. *J. Cell Biol. 51*:26–51.

Weiss, P. 1967. Neuronal dynamics. *Neurosci. Res. Progr. Bull. 5*:371–400.

Weiss, P. 1969. Neuronal dynamics and neuroplasmic (axonal) flow. *Symp. Int. Soc. Cell Biol. 8*:3–34.

Weiss, P. 1970. Neuronal dynamics and neuroplasmic flow. In: *The Neurosciences. Second Study Program.* F. O. Schmitt, Ed. New York, The Rockefeller University Press, pp. 840–850.

Weiss, P., and Hiscoe, H. B. 1948. Experiments on the mechanism of nerve growth. *J. Exp. Zool. 107*:315–393.

Weiss, P., and Pillai, P. A. 1965. Convection and fate of mitochondria in nerve fibers: axonal flow as vehicle. *Proc. Natl. Acad. Sci. U.S.A. 54*:48–56.

Weiss, P., Taylor, A. C., and Pillai, P. A. 1962. The nerve fiber as a system in continuous flow: microcinematographic and electronmicroscopic demonstrations. *Science 136*:330.

Weiss, P., and Wang, H. 1936. Neurofibrils in living ganglion cells of the chick, cultivated in vitro. *Anat. Rec. 67*:105–117.

Welch, K., and Friedman, V. 1960. The cerebrospinal fluid valves. *Brain 83*:454–469.

Welch, K., and Pollay, M. 1961. Perfusion of particles through arachnoid villi of the monkey. *Am. J. Physiol. 201*:651–654.

Wendell-Smith, C. P., Blunt, M. J., and Baldwin, F. 1966. The ultrastructural characterization of macroglial cell types. *J. Comp. Neurol. 127*:219–239.

Wersäll, J., Flock, A., and Lundquist, P. G. 1965. Structural basis for directional sensitivity in cochlear and vestibular sensory receptors. *Cold Spring Harb. Symp. Quant. Biol. 30*:115–132.

Wesemann, W., Henkel, R., and Marx, R. 1971. Receptors of neurotransmitters. V. Sialic acid distribution and characterization of the 5-hydroxytryptamine receptor in synaptic structures. *Biochem. Pharmacol. 20*:1961–1966.

Wessells, N. K., Spooner, B. S., Ash, J. F., Bradley, M. O., Luduena, M. A., Taylor, E. L., Wrenn, J. J., and Yamada, K. M. 1971. Microfilaments in cellular and developmental processes. *Science 171*:135–143.

West, R. W. 1972. Superficial warming of epoxy blocks for cutting of 25–150 μm sections to be resectioned in the 40–90 nm. range. *Stain Technol. 47*:201–204.

Westergaard, E. 1970. The Lateral Cerebral Ventricles and the Ventricular Walls. Doctoral dissertation, University of Aarhus. I kommission hos Andelsbogtrykkeriet i Odense.

Westergaard, E. 1972. The fine structure of nerve fibers and endings in the lateral cerebral ventricles of the rat. *J. Comp. Neurol. 144*:345–354.

Westergaard, E., and Brightman, M. W. 1973. Transport of proteins across normal cerebral arterioles. *J. Comp. Neurol. 152*:17–44.

Westrum, L. E. 1965. On the origin of synaptic vesicles in the cerebral cortex. *J. Physiol. (Lond.) 179*:4P–6P.

Westrum, L. E. 1966. Synaptic contacts on axons in the cerebral cortex. *Nature (Lond.) 210*:1289–1290.

Westrum, L. E. 1970. Observations on initial segments of axons in the prepyriform cortex of the rat. *J. Comp. Neurol. 139*:337–356.

Westrum, L. E. 1973. Early forms of terminal degeneration in the spinal trigeminal nucleus following rhizotomy. *J. Neurocytol. 2*:189–215.

Westrum, L. E., and Blackstad, T. W. 1962. An electron microscopic study of the stratum radiatum of the rat hippocampus (regio superior, CA 1) with particular emphasis on synaptology. *J. Comp. Neurol. 119*:281–309.

Westrum, L. E., and Gray, E. G. 1976. Microtubules and membrane specializations. *Brain Res.* (in press).

Westrum, L. E., White, L. E., and Ward, A. A. 1964. Morphology of the experimental epileptic focus. *J. Neurosurg. 21*:1033–1046.

White, E. L. 1972. Synaptic organization in the olfactory glomerulus of the mouse. *Brain Res. 37*:69–80.

Whitear, M. 1952. Internodal length in the skin plexuses of fish and the frog. *Q. J. Microsc. Sci. 93*:307–313.

Whittaker, V. P. 1965. The application of subcellular fractionation techniques to the study of brain function. *Progr. Biophys. 15*:39–96.

Whittaker, V. P. 1969. The nature of the acetylcholine pools in brain tissue. In: *Progress in Brain Research*, Vol. 31, *Mechanisms of Synaptic Transmission.* K. Akert and P. G. Waser, Eds. Amsterdam, Elsevier, pp. 211–222.

Whittaker, V. P. 1972. The use of synaptosomes in the study of synaptic and neural membrane function. In: *Structure and Function of Synapses.* G. D.

Pappas and D. P. Purpura, Eds. New York, Raven Press, pp. 87–100.

Whittaker, V. P., and Gray, E. G. 1962. The synapse: Biology and morphology. *Br. Med. Bull. 18*:223–228.

Whittaker, V. P., Michaelson, I. A., and Kirkland, R. J. A. 1964. The separation of synaptic vesicles from disrupted nerve ending particles ('synaptosomes'). *Biochem. J. 90*:293–303.

Whittaker, V. P., and Zimmerman, H. 1974. Biochemical studies on cholinergic synaptic vesicles. In: *Synaptic Transmission and Neuronal Interactions.* M. V. L. Bennett, Ed. New York, Raven Press, pp. 217–238.

Wilcox, H. H. 1959. Structural changes in the nervous system related to the process of aging. Present status of knowledge. In: *The Process of Aging in the Nervous System.* J. E. Birren, H. Imus, and W. Windle, Eds. Springfield, Ill., Charles C Thomas, pp. 16–23.

Wilder, B. J., Schimpff, B. D. and Collins, G. H. 1972. Ultrastructure study of the chronic experimental epileptic focus. *Epilepsia 13*:341–355.

Willey, T. J. 1973. The ultrastructure of the cat olfactory bulb. *J. Comp. Neurol. 152*:211–232.

Willey, T. J., and Schultz, R. L. 1971. Intranuclear inclusions in neurons of the cat primary olfactory system. *Brain Res. 29*:31–45.

Williams, P. L., and Hall, S. M. 1971a. Prolonged *in vivo* observations of normal peripheral nerve fibres and their acute reactions to crush and deliberate trauma. *J. Anat. 108*:397–408.

Williams, P. L., and Hall, S. M. 1971b. Chronic Wallerian degeneration—an *in vivo* and ultrastructural study. *J. Anat. 109*:487–503.

Williams, P. L., and Kashef, R. 1968. Asymmetry of the node of Ranvier. *J. Cell Sci. 3*:341–356.

Williams, P. L., and Wendell-Smith, C. P. 1971. Some additional parametric variations between peripheral nerve fibre populations. *J. Anat. 109*:502–526.

Williams, V., and Grossman, R. G. 1970. Ultrastructure of cortical synapses after failure of presynaptic activity in ischemia. *Anat. Rec. 166*:131–142.

Windle, W. F., Ed. 1958. *Biology of Neuroglia.* Springfield, Ill., Charles C Thomas.

Wischnitzer, S. 1960. The ultrastructure of the nucleus and nucleocytoplasmic relations. *Int. Rev. Cytol. 10*:137–162.

Wislocki, G. B., and Ladman, A. J. 1958. The fine structure of the mammalian choroid plexus. In: *Ciba Foundation Symposium on Cerebrospinal Fluid.* G. E. W. Wolstenholme and C. M. O'Connor, Eds. Boston, Little, Brown and Co., pp. 55–79.

Wiśniewski, H. M., Ghetti, B., and Terry, R. D. 1973. Neuritic (senile) plaques and filamentous changes in aged rhesus monkeys. *J. Neuropathol. Exp. Neurol. 32*:566–584.

Wiśniewski, H., and Morell, P. 1971. Quaking mouse: Ultrastructural evidence for the arrest of myelinogenesis. *Brain Res. 29*:63–73.

Wiśniewski, H., Shelanski, M. L., and Terry, R. D. 1968. Effects of mitotic spindle inhibitors on neurotubules and neurofilaments in anterior horn cells. *J. Cell Biol. 38*:224–229.

Wittkowski, W. 1969. Ependymokrinie und Rezeptoren in der Wand des Recessus infundibularis der Maus und ihre Beziehung zum kleinzelligen Hypothalamus. *Z. Zellforsch. Mikrosk. Anat. 93*:530–546.

Wohlfarth-Bottermann, K. E. 1963. Differentiations of the ground cytoplasm and their significance for the generation of amoeboid movement. In: *Primitive Motile Systems in Cell Biology.* R. D. Allen and N. Kamiya, Eds. New York, Academic Press, pp. 79–110.

Wolfe, D. E. 1961. Electron microscopic criteria for distinguishing dendrites from preterminal nonmyelinated axons in the area postrema of the rat, and characterization of a novel synapse. *Abstracts, First Annual Meeting of the American Society for Cell Biology,* p. 228.

Wolfe, D. E. 1965. The epiphyseal cell: An electron microscopic study of its intercellular relationships and intercellular morphology in the pineal body of albino rat. In: *Progress in Brain Research,* Vol. 10, *Structure and Function of the Epiphysis Cerebri.* J. A. Kappers and J. P. Schadé, Eds. Amsterdam, Elsevier, pp. 332–388.

Wolfe, D. E., Potter, L. T., Richardson, K. C., and Axelrod, J. 1962. Localizing tritiated norepinephrine in sympathetic axons by electron microscopic autoradiography. *Science 138*:440–441.

Wolff, J. 1963. Beiträge zur Ultrastruktur der Kapillaren der normalen Grosshirnrinde. *Z. Zellforsch. Mikrosk. Anat. 60*:409–431.

Wolff, J. R., and Bär, T. 1972. "Seamless" endothelia in brain capillaries during development of the rat's cerebral cortex. *Brain Res. 41*:17–24.

Wong, M. T. 1970. Somato-dendritic and dendro-dendritic synapses in the squirrel monkey lateral geniculate nucleus. *Brain Res. 20*:135–139.

Wong-Riley, M. T. T. 1972. Neuronal and synaptic organization of the normal dorsal lateral geniculate nucleus of the squirrel monkey, *Saimiri sciureus. J. Comp. Neurol. 144*:25–60.

Wood, J. G., McLaughlin, B. J., and Barber, R. P. 1974. The visualization of concanavalin A binding sites in Purkinje cell somata and dendrites of rat cerebellum. *J. Cell Biol. 63*:541–549.

Woollard, H. H. 1924. Vital staining of the leptomeninges. *J. Anat. 58*:89–100.

Worthington, W. C., and Cathcart, R. S. 1963. Ependymal cilia; distribution and activity in the adult human brain. *Science 139*:221–222.

Wrenn, J. T., and Wessells, N. K. 1969. An ultrastructural study of lens invagination in the mouse. *J. Exp. Zool. 171*:359–368.

Wuerker, R. B. 1970. Neurofilaments and glial filaments. *Tiss. Cell 2*:1–10.

Wuerker, R. B., and Kirkpatrick, J. B. 1972. Neuronal microtubules, neurofilaments, and microfilaments. *Int. Rev. Cytol. 33*:45–75.

Wuerker, R., and Palay, S. L. 1969. Neurofilaments and microtubules in anterior horn cells of the rat. *Tiss. Cell 1*:387–402.

Wyburn, G. M. 1958. The capsule of spinal ganglion cells. *J. Anat. 92*:528–533.

Wyckoff, R. W. G., and Young, J. Z. 1956. The motoneuron surface. *Proc. R. Soc. Ser. B 144*:440–450.

Yamada, K. M., Spooner, B. S., and Wessells, N. K. 1971. Ultrastructure and function of growth cones and axons in cultured nerve cells. *J. Cell Biol. 49*:614–635.

Yamauchi, A., Fujimaki, Y., and Yokota, R. 1975. Reciprocal synapses between cholinergic postganglionic axon and adrenergic interneuron in the cardiac ganglion of the turtle. *J. Ultrastruct. Res. 50*:47–57.

Yamauchi, A., Yokota, R., and Fujimaki, Y. 1975. Reciprocal synapses between cholinergic axons and small granule-containing cells in the rat cardiac ganglion. *Anat. Rec. 181*:195–210.

Yasuzumi, G., and Tsubo, I. 1966. The fine structure of nuclei as revealed by electron microscopy. III. Adenosine triphosphatase activity in the pores of nuclear envelope of mouse choroid plexus epithelial cells. *Exp. Cell Res. 43*:281–292.

Young, J. Z. 1942. The functional repair of nervous tissue. *Physiol. Rev. 22*:318–374.

Young, J. Z. 1945. History of the shape of a nerve fibre. In: *Essays on Growth and Form, presented to d'Arcy Wentworth Thompson.* W. E. leGros Clark and P. B. Medawar, Eds. Oxford, Clarendon Press, pp. 41–94.

Yu, R. C.-P., and Bunge, R. P. 1975. Damage and repair of the peripheral myelin sheath and node of Ranvier after treatment with trypsin. *J. Cell Biol. 64*:1–14.

Zampighi, G., and Robertson, J. D. 1973. Fine structure of the synaptic discs separated from the goldfish medulla oblongata. *J. Cell Biol. 56*:92–105.

Zelená, J. 1970. Ribosome-like particles in myelinated axons of the rat. *Brain Res. 24*:359–363.

Zelená, J. 1971. Neurofilaments and microtubules in sensory neurons after peripheral nerve section. *Z. Zellforsch. Mikrosk. Anat. 117*:191–211.

Zelená, J. 1972. Ribosomes in myelinated axons of dorsal root ganglia. *Z. Zellforsch. Mikrosk. Anat. 124*:217–229.

Zenker, W., and Högl, E. 1976. The prebifurcation section of the axon of the rat spinal ganglion cell. *Cell Tiss. Res. 165*:345–363.

Zenker, W., and Hohberg, E. 1973. A-α-nerve-fibre: number of neurotubules in the stem fibre and in the terminal branches. *J. Neurocytol. 2*:143–148.

INDEX

Page numbers in italics indicate illustrations; page numbers followed by (t) indicate tables.